Clinical Nutrition

The Nutrition Society Textbook Series

Introduction to Human Nutrition

Introduction to human nutrition: a global perspective on food and nutrition
Body composition
Energy metabolism
Nutrition and metabolism of proteins and amino acids
Digestion and metabolism of carbohydrates
Nutrition and metabolism of lipids
Dietary reference standards
The vitamins
Minerals and trace elements
Measuring food intake
Food composition
Food and nutrition: policy and regulatory issues
Nutrition research methodology
Food safety: a public health issue of growing importance
Food and nutrition-related diseases: the global challenge

Public Health Nutrition

An overview of public health nutrition
Nutrition epidemiology
Food choice
Assessment of nutritional status at individual and population level
Assessment of physical activity
Overnutrition
Undernutrition
Eating disorders, dieting and food fads
PHN strategies for nutrition: intervention at the level of individuals
PHN strategies for nutrition: intervention at the ecological level
Food and nutrition guidelines
Fetal programming
Cardiovascular disease
Cancer
Osteoporosis
Diabetes
Vitamin A deficiency
Iodine deficiency
Iron deficiency
Maternal and child health
Breast feeding
Adverse outcomes in pregnancy

Nutrition and Metabolism

Core concepts of nutrition
Molecular aspects of nutrition
Integration of metabolism 1: Energy
Integration of metabolism 2: Macronutrients
Integration of metabolism 3: Protein and amino acids
Pregnancy and lactation
Growth and aging
Nutrition and the brain
The sensory systems and food palatability
The gastrointestinal tract
The cardiovascular system
The skeletal system
The immune and inflammatory systems
Phytochemicals
The control of food intake
Overnutrition
Undernutrition
Exercise performance

Sport and Exercise Nutrition

Nutrient basics
Exercise physiology
Exercise biochemistry
Carbohydrate
Protein and amino acids
Fat metabolism
Fluids and electrolytes
Micronutrients
Supplements and ergogenic aids
Nutrition for weight and resistance training
Nutrition for power and sprint training
Nutrition for middle-distance and speed-endurance training
Nutrition for endurance and ultra-endurance training
Nutrition for technical and skill-based training
Nutrition for disability athletes
Competition nutrition
Losing, gaining and making weight for athletes
Eating disorders and athletes
Bone health
Nutrition and the gastrointestinal tract for athletes
Immunity
Travel
Population groups: I
Population groups: II
Training and competition environments

Clinical Nutrition

Second Edition

Edited on behalf of The Nutrition Society by

Professor Marinos Elia
Institute of Human Nutrition
University of Southampton
UK

Professor Olle Ljungqvist
Department of Surgery
Örebro University Hospital and Karolinska Institutet
Sweden

Dr Rebecca J Stratton
Institute of Human Nutrition
University of Southampton
UK

Editor-in-Chief

Professor Susan A Lanham-New
Department of Nutritional Sciences
University of Surrey
UK

Foreword by Professor Dame Sally C. Davies

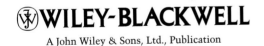

WILEY-BLACKWELL
A John Wiley & Sons, Ltd., Publication

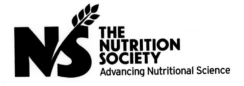

THE NUTRITION SOCIETY
Advancing Nutritional Science

This edition first published 2013
First edition published 2005
© 2005, 2013 by The Nutrition Society

Wiley-Blackwell is an imprint of John Wiley & Sons, formed by the merger of Wiley's global Scientific, Technical and Medical business with Blackwell Publishing.

Registered Office
John Wiley & Sons, Ltd, The Atrium, Southern Gate, Chichester, West Sussex, PO19 8SQ, UK

Editorial Offices
9600 Garsington Road, Oxford, OX4 2DQ, UK
The Atrium, Southern Gate, Chichester, West Sussex, PO19 8SQ, UK
2121 State Avenue, Ames, Iowa 50014-8300, USA

For details of our global editorial offices, for customer services and for information about how to apply for permission to reuse the copyright material in this book please see our website at www.wiley.com/wiley-blackwell.

Library of Congress Cataloging-in-Publication Data

Clinical nutrition / edited on behalf of the Nutrition Society by Marinos Elia ... [et al.]. – 2nd ed.
  p. ; cm.
  Includes bibliographical references and index.
  ISBN 978-1-4051-6810-6 (pbk. : alk. paper)
  I. Elia, Marinos. II. Nutrition Society (Great Britain)
  [DNLM: 1. Nutrition Therapy. 2. Nutritional Physiological Phenomena. WB 400]
  615.8′54–dc23
                                2012022785
A catalogue record for this book is available from the British Library.

Wiley also publishes its books in a variety of electronic formats. Some content that appears in print may not be available in electronic books.

Cover image: courtesy of iStockphoto/skystardream
Cover design by Sophie Ford (www.hisandhersdesign.co.uk)

Set in 10/12pt Minion by SPi Publisher Services, Pondicherry, India
Printed in Singapore by Ho Printing Singapore Pte Ltd

1   2013

Contents

Visit the supporting companion website for this book:
www.wiley.com/go/elia/clinicalnutrition

Contributors

Dr Isabelle Aeberli
St John's Research Institute, India
ETH Zurich, Switzerland

Professor Simon P Allison
Formerly University of Nottingham
and Queen's Medical Centre
UK

Professor Bruce R Bistrian
Beth Israel Deaconess Medical Center
USA

Professor Federico Bozzetti
University of Milan
Italy

Dr Eduard Cabré
Hospital Universitari Germans Trias i Pujol
Spain

Dr Saveria Capria
La Sapienza University of Rome
Italy

Abeed H Chowdhury
Nottingham University Hospitals
Queen's Medical Centre, Nottingham
UK

Peter Collins
Queensland University of Technology
Australia

Professor John A Dodge
University of Swansea
UK

Professor Marinos Elia
University of Southampton
UK

Professor Filippo Rossi Fanelli
La Sapienza University of Rome
Italy

Professor Ken Fearon
University of Edinburgh
UK

Professor Gema Frühbeck
Clinica Universidad de Navarra-CIBERobn
Spain

Professor Miquel A Gassull
Hospital Universitari Germans Trias i Pujol
Spain

Dr Kate Gatenby
University of Leeds
UK

Professor Robert F Grimble
University of Southampton
UK

Professor Gianfranco Guarnieri
University of Trieste
Italy

Dr Anna Paola Iori
La Sapienza University of Rome
Italy

Cora F Jonkers-Schuitema
Academic Medical Centre, Amsterdam
The Netherlands

Professor Mark Kearney
University of Leeds
UK

Professor Anura V Kurpad
St John's Research Institute
India

Professor Olle Ljungqvist
Örebro University Hospital and Karolinska Institutet
Sweden

Professor Dileep N Lobo
Nottingham University Hospitals
Queen's Medical Centre, Nottingham
UK

Professor John MacFie
Scarborough Hospital
UK

Dr Paula McGurk
University Hospital Southampton
NHS Foundation Trust
UK

Dr Clare McNaught
Scarborough Hospital
UK

Professor Simon H Murch
Warwick Medical School, University of Warwick
UK

Associate Professor Maurizio Muscaritoli
La Sapienza University of Rome
Italy

Dr Nicholas I Paton
National University of Singapore
Singapore

Professor Mathias Plauth
Staedtisches Klinikum Dessau (Municipal
Hospital Dessau)
Germany

Associate Professor Christine Rodda
Monash University
Australia

Dr Tatjana Schütz
Leipzig University Medical Centre
Germany

Professor Jean-Marc Schwarz
Touro University California
USA

Roberta Situlin
University of Trieste
Italy

Dr Rebecca J Stratton
University of Southampton
UK

Professor Luc Tappy
University of Lausanne
Switzerland

Dr Marian AE van Bokhorst-de van der Schueren
VU University Medical Centre
The Netherlands

Esther van den Hogen
Maastricht UMC
The Netherlands

Dr Stephen Wheatcroft
University of Leeds
UK

Dr Anthony F Williams
St George's, University of London
UK

Kate Williams
South London and Maudsley NHS Foundation Trust
UK

Dr Jean-Fabien Zazzo
Hôpital Antoine-Béclère (Assistance
Publique-Hôpitaux de Paris)
France

Series Foreword

The Nutrition Society was established in 1941 as a result of a group of leading physiologists, biochemists and medical scientists recognising that the emerging discipline of nutrition would benefit from its own Learned Society. The Nutrition Society's mission was, and firmly remains, *"to advance the scientific study of nutrition and its application to the maintenance of human and animal health"*. It is the largest Learned Society for Nutrition in Europe and has over 2,700 members worldwide. For more details about the Society and how to become a member, visit the website at www.nutritionsociety.org.

Throughout its history, a primary objective of the Society has been to encourage nutrition research and to disseminate the results of such research. This is reflected in the several scientific meetings with the Nutrition Society, often in collaboration with sister Learned Societies in Europe, Africa, Asia and the USA, organised each year.

The Society's first journal, *The Proceedings of the Nutrition Society* published in 1944, records the scientific presentations made to the Society. Shortly afterwards, in 1947, the *British Journal of Nutrition* was established to provide a medium for the publication of primary research on all aspects of human and animal nutrition by scientists from around the world. Recognising the needs of students and their teachers for authoritative reviews on topical issues in nutrition, the Society began publishing *Nutrition Research Reviews* in 1988. The journal *Public Health Nutrition*, the first international journal dedicated to this important and growing area, was subsequently launched in 1998. The Society is constantly evolving and has most recently launched the *Journal of Nutritional Science* in 2012. This is an international, peer-reviewed, online only, open access journal.

Just as in research, having the best possible tools is an enormous advantage in both teaching and learning. The Nutrition Society Textbook Series was established by Professor Michael Gibney (University College Dublin) in 1998. It is now under the direction of the second Editor-in-Chief, Professor Susan Lanham-New (University of Surrey), and continues to be an extraordinarily successful venture for the Society. This series of Human Nutrition textbooks is designed for use worldwide and this was achieved by translating the Series in multiple languages including Spanish, Greek, Portuguese and Indonesian. The sales of the textbook (>30,000 copies) are a tribute to the value placed on the textbooks both in the UK and worldwide as a core educational tool.

This Second Edition of *Clinical Nutrition* focuses on the metabolically compromised patient and provides a most thorough review of the importance of nutrition across the clinical spectrum. The textbook is aimed at those with an interest in nutrition in the clinical setting, including students, nutritionists, dietitians, medics, nursing staff or other allied health professionals.

In my capacity as the Chief Medical Officer (CMO) for England, and the UK Government's Principal Medical Adviser, the professional lead for all Directors of Public Health and Chief Scientific Adviser for the Department of Health, it gives me great pleasure to write the Foreword for the Second Edition of *Clinical Nutrition*. I have been actively involved in NHS Research and Development from its establishment and I understand how important clinical nutrition is to the patient and the medical team. This textbook brings together science and clinical practice and is a valuable resource to all those working in the field.

Professor Dame Sally C. Davies
Chief Medical Officer
Chief Scientific Adviser

Preface

The Nutrition Society's Textbook Series continues to go from strength to strength following its development over 10 years ago. The forward thinking focus that Professor Michael Gibney (University College Dublin) had at that time is to be especially noted. My task as the new Editor-in-Chief since 2009 is much easier than the visionary one that Professor Gibney had back in the late 1990s and it remains a tremendous honour for me to be following in his footsteps.

The first and second textbooks in the Series, *Introduction to Human Nutrition* (IHN) and *Nutrition and Metabolism* (N&M), are now out in Second Editions and sales continue apace. We are currently working on the Second Edition of the third textbook in the Series, *Public Health Nutrition* (PHN), and we are absolutely delighted now to present to the field of Nutritional Sciences, Elia *et al*'s *Clinical Nutrition* Second Edition. This follows our publication last year of the fifth textbook in the Series, *Sport and Exercise Nutrition* First Edition (SEN1e). The sales of SEN1e have surpassed all expectations and we were most grateful to Dr Richard Budgett OBE, Chief Medical Officer for the London 2012 Olympic and Paralympic Games, for his enthusiasm, support and most generous Foreword.

Clinical Nutrition Second Edition (CN2e) is a great strength of the Textbook Series and the Nutrition Society is indebted to the Senior Editor, Professor Marinos Elia (University of Southampton), for his careful planning and editorial leadership of the book following the critical role he played with the development of the First Edition of *Clinical Nutrition*. Sincerest of thanks are also due to the Editors, Professor Olle Ljungqvist (Örebro University Hospital and Karolinska Institutet, Sweden) and Dr Rebecca Stratton (University of Southampton) for their immense work on this Second Edition.

This Second Edition is intended for those with an interest in nutrition in the clinical setting, whether they are dietitians or medics, nursing staff or other allied health professionals. The book starts by setting the scene in assessing nutritional status and discusses the clinical consequences and current management options with under-nutrition and over-nutrition, and eating disorders and metabolic disease. The subsequent later chapters deal with the different organ systems of the body, setting out the most up-to-date thinking on the role of nutrition, whether it involves nutritional support, nutritional education or a combination of both.

We are extremely honoured that the Foreword for the Second Edition has been written by Dame Sally Davies, Chief Medical Officer (CMO) for England, and the UK Government's Principal Medical Adviser. It gives us great confidence in this Textbook to have such a seal of approval from someone so eminent in the clinical field. Our sincerest of thanks indeed for Dame Sally's help and support.

The Society is most grateful to the textbook publishers Wiley-Blackwell for their continued help with the production of the textbook and in particular Nick Morgan, Sara Crowley-Vigneau and Marilyn Pierro, as well as Aravinthakumar Ranganathan, the project manager at SPi Publisher Services. In addition, many grateful thanks to Professor Lisa Roberts, Dean of the Faculty of Health and Medical Sciences, University of Surrey for her great encouragement of the Textbook Series production.

Finally, sincerest of thanks indeed to the Nutrition Society President, Professor Sean J.J. Strain (University of Ulster), for all his belief in the Textbook Series and to Professor David Bender, Honorary Publications Officer, for being such a great sounding board. The Series remains indebted to Sharon Hui (Assistant Editor, NS Textbook Series) and Jennifer Norton (NS Business Development Manager) for their huge contribution to the development of the Series and for making the textbooks such an enjoyable journey.

I do hope that you will find the textbook a great resource. Happy reading indeed!

With my warmest of wishes.

Professor Susan A. Lanham-New
Head, Department of Nutritional Sciences
Faculty of Health and Medical Sciences
University of Surrey
and Editor-in-Chief, Nutrition Society Textbook Series

The Nutrition Society Textbook Series Editorial Team

Editor-in-Chief
Susan A Lanham-New
University of Surrey, UK

Assistant Editor
Sharon S Hui
The Nutrition Society, UK

Business Development Manager
Jennifer Norton
The Nutrition Society, UK

First Edition Acknowledgements

Editor-in-Chief
Michael J Gibney

Editors
Marinos Elia
Olle Ljungqvist
Julie Dowsett

Authors

Chapter 1: Principles of Clinical Nutrition
Marinos Elia

Chapter 2: Nutritional Assessment
Khursheed Jeejeebhoy
Mary Keith

Chapter 3: Overnutrition
Gema Frühbeck

Chapter 4: Undernutrition
Anura Kurpad

Chapter 5: Metabolic Disorders
Luc Tappy
Jean-Marc Schwarz

Chapter 6: Eating Disorders
Janet Treasure
Tara Murphy

Chapter 7: Adverse Reactions to Foods
Simon Murch

Chapter 8: Nutritional Support
Karin Barendregt
Peter Soeters

Chapter 9: Ethics and Nutrition
John Macfie

Chapter 10: The Gastrointestinal Tract
Miguel A Gassull
Eduard Cabré

Chapter 11: Nutrition in Liver Disease
Marietjie Herselman
Demetre Labadarios
Christo Van Rensburg
Aref Haffejee

Chapter 12: Nutrition and the Pancreas
Jean Fabien Zazzo

Chapter 13: The Kidney
Gianfranco Guarnieri
Roberta Situlin
Gabriele Toigo

Chapter 14: Nutritional and Metabolic Support in Hematologic Malignancies and Hematopoietic Stem Cell Transplantation
Maurizio Muscaritoli
Gabriella Grieco
Filippo Rossi Fanelli
Zaira Aversa

Chapter 15: The Lung
Annemie Schols
Emiel FM Wouters

Chapter 16: Nutrition and Immune and Inflammatory Systems
Bruce Bistrian
Bob Grimble

Chapter 17: The Heart and Blood Vessels
Stephen Wheatcroft
Brian Noronha
Mark Kearney

Chapter 18: Nutritional Aspects of Disease Affecting the Skeleton
Christine Rodda

Chapter 19: Nutrition in Surgery and Trauma
Olle Ljungqvist
Kenneth Fearon
Roderick Little

Chapter 20: Infectious Diseases
Nicholas Paton
Miguel A Gassull
Eduard Cabré

Chapter 21: Nutritional Support in Patients with Cancer
Federico Bozzetti

Chapter 22: Pediatric Nutrition
Anthony F Williams

Chapter 23: Cystic Fibrosis
Olive Tully
Julie Dowsett

Chapter 24: Water and Electrolytes
Meritxell Girvent
Guzman Franch
Antonio Stiges-Serra

Chapter 25: Illustrative Cases
Simon Allison

1

Principles of Clinical Nutrition: Contrasting the Practice of Nutrition in Health and Disease

Marinos Elia

Institute of Human Nutrition, University of Southampton, Southampton, UK

Key messages

- To understand how to best meet the nutritional needs of an individual, the distinction between physiology in health and pathophysiology in disease needs to be carefully considered.
- For some groups of patients, the requirements are higher than those in health, while for other groups of patients they are lower. If recommendations for healthy individuals are applied to patients with certain types of disease, they may produce harm.
- In health, only the oral route is used to provide nutrients to the body. In clinical practice, other routes can be used. The use of the intravenous route for feeding raises a number of new issues.
- Alterations in nutritional therapy during the course of an acute disease may occur because the underlying disease has produced new complications or because it has resolved. Similarly, in more chronic conditions there is a need to review the diet at regular intervals.

1.1 Introduction

Clinical nutrition focuses on the nutritional management of individual patients or groups of patients with established disease, in contrast to public health nutrition, which focuses on health promotion and disease prevention in the general population. The two disciplines overlap, however, especially in older people, who are often affected by a range of disabilities or diseases. Working together, instead of independently, the two disciplines are more likely to facilitate successful implementation of local, national, and international policies on nutrition. To understand the overlap between them, it is necessary to consider not only some of the principles of nutrition that apply to health, but also special issues that apply to the field of clinical nutrition. These include altered nutritional requirements associated with disease, disease severity and malnutrition, and nonphysiological routes of feeding using unusual feeds and feeding schedules. This introductory chapter provides a short overview of these issues, partly because they delineate qualitative or quantitative differences between health and disease, and partly because they form a thread that links subsequent sections of this book, which is divided into discrete chapters addressing specific conditions.

It is now possible to feed all types of patients over extended periods of time, including those who are unconscious, unable to eat or swallow, or have little or no functional gastrointestinal tract. It is possible to target specific patient groups with special formulations, and even to change the formulation in the same patient as nutritional demands alter during the course of an illness. Since some of these formulations may be beneficial to some patient groups and detrimental to other groups or to healthy subjects, the distinction between physiology in health and pathophysiology in disease needs to be considered carefully. It is hoped that some of the principles outlined here will help to establish a conceptual framework for considering some of the apparently diverse conditions discussed in this textbook.

1.2 The spectrum of nutritional problems

Clinical nutrition aims to treat and prevent suffering from malnutrition. However, there is no universally accepted definition for 'malnutrition' (literally, 'bad nutrition'). The following definition, which encompasses both under- and over-nutrition, is offered for the purposes of this chapter.

Malnutrition is a state of nutrition in which a deficiency or excess (or imbalance) of energy, protein, and other nutrients causes measurable adverse effects on tissue/body function (shape, size, and composition) and clinical outcome.

In this chapter and elsewhere, however, the term 'malnutrition' is mainly used to refer to under- rather than over-nutrition.

Both under- and over-nutrition have adverse physiological and clinical effects. Those relating to under-nutrition (Table 1.1) are diverse, which

explains why malnourished patients may present to a wide range of medical disciplines. Several manifestations may occur simultaneously in the same individual, although some predominate. They may be caused by multiple deficiencies. Specific nutrient deficiencies may also have diverse effects, affecting multiple systems, but it is not entirely clear why the same deficiency can present in a certain way in one subject and a different way in another. For example, it is not clear why some patients with deficiency of vitamin B_{12} present to the haematologist with megaloblastic anaemia, others to the neurologist with neuropathy and other neurological manifestations (e.g. subacute combined degeneration of the cord), and still others to the geriatrician with cognitive impairment or dementia.

The spectrum of presentations is more diverse than this would indicate because protein–energy malnutrition frequently coexists with various nutrient deficiencies. For example, patients with gastrointestinal problems are frequently underweight and at the same time exhibit magnesium, sodium, potassium, and zinc deficiencies, due to excessive losses of these nutrients in diarrhoea or other gastrointestinal effluents. There may also be problems with absorption; for example, patients with Crohn's disease affecting the terminal ileum, where vitamin B_{12} is absorbed, are at increased risk of developing B_{12} deficiency. Patients who have had surgical removal of their terminal ileum or stomach, which produces the

Table 1.1 Physical and psychosocial effects of under-nutrition.

Adverse effect	Consequence
Physical	
Impaired immune responses	Predisposes to infection
Reduced muscle strength and fatigue	Inactivity, inability to work effectively, and poor self-care. Abnormal muscle (or neuromuscular) function may also predispose to falls or other accidents
Reduced respiratory muscle strength	Poor cough pressure, predisposing to and delaying recovery from chest infection
Inactivity, especially in bed-bound patient	Predisposes to pressure, sores, and thromboembolism
Impaired thermoregulation	Hypothermia, especially in the elderly
Impaired wound-healing	Failure of fistulae to close, un-united fractures, increased risk of wound infection resulting in prolonged recovery from illness, increased length of hospital stay, and delayed return to work
Foetal and infant programming	Predisposes to common chronic diseases, such as cardiovascular disease, stroke, and diabetes in adult life
Growth failure	Stunting, delayed sexual development, and reduced muscle mass and strength
Psychosocial	
Impaired psychosocial function	Even when uncomplicated by disease, undernutrition causes apathy, depression, self-neglect, hypochondriasis, loss of libido, and deterioration in social interactions. It also affects personality and impairs mother–child bonding

intrinsic factor necessary for B_{12} absorption, fail to absorb vitamin B_{12}. Isolated nutrient deficiencies may also occur, for example iron deficiency due to heavy periods in otherwise healthy women.

Another complexity is the interaction between nutrients, which may occur at the level of absorption, metabolism within the body, or excretion. One nutrient may facilitate the absorption of another; for example, glucose enhances the absorption of sodium (on the glucose–sodium co-transporter). This is the main reason why oral rehydration solutions used to correct salt deficiency due to diarrhoea (or fluid losses due to other gastrointestinal diseases) contain both salt and glucose. In contrast, other nutrients compete with each other for absorption. For example, because of competition between zinc and copper for intestinal absorption, administration of copper may precipitate zinc deficiency, especially in those with borderline zinc status. Other nutrients interact with each other during tissue deposition. Accretion

of lean tissue requires multiple nutrients, and lack of one of them, such as potassium or phosphate, can limit its deposition, even when adequate amounts of protein and energy are available (Figure 1.1). This emphasises the need to provide all necessary nutrients in appropriate amounts and proportions.

1.3 Nutritional requirements

Effect of disease and nutritional status

Fluid and electrolytes

The principles of nutrient requirements in healthy individuals are described in *Introduction to Human Nutrition* (Gibney *et al.*, 2009), an earlier volume in this textbook series. The average nutrient intake refers to the average intake necessary to maintain nutrient balance. The reference nutrient intake (RNI) refers to the intake necessary to satisfy the requirements of 97.5% of the healthy population (+2 standard deviations from the average nutrient intake). In patients with a variety of diseases, the requirements are more variable (Figure 1.2): for some groups of patients, they are higher than for those in health, while for other groups they are lower. For example, in patients with gastrointestinal fluid losses, the requirement for sodium may be double the RNI, while in patients with severe renal or liver disease who retain salt and water, the requirements may be well below the average nutrient requirement for healthy subjects ingesting an oral diet. The requirements for potassium and phosphate may also be well below the RNI for patients with severe renal disease in whom there is failure of excretion. Therefore, if recommendations

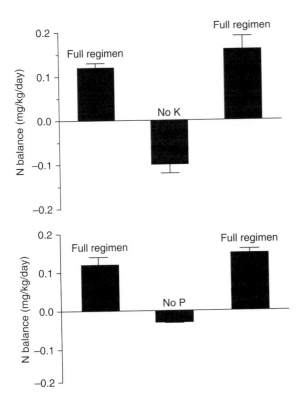

Figure 1.1 Effect of omitting potassium (K) and phosphate (P) from a parenteral nutrition regimen on the nitrogen (N) balance of depleted patients receiving hypercaloric feeding. Data from Rudman *et al.* (1975).

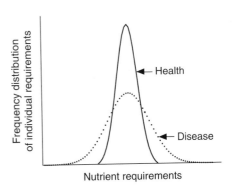

Figure 1.2 Frequency distribution of nutrient requirements in health and disease.

for healthy individuals are applied to patients with certain types of disease, they may produce harm. A general guide to the requirements for sodium and potassium in patients with gastrointestinal fluid loss (above those for maintenance) is provided in Table 1.2, which shows the electrolyte content of various fluids. A person with a loss of 1.5 litres of small-intestinal fluid may require ~150 mmol of sodium above maintenance (the RNI for sodium is 70 mmol/day according to UK reference standards), whereas loss of the same volume of nasogastrically aspirated fluid requires only ~90 mmol extra sodium. Note that the requirements for potassium in patients losing gastrointestinal fluids are generally much lower than those for sodium (Table 1.2).

Excessive salt and fluid administration can be just as detrimental as inadequate intake, causing fluid retention and heart failure in some individuals. Fluid retention is often detected clinically by noting pitting oedema at the ankles or over the sacrum, but oedema can also affect internal tissues and organs, causing a variety of problems. Some of these problems are shown in Table 1.3. A recent study has questioned the routine clinical practice of administering large amounts of fluid in the early postoperative period in an attempt to reduce the risk of hypotension. In a randomised controlled trial carried out in Denmark, routine fluid administration was compared with a fluid-restricted regimen that aimed to approximately maintain body weight. In those receiving routine fluid therapy, not only did body weight increase significantly more than in the fluid-restricted group, but it significantly increased a variety of complications, including tissue-healing and cardiopulmonary complications. It also increased mortality, but this did not

reach statistical significance, possibly because only a small number of subjects died during the course of the study. Acute accidental and elective surgical trauma is associated with a tendency to retain salt and water, at least partly because of increased secretion of mineralocorticoids and antidiuretic hormone. Therefore, administration of excess salt and water as in protein–energy malnutrition may lead to fluid retention that would not occur in normal subjects.

Protein

Another difference between nutritional requirements in health and disease concerns body composition and nutrient balance. In healthy adults, nutritional intake aims to maintain body composition (lean body mass and fat mass) within a desirable range, but this may not be the case in subjects with disease-related malnutrition in whom there is a need to replete tissues so that body function can improve. The response of the body to nutritional support also varies between health and disease with or without malnutrition. Consider the effect of increasing protein intake in normal, depleted, and catabolic subjects (severe acute disease), all of whom are close to energy balance (Figure 1.3). In healthy subjects, nitrogen (N) (1 g N = 6.25 g protein) balance is achieved with an intake of 0.105 g N/kg/day (the RNI necessary to achieve balance in 97.5% of the population is ~0.13 g N/kg/day according to World Health Organization (WHO) reference data). Increasing the N intake above this amount leads to little or no further net protein deposition. Depleted subjects continue to deposit protein (positive N balance) when intake is increased above 0.1 (and above 0.13) g N/kg/day, while catabolic patients show

Table 1.2 Electrolyte contents of some body secretions (mmol/l).

Secretion/excretion	Na	K
Gastric	60	10
Pancreatic	140	5
Biliary	140	5
Small-intestinal	100	10
Diarrhoea	60[a]	20
Faeces	25	55
Sweat		
insensible	10	10
visible	60	10

[a] Variable (30–140 mmol/l)

Table 1.3 Some problems caused by oedema.

Site of oedema	Consequence
Liver	Abnormal liver-function tests
Gastrointestinal tract	Impaired gastric motility with subsequent delay in the time taken to tolerate oral food and recover from abdominal surgery; impaired absorption
Brain	Impaired consciousness in those with a head injury associated with some preexisting cerebral oedema
Wounds	Delayed healing

a negative N balance, with little improvement above an intake of ~0.25 g N/kg/day. With this in mind, protein requirements take into account the need to limit, but not necessarily abolish, N losses in catabolic patients, and the need to replete tissues in malnourished patients so that their function improves.

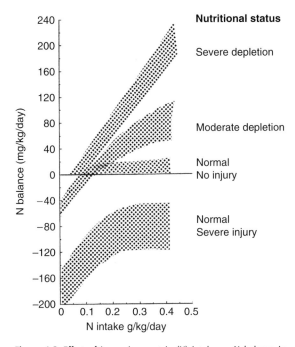

Figure 1.3 Effect of increasing protein (N) intake on N balance in depleted, healthy, and catabolic patients close to energy balance.

These criteria differ from those in healthy, well-functioning adults, who have no need to change their body composition. In contrast, in healthy children it is necessary to cater for growth and development, which is associated with deposition of tissue and a positive N balance. Similar considerations apply to calculating the requirements of other nutrients and of energy, but metabolism in health and disease differs in a number of ways, which affects concepts about requirements.

Energy

In healthy subjects the energy requirements necessary to maintain energy stores are often calculated as multiples of basal metabolic rate (BMR). However, in many acute diseases (Figure 1.4) and a number of chronic diseases BMR has been found to be increased, which led to the view that the energy requirements in such states were also usually increased. This conclusion failed to take into account the decrease in physical activity that occurs as a result of many diseases and disabilities. This decrease counteracts or more than counteracts the increase in BMR, so that total energy expenditure in most disease states (and hence the energy intake necessary to maintain balance) is actually close to normal, or even decreased. As previously noted, there is also the need to consider changes in energy stores. In obese individuals it is desirable to reduce the energy stores by providing hypocaloric feeding, and in depleted patients to increase energy stores by providing

Figure 1.4 Effect of acute disease severity (expressed as multiples of normal BMR) on total energy expenditure (shaded area). The difference between total energy expenditure and BMR is due to physical activity (and some thermogenesis, which typically accounts for ~10% of energy intake). The increase in BMR is counteracted by a decrease in physical activity. (a) Infection, persistent fever (1 °C); (b) infection, persistent fever (2 °C); (c) burns 10% (first month), single fracture (first week), postoperative (first 4 days); (d) burns 10–25% (first month), multiple long-bone fractures (first week); (e) severe sepsis/multiple trauma (patient on respirator); (f) burns 25–95% (first month).

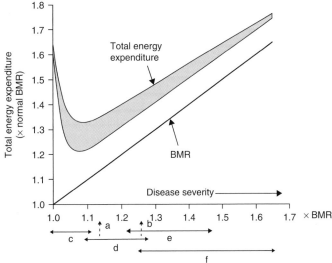

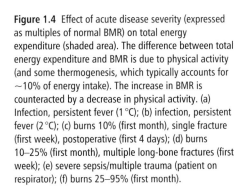

hypercaloric feeding. In both cases, it is usually better to do this during the recovery phase of illness rather than the acute and more unstable phase of illness (see later in this chapter).

In estimating the energy requirements of a hospitalised patient, it is worth considering the energy contribution from nondietary sources, such as intravenous dextrose 5% (~200 kcal/l), dialysate, and fat-based drugs such as propofol (~1.1 kcal/ml) and drugs that may need to be administered with saline.

Metabolic blocks and nutritional requirements

Inborn errors of metabolism

When there is a block in a metabolic pathway that involves conversion of substance A to B, there is an accumulation of substance A, which may be toxic (either directly or via its products), and a depletion in substance B, which needs to be either formed within the body by alternative pathways or provided by the diet. An alternative strategy is to replace the enzyme responsible for the block, for example by organ transplantation, although this has only been used for a few metabolic disorders. One of the best known examples of a metabolic block occurs in phenylketonurea (PKU), due to deficiency of the enzyme phenylalanine hydroxylase, the gene of which is located on chromosome 12 (12q). In the absence of phenylalanine hydroxylase, the gene of which normally converts the amino acid phenylalanine to tyrosine in the liver, there is an accumulation of phenylalanine and its metabolites, which causes brain damage, mental retardation, and epilepsy. Tyrosine, which is distal to the block, is provided by the diet so the treatment for PKU is to ingest a low-phenylalanine diet (some phenylalanine is required for protein synthesis) (see later in this chapter for the duration of treatment). The diet, which is not found in nature, is specifically manufactured to restrict the intake of phenylalanine. Other metabolic blocks may require exclusion of other individual nutrients, for example restriction of galactose and lactose in children with galactosemia. Some diets may exclude whole proteins, which can cause food allergy or sensitivity. In the case of coeliac disease, which is responsible for a small-bowel enteropathy with malabsorption, this means avoiding gluten, which is found in wheat and wheat products (see Chapter 8). However, the problem here is not due to

a block in a metabolic pathway, but to an abnormal reaction to food, which appears to be acquired.

Acquired metabolic blocks

Not all metabolic blocks are inherited as inborn errors of metabolism. For example, deficiency of phenylalanine hydroxylase can occur as a result of cirrhosis. Since in healthy subjects tyrosine can be formed from phenylalanine, some feed manufacturers have added little or no tyrosine to parenteral nutrition regimens, especially since tyrosine has a low solubility. However, a few patients with severe liver disease lose the ability to synthesise sufficent tyrosine, with the result that it becomes rate-limiting to protein synthesis, even in the presence of all other necessary amino acids (i.e. the enzymatic deficiency is ultimately responsible for the metabolic block in protein synthesis, which can be reversed by administering tyrosine). Other examples of acquired metabolic blocks due to amino acids involve histidine in some patients with renal disease, and cystine in liver disease. It is therefore essential that these amino acids (described as conditionally essential) are provided in the diet (oral or intravenous) of such patients, even though they are not essential for healthy subjects.

Acquired metabolic blocks may involve other types of nutrients. An interesting example concerns vitamin D, which is hydroxylated in the liver to produce 25-hydroxy vitamin D and further hydroxylated in the kidney to produce the active metabolite 1,25-dihydroxy vitamin D (Figure 1.5). Some patients with chronic renal failure are unable to produce sufficient amounts of 1,25-dihydroxy vitamin D, due to loss of activity of the enzyme 1 alpha hydroxylase in the kidney. Such patients may suffer from metabolic bone disease, which is at least partly due to deficiency of 1,25-dihydroxy vitamin D. This metabolic block can be bypassed by providing either synthetic 1,25-dihydroxy vitamin D or synthetic 1-hydroxy vitamin D, which is converted to 1,25-dihydroxy vitamin D in the liver (Figure 1.5). Such therapy differs from that used in the treatment of PKU in at least two ways: it involves administration of substance distal to the block (cf. restriction of phenylalanine, which is proximal to the block) and it is not found in the normal diet in any significant amounts. It is an example of nutritional pharmacology involving administration of a bioactive substance.

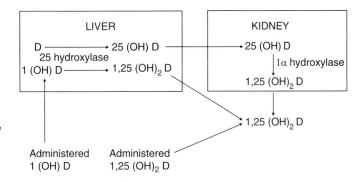

Figure 1.5 Metabolism of vitamin D in the liver and kidney. In renal failure, the formation of 1,25-dihydroxy vitamin D (1,25 (OH)$_2$ D) in the kidney may be inadequate, in which case 1,25-dihydroxy vitamin D or 1-hydroxy vitamin D (25 (OH) D) can be prescribed.

Table 1.4 Some examples of nutritional pharmacology.

Type I (prenutrients)	
Organic phosphates	The amount of calcium and phosphate that can be added to parenteral nutrition solutions is limited by the solubility of calcium phosphate, which can precipitate. Organic phosphates, such as glycerol-phosphate or glucose-phosphate, are soluble and do not precipitate in the presence of calcium. The organic phosphate is hydrolysed within the body to yield free phosphate
Dipeptides	Glutamine degrades during heat sterilisation and storage of parenteral amino acid solutions. It can be provided as a dipeptide (e.g. alanylglutamine), which is stable and can be stored for extended periods of time. Poorly soluble amino acids can be provided as soluble dipetides, such as glycyltyrosine or alanylcystine. The dipeptides are hydrolysed within the body to yield free amino acids
Type II (pharmacological doses)	
Glycerol	Free glycerol is used as an emulsifying agent in intravenous fat solutions
Medium-chain triglycerides	Medium-chain triglycerides (up to 50% of total lipid) may be better absorbed and tolerated than long-chain triglyceride. In intravenous use, these may avoid infusional hyperlipidaemia
Glutamine	Glutamine may be given in large amounts (12–30 g), with the aim of improving clinical outcome (e.g. in intensive care units)
Oligofructose	Bifidobacteria or oligofructose, which is a fermentable bifidogenic substrate, can be given orally with the aim of changing intestinal microflora and reducing the growth of potentially pathogenic organisms
Type III (bioactive substances)	
Erythropoietin	Increases utilisation of iron and Hb synthesis in anaemic patients with end-stage renal failure
1,25-dihydroxy and 1-hydroxy vitamin D	Used in renal failure when there is a block in 1α hydroxylation of 25-hydroxy vitamin D
Growth hormone	Aims to improve N balance

A variety of other bioactive substances have been used in clinical nutrition with the aim of improving outcome. Some products of metabolism require more than one class of substrate for their synthesis. For example, haemoglobin (Hb) comprises a variety of amino acids and iron, which forms part of the haem component. All the substrates may be available in adequate quantities, but a block in Hb synthesis can still occur as a result of a deficiency of erythropoietin, a bioactive substance produced by the kidney that stimulates Hb synthesis. Erythropoietin synthesis is upregulated during hypoxia, which explains the high Hb concentrations in people living at high altitudes. In contrast, lack of erythropoietin leads to anaemia. One of the features of end-stage renal failure is severe anaemia, which is at least partly due to the inability of the damaged kidney to produce enough erythropoietin. Traditionally, this anaemia was treated by repeated blood transfusions. Now that recombinant erythropoietin is available, it can be used to treat the anaemia and to eliminate or dramatically reduce the need for repeated blood transfusions, which carry the risk of transmitting infections, such as HIV and hepatitis, and which require admission of patients to special healthcare facilities. Importantly, injections of recombinant erythropoietin have also been shown to improve quality of life in patients with severe renal disease. Other examples of nutritional pharmacology, shown in Table 1.4, are divided into those involving administration of prenutrients, pharmacological doses of normal nutrients, and bioactive substances (see Table 1.4 for the rationale for specific types of nutritional pharmacology).

The uncritical use of bioactive substances can produce unpredictable serious side effects, including death. An example involves injections of pharmacological doses of growth hormone (GH) in critically ill patients. It was thought that GH might be beneficial in limiting the marked N loss that frequently occurs in such patients (equivalent to overcoming a metabolic block in net protein synthesis). GH is known to stimulate protein synthesis, and had previously been shown to improve N balance in a wide range of clinical conditions. However, in a large multicentre trial involving patients admitted to intensive care units, pharmacological doses of GH doubled mortality compared with the placebo group (from about 20 to 40%), sending a signal to the scientific and clinical community about the dangers of such interventions, especially when the mechanisms of action have not been previously evaluated.

The mechanism(s) responsible for the increased mortality with GH is still uncertain, but several suggestions have been made. One is that large doses of GH have detrimental effects on immune cells, which play a key role in host defence in critical illness. Another concerns the fluid-retaining properties of GH (see earlier for the detrimental effects of fluid overload). Yet another concerns the protein-stimulating properties of GH, which were, paradoxically, the main reason for using GH in the first place. Since muscle is thought to be a major site of action of GH, it is possible that stimulation of protein synthesis here may limit the availability of amino acids, including glutamine, to other tissues. These amino acids would normally be used for synthesis of proteins, for example the acute-phase proteins in the liver, which participate in the response to infection and inflammation. They are also normally used as fuel for a variety of cells, including immune cells (some preferentially utilising glutamine as a fuel), which play an important role in combating infection.

It has also been suggested that some of the detrimental effects of GH are due to cardiac arrhythmias from high concentrations of non-esterified fatty acids produced by the lipolytic effect of GH. Another suggestion is that the mortality is partly due to disturbances in glucose homeostasis, since GH produces significantly higher circulating glucose concentrations than the placebo. Hyperglycaemia in critically ill patients can have a range of detrimental effects, including predisposition to catheter-related sepsis in those receiving intravenous nutrition.

Effect of the route of feeding on nutrient requirements

In health, only the oral route is used to provide nutrients to the body; in clinical practice, other routes (or a combination) can be used. Before discussing their effect on nutrient requirements, it is necessary to briefly consider the type of nutritional support and feeding route. In general, food is the first line of treatment, but if this is inadequate to meet the needs of patients, oral supplements may be used, followed by enteral tube feeding and then intravenous feeding (parenteral nutrition). However, this linear sequence is inadequate in a number of situations. The first-line treatment for someone who has acutely developed short bowel syndrome is parenteral nutrition, not oral nutrition, oral supplements, or even enteral tube feeding. Similarly, tube feeding may be the first-line treatment for a patient with a swallowing problem – not oral food or supplements, which can cause detrimental effects. In some situations (e.g. cerebral palsy), oral feeding is possible, but this can take several hours per day and so it may be more practical to tube feed. In essence, the simplest, most physiological, and safest route to provide a patient's nutritional requirements should be sought, while taking into account the practicalities of feeding. Occasional unusual and unsuspected routes deliver nutrients into the body (see below). The route of feeding can have major effects on nutrient requirements, particularly parenteral nutrition.

Parenteral nutrition

The use of the intravenous route for feeding raises a number of new issues, especially in relation to nutrients which are poorly absorbed by the gut. For some nutrients, such as sodium, potassium iodide, fluoride, and selenium, which are well absorbed, the intravenous requirements are similar to the oral requirements. For nutrients that are poorly absorbed, such as iron, calcium, and especially chromium and manganese, the intravenous requirements are considerably lower than the oral requirements, sometimes up to 10-fold lower (Figure 1.6). If the doses of some

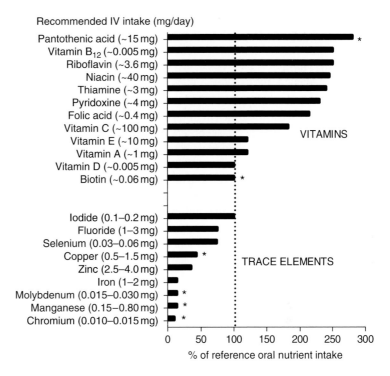

Recommended IV intake (mg/day)

VITAMINS

TRACE ELEMENTS

% of reference oral nutrient intake

Figure 1.6 Recommended doses of vitamins and trace elements for intravenous (IV) nutrition expressed as a percentage of the recommended nutrient intake (UK values). Those marked with an asterisk indicate nutrients for which there was inadequate information to establish a reference nutrient intake (RNI). For these nutrients, the midpoint of the estimated average oral intake is used for comparative purposes.

of these trace elements or minerals recommended for oral nutrition were to be used intravenously over prolonged periods of time, they would probably produce toxic effects.

This consideration highlights the key role of the gut in regulating the amount of micronutrients absorbed in health. Sometimes the gut plays the only important role in controlling the status of nutrients within the body. For example, there is no effective physiological way of eliminating excess iron once it is within the body. In contrast to the recommended intakes of intravenous trace elements, those for intravenous vitamins are usually higher than the RNI for oral nutrition (Figure 1.6). There are several reasons why this is so. First, patients receiving parenteral (intravenous) nutrition usually have severe disease, which may increase the requirements for some vitamins. Second, patients are often affected by preexisting malnutrition and are in need of repletion. Third, the prescribed nutrients may not be delivered to the patient because they are lost during preparation or storage (e.g. vitamin C may be oxidised by oxygen present in the bag, a process catalysed by copper; vitamin A may be destroyed by sunlight; and some nutrients

may be adsorbed on to the plastic bag containing the parenteral nutrition solution).

Gastric and jejunal feeding

Feed may be delivered directly into the stomach using a nasogastric tube, or a gastrostomy tube for long-term feeding in patients with swallowing difficulties. Jejunal feeding (e.g. jejunostomy or nasojejunal tube feeding) can be used in patients with poor gastric emptying, those at risk of regurgitation and aspiration pneumonia, and those with abnormal gastric anatomy and function. Nutrient requirements associated with these routes of feeding when the bowel is functioning normally are generally similar to those for oral feeding, although many patients on long-term tube feeding are physically inactive due to the underlying disease, and therefore their energy requirements may be less than in healthy subjects. An unusual complication of enteral tube feeding concerns the neurological control of eating. A few children who start tube feeding when young and continue receiving it for prolonged periods may 'forget' how to eat. They may have to relearn how to eat when tube feeding is terminated. In contrast, some patients with dementia appear to forget how to eat, have difficulty in relearning, and thus need to start tube feeding.

Cutaneous (skin)

Essential fatty acid deficiency can be treated or prevented by topical skin application of corn oil or safflower oil, which allows sufficient uptake of essential fatty acids into the body. These observations are of more scientific/historical than practical clinical interest, since essential fatty acids can usually be delivered into the gut or directly into veins. Irradiation of the skin with ultraviolet light can also be used to prevent vitamin D deficiency in housebound patients not exposed to direct sunlight. Alternatively, vitamin D tablets can be prescribed, especially since the amount of vitamin in the normal diet is unlikely to be sufficient to meet the RNI (10 μg/day for subjects aged over 50 years, according to UK recommendations).

Subcutaneous

Subcutaneous infusions of saline/dextrose may be given to maintain comfort and hydration in some terminally ill patients requiring palliative care who cannot drink or eat and who have poor venous access.

Rectal

One of the physiological functions of the large bowel is to absorb salt and water, a property that can be utilised by a rectal infusion of saline in terminally ill patients who are unable to eat/drink and have poor venous access. In the past, rectal feeding was used to provide a range of other nutrients, including alcohol, which is relatively well absorbed from the large bowel. In 1881, American President James A. Garfield received rectal feeding, which included alcohol, during his terminal illness following a gunshot wound inflicted by an assassin.

Peritoneal

During peritoneal dialysis with solutions of hypertonic glucose, which can cross the peritoneal membrane, several hundred calories may enter the systemic circulation. This is a side effect of treatment that is often not appreciated.

It is useful to remember that tissues that are used to provide nutritional access to the body can also be sites of abnormal nutrient losses; for example, loss of protein, loss of trace elements from burned skin, loss of protein from the kidney of patients with nephrotic syndrome, and loss of a variety of nutrients from the gut in patients with inflammatory bowel disease or diarrhoea.

Effect of the phase of disease on nutritional requirements

One of the first steps in the management of patients with severe acute disease is to resuscitate them to establish adequate oxygenation and acid–base status, as well as cardiovascular and metabolic stability. This may involve correcting dehydration or overhydration, and treating any hypoglycaemia or hypothermia. Aggressive nutritional support before this stability is established can precipitate further problems with adverse clinical outcomes. For example, a common consequence of major abdominal surgery or systemic illness is ileus or slow gastric emptying. To facilitate oral feeding after surgery, several actions are useful. These include:

- Using appropriate analgaesia, including local anaesthetics given via a continuous epidural catheter during the first few days after surgery (this minimises the need for opiates, which have inhibitory effects on gastrointestinal motility).
- Avoiding overhydration, which predisposes to postoperative ileus.
- Ensuring that the patient is fully informed that they should eat.

For some patients, there are risks with giving normal food or oral nutrition shortly after surgery. Aggressive feeding by mouth or by a nasogastric tube may still lead to gastric pooling, predisposing to nausea, vomiting, regurgitation, or aspiration pneumonia. This is more likely to happen in patients who have swallowing problems or preexisting reflux problems (e.g. in association with a hiatus hernia), or who are nursed in a horizontal position.

Aggressive intravenous nutrition with copious amounts of glucose in the early phase of an acute illness, when there is insulin resistance, can result in hyperglycaemia, hyperosmolarity, and exacerbation of existing metabolic instability. During the early phase of a severe acute illness, it may therefore sometimes be necessary to start with hypocaloric nutrition and increase this over a period of time. This is to ensure metabolic stability and tolerance to nutrients, while maintaining adequate tissue function and limiting excess N loss.

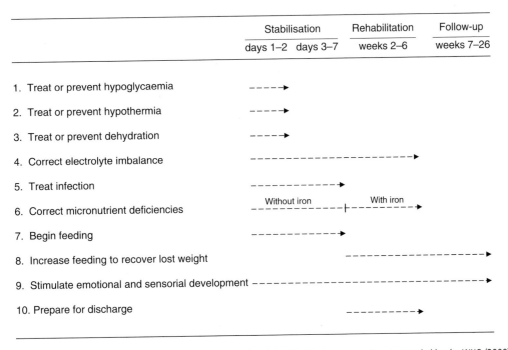

	Stabilisation		Rehabilitation	Follow-up
	days 1–2	days 3–7	weeks 2–6	weeks 7–26
1. Treat or prevent hypoglycaemia				
2. Treat or prevent hypothermia				
3. Treat or prevent dehydration				
4. Correct electrolyte imbalance				
5. Treat infection				
6. Correct micronutrient deficiencies				
7. Begin feeding				
8. Increase feeding to recover lost weight				
9. Stimulate emotional and sensorial development				
10. Prepare for discharge				

Figure 1.7 Time frame for the management of a child with severe malnutrition (the 10-step approach recommended by the WHO (2000)).

Tissue repletion is mainly recommended during the recovery phase of an acute illness. Similarly, in obese patients the focus on long-term weight loss usually occurs after the acute phase of illness.

The WHO has provided a 10-step guide to the nutritional management of malnourished children, which reemphasises the need to consider nutritional support according to the phase of disease. Again, this begins with the stabilisation phase, associated with resuscitation, which is followed by the rehabilitation phase, which can take several weeks, and finally the follow-up phase (Figure 1.7). It is notable that the guidelines suggest withholding iron supplementation during the early phase of illness. This is because of concern about the possible adverse effects of iron, which has prooxidant properties that facilitate formation of free radicals, which in turn produce cellular damage. The risk is considered to be greater during the early phase of disease, when oxidant stresses are high and antioxidant defences are frequently low as a result of preexisting malnutrition.

A particular complication of aggressive refeeding of malnourished individuals is the refeeding syndrome. Rapid refeeding of such individuals can precipitate respiratory, cardiovascular, and metabolic problems, which may result in sudden death. For example, sudden death was reported when victims of World War II concentration camps were rapidly refed, especially with high-carbohydrate diets. The metabolic abnormalities of the refeeding syndrome include low circulating concentrations of potassium, magnesium, and phosphate, which enter lean tissue cells during the process of repletion under the influence of insulin. The low circulating concentrations of these nutrients can precipitate cardiac arrhythmias and sudden death. Slow initial refeeding while monitoring the circulating concentration of these nutrients can reduce the risk of developing the refeeding syndrome. Precise feeding schedules vary from centre to centre, but they may begin with half or less than half of the requirements in severely depleted individuals.

Alterations in nutritional therapy during the course of an acute disease may occur because the underlying disease has produced new complications or because it has resolved. Similarly, in more chronic conditions there is a need to review the diet at regular intervals. A therapeutic diet lacking particular dietary components may no longer be needed if, for example, a specific food allergy or sensitivity has resolved. Another consideration is whether a vulnerable developmental period has passed. It used to be thought that cerebral damage due to PKU did not occur after the early developmental period and that it would thus be possible to replace the phenylalanine-poor diet with a more normal diet during later childhood, despite persistence of the underlying metabolic abnormality. Children who reverted to a normal diet, especially during early childhood, were however found to be particularly vulnerable to regression of the developmental quotient (IQ) and development of other neurological symptoms. Children who stopped the phenylalanine-poor diet at or after the age of 15 were generally not affected in this way, but few long-term follow-up studies (e.g. 20–30 years) have examined effects on IQ. Many centres therefore recommend some restriction of phenylalanine throughout life.

Feeding schedules

In healthy people, food is normally ingested during a small number of meals, usually two to three per day, although additional snacks may also be taken. Most patients with disease follow similar patterns of eating, but some may require different feeding schedules. For example, children with certain forms of glycogen storage disease need to ingest small, frequent meals rich in carbohydrate to prevent hypoglycaemia. In patients receiving artificial nutritional support (enteral tube feeding or parenteral nutrition), less physiological feeding schedules may be employed, out of either necessity or convenience. Continuous feeding over prolonged periods of time, up to 24 hours per day, is simple and convenient to carers managing bed-bound patients, including those who are unconscious. Continuous feeding over prolonged periods may also be necessary when only slow rates of feeding are tolerated. For example, patients with certain intestinal problems, such as the short bowel syndrome, may be able to tolerate and absorb sufficient nutrients to meet their needs only if the gut is infused slowly with nutrients over a prolonged period of time during the day and the night. Such an enteral feeding schedule may avoid the need for parenteral nutrition, which is less physiological, more costly, and often associated with a greater number of serious complications.

Many patients on home parenteral nutrition and enteral tube feeding may be able to receive adequate amounts of feed during 12–16 hours per day. This means that they receive continuous pump-assisted infusion during the night (and part of the day), which is again unphysiological. During the day, such patients can disconnect themselves from the feeding equipment to undertake activities of normal daily living, including exercise. This practice can have both physical and psychological benefits. It is also associated with some disadvantages, however, including dependency on the feeding equipment and in some cases abnormal appetite sensations. Although lack of appetite is typical during acute illness, some patients with little or no inflammatory disease who are on long-term artificial nutrition may suffer from hunger and desire to eat, even when sufficient nutrients are delivered artificially by tube into the stomach or by catheter into a vein. These abnormal and sometimes distressing and persisting appetite sensations may be due to provision of liquid rather than solid food, to bypassing of part of the gut (gastric feeding) or the entire gut (parenteral nutrition), or to lack of or reduced gastric distension. They may also be the result of psychosocially conditioned responses, such as those stimulated by observing others eating. The physiological responses to normal food intake, which are associated with fluctuating hormonal and substrate responses, are either attenuated or absent when continuous feeding is provided. The clinical significance of these changes is unclear.

Structure and function

Several bodily functions are related to body composition, specifically the mass of tissue or tissue components. For example, the risk of fracture is greater in individuals with a low bone mineral mass (osteoporosis). Muscle strength is related to muscle mass, and body mass index (BMI = (weight in kg)/(height in m)^2) has been found to be a useful marker for a wide range of bodily functions and for wellbeing, including quality of life. Repletion of tissues is often associated with improvements in bodily functions, including muscle strength and fatigue, reproductive function, and psychological behavior. However, improvements in physiological function and clinical outcome can also occur in the presence of little or no change in gross body composition, and vice versa. Nutritional intervention during key phases of an illness can have an important effect on outcome. Examples include fluid balance (avoiding

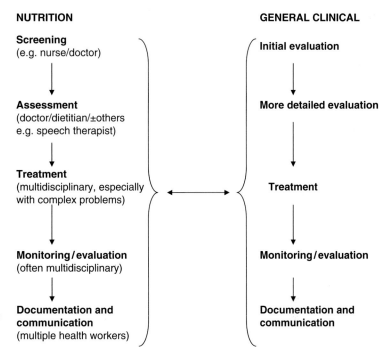

NUTRITION

Screening
(e.g. nurse/doctor)

Assessment
(doctor/dietitian/±others
e.g. speech therapist)

Treatment
(multidisciplinary, especially
with complex problems)

Monitoring/evaluation
(often multidisciplinary)

**Documentation and
communication**
(multiple health workers)

GENERAL CLINICAL

Initial evaluation

More detailed evaluation

Treatment

Monitoring/evaluation

**Documentation and
communication**

Figure 1.8 Similarities in nutritional and general clinical management pathways and the interaction between the two. Based on Elia (2003).

high fluid intake in the early postoperative period; see earlier in this chapter), oral nutritional supplementation in the perioperative period, and control of blood glucose concentration with insulin in critically ill patients (see earlier). The administration of GH to critically ill patients to improve N balance has been associated with detrimental effects, illustrating a dissociation between gross body composition and function.

1.4 Management pathways

Although resources vary in different countries, in different places in the same country, and at different times in the same place in the same country (e.g. during famines), there are common overarching management pathways. These begin with nutritional screening and assessment, which should be linked to care plans (Figure 1.8). The care plans may involve different healthcare settings (e.g. hospital, community care homes). Since the time spent in hospital may be short (<5% of the duration of an acute illness from onset to complete recovery), treatment initiated there may need to continue and be assessed in the community. It is disturbing that

malnutrition is underrecognised and undertreated, and that there is frequent lack of continuity of care. The initial recognition of malnutrition or of risk of malnutrition is an essential first step in the management pathway and is discussed in the next chapter. Chapter 25 illustrates using case studies how the nutritional screening test becomes an integral part of management.

1.5 Concluding remarks

The science of clinical nutrition is rapidly expanding and includes an appreciation of medicine, pharmacology, and nursing disciplines. As you read this book, you will appreciate the link between nutritional needs and outcome, including quality of life, in a wide range of disease states. It is essential that clinicians provide education and nutrition support to patients, centred on the most up-to-date and sound evidence-based practices.

Whether physiological or nonphysiological interventions are used, the practice of clinical nutrition is guided by improvements in bodily functions and clinical outcomes, especially if these are also cost-effective.

References and further reading

Elia M, chairman and editor. The 'MUST' report. Nutritional screening for adults: a multidisciplinary responsibility. Development and use of the 'Malnutrition Universal Screening Tool' ('MUST') for adults. A report by the Malnutrition Advisory Group of the British Association for Parenteral and Enteral Nutrition, 2003.

Elia M. Nutrition. In: Clinical Medicine, 8th edn (P Kumar, M Clark, eds). London: Saunders Elsevier, 2012.

Elia M, Russell CA. Combating malnutrition: recommendations for action. A report from the Advisory Group on Malnutrition, led by BAPEN. London, 2009.

Gibney MJ, Lantham SA, Cassidy A, Voster HH, editors. Introduction to Human Nutrition, 2nd edn . Oxford: Wiley-Blackwell, 2009.

Keys A, Brozek J, Henschel A, Mickelsen O, Taylor HL. The Biology of Human Starvation, Vol. 1. Minneapolis, MN: University of Minnesota Press, 1950, pp. 81–535.

Leyton GB. The effects of slow starvation. Lancet 1946; ii: 73–79.

Rudman D, Millikan WJ, Richardson TJ, Bixler TJ II, Stackhouse WJ, McGarity WC. Elemental balances during intravenous hyperalimentation of underweight adult subjects. J Clin Invest 1975; 55: 94–104.

Scientific Advisory Committee on Nutrition. Dietary reference values for enery, 2011. London: The Stationary Office, 2013.

Sobotka L, editor. Basics in Clinical Nutrition, 4th edn. Prague: Galen, 2011.

Stratton RJ, Green CJ, Elia M. Disease-related Malnutrition. An Evidence-based Approach to Treatment. Oxford: CABI Publishing, 2003.

WHO. Management of Severe Malnutrition: A Manual for Physicians and Other Senior Health Workers. Geneva: WHO, 1999.

WHO. Management of the Child with Serious Infection or Severe Malnutrition. Geneva: WHO, 2000. Available from http://whqlibdoc.who.int/hq/2000/WHO_FCH_CAH_00.1.pdf.

WHO Technical Report Series: no 935. Protein and amino acid requirements in human nutrition. Report of a joint WHO/FAO/UNU expert consultation. Geneva, 2007.

2
Nutritional Screening and Assessment

Marinos Elia and Rebecca J Stratton

Institute of Human Nutrition, University of Southampton, Southampton, UK

Key messages

- An evaluation of a person's nutritional status is a key step in the management of malnutrition.
- Many screening instruments for malnutrition exist and the choice depends on the purpose for which they were designed, the target population, and the characteristics of the tools, such as reliability, validity, and user-friendliness. The use of the same consistent criteria within and between settings can facilitate care during the patient journey.
- In contrast to nutritional screening, which is a rapid procedure, often undertaken at the bedside or in the field, a more detailed
- nutritional assessment of nutritional status, including the status of individual nutrients, is more time-consuming and may involve a variety of different approaches, ranging from a detailed clinical and dietary history to a physical examination, and an array of investigations, ranging from body composition tests to laboratory measurements of nutrient concentrations in physiological fluids.
- The results of nutritional screening and assessments should be linked to a care plan, with clearly defined goals for treatment where appropriate, which should be re-evaluated at intervals.

2.1 Introduction

Considerable emphasis is placed on the identification of malnutrition, because it is the first step in the management of malnutrition. Ultimately, the aim is to provide effective treatment to individuals who need nutritional support and not to provide it to those who do not need it. Without identification, no effective treatment can occur. Inappropriate identification can be counterproductive, since treatment may be given to those who do not need it, and thus withheld from those who would stand to benefit from it.

For practical reasons, nutritional screening is often distinguished from nutritional assessment:

- *Nutritional screening* is a simple, quick, and general procedure used by nursing, medical, or other staff, often at first contact with a patient, to detect significant risk of nutritional problems, so that a clear action plan can be implemented. This may involve referral to a dietitian or another expert.
- *Nutritional assessment* is a more detailed and specific evaluation of a patient's nutritional status, usually undertaken by an individual with some nutritional expertise (e.g. dietitian, clinician with an interest in nutrition or nutrition nurse specialist). Assessment is usually carried out when serious nutritional problems are identified by the screening process, or when there is uncertainty about the appropriate course of action. It allows specific nutritional care plans to be developed for individual patients. It can also be used to identify micronutrient status, although this frequently requires confirmation by laboratory investigations.

Clinical Nutrition, Second Edition. Edited by Marinos Elia, Olle Ljungqvist, Rebecca J Stratton and Susan A Lanham-New.
© 2013 The Nutrition Society. Published 2013 by Blackwell Publishing Ltd.

It is also useful to distinguish between a nutritional screening test and a screening programme:

- A *screening test*, typically a recognised screening tool or instrument, is the test used to identify a disease or a condition (e.g. malnutrition or obesity).
- A *screening programme* is the full range of activities from identification of risk using a screening test to definitive diagnosis and treatment of the disease or condition.

This chapter focuses predominantly on nutritional screening and assessment in adults, although the general principles also apply to children (for paediatric aspects, especially anthropometry, see Chapter 23).

2.2 Nutritional screening

The screening test (or screening tool) should be simple and quick to perform, valid and reliable, and acceptable to both patient and health worker. Ideally it should also be able to identify risk of malnutrition in those who are unconscious or confused, and in those in whom weight or height cannot be measured. Furthermore, a screening test that is portable will facilitate care during the patient journey. Use of multiple screening tests based on different principles during the patient journey, either within care settings (e.g. transfer of patients from one ward to another or from one hospital to another) or between care settings, can be confusing and counterproductive. Since nutritional problems exist in all care settings, there would be several practical advantages if the same screening principles could be applied to all types of patients by a range of care workers. These advantages include facilitation of audits, economic evaluations, and comparisons of malnutrition prevalence between different groups of patients using consistent criteria. Furthermore, screening tools that simultaneously address both under- and over-nutrition would help bridge the gap between clinical and public health nutrition. Some screening tools have been developed for very specific applications, but unless they have demonstrable advantages over more general tools, there is likely to be some resistance to adopting them for routine clinical care, especially in care settings where the target population forms only a small proportion of the total population. The need

to use different screening tools for different population groups would increase organisational complexity.

The choice of screening tool may not be easy, especially since some screening tools have poor agreement with others. There are a large number of screening instruments: some for children, others for adults, and some for both adults and children. In addition, many tools have been developed for use in specific subgroups of patients. Some adult screening tools have been specifically developed for older people and others for adults of all ages. Certain tools have been developed for particular care settings, such as hospitals and care homes, while others have been developed for all care settings. Some screening tools have been developed for use in specific clinical conditions, such as liver transplantation, renal dialysis, and learning difficulties, while others have been developed for all types of conditions. Screening tools have also been developed for use by specific healthcare workers, such as doctors (e.g. Subjective Global Assessment, SGA), nurses, or dietitians, or a combination of all three (e.g. the 'Malnutrition Universal Screening Tool', 'MUST'). Some have even been developed for members of the public, such as carers or the patients themselves, who are expected to self-screen (e.g. Screen I and II and DETERMINE). Some screening tools have been developed with other aims in mind, including: to identify nutritional status, to identify the need for nutritional intervention, to predict clinical outcomes without nutritional intervention, to predict healthcare use, and to predict clinical outcomes of nutritional interventions. This wide array of screening tools, coupled with the lack of a universally accepted definition for malnutrition and the wide variability between tools in validity, reliability, and ease of use, can create difficulties in choosing a screening tool that is fit for purpose. Figure 2.1 provides a framework for screening-tool selection that takes into account the aims, applications, and processes associated with particular screening tools, the principles on which they are based, and the overall purpose of the screening programme.

Although several examples of nutrition screening tools can be used to illustrate the underlying principles, details of only three are provided here (Subjective Global Assessment (SGA)) (Figure 2.2), Mini Nutritional Assessment (short form)

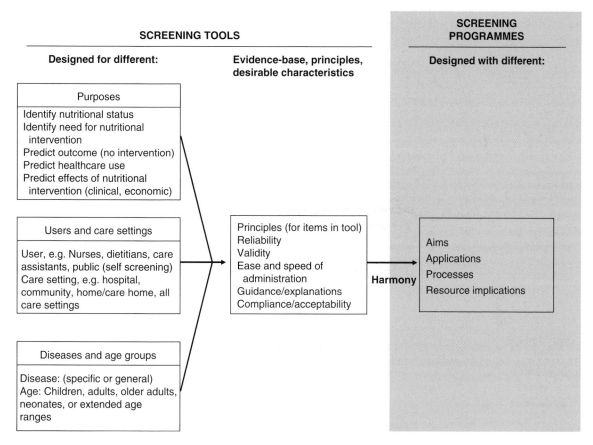

Figure 2.1 A framework for screening-tool selection. Reprinted from Elia & Stratton (2012), © BioMed Central.

(MNA, www.mna-elderly.com) (Figure 2.3), and 'Malnutrition Universal Screening Tool' ('MUST', www.bapen.org.uk) (Figure 2.4). These were chosen partly because they are commonly cited or widely used, and partly because they illustrate the diversity of purpose and target populations. The SGA (Figure 2.2) was developed for use by clinicians in the late 1980s to predict clinical outcome without nutritional intervention, initially in hospitalised patients with gastrointestinal problems, and later in other groups of patients within the hospital setting. It is applicable to adults of all ages, although it may not be easy to administer for untrained nonmedical practitioners, who are required to identify certain signs including the presence of ascites and then integrate their overall findings into an overall subjective category of risk. Since it is a subjective tool, it does not involve measurement of weight or

height. There is no clear guidance about how the results of the SGA are linked to a care plan. The MNA was developed in the early 1990s for use in older people (>65 years), and it is now used in different care settings. The original tool, with 18 items, took considerable time to complete (and as such can be regarded more like an assessment than a screening tool, according to the criteria indicated above), and over time shorter versions have been produced (Figure 2.3). If the short version of the tool indicates 'possible malnutrition' ('malnutrition' or 'at risk of malnutrition'), it is recommended that a more detailed assessment be performed using the full version of the MNA. The tool involves measurement of weight and height to establish body mass index (BMI). A BMI <23 kg/m² contributes to the final malnutrition score (greater contributions to 'possible malnutrition' occur at BMI <21 kg/m², and

(Select appropriate category with a check mark, or enter numerical value where indicated by "#")

A. History

1. Weight change

Overall loss in past 6 months: amount = #_____kg; % loss = #_____

Change in past 2 weeks: _____increase

_____no change

_____decrease

2. Dietary intake change (relative to normal)

_____No change

_____Change   _____duration = #_____weeks

_____type: _____suboptimal solid diet   _____full liquid diet

_____hypocaloric liquids   _____starvation

3. Gastrointestinal symptoms (that persisted for >2 weeks)

_____none _____nausea _____vomiting _____diarrhoea _____anorexia

4. Functional capacity

_____No dysfunction (e.g. full capacity)

_____Dysfunction _____duration = #_____weeks

_____type: _____working suboptimally

_____ambulatory

_____bedridden

5. Disease and its relation to nutritional requirements

Primary diagnosis (specify)_____

Metabolic demand (stress):   _____no stress   _____low stress

_____moderate stress _____high stress

B. Physical (for each trait specify: 0 = normal, 1+ = mild, 2+ = moderate, 3+ = severe)

#_____loss of subcutaneous fat (triceps, chest)

#_____muscle wasting (quadriceps, deltoids)

#_____ankle oedema

#_____sacral oedema

#_____ascites

C. SGA rating (select one)

_____A = Well nourished

_____B = Moderately (or suspected of being) malnourished

_____C = Severely malnourished

Figure 2.2 Subjective Global Assessment (SGA) Detsky AS *et al*. J Parenter Enteral Nutr (Vol. 11, No. 1) pp. 8–13, copyright © 1987 by SAGE Publications. Reprinted by permission of SAGE Publications.

even greater contributions at BMI <19 kg/m²). The MNA was developed to establish nutritional status but, as with the SGA, clear guidance linking the results to a care plan is not provided. The 'MUST', developed in the UK, was launched in 2003 after field testing in over 200 centres. Its purpose was to establish the need for nutritional support according to nutritional status, including obesity, in adults of all ages in all care settings. Objective criteria, such as measurements of weight and height, are used whenever possible, and subjective criteria when necessary. The BMI cut-off point for malnutrition is

<18.5 kg/m² (or <20 kg/m² for possible malnutrition in those without other criteria). BMI, together with the other two 'MUST' criteria (unintentional weight loss and an acute disease effect that has produced or is likely to produce no intake for more than 5 days), can be considered to represent a nutritional journey beginning in the past (history of weight loss), through the present (current weight status in the form of BMI), and continuing into the future (likely future weight change during the course of a disease) (Figure 2.4). This resonates with standard principles associated with establishing an overview of a patient

Mini Nutritional Assessment
MNA®

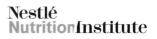

Last name: _____   First name: _____

Sex: _____   Age: _____   Weight, kg: _____   Height, cm: _____   Date: _____

Complete the screen by filling in the boxes with the appropriate numbers. Total the numbers for the final screening score.

Screening

A Has food intake declined over the past 3 months due to loss of appetite, digestive problems, chewing or swallowing difficulties?
0 = severe decrease in food intake
1 = moderate decrease in food intake
2 = no decrease in food intake   ☐

B Weight loss during the last 3 months
0 = weight loss greater than 3 kg (6.6 lbs)
1 = does not know
2 = weight loss between 1 and 3 kg (2.2 and 6.6 lbs)
3 = no weight loss   ☐

C Mobility
0 = bed or chair bound
1 = able to get out of bed/chair but does not go out
2 = goes out   ☐

D Has suffered psychological stress or acute disease in the past 3 months?
0 = yes   2 = no   ☐

E Neuropsychological problems
0 = severe dementia or depression
1 = mild dementia
2 = no psychological problems   ☐

F1 Body Mass Index (BMI) (weight in kg) / (height in m²)
0 = BMI less than 19
1 = BMI 19 to less than 21
2 = BMI 21 to less than 23
3 = BMI 23 or greater   ☐

IF BMI IS NOT AVAILABLE, REPLACE QUESTION F1 WITH QUESTION F2.
DO NOT ANSWER QUESTION F2 IF QUESTION F1 IS ALREADY COMPLETED.

F2 Calf circumference (CC) in cm
0 = CC less than 31
3 = CC 31 or greater   ☐

Screening score (max. 14 points)

12–14 points: Normal nutritional status
8–11 points: At risk of malnutrition
0–7 points: Malnourished   ☐ ☐

References
1. Vellas B, Villars H, Abellan G, et al. Overview of the MNA® - Its History and Challenges. *J Nutr Health Aging*. 2006; **10:**456–465.
2. Rubenstein LZ, Harker JO, Salva A, Guigoz Y, Vellas B. Screening for Undernutrition in Geriatric Practice: Developing the Short-Form Mini Nutritional Assessment (MNA-SF). *J. Geront*. 2001; **56A:** M366–377.
3. Guigoz Y. The Mini-Nutritional Assessment (MNA®) Review of the Literature - What does it tell us? *J Nutr Health Aging*. 2006; **10:**466–487.
4. Kaiser MJ, Bauer JM, Ramsch C, *et al.* Validation of the Mini Nutritional Assessment Short-Form (MNA®-SF): A practical tool for identification of nutritional status. *J Nutr Health Aging*. 2009; **13:**782–788.

® Société des Produits Nestlé, S.A., Vevey, Switzerland, Trademark Owners © Nestlé, 1994, Revision 2009. N67200 12/99 10M
For more information: www.mna-elderly.com

Figure 2.3 Short-form Mini Nutritional Assessment (NMA) (Guigoz, 2006; Kaiser *et al.*, 2009; Rubenstein *et al.*, 2001; Vellas *et al.*, 2006). ® Société des Produits Nestlé, S.A., Vevey, Switzerland; Trademark Owners © Nestlé, 1994, Revision 2009. N67200 12/99 10 M. For more information: www.mna-elderly.com.

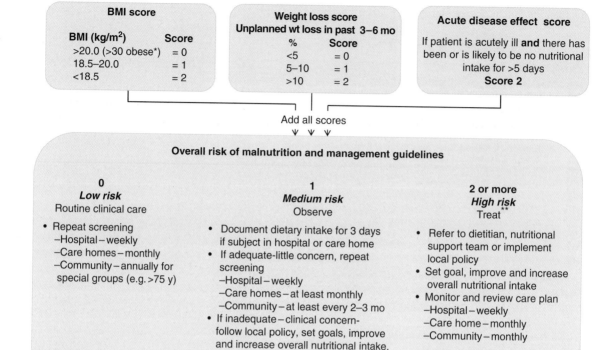

BMI score

BMI (kg/m²)	Score
>20.0 (>30 obese*)	= 0
18.5–20.0	= 1
<18.5	= 2

Weight loss score
Unplanned wt loss in past 3–6 mo

%	Score
<5	= 0
5–10	= 1
>10	= 2

Acute disease effect score

If patient is acutely ill **and** there has been or is likely to be no nutritional intake for >5 days
Score 2

Add all scores

Overall risk of malnutrition and management guidelines

0
Low risk
Routine clinical care

- Repeat screening
  –Hospital–weekly
  –Care homes–monthly
  –Community–annually for special groups (e.g. >75 y)

1
Medium risk
Observe

- Document dietary intake for 3 days if subject in hospital or care home
- If adequate-little concern, repeat screening
  –Hospital–weekly
  –Care homes–at least monthly
  –Community–at least every 2–3 mo
- If inadequate–clinical concern- follow local policy, set goals, improve and increase overall nutritional intake, monitor and review care plan regularly

2 or more
High risk
Treat**

- Refer to dietitian, nutritional support team or implement local policy
- Set goal, improve and increase overall nutritional intake
- Monitor and review care plan
  –Hospital–weekly
  –Care home–monthly
  –Community–monthly

** Unless detrimental or no benefit is expected from nutritional support, e.g. imminent death.

Record malnutrition risk category, presence of obesity and/or need for special diets and follow local policy. Re-assess those identified at risk as they move through care settings. If unable to obtain height and weight, alternative measurements and subjective criteria are provided.
* in the obese, underlying acute conditions are generally controlled before the treatment of obesity.

Figure 2.4 'Malnutrition Universal Screening Tool' ('MUST'). The 'Malnutrition Universal Screening Tool' ('MUST') is adapted and reproduced here with the kind permission of BAPEN (British Association for Parenteral and Enteral Nutrition). For further information on 'MUST' see www.bapen.org.uk.

in routine clinical practice. The tool can be administered by a variety of healthcare workers for clinical as well as public health purposes.

All of the aforementioned screening tools were developed for use in Western societies and therefore caution should be exercised in using them in developing countries with predominantly non-Caucasian populations.

A variety of other screening tools incorporating special features also exist. Some tools require information about dietary intake and requirements. For example, Nutritional Risk Screening – 2002 (NRS-2002), which was developed for hospital use, requires specific information about the extent to which dietary intake meets requirements. This may not always be easy to establish, partly because an accurate assessment of dietary intake can be difficult, and partly because dietary requirements vary with the type,

severity, and stage of disease, the degree of existing malnutrition, and the type of nutrient. Total energy requirements are typically not increased in acute and chronic diseases. However, the requirement for specific nutrients may increase or decrease depending on the nutrient (see Chapter 1), sometimes simultaneously in the same patient. Another special feature of some screening tools is that they require blood tests. For example, the Geriatric Nutritional Risk Index, developed by French workers as a modification of Buzby's Nutritional Risk Index, which is applicable to adults of all ages, incorporates a blood test. In order to be rapid, so that a category for malnutrition risk can be produced almost immediately at the bedside or in the field, screening tools do not generally incorporate blood tests (although these may feature in nutritional assessment (see Section 2.3)). Chapter 25 uses case studies to illustrate how the nutritional screening test can become an integral part of management from the outset. In some centres, where certain blood tests are taken routinely and the results are reported quickly using electronic systems, there may be little delay in obtaining the results as part of nutritional screening. However, it is important to remember that the circulating concentration of proteins such as albumin, which is a component of some screening tools, is more likely to be affected by trauma, elective surgery, inflammatory status, and hydration status than by nutritional status *per se*.

Nutrition screening tools were largely developed to detect protein–energy malnutrition, rather than specific nutrient deficiencies. Although the presence of protein–energy malnutrition is often associated with specific nutrient deficiencies, this is not invariably the case. The issue of nutrient deficiencies is addressed in Section 2.3. In the end, all the information is considered and a care plan with goals is implemented, and is followed up with repeat nutritional screening/assessment as required.

2.3 Nutritional assessment

Nutritional assessment can take many forms, ranging from clinical history to detailed or sophisticated measurements of body composition, laboratory tests for protein–energy malnutrition and specific nutrient deficiencies, measurement of nutrient turnover using isotopes, and functional tests such as muscle function tests. Although the results obtained from such procedures can be, and often are, combined to build an overall picture of nutritional status, this chapter largely focuses on the clinical considerations. The clinical assessment typically begins with a well-structured history to identify conditions likely to be associated with nutritional deficiencies, and a dietary history to indicate unusual dietary patterns or major changes in dietary intake.

Clinical history

Protein–energy malnutrition

Weight loss: the clinical history can establish the extent of recent unintentional weight loss (or weight gain). Unplanned weight loss of >10% of body weight over 3–6 months is generally considered to be clinically significant, and 5–10% may also be clinically significant and deserves further observation, especially if the weight loss is accelerating and is associated with deteriorating body function. In the absence of reliable information on weight change, the history may still be helpful if it indicates that clothes or belts and finger rings have become looser (or tighter). Patients may have also noticed that they have lost muscle bulk and that their skin has become more thin and friable.

Anorexia: major and persistent changes in subjective impression of appetite may also indicate risk of malnutrition.

Other symptoms: persistent swallowing difficulties, vomiting and diarrhoea, poor- or ill-fitting dentures, and painful mouth conditions can also mark the development of protein-energy malnutrition.

Socio-economic: the history may elicit poverty, social isolation, and difficulties with shopping. These can be particularly problematic in patients who have become weak and unable to shop or cook as a result of their malnutrition. The history may also identify other problems suggestive of poor dietary intake, such as the inadvertent failure of relatives or the social services to provide necessary support, including delivery of food.

Underlying disease: a known history of a specific disease or the likely development of a new disease may coincide with the development of protein–energy malnutrition. Indeed, weight loss can be a presenting symptom of many diseases.

Specific nutrient deficiencies

The symptoms (and signs) of individual nutrient deficiencies, such as vitamin and trace-element deficiencies, are often nonspecific and often do not manifest themselves until the deficiencies are at an advanced stage. Nevertheless, the clinical history can point towards the possibility of deficiency and may also identify the predisposing causes. Examples include:

- Thiamine deficiency in alcoholics with poor dietary intake.
- Vitamin D deficiency in older people or those with disease who are not exposed to sunlight.
- Vitamin B_{12} deficiency in patients with a gastrectomy (site of intrinsic factor production) and resection of the terminal ileum (site of B_{12} absorption).

- Iron deficiency in women with heavy periods, subjects with gastrointestinal blood loss, and those taking nonsteroidal anti-inflammatory drugs.
- Sodium, potassium, and magnesium deficiency in patients with persistent diarrhoea, vomiting, and excessive gastrointestinal fluid losses, which may occur in patients with fistulae (e.g. dizziness on standing, especially if coupled by postural hypotension on examination in patients with large gastrointestinal fluid losses, suggests the presence of dehydration and/or sodium deficiency).
- Multiple vitamin deficiencies in patients with malabsorption syndromes, such as coeliac disease or short bowel syndromes.
- Fluid disturbances in patients who drink little, have large gastrointestinal effluents, and take large quantities of diuretics (predisposing to dehydration), or excessive fluid intake in patients with heart or renal failure and other conditions associated with impaired capacity to excrete fluid.

Dietary history

There are a variety of methods for assessing dietary intake (e.g. 24-hour dietary history, food diary or record charts, food-frequency questionnaire, and weighed food intake), but even if this can be done accurately using the weighed food intake method, assessments over a day or two may be of little value in assessing the average dietary intake of certain nutrients because of substantial day-to-day variation. Table 2.1 indicates that the duration of dietary intake assessment necessary to produce a result that is within ±10% of the average intake varies considerably with different dietary components.

However, in clinical practice the dietary history can be of value in the assessment of nutritional status by identifying the following:

- Major reduction in dietary intake, especially if coupled with the onset of anorexia, which is often associated with substantial weight loss.
- Unusual patterns of dietary intake over long periods of time, which may increase risk of nutrient deficiencies (e.g. strict vegans are at risk of developing B$_{12}$ deficiency).
- Adverse reactions to specific food items, which can in themselves induce nutritional problems (see Chapter 8).

Table 2.1 Number of days necessary to obtain estimates of dietary intake within 10% of average intake in healthy people using weighed food intakes. Data from Bingham (1987).

Dietary component	Number of days
Energy	5
Carbohydrate	6
Fat	7
Dietary fibre	10
Calcium	10
Iron	12
Thiamin	15
Riboflavin	19
Cholesterol	27
Vitamin C	36

Such a history can be undertaken by clinicians as part of the general clinical history, but a more detailed evaluation can be undertaken by dietitians.

Clinical examination

Protein–energy malnutrition

Clinical examination can reveal evidence of chronic protein energy malnutrition:

- *Muscle*: muscle wasting is often visible, particularly in certain parts of the legs (quadriceps in proximal leg), proximal arms (deltoids), and face (temporalis muscle).
- *Fat*: loss of fat is evident from the presence of loose skinfolds and from little or absent clinically detectable subcutaneous fat.
- *Fat and muscle*: loss of fat and muscle is responsible for the appearance of hollow cheeks and buttocks, and prominent bony outlines and protrusions.
- *Skin*: the skin is thin and friable and may also show signs of dehydration or oedema.

Specific nutrient deficiencies

Signs of specific nutrient deficiencies generally occur at an advanced stage of the deficiency, but similar signs may arise from other causes. The key is to think about signs that may be due to nutrient deficiencies, in the light of the clinical history and underlying disease. To assist in this thought process, Table 2.2 summarises clinical signs according to nutritional causes, Table 2.3 the signs due to specific vitamin

Table 2.2 Clinical signs and nutritional causes.

Sign	Nutritional causes
Skin	
Easy bruising	Vitamin C (positive Hess test); Vitamin K (negative Hess test) (may also occur with steroids and anticoagulants)
Dry scaly skin	Essential fatty acid deficiency (much more often it is a nonspecific feature of other conditions)
Depigmented thin and easily plucked hair with depigmentation of the skin	Kwashiorkor
Nails	
Koilonychia	Iron (but occasionally of genetic origin)
Leuconychia	Protein (but may occur with many chronic diseases associated with reduced synthesis of the protein keratin in nails)
Eyes	
Keratomalacia and xerophthalmia	Vitamin A
Neck	
Goitre	Iodine deficiency (but may be due to other types of thyroid disease)
Mouth	
Angular stomatitis	Iron and some B vitamins (but also occurs with ill-fitting dentures)
Atrophic tongue	Iron, vitamin B_{12}, folic acid, other B vitamins (but also occurs after administering some broad-spectrum antibiotics)
Aphthous ulcers	Linked to B vitamin and iron deficiencies (but is also a nonspecific feature of several conditions, such as inflammatory bowel disease and coeliac disease)
Varicose venules under the tongue	Vitamin C

Table 2.3 Some vitamin deficiencies and their manifestations.

Vitamin	Physical signs of deficiency
Water-soluble vitamins	
Thiamine	Peripheral neuropathy (dry form of beri-beri) and oedema (wet form of beri-beri), ophthalmolegia, Wernicke–Korsakoff syndrome
Folic acid	Anaemia (megaloblastic and macrocytic[a]), atrophic tongue
Vitamin B_{12}	Anaemia (megaloblastic and macrocytic[a]), peripheral neuropathy, subacute combined degeneration of the cord (may lead to absent ankle jerks and up-going toes in response to the plantar reflex)
Vitamin C	Easy bruising, perifollicular haemorrhages, ecchymosis (positive Hess test), painful legs (due to subperiosteal haemorrhages), corkscrew hair
Fat-soluble vitamins	
Vitamin A	Xerophthalmia, keratomalacia, hyperkeratosis of the skin, Bitot's spots
Vitamin D	Rickets in children (e.g. swollen wrists, rickety rosary, knock knees), tetany, positve Trousseau's sign (hypocalcaemia) proximal myopathy
Vitamin E	Myelopathy, ataxia, loss of position sense in legs, retinopathy, blindness
Vitamin K	Bleeding and easy bruising (negative Hess test)

[a]The macrocytic and megaloblastic nature of the anaemia requires confirmation by laboratory tests (iron deficiency produces a microcytic, hypochromic anaemia, which is not megaloblastic).

Table 2.4 Trace-element deficiencies and their manifestations.

Trace element	Features of deficiency
Chromium[a]	Hyperglycaemia, peripheral neuropathy, confusion
Cobalt (vitamin B$_{12}$)	Anaemia (macrocytic and megaloblastic), peripheral neuropathy, subacute combined degeneration of the spinal cord
Copper	Anaemia with megaloblastic features and neutropaenia (Menke's kinky hair syndrome is a rare condition in children due to copper malabsorption)
Iodine	Hypothyroidism, goitre
Iron	Hypochromic anaemia, angular stomatitis, koilonychias, aphthous ulcers
Manganese[a]	Dermatitis, changes of hair colour, hypothrombinaemia
Molybdenum[a]	Impaired consciousness, hypouricaemia, intolerance to sulphite and amino acids
Selenium	Myopathy, cardiomyopathy (Keshan disease)
Zinc	Rash (often peristomal and acral dermatitis), alopecia, impaired taste and smell, diarrhoea

[a]Deficiencies are rare but have been reported in patients receiving long-term parenteral nutrition.

deficiencies, and Table 2.4 signs due to specific trace-element deficiencies.

The relevant history and signs associated with nutritional problems are considered together to establish an overall assessment of nutritional status, in the light of the known (or likely) underlying diseases or other predisposing causes. While protein–energy malnutrition is usually diagnosed at the bedside or in the field, micronutrient deficiencies often rely heavily on the laboratory. In some cases, specific absorption tests are required, as in the case of vitamin B$_{12}$ deficiency due to pernicious anaemia. Body-composition measurements can help assess nutritional status but are not generally used in routine clinical practice, with the exception of dual-energy X-ray absorptiometry (DXA), which is used to identify and manage osteoporosis in many centres. Some studies suggest that simple measurements of body composition using bedside techniques may be superior to BMI in predicting clinical outcomes, in the absence of specific nutritional interventions. Among the bedside body-composition techniques are anthropometry and bioelectrical impedance.

Box 2.1 Calculating the cross-sectional area of muscular and nonmuscular limb tissues

The formulas assume circular limb and muscle configurations. A correction can be made for the cross-sectional areas of bone at the mid-upper arm (10 cm^2 for men and 6.5 cm^2 for women).

1. Limb muscle circumference = limb circumference – $\pi \times$ skinfold thickness

2. Limb muscle cross-sectional area

$$= \frac{(\text{limb muscle circumference})^2}{4\pi}$$

3. Nonmuscle limb area = limb cross-sectional area – muscle cross-sectional area

4. Limb cross-sectional area = $\dfrac{(\text{limb circumference})^2}{4\pi}$

Anthropometry in the form of limb circumferences is incorporated into certain screening tools; for example, upper-arm circumference in 'MUST' and calf circumference in MNA. In 'MUST', upper-arm circumference may be used when the BMI cannot be established (a circumference of <23.5 cm suggests that a BMI <20 kg/m^2 is likely, whereas a value >32 cm suggests that obesity (BMI >30 kg/m^2) is likely. However, since limb-circumference measurements depend on the presence of several tissues, mainly muscle, adipose tissue, and bone, this cannot be used to accurately assess the composition of the limb. An indication of the proportion of fat and muscle in the arm can be obtained by combining measurements of arm circumference and skinfold thickness (Box 2.1), which should be undertaken by a trained worker.

The use of body-composition measurements in the routine assessment of nutritional status would be facilitated by the following:

- Establishment of generally agreed reference standards and cut-off points for lean tissue mass or muscle mass (several definitions for sarcopenia are currently available using different criteria, based on different population groups, which may or may not include functional components).

- Robust validation of the accuracy of body-composition techniques in patients with disease, rather than relying on extrapolations and relationships obtained in healthy populations.

- Demonstrations that body-composition measurements are superior to other routinely used indices of nutritional status, such as BMI, in predicting clinical outcomes both with and without nutritional support.

It is beyond the scope of this chapter to consider the advantages and disadvantages of different body-composition techniques, or to consider kinetic studies and other methods of assessing the stores of individual nutrients. However, in clinical practice the assessment of nutrient status often relies on the laboratory. For example, circulating folic acid and B_{12} concentrations are routinely used to assess the status of these vitamins. The excretion of sodium in urine may be used to confirm the presence of sodium deficiency, especially in patients without renal impairment or during the early period of an acute and severe disease, which tend to independently reduce urine sodium excretion. In some cases, confirmation of a deficiency arises from a therapeutic trial. For example, when thiamine deficiency is suspected, large therapeutic doses of thiamine may be given before (or in the absence of) a laboratory test, because reliance on the results of a blood test undertaken by a specialised laboratory may be associated with unwarranted delays, since severe untreated thiamine deficiency can produce irreversible brain damage. While the laboratory can make very valuable contributions to the diagnosis of nutrient deficiencies (or toxicities), certain laboratory tests need to be interpreted with caution. For example, a low plasma zinc concentration may occur during the acute phase of injury as a result of a reduction in the concentration of circulating proteins that bind zinc (mainly albumin and alpha 2 macroglobulin). A low circulating retinol (vitamin A) concentration may be due to a low retinol-binding protein, which is also a negative acute-phase protein, declining in concentration during the acute phase of an illness. Results are easier to interpret when there is little or no acute-phase reaction. The circulating concentration of nutrients is also affected by hydration status. For example, dehydration increases the cirulating concentration of nutrients. In the case of some nutrients, more accurate assessment of status can be obtained after applying correction factors that take into account the concentration of the carrier molecules. For example, the circulating calcium concentration is corrected for albumin concentration, which binds calcium, in order to establish the free calcium concentration. In the case of the fat-soluble vitamin E, which circulates

in association with lipoproteins, its status is typically assessed as a ratio to triacylgycerol or cholesterol concentrations.

In the end, all the information from the history, examination, and results of investigations is considered together, to help establish an overall picture of nutritional status so that appropriate nutritional care plans can be implemented. If nutritional support is required as part of the care plan, the goals of treatment should be set and reviewed intermittently in light of the changes in nutritional status which occur once nutritional support is implemented. The underlying causes and complications of disease are treated simultaneously.

2.4 Concluding remarks

Since nutritional screening is the first step in the management of malnutrition, it has become an important routine procedure in the hospitals and care homes of some countries. Screening can be audited, inspected, and regulated, but practice varies widely between countries. It is hoped that in the future more countries will adopt mandatory screening policies that employ valid, reliable, and user-friendly screening tools. However, screening by itself is of little or no value if the results are not linked to a care plan which allows malnutrition to be effectively managed. Policies to address both issues would be more effective than just screening. In settings where the prevalence of malnutrition is low, the likelihood of screening is also low, and staff are often under considerable pressure to undertake other tasks. In some situations it may be possible for patients to screen themselves. Preliminary work in hospital outpatient clinics suggests that patient self-screening using electronic versions of 'MUST' can be undertaken easily and reliably, and at the same time predict clinical outcome. More such studies need to be undertaken in different settings, including general practice, where the prevalence of malnutrition is lower than in hospital outpatients, need to be undertaken, and the potential implementation of self-screening in routine clinical practice needs to be evaluated.

Validation of new methods to assess protein-energy status and specific nutrient deficiencies are also expected. For example, new body-composition techniques may become powerful tools in the future.

In addition, new methods for accurately assessing stores of individual nutrients may also become powerful tools which find their way into routine clinical practice.

References and further reading

Bauer JM, Kaiser MJ, Sieber CC. Evaluation of nutritional status in older persons: nutritional screening and assessment. Curr Opin Clin Nutr Metab Care 2010; 13: 8–13.

Bingham S. The dietary assessment of individuals; methods, accuracy, new techniques and recommendations. Nutrition Abstracts and Reviews 1987; 57: 705–742.

Buzby GP, Knox LS, Crosby L, *et al.* Study protocol: a randomized clinical trial of total parenteral nutrition in malnourished surgical patients. Am J Clin Nutr 1988; 47: 366–381.

Detsky AS, McLaughlin JR, Baker JP, *et al.* What is subjective global assessment of nutritional status? J Parenter Enteral Nutr 1987; 11: 8–13.

Elia M, chairman and editor. The 'MUST' report. Nutritional screening for adults: a multidisciplinary responsibility. Development and use of the 'Malnutrition Universal Screening Tool' ('MUST') for adults. A report by the Malnutrition Advisory Group of the British Association for Parenteral and Enteral Nutrition, 2003.

Elia M, Stratton RJ. Considerations for screening tool selection and role of predictive and concurrent validity. Curr Opin Clin Nutr Metab Care 2011; 14: 425–433.

Elia M, Stratton RJ. An analytic appraisal of nutrition screening tools supported by original data with particular reference to age. Nutrition 2012; 28(5): 477–494.

Gibson R. Principles of Nutritional Assessment. 2nd edn. Oxford: Oxford University Press, 2005.

Guigoz Y. The Mini-Nutritional Assessment (MNA®) review of the literature – what does it tell us? J Nutr Health Aging 2006; 10: 466–487.

Heymsfield SB, Lohman TG, Wang W, Going SB. Human Body Composition. 2nd edn. Champaign, IL: Human Kinetics, 2005.

Kaiser MJ, Bauer JM, Ramsch C, *et al.* Validation of the Mini Nutritional Assessment Short-Form (MNA®-SF): a practical tool for identification of nutritional status. J Nutr Health Aging 2009; 13: 782–788.

Kondrup J, Rasmussen HH, Hamberg O, Stanga Z, Ad Hoc ESPEN Working Group. Nutritional risk screening (NRS 2002): a new method based on an analysis of controlled clinical trials. Clin Nutr 2003; 22: 321–336.

Rubenstein LZ, Harker JO, Salva A, Guigoz Y, Vellas B. Screening for undernutrition in geriatric practice: developing the Short-Form Mini Nutritional Assessment (MNA-SF). J Geront 2001; 56A: M366–377.

Stratton RJ, Green CJ, Elia M. Disease-related malnutrition: an evidence-based approach to treatment. Oxford: CABI Publishing, 2003.

Vellas B, Garry PJ, Guigoz Y. Mini Nutritional Assessment (MNA): research and practice in the elderly. Karger, Basel: Nestle Nutrition Services, 1999.

Vellas B, Villars H, Abellan G, *et al.* Overview of the MNA® – its history and challenges. J Nutr Health Aging 2006; 10: 456–465.

3
Water and Electrolytes

Abeed H Chowdhury and Dileep N Lobo
Nottingham University Hospitals, Queen's Medical Centre, Nottingham, UK

Key messages

- Nutrition and fluid/electrolyte balance are closely linked.
- Starvation, injury, or surgical stress can lead to disturbed fluid and electrolyte balance.
- Fluid can shift to the interstitial compartment during starvation, injury, or surgical stress and lead to tissue oedema.
- The regulation of fluid within body water compartments is achieved through the control of ECF osmolarity.
- Thirst is a behavioral response to loss of body fluid. Together with reflex endocrine and neural responses, thirst is responsible for maintaining the homeostasis of body

fluids, and more specifically for the regulation of the ECF compartment.
- Starvation, severe trauma, sepsis, and other disease processes can cause alterations in the sizes of the body water compartments and in exchangeable ions, and may acutely alter the volume and composition of the ICF.
- Intravenous fluid therapy can cause morbidity when associated with fluid overload. Harmful effects on the cardiorespiratory, gastrointesinal, and renal organ systems can be avoided with a balanced approach to supplementary fluid volume and composition.

3.1 Introduction

Starvation affects a number of metabolic processes central to homeostasis and these effects may be exacerbated by the presence of critical illness and surgical or traumatic stress. Furthermore, the control of metabolism and that of fluid/electrolyte balance are closely linked. In normal circumstances, the absorption of fluid and nutrients from the gastrointestinal tract counters the losses incurred during metabolism and cellular respiration. As such, the disruption of homeostatic mechanisms during starvation or injury has consequences not only for nutritional status but for the regulation of fluid and electrolytes. In this chapter, the principles of water/electrolyte balance and their impact on metabolic processes relevant to clinical nutrition will be discussed.

3.2 Fluid compartments of the body

As total body water makes up about 60% of body weight, an appreciation of the body water compartments (Figure 3.1) and the processes by which they are maintained is vital for an understanding of water/electrolyte balance. The intracellular fluid (ICF) compartment accounts for ~40% of total body weight (TBW), with cells separated from the extracellular fluid (ECF) (~20% of TBW), in which they are bathed, by the cell membrane. The ECF is divided into two further compartments by the capillary membrane: intravascular fluid (~5% of TBW) and interstitial fluid, which is intercellular (~15% of TBW).

Although impermeable to most molecules and proteins, some substances, such as water, carbon dioxide, and oxygen, can diffuse freely across the cell

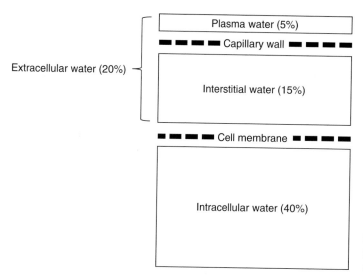

Figure 3.1 The body water compartments. Figures are approximate percentages of body weight in the average individual.

Table 3.1 Electrolyte concentrations in body water compartments. ECF, extracellular fluid; ICF, intracellular fluid.

Electrolyte	ECF (mmol/l)	ICF (mmol/l)	Total in body (mmol)
Sodium	140–155	10–18	3000–4000
Potassium	4.0–5.5	120–145	3000–4000
Calcium	2.2–2.5	2.2–2.5	25 000–27 000
Ionised calcium	0.9–1.3	1×10^{-4}	–
Magnesium	0.7–1.2	15–25	900–1200
Chloride	98–106	2–6	3000–4000
Phosphate	0.7–1.3	8–20	30 000–32 000

membrane. In addition, the cell membrane houses transport mechanisms to facilitate the inward transport of nondiffusible nutrients required for cellular metabolism as well as the selective expulsion of molecules to maintain a stable internal environment. Central to this vital process is the Na$^+$/K$^+$-ATPase pump, which maintains intracellular concentrations of sodium and potassium at 8 and 150 mmol/l respectively, in contrast to the concentrations of 140 and 5 mmol/l typically found in the ECF. The electrolyte concentrations found in body water compartments are outlined in Table 3.1.

The negative charges on intracellular protein molecules also help retain potassium within the cell (Gibbs–Donnan equilibrium). Correspondingly, shifts of water into or out of the cell are dependent on the osmotic gradient between the ECF and the ICF. With increased osmolarity of the ECF, water moves from the ICF to the ECF, resulting in cellular dehydration. Conversely, if salt is lost from or water added to the ECF to cause a hypotonic environment, water shifts from the ECF into the cell.

In blood vessels, the pores in the capillary membrane allow water, electrolytes, nutrients, and some macromolecules to cross from the circulation to the tissues. This movement of fluid across the capillary membrane is largely determined by the forces described by Starling's equation:

$$J_v = K_f ([P_c - P_i] - \sigma[\pi_c - \pi_i])$$

where:

- $([P_c - P_i] - \sigma[\pi_c - \pi_i])$ is the net driving force;
- K_f is the proportionality constant;
- J_v is the net fluid movement between compartments.

According to Starling's equation, the movement of fluid depends on six variables:

(1) capillary hydrostatic pressure (P_c);
(2) interstitial hydrostatic pressure (P_i);
(3) capillary oncotic pressure (π_c);
(4) interstitial oncotic pressure (π_i);
(5) filtration coefficient (K_f);
(6) reflection coefficient (σ).

Increased vascular hydrostatic pressure or decreased plasma oncotic pressure (Figure 3.2) facilitates the outward flow of water from blood vessels.

(a) *Hydrostatic pressure*

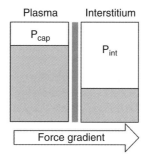

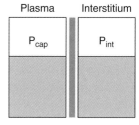

(b) *Oncotic (colloid osmotic) pressure*

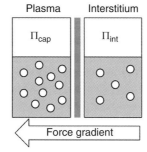

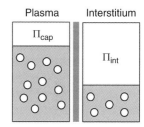

Figure 3.2 Diagrammatic model showing the effect of hydrostatic and oncotic pressure gradients on fluid movements across the capillary wall. P, hydrostatic pressure; Π, oncotic pressure; cap, capillary; int, interstitial.

In tissues, the interstitial space is separated from the circulation by the capillary membrane and from the ICF by the cell membrane. The interstitial space acts as a buffer for changes which occur in plasma volume. Regulation of the interstitial volume is governed by local factors, which include Starling's forces, but also the adequacy of lymphatic drainage, enabling fluid, and colloid molecules to be returned to the circulation. In health, there is continual leakage of albumin from the intravascular space, which occurs at a rate of about 5% per hour (Figure 3.3a). This rate can increase up to fourfold in critical illness, causing a shift of fluid towards the interstitium. Return of albumin to the circulation occurs via the lymphatic system, and as the rate of lymphatic drainage from the interstitium remains largely stable or is reduced by pressure generated by muscle contraction, excessive fluid transfer to the interstitium can cause tissue oedema (Figure 3.3b). This form of fluid transfer between the plasma and interstitium accounts for the rapid swelling of acutely inflamed tissues and the oedematous swelling characteristic of limb venous thrombosis.

Factors that influence the escape of plasma proteins from the intravascular space, thereby lowering the plasma oncotic pressure, include the size of membrane pores and properties of the endothelial glycocalyx – a complex structure comprising membrane-bound proteoglycans, glycoproteins, and bound plasma constituents. The endothelial glycocalyx forms a protective layer against the shear forces of blood cells on the luminal surface of the endothelium and has been shown to play an important role in barrier function, leukocyte adherence, and platelet aggregation. In capillaries, the layer is 0.5 μm thick; however, with greater vascular diameter, the glycocalyx layer increases in thickness. This thickness may be important as a determinant of vascular permeability and may become denuded with the interaction of drugs, enzymes, cytokines, or ischaemia and reperfusion, thereby reducing intravascular oncotic pressure and promoting tissue oedema.

The mechanism by which macromolecules escape from the intravascular space is described by the two-pore theory. In this model, small solutes are able to pass through small pores (radius: 2.5–3.0 nm) in the capillary membrane, present throughout the entire

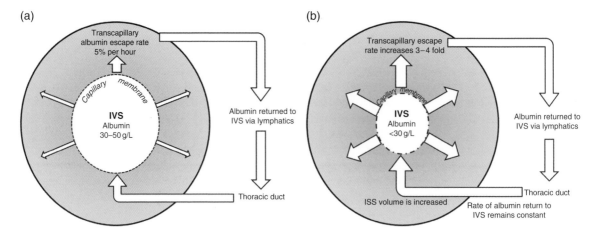

Figure 3.3 Capillary permeability and albumin flux in (a) health and (b) critical illness. ISS, interstitial space; IVS, intravascular space.

microvascular bed. Conversely, larger molecules can only pass through larger pores (radius: 10–11 nm) sited on the venous side of the capillary network. The small pores outnumber the large pores by 3000–3600:1. The transit of macromolecules across the pores occurs mainly by convection. Hence, an increase in capillary hydrostatic pressure caused by an expansion of plasma volume can result in leakage of larger molecules to the extravascular space, leading to the appearance of tissue oedema.

Further to the aforementioned compartments, it has been a traditionally held belief that a supplementary internal compartment, termed the 'third space', can arise in circumstances of trauma or blood loss. Fluid transfer to this compartment had been deemed distinct from the anatomical fluid shifts known to occur during illness, where fluid can accumulate within peritoneal or pleural cavities or the interstitial space of traumatised tissue but is ultimately subject to redistribution to the circulation. This model of fluid transfer to a proposed 'third space' has been the subject of controversy, with many highlighting the lack of firm evidence to support the concept. Since the anatomical location of the 'third space' has remained unclear, direct measurement of its volume has proved difficult, leading to questions over its exact nature.

Notwithstanding controversy over the existence of a 'third space', compartmentalisation is of major importance to maintaining the stability of the intracellular environment in the face of changes in both the intravascular and extracellular environments. It also allows the renal and gastrointestinal tracts to play

an integral role in fluid and electrolyte balance, systems which effect responses to fluctuations in intra- and extravascular fluid composition. This is achieved through complex neuroendocrine interactions, which in due course promote the secretion or excretion of water with a different osmolality to that found in plasma.

3.3 Flux of fluid through the kidney and gastrointestinal tract

The kidneys and gastrointestinal tract play key roles in the maintenance of ECF volume and electrolyte balance in the face of variable daily fluid intake. This is important because mammalian tissues require a medium of fairly constant salt and water composition for normal function. Of equal importance, however, is the need to preserve enough fluid within the circulation to maintain blood pressure. It is clear that systemic blood pressure is dependent on the volume of blood within the vascular system and is a product of cardiac output and systemic vascular resistance. Cardiac output is related to the effective circulatory volume, and variations in these parameters normally parallel changes affecting the ECF volume. Accordingly, the regulation of blood pressure by the kidneys is accomplished by the control of ECF volume. This is an impressive feat when one considers that in a period of 24 hours, the two kidneys filter approximately 180 litres of ECF, with all but 1–2 litres of water and 50–100 mmol of sodium being reabsorbed.

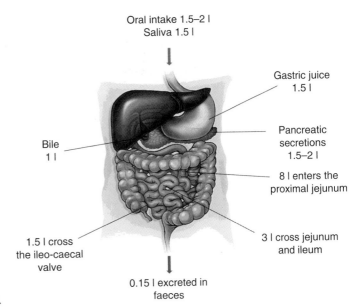

Oral intake 1.5–2 l
Saliva 1.5 l

Gastric juice
1.5 l

Pancreatic
secretions
1.5–2 l

8 l enters the
proximal jejunum

Bile
1 l

3 l cross jejunum
and ileum

1.5 l cross
the ileo-caecal
valve

0.15 l excreted in
faeces

Figure 3.4 Flux of fluid across the gastrointestinal tract.

The volume of the ECF is influenced by its osmolarity and can be derived from the relationship:

$$ECF\ volume = total\ osmoles/osmolarity$$

Therefore, in regulating the osmolarity of the ECF, the kidneys are, in essence, able to regulate ECF volume and hence effective circulatory volume. In addition, the kidneys are able to detect changes in afferent arteriolar pressure using pressure detectors at the juxtaglomerular apparatus and subsequently to direct renal responses to the excretion or reabsorption of sodium and water through the renin–angiotensin–aldosterone system (RAAS). In this way, the kidneys are able to integrate information derived from both pressure and osmoreceptors to infer changes in blood volume status and execute the appropriate responses to modify ECF volume.

Cooperating with the kidneys in the control of fluid and electrolyte balance is the gastrointestinal tract, with 9 litres of fluid, containing a sodium load of 110–120 mmol/l, passing through the small bowel daily and only 150 ml being lost in stool (Figure 3.4).

Most of the fluid that passes through the gastrointestinal tract is derived from the secretions of the ECF rather than oral ingestion, and as such, small changes in absorptive capacity can have a profound effect on fluid and electrolyte balance. Nearly all of this fluid is reabsorbed from the gastrointestinal tract, facilitated by a Na^+/K^+-ATPase-generated osmotic gradient, as well as the co-transport of sodium with organic solutes, such as glucose, amino acids, or bile acids, in the small intestine and short-chain fatty acids in the colon.

In circumstances where there is deficit in effective circulatory volume, the reabsorption of both sodium and water from the gastrointestinal tract is enhanced. This is facilitated by the action of components of the RAAS on the small bowel mucosa, where receptors for aldosterone, angiotensin I, and angiotensin II are known to exist. In this way, the kidneys and gastrointestinal tract are able to integrate their roles in fluid and electrolyte balance.

3.4 Body electrolyte content and concentration

As mentioned previously, intravascular and ECF volumes are essentially preserved by the factors controlling body sodium, the predominant cation found within these compartments. For mammals, evolutionary pressures have led to the development of efficient mechanisms to preserve sodium and water, allowing survival in environments where these nutritional commodities might be scarce. On the other

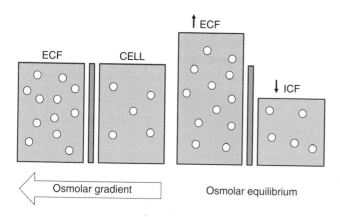

Osmolar gradient   Osmolar equilibrium

Figure 3.5 Diagrammatic model showing the effect of the osmotic pressure gradient on water movement across the cell membrane.

hand, there have been few evolutionary precedents demanding a sustained response to water and sodium excess. Thus, in the main, water- and sodium-retaining mechanisms are much more developed and powerful than those designed for water and electrolyte excretion.

Total body sodium equates to approximately 3000–4000 mmol, with 53% of this available as an exchangeable fraction. The remaining 47% is considered part of a non-exchangeable fraction and exists within bone. Furthermore, most of the exchangeable fraction is located within the ECF, contrasting with an intracellular fraction of only 9%. Daily sodium intake varies, but on average amounts to 1 mmol/kg, and is equivalent to the amount excreted in the urine and faeces. In health, daily sodium losses are readily compensated for by the substantial reserves of the exchangeable fraction.

The body contains an equivalent amount of potassium as sodium, but in contrast to sodium the majority of the exchangeable fraction of potassium is intracellular. Furthermore, extracellular concentrations of potassium are under stringent control, as even small fluctuations can be clinically harmful. Any excess is usually excreted by the kidneys, but in critical illness, elevated potassium concentration within the ECF is compounded by the cellular efflux of amino acids and glucose, which are accompanied by potassium to maintain electrical neutrality.

Fluid shifts between ECF and ICF compartments

Water is able to move freely across most cell membranes, facilitated by transmembrane water channels known as aquaporins. Except for brief periods, the ECF and ICF remain in osmotic equilibrium. Hence, a measurement of plasma osmolarity provides a reasonable measure of both ECF and ICF osmolarity. On the other hand, the movement of ions across cell membranes depends on the presence of specific transporters. These transporters maintain a stable intracellular environment and counter minor fluctuations in ion concentration. In real terms, there is no appreciable inward shift of ions across the cell membrane. It can, therefore, be assumed that equilibration between ECF and ICF osmolarity occurs principally by the movement of water, and not by the movement of osmotically active solutes. In the main, these water shifts occur only when the ECF osmolarity is altered significantly (Figure 3.5).

3.5 Regulation of body water compartments

Physiological mechanisms to match the intake of water to output have evolved with the specific aims of maintaining extracellular osmolarity and protecting effective circulatory volume. These mechanisms detect changes in the volume of body water compartments and then signal the appropriate response in terms of excretion of sodium and water.

Coupled to these detectors are neuroendocrine pathways which promote the intake and retention of water from the kidneys and gastrointestinal tract, and complementary pathways, in order to promote the secretion and excretion of fluid when necessary. These pathways are discussed further in this section.

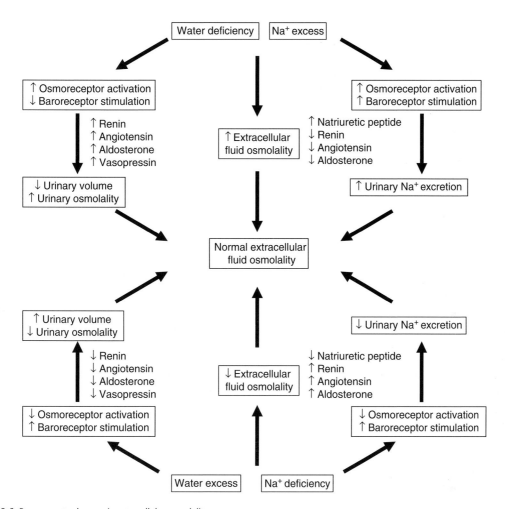

Figure 3.6 Responses to changes in extracellular osmolality.

Control of body fluid osmolality

The ability to excrete urine with a different osmolality from plasma plays a central role in the regulation of water balance. When plasma osmolality is decreased, vasopressin secretion from the posterior pituitary is inhibited and results in the excretion of dilute urine, with subsequent return of the plasma osmolality to normal values. When plasma osmolality is increased, vasopressin release and thirst are stimulated and the combination of decreased urinary water loss and increased water intake results in decreased plasma osmolality. The influence of sodium/water balance on extracellular osmolality and the responses that aim to return osmolality toward normal values are shown in Figure 3.6.

In order to preserve a stable internal environment, there is a minimum volume of water that must be excreted by the kidneys, termed the *volume obligatoire*. This obligatory renal water loss is directly related to the excretion of solutes. If 800 mOsm of solute has to be excreted per day to maintain the steady state, and the maximum urinary osmolality is 1200 mOsm/kg, a minimum of 670 ml/day of urine will be required to excrete the 800 mOsm solute load. In the clinical setting of critical illness, where the concentrating ability of the kidneys may be compromised, it can be recognised that the *volume obligatoire* must increase in order to excrete an excess solute load.

The normal kidney responds to water or sodium excess or deficit, via osmo- and volume receptors, acting through vasopressin and the RAAS to restore effective circulatory volume and ECF osmolality. The receptors which facilitate the release of vasopressin include those sensitive to changes in osmolality located in the anterior hypothalamus, as well as pressure receptors relaying information from cardiovascular afferents to the nucleus of the tractus solitarius. Maintenance of volume always overrides maintenance of osmolality if hypovolaemia and hypoosmolality coexist. Vasopressin secretion from the magnocellular neurones of the supraoptic and paraventricular nuclei acts primarily on the kidney to increase urine osmolality. It achieves this through two main effects:

(1) Vasopressin increases permeability of the distal tubule and collecting duct cells to water. This is facilitated through the insertion of water channels (aquaporin-2) into the apical membrane of distal tubule and collecting-duct epithelial cells. Insertion of aquaporin-2 water channels occurs by exocytosis of intracellular vesicles and is initiated via a G-protein coupled process on the binding of vasopressin to V2 receptors. These aquaporin channels allow water to move down their osmotic gradient out of the nephron, resulting in a more concentrated filtrate.

(2) Vasopressin increases permeability of the inner medullary portion of the collecting duct to urea, which facilitates its reabsorption into the medullary interstitium as it travels down the concentration gradient created by removing water from the connecting tubule, cortical collecting duct, and outer medullary collecting duct.

In addition to the actions of vasopressin, the RAAS works in parallel to conserve sodium and water. Synthesised and stored in the juxtaglomerular cells of the kidney, renin is released in response to low blood pressure in afferent arterioles, decreased tubular chloride concentration reaching the macula densa, or excitation of sympathetic nerves innervating the juxtaglomerular cells. The primary role of renin is to cleave angiotensinogen to angiotensin I. This in turn is cleaved to angiotensin II by angiotensin-converting enzyme. The physiological effects of angiotensin II are wide-ranging, but important actions for the control of sodium/water balance include the stimulation of aldosterone release from the adrenal cortex,

reduction of renal blood flow, increased tubular sodium reabsorption, and the stimulation of thirst. Aldosterone is a steroid hormone which stimulates sodium and water reabsorption from the distal tubule and collecting-duct segments of the nephron. Providing negative feedback to inhibit renin release, and in turn the RAAS as a whole, are high circulating levels of angiotensin II, increased intrarenal arterial pressure, elevated tubular solute load, and tubuloglomerular feedback.

In addition to established roles in the control of blood pressure and circulatory volume, diverse effects of RAAS activation are increasingly being recognised, including those on the gastrointestinal system, where components of the RAAS influence the uptake and secretion of fluid and electrolytes. There also exist compounds derived from the intestine which are known to act on the kidney, principally to cause natriuresis, such as guanylin and uroguanylin.

Another peptide, urodilatin, which is produced by the renal distal tubules in a paracrine fashion, also stimulates natriuresis and has been shown to play a greater role in the response to elevations in sodium concentrations than atrial natriuretic peptide (ANP), which has been shown to respond primarily to changes in blood volume.

Control of effective circulatory volume

For the most part, mechanisms to control arterial volume involve the detection of pressure changes within blood vessels, used as an indirect method of estimating blood volume. These sensor mechanisms can be considered to be of broadly two types: neural mechanoreceptors and nonneural mechanoreceptors. A third mechanism specific to the kidney includes the physical effects of blood volume on renal tubuloglomerular function.

Mechanical stretch receptors are present in the walls of certain blood vessels, such as the baroreceptors of the carotid sinus and aorta, as well as those present in the wall of the cardiac atria. These receptors transduce pressure changes in the cardiovascular system and effect specific responses through neural mechanisms, in particular the inhibition of vasopressin release and the reduction in renal sympathetic tone.

Stretch-induced release of ANP results in nonneural effects on vascular tone and an increase in the renal excretion of sodium. The results of this are decreased

Table 3.2 Efferent signals as a response to changes in blood volume/pressure, and their actions on renal sodium excretion. ADH, antidiuretic hormone.

Renal sympathetic nerves ($\uparrow$ activity = $\downarrow$ Na$^+$ excretion)	$\downarrow$ Glomerular filtration rate
	$\uparrow$ Renin secretion
	$\uparrow$ Proximal and distal nephron sodium reabsorption
	$\uparrow$ Angiotensin II levels $\uparrow$ proximal nephron Na$^+$ reabsortion
Renin–angiotensin–aldosterone ($\uparrow$ secretion = $\downarrow$ Na$^+$ excretion)	$\uparrow$ Aldosterone levels $\uparrow$ distal nephron Na$^+$ reabsorption
	$\uparrow$ Angiotensin II levels $\uparrow$ ADH secretion
	$\uparrow$ Glomerular filtration rate
Atrial natriuretic peptide ($\uparrow$ secretion = $\uparrow$ Na$^+$ excretion)	$\downarrow$ Renin secretion
	$\downarrow$ Aldosterone secretion
	$\downarrow$ Distal nephron Na$^+$ reabsorption
	$\downarrow$ ADH secretion and action on distal nephron

blood pressure – achieved through natriuresis and diuresis – vasodilatation, increased endothelium permeability, and antagonism of the RAAS. Recent healthy-volunteer studies, using 1 litre infusions of 0.9% saline or colloid, have suggested that the natriuretic peptide response is actually more volume- than sodium-dependent, as the excretion of sodium loads is more reliant on a slow and sustained suppression of the RAAS. A summary of efferent signals and their effect on sodium excretion is provided in Table 3.2.

Thirst regulation and water balance

As previously mentioned, there is an obligatory volume of water that is lost depending on the quantity of solute that must be excreted by the kidneys. Added to this are losses incurred through perspiration – to control body temperature – and water – which passes through the gastrointestinal tract and is lost in faeces (insensible losses). Although the loss of water from the renal tract can be stemmed, countering a deficit in body water can only be achieved in nature by the ingestion of water via the gastrointestinal tract.

The appropriate intake of oral fluid when total body water is depleted is achieved through the activation of thirst. This can be defined as a strong motivation to seek, obtain, and consume water in response to deficits in body water, and is stimulated primarily through changes in plasma osmolarity and plasma volume. In general, two types of stimulus independently activate thirst. The primary stimulus is an increase in the osmolarity of the ECF; a secondary and less powerful stimulus occurs with a decrease in ECF volume and is termed 'hypovolaemic thirst'.

Thirst stimulated by plasma osmolarity and sodium concentration

Experiments conducted over 25 years ago have provided insights into the neural mechanisms of osmotically stimulated thirst. A central component of water-seeking behaviour is the median preoptic nucleus (MnPO), which stimulates or abolishes drinking following the integration of afferent signals from osmoreceptors located outside the blood–brain barrier, including the anteroventral region of the third ventricle, the organum vasculosum of the lamina terminalis (OVLT), and the subfornical organ (SFO). Although it is clear that the MnPO is the site where afferent signals converge, efferent pathways from this region are still not clearly defined. Recent investigations using positron-emission tomography in healthy volunteers have identified areas of the brain which might be involved in downstream signalling from the MnPO, such as the anterior and posterior regions of the cingulate cortex, which seem to be activated in association with the sensation of thirst in response to infusions of hypertonic saline.

Thirst stimulated by hypovolaemia

Thirst can be stimulated by a reduction in effective circulatory volume, involving a mechanism similar to that stimulated by changes in ECF osmolality, and is mediated by both neural and endocrine-mediated responses. Activation of the RAAS, and specifically the release of angiotensin II, stimulates drinking behaviour by acting on the SFO in the hypothalamus. In this way, information derived from volume and pressure sensors, such as the juxtaglomerular apparatus, can be integrated with responses that stimulate the intake of water.

Inhibition of thirst is proposed to involve hindbrain networks, such as the area postrema and the nucleus of the tractus solitarius. These neurons project to the lateral parabrachial nucleus and may be involved in the inhibition of drinking observed in response to hormones such as ANP.

Thus, dipsogenic responses to hypovolaemia involve the integration of stimulatory input from baroreceptors and the RAAS acting on the forebrain, as well as inhibitory hormonal influences derived from the cardiopulmonary system acting on the hindbrain to promote or inhibit water-seeking behaviour.

3.6 The metabolic response to starvation and injury

Patients with critical illness may be subject to starvation, injury, or both, and although many features are shared, the metabolic responses to these physiological insults are distinct. Furthermore, these responses have consequences for fluid and electrolyte balance, which in the clinical setting may have an impact on morbidity. Starvation is characterised by a low-insulin state with a global reduction in metabolism and eventually catabolism. Injury, on the other hand, potentiates a phased metabolic response in a scheme originally described by Sir David Cuthbertson. This is typified by pituitary hormone release and the activation of the sympathetic nervous system. The net result of these responses in both starvation and injury is to promote catabolism and the retention of both sodium and water. With refeeding or recovery from injury during the convalescent phase, the ability to excrete sodium and water loads returns and net anabolic activity is restored.

Starvation

Without intervention, absolute starvation leads ultimately to death. However, a number of adaptive metabolic processes have evolved in order to postpone this outcome for as long as possible, with the primary aim of maintaining the function of vital organs and skeletal muscle. During the initial stages of starvation, carbohydrate present in the circulation and within the ECF is broken down and used preferentially to preserve muscle, which is required for the search for food. However, as starvation progresses, adaptation occurs to reduce the metabolic rate (by up to 25%) and prepare the brain and kidney to use alternative fuel sources. Although the oxidation of free fatty acids (FFAs) by the liver leads to ketone body formation, which can be utilised by the brain,

prolonged starvation leads to a loss of both lean and fat body mass and significant reduction in TBW due to the catabolism of skeletal muscle.

Injury

The metabolic response to injury is broadly similar to that seen in starvation, and in many cases of traumatic injury starvation may also be present to varying degrees. Uncomplicated surgery or moderate trauma is usually followed by a brief period of starvation, but little catabolism occurs during this time. Major trauma or surgery, on the other hand, can result in marked catabolism, especially if the clinical course is complicated by sepsis. This is brought about by the release of counter-regulatory hormones, including catecholamines, insulin, cortisol, and glucagon, such that the basal metabolic rate is increased and the breakdown of glycogen, fat, and protein is enhanced. Fat catabolism is promoted by cortisol, which is released in response to stress or injury and can result in the loss of up to 500 g of adipose tissue per day.

In severe trauma, the breakdown of skeletal muscle also provides a source of amino acids for gluconeogenesis. Nitrogen balance during this phase of injury is often disturbed, with oral intake reduced in the face of marked urinary losses, amounting to up to 20–30 g/day in patients with severe trauma or sepsis. In fact, patients undergoing abdominal surgery can expect to lose about 600 g of skeletal muscle protein, even in the absence of complicating factors.

This loss of lean and fat body mass, the counter-regulatory hormone response, and the production of inflammatory mediators all have important consequences for the balance of fluid and electrolytes between the ECF, ICF, and interstitium.

3.7 Body water compartments and electrolytes in starvation and injury

Extracellular fluid

Starvation is known to cause reductions in both body fat and lean body mass. Keys and colleagues, however, demonstrated that despite this loss of fat and muscle, the ECF volume remains at the prestarvation level. Thus, as starvation continues, ECF volume increases as a proportion of TBW in relative terms.

Injury produces a similar outcome, with retention of sodium and water and an expansion of ECF volume. These changes occur primarily as a result of vasopressin release and subsequent activation of the RAAS, but the situation is compounded by an increase in capillary permeability. In the first few days following injury, sodium and water are retained in preference to potassium. This may in part be due to the effect of mineralocorticoid, but also reflects the release of potassium from the intracellular compartment as protein and glycogen are catabolised. As plasma potassium concentrations must be kept within a narrow physiological range, some potassium is excreted in the urine.

It has also been shown that injury causes an increase in ECF osmolarity, especially in the setting of haemorrhage. This effect is produced by the release of hepatic glucose as well as by reduced glucose clearance, which results from decreased insulin sensitivity. The net effect is to promote a shift of fluid from the ICF to the ECF, and this is more pronounced with greater degrees of haemorrhage as a proportion of total blood volume. This effect may have evolved as an additional mechanism to protect effective circulating volume in the face of fluid depletion from the vascular compartment.

Eventually, sodium and water retention give way to diuresis, and the ability to excrete sodium and water loads is reestablished. However, this phase may be delayed in the presence of severe injury or sepsis and may be complicated by the administration of salt-containing fluids during resuscitation, which increase the ECF volume and may not be excreted as effectively as fluids of more balanced composition.

Starvation is known to affect the function of a number of organ systems, not least the kidneys, and although these changes have implications for fluid and electrolyte balance, they are not yet completely understood. Complicating the issue are the differing responses observed for complete and partial starvation. Complete starvation is characterised in the initial phase by diuresis and natriuresis, however this is often short-lived and eventually gives way to vasopressin- and aldosterone-mediated sodium and water retention. Also, this diuretic and natriuretic phase may be absent for individuals affected by partial starvation, which, in the main, is observed more frequently than complete starvation in the clinical setting.

Recent animal experiments suggest that food deprivation impairs water handling by the kidney via mechanisms independent of vasopressin, ultimately depressing glomerular filtration rate (GFR) and expanding the ECF. In the presence of malnutrition, these changes lead to reductions in both cardiac output and arterial pressure. Hypoalbuminaemia as a consequence of increased catabolism and decreased hepatic synthesis lowers capillary oncotic pressure. In accordance with Starling's principle, fluid shifts out of blood vessels into the interstitial compartment, thereby reducing venous return. This has the cumulative effect of reducing renal plasma blood flow and hence GFR. Furthermore, protein–energy malnutrition is known to impair renal concentrating capacity by a mechanism which spares the ability to produce dilute urine. Experimental studies indicate that malnutrition may diminish medullary interstitial urea concentration and reduce the tubular-to-interstitium gradient required for urine concentrating capacity. This can result in profound hypovolaemia, although renal concentrating capacity is usually restored after refeeding and rehydration has commenced.

Intracellular fluid

During injury, expansion of the ECF volume with the retention of sodium affects the ICF volume only if there is a change in ECF osmolarity. In starvation, glycogenolysis and protein catabolism lead to the efflux of potassium from the cell. Moreover, in severe illness or starvation, the metabolic activity of cells may be reduced, and sodium is removed less efficiently by the Na^+/K^+-ATPase in what is termed the 'sick cell syndrome'. In these circumstances, water, sodium, and chloride tend to accumulate within the cell, causing ICF expansion.

On the other hand, there may exist a healthy 'cell swelling', promoted by anabolic agents, which determine the increase in the ICF compartment associated with an anabolic process. During refeeding or convalescence from injury, metabolic activity and the intracellular demand for potassium increase, which can result in clinically harmful hypokalaemia if supplementary potassium is not provided (see Chapters 5 and 9).

Interstitial fluid

In circumstances of starvation or injury, expansion of fluid within the tissues can result in oedema. Factors

Table 3.3 Properties of commonly prescribed crystalloids. From Queen's Medical Centre, Nottingham, UK.

	Plasma[a]	0.9% NaCl	0.45% NaCl	Hartmann's solution	Ringer's lactate	Ringer's acetate	Plasma-Lyte 148	Sterofundin ISO	0.18% NaCl/4% dextrose	5% dextrose
Na$^+$ (mmol/l)	135–145	154	77	131	130	130	140	140	31	–
Cl$^-$ (mmol/l)	95–105	154	77	111	109	110	98	127	31	–
[Na$^+$]:[Cl$^-$] ratio	1.28–1.45:1	1:1	1:1	1.18:1	1.19:1	1.18:1	1.43:1	1.10:1	1:1	–
K$^+$ (mmol/l)	3.5–5.3	–	–	5	4	4	5	4	–	–
HCO$_3^-$ (mmol/l)	24–32	–	–	29	–	–	–	–	–	–
Ca^{2+} (mmol/l)	2.2–2.6	–	–	4	3	2	–	2.5	–	–
Glucose (mmol/l)	3.5–5.5	–	–	–	–	–	–	–	222.2 (40 g)	277.8 (50 g)
Lactate (mmol/l)	–	–	–	29	28	–	–	–	–	–
Acetate (mmol/l)	–	–	–	–	–	30	27	24	–	–
Gluconate (mmol/l)	–	–	–	–	–	–	23	–	–	–
pH	7.35–7.45	5.0–5.5	5.6	6.5	6.6	7.4	7.4	4.6–5.4	4.5	4.0
Osmolality (mOsm/l)	275–295	308	154	274	274	270	295	304	286	280

[a] Normal laboratory range.

which determine the degree of interstitial fluid accumulation include the magnitude of the metabolic response to injury, the underlying nutritional status, the adequacy of lymphatic drainage, and the volume and type of supplementary fluid administration. In critically ill patients, this is of major significance, as oedema can interfere with the normal physiological processes of many specialised tissues, including the lungs, heart, and gastrointestinal tract. In clinical studies with patients undergoing abdominal surgery, it has been shown that a positive fluid balance is more likely to produce interstitial oedema and perioperative weight gain. Furthermore, when oedema is present, the frequency of postoperative complications is significantly increased. These findings have since been validated by a number of randomised studies, demonstrating an increase in postoperative complications in the presence of fluid overload and perioperative weight gain above 2.5 kg.

As well as volume, it is clear that the composition of supplementary intravenous fluid may increase the risk of interstitial oedema, particularly with 0.9% saline infusion. Even for healthy subjects, infusion of 2 l of 0.9% saline is retained for longer and results in greater expansion of the extravascular fluid compartment than fluids more balanced in composition. Furthermore, a significant increase in serum chloride as a result of 0.9% saline infusion is associated with reductions in both renal artery flow velocity and renal cortical perfusion, illustrating the potentially harmful effects of solutions unbalanced in composition.

3.8 Effects of salt and water overload

Intravenous crystalloids or colloids are often used to expand the intravascular volume, and for a given volume, colloids are more effective than crystalloids (Table 3.3). The effectiveness of a given crystalloid in expanding the plasma volume is dependent on two main factors: the volume of distribution and the metabolic fate of the solute. For instance, dextrose-containing solutions tend to distribute throughout total body water once the dextrose has been metabolised or taken up by cells and is rapidly diuresed. Hence, this fluid type has only very limited and transient plasma volume-expanding properties, and when given in large volumes may actually decrease plasma

sodium concentration and osmolality, to an extent that may be harmful. Increased plasma expansion is achieved with sodium-containing crystalloid solutions, although this expansion is modest in comparison to that of colloids. Sodium-containing crystalloids tend to distribute within the interstitium as well as plasma, expanding the latter by about 20–25%, such that 4–5 l needs to be infused to expand the plasma volume by 1 l. Colloid solutions, on the other hand, contain high-molecular-weight constituents that are relatively resistant to enzymatic breakdown, and as such remain in the vascular space for longer. This property is also related to the number of molecules contained in the solution and the particle size. Small particles with low molecular weight exert a greater oncotic effect for a given number of molecules. Larger molecules, however, have a greater intravascular persistence but generate a lower oncotic gradient due to having fewer particles. Nevertheless, most modern colloid preparations produce a plasma expansion in the order of 65–90% of infused volumes. For some colloids, this increase in oncotic pressure may actually lead to a net decrease in interstitial fluid volume as water is drawn out of the tissues and into the intravascular space.

The harmful effects of salt and water overload due to the administration of sodium-containing solutions for resuscitation and maintenance have long been recognised. However, only recently have the physiological effects on organ systems been determined in any detail. Studies in both normal subjects and patients have improved our understanding of the response to infusions of crystalloids and colloids and their distribution within body fluid compartments.

From an evolutionary perspective, mechanisms to conserve sodium and water are much more developed than those dealing with excess. In this regard, infusion of 0.9% saline is excreted much more slowly than solutions with a lower sodium and chloride content and results in prolonged dilution of the haematocrit and albumin. Retention of fluid can result in weight gain that persists, in comparison with solutions of more balanced electrolyte composition, which generally are diuresed more rapidly.

Furthermore, a greater proportion of high salt-containing fluids are distributed within the extravascular space compared to balanced solutions, which tend to be excreted more rapidly.

These differences in fluid distribution may explain the greater tendency to form tissue oedema following 0.9% saline infusion and may be a factor in the aetiology of postoperative complications. In fact, a significant increase in postoperative complications is observed for patients who experience a postoperative weight gain of greater than 2.5 kg and it is likely that a narrow range exists where minimal weight gain or loss results in fewer complications. In a recent metaanalysis of randomised studies involving patients undergoing abdominal surgery, it was shown that patients who received less than 1.75 l or greater than 2.75 l per day in the postoperative period had an increase in complications and a greater length of hospital stay. In current practice, large volumes of 0.9% saline are still frequently prescribed in the perioperative period, despite evidence suggesting that a balance should be sought in terms of both infusion volume and fluid composition. Fluid overload and deficit are both detrimental to outcome, especially in surgical patients.

Gastrointestinal function

A number of investigators have examined the impact of fluid therapy on gastrointestinal function, with the overriding conclusion that fluid overload affects gastrointestinal function in an adverse manner.

In patients undergoing colorectal surgery, positive salt and water balance sufficient to cause 3 kg perioperative weight gain was shown to delay return to normal bowel function and prolong hospital stay. These effects are likely to be the result of intestinal oedema as a consequence of salt and water excess. Results from experimental studies have supported this concept and mechanisms to explain these effects have now been provided, highlighting the negative effect of fluid overload on the myosin light chain apparatus, a complex central to smooth-muscle contraction and intestinal transit.

Another important gastrointestinal consequence of fluid therapy may be its impact on intestinal anastomoses, with a number of studies reporting higher rates of leak associated with fluid overload. In the setting of elective colorectal resection, Brandstrup and colleagues observed an increased rate of anastomotic leakage when the mean fluid intake on the day of operation was 5.4 l compared to 2.7 l. In a more recent retrospective study of trauma patients undergoing primary colorectal resection and anastomosis, it was

also established that anastomotic dehiscence was associated with larger volumes of postoperative crystalloid infusion. Experimental studies in rodents have provided a mechanism for these observed effects. Small bowel anastomoses were more likely to burst under pressure following infusions designed to produce fluid overload. Furthermore, resected anastomotic segments from the overload rodents had significantly lower hydroxyproline concentrations, which may indicate poorer anastomotic healing.

Renal function

Renal failure due to hypovolaemia, sepsis, or the toxicity of drugs can add significantly to perioperative morbidity, with some patients requiring dialysis in the critical care setting. Intravenous fluids can be used to promote diuresis, but the administration of fluids with high sodium and chloride content may produce disturbances in fluid and electrolyte balance, which may adversely affect renal function. It has long been established that infusion of high salt-containing solutions increases plasma chloride concentration and leads to a disturbance in acid–base balance, termed 'hyperchloraemic acidosis'. Animal studies have suggested that hyperchloraemia causes a reduction in renal blood flow and perfusion, and ultimately GFR. The idea that elevated plasma chloride may not be benign has recently been supported by a study in humans, in which healthy subjects who received 2 l of 0.9% saline over 60 minutes experienced hyperchloraemic acidosis associated with a 9% reduction in renal artery blood flow velocity and a 12% reduction in renal cortical perfusion. These effects were absent following the infusion of a balanced crystalloid and support the view that excess chloride imparted by 0.9% saline infusion may have a detrimental effect on renal blood flow and should be avoided in patients with renal impairment.

Low serum albumin concentrations

Serum albumin concentration is an important prognostic marker in critical illness and hypoalbuminaemia is known to be associated with poor clinical outcomes. The metabolic response to injury increases the permeability of the capillary membrane to proteins, causing the typical swelling and inflammation at the site of injury and a more generalised increase

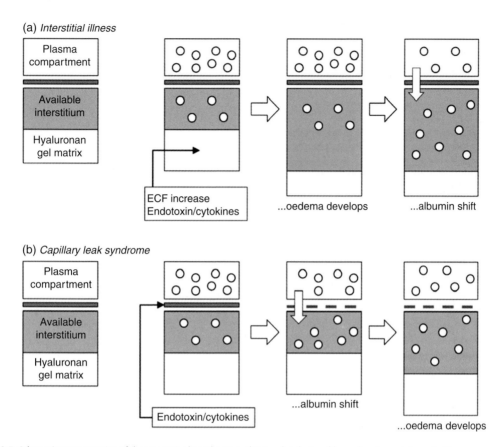

Figure 3.7 Schematic representation of the two major hypotheses explaining distributional hypoalbuminaemia in acute illness.

in capillary permeability throughout the body. The transcapillary escape rate of albumin, as measured by plasma disappearance of labelled albumin, is increased up to fourfold, and as such, albumin is redistributed from the intravascular to the interstitial space, contributing to the fall in serum albumin concentration during illness. Two major hypotheses have been advanced in order to explain this phenomenon (Figure 3.7): increased available space in the interstitial compartment due to matrix degradation and increased capillary permeability to macromolecules.

3.9 Fluid therapy: practical aspects

Assessment

Although many indications exist, fluid therapy is usually given for resuscitation, replacement, or maintenance purposes. These distinctions are important because the composition, volume, and rate of fluid administered in these settings will differ quite markedly. Prior to commencing fluid therapy, an assessment of a patient's individual requirements is vital to the process of correcting fluid and electrolyte disorders, and is achieved with a detailed history, examination, and the interpretation of fluid charts and investigations.

The presence of vomiting, diarrhoea, gastrointestinal fistulae, or obstruction in the clinical history may point to the likelihood of fluid and electrolyte disturbance, and patients with these features may be both salt- and water-depleted, or in severe cases, hypovolaemic. Similarly, patients who have lost blood may demonstrate physiological signs of low circulatory volume, including pallor, sweating, tachycardia, hypotension, and oliguria. The clinical features of salt and water depletion are summarised in Box 3.1.

Fluid deficits may be revealed by an increase in urine osmolality or specific gravity. However, in patients with renal failure, assessment of urine

> **Box 3.1   Clinical features and consequences of salt and water depletion**
>
> - Dry mouth and reduced production of saliva.
> - Diminished skin turgor.
> - Postural hypotension.
> - Oliguria.
> - Tachycardia.
> - Reduced stroke volume.
> - Impaired renal perfusion.
> - Increased viscosity of pulmonary secretions.
> - Increased blood viscosity.

osmolality may not be a reliable indicator of fluid deficit, as the concentrating capacity of the kidneys is impaired. Blood concentrations of creatinine and urea are usually elevated in the presence of a fluid deficit and although haemoglobin concentrations may similarly be increased, this may not accurately predict a fluid deficit, especially in the presence of blood loss or anaemia. Concentrations of both sodium and potassium may change in the presence of fluid overload and fluid deficit, as well as critical illness, making the interpretation of these parameters in regard to fluid and electrolyte balance difficult. Low plasma sodium can be the result of plasma dilution with non-sodium-containing fluids, such as 5% dextrose, where there is fluid excess. However, significant loss of gastrointestinal fluid can also cause low plasma sodium with fluid deficit, and is commonly precipitated by severe diarrhoea or loss of electrolyte-rich fluid from a gastrointestinal fistula or ileostomy. Plasma sodium may become elevated with fluid deficit but may also be the result of sodium excess. In contrast, plasma potassium concentrations are a poor indicator of hydration, as any excess is usually excreted by the kidneys. Furthermore, critical illness can affect renal function as well as the activity of the Na^+/K^+-ATPase pump and may give rise to clinically harmful hyperkalaemia.

Charts for parameters such as weight and urine output can be used to assess the response to fluid therapy. Weight change is a very sensitive indicator of fluid balance, except in the setting of gastrointestinal obstruction, where fluid can be sequestered and remain unavailable for redistribution to the ECF compartment. As this fluid is incorporated when weight is measured, interpretation in this setting requires a degree of clinical judgment.

The urine output is often used as an indicator of organ perfusion and is dependent on adequate blood volume and normal functioning kidneys. Although a rate of urine production of less than 0.5 ml/kg/h has traditionally triggered intravenous fluid supplementation, there are many clinical scenarios where urine output may not accurately reflect fluid status. Reduced urine output may be observed following surgery, injury, or illness, but this is usually the result of mineralocorticoid release as part of a normal metabolic response. A reasonable guide to adequate urine production is the blood-urea concentration, which remains in the normal range unless low effective circulatory volume prevents sufficient urine from being produced for waste excretion.

Treatment

Intravenous fluid therapy can be harmful, and as such should be given the same careful consideration as the prescription of any drug. Injudicious fluid prescribing due to lack of or overzealous therapy can cause significant morbidity, most of which is avoidable. In general, patients will require supplementary fluid in several specific clinical situations. These are for the treatment of hypovolaemic shock, replacement of ongoing loss of fluid and electrolytes, or supply of maintenance fluid for patients unable to replenish orally.

Resuscitation

In the setting of resuscitation for hypovolaemia, it is important to consider the cause of the haemodynamic insult. For patients suffering haemorrhage, fluid therapy may well be indicated, but of greater importance is the control of haemorrhage, which itself may be considered a fundamental part of resuscitation. Fluid therapy given alongside haemorrhage control should be initiated with balanced crystalloids, such as Hartmann's solution. The use of balanced solutions with more physiological chloride content avoids hyperchloraemic acidosis, which may compound acidosis already present due to trauma, sepsis, or poor tissue perfusion. In addition, therapy with balanced solutions avoids the negative effects on renal blood flow associated with hyperchloraemia. Dextrose-containing solutions should also be avoided, due to poor plasma expansion and the risk of hyponatraemia. Colloids in this regard perform better and will expand the intravascular compartment to a greater extent for a given volume. However, one should also bear in mind that even in the course of resuscitation, there remains the potential for fluid overload, and the aim should be the restoration of normal physiology as the clinical endpoint. Ultimately patients who have suffered significant haemorrhage may require blood transfusion. Large amounts of blood transfusion may necessitate clotting factors (e.g. fresh frozen plasma) and platelets as well.

Maintenance fluid

Occasionally, patients may be unable to meet their daily requirement of fluid and electrolytes using the oral route. This can be due to a variety of reasons, but most commonly occurs in the critical care setting, where patients are often unconscious and/or have gastrointestinal dysfunction. In normal circumstances, humans require 25–35 ml/kg/day of water, 0.9–1.5 mmol/kg/day of sodium, and approximately 1 mmol/kg/day of potassium. In addition, 400 calories are required to prevent the production of ketones, characteristic of starvation. In an average 70 kg patient, the daily requirement of 1.7–2.5 l of water, 60–105 mmol of sodium, and 70 mmol of potassium can be readily met with a regimen consisting of 1 l of Hartmann's or Plasma-Lyte 148 and 1–1.5 l of 5% dextrose. However, this practice of fluid administration for maintenance should not be considered routine, and both fluids and food should be commenced orally when this route becomes available with the discontinuation of intravenous fluids once sufficient oral intake has been achieved.

Fluid therapy for ongoing losses

Patients suffering substantial loss of fluid from the gastrointestinal tract, such as that lost from nasogastric aspirate, diarrhoea, intestinal stoma, or intestinal fistulae, require supplementary fluid over and above that prescribed for daily maintenance. In addition, fluid may be lost insensibly through hyperventilation, the use of nonhumidified face masks, open wounds, or excessive sweating. It can be seen, therefore, that the appropriate type of fluid replacement may vary with the electrolyte content of the fluid lost. An accurate measure of the volume of replacement should be made in order to provide like-for-like replacement. A summary of the electrolyte content of gastrointestinal secretions is given in Table 3.4.

Table 3.4 Approximate electrolyte content of gastrointestinal secretions.

Secretion	Sodium (mmol/l)	Potassium (mmol/l)	Chloride (mmol/l)
Saliva	44	20	–
Gastric juice	70–120	10	100
Bile	140	5	100
Pancreatic juice[a]	140	5	75
Small intestine	110–120	5–10	105
Diarrhoea (adult)	120	15	90

[a]Pancreatic juice contains 50–70 mmol HCO_3^-/l.

3.10 Goal-directed fluid therapy

In the perioperative setting, it is clear that adverse effects may be precipitated by fluid administration causing a deviation from zero fluid balance. This is evidenced by an increase in postoperative complications for patients who experience a perioperative weight increase of greater than 2.5 kg. On the other hand, it is important not to ignore the detrimental effects of underhydration, which can result in decreased venous return, cardiac output, tissue perfusion, and oxygen delivery. Traditionally, perioperative fluid-administration strategies were based on fixed infusion-rate strategies, using general estimations of perioperative fluid losses. Recent technological advances have allowed cardiovascular parameters to be monitored in much more detail than before and have led to the development of individualised goal-directed fluid therapy (GDFT) to improve cardiac output, optimise blood flow, and enhance end-organ oxygen delivery. The rationale forming the basis of GDFT is that patients have disparities in preoperative volume status and that deficits in tissue perfusion occur despite an absence of discernable changes in conventional intraoperative monitoring, such as in heart rate or arterial blood pressure. Improvements in postoperative gastrointestinal function and reductions in morbidity when employing GDFT include a quicker return of normal gastrointestinal function and lower rates of nausea and vomiting. Most studies evaluating the effectiveness of GDFT have used the oesophageal Doppler for optimisation of cardiac parameters, but other techniques including noninvasive cardiac-output monitoring (PiCCO and LiDCO) continue to evolve and are likely to be incorporated into GDFT in the future.

3.11 Implications of water and sodium metabolism in nutrition therapy for specific clinical conditions

Diarrhoeal illness

Diarrhoeal illness is one of the most common causes of disturbed fluid and electrolyte balance, and worldwide is responsible for significant morbidity and mortality. Diarrhoea, as a result of gastrointestinal infection, is usually the response to stimulation of intestinal secretory capacity. In contrast, a reduction in absorptive capacity is the predominant mechanism of diarrhoea in short bowel syndrome and inflammatory bowel disease.

The absorption of water from the gastrointestinal tract is dependent on an osmotic gradient, created by the coupling of sodium with the co-transport of glucose, amino acids, bile acids, or short-chain fatty acids. This coupling of sodium with organic solutes provides the therapeutic rationale behind oral rehydration in severe diarrhoea.

Osmotic diarrhoeas can occur with a significant ingestion of osmotically active substances of low molecular weight, such as lactulose, sorbitol, or magnesium, countering the osmotic gradient created by the coupled transport of sodium and resulting in shift of fluid into the gut. Poor absorption of carbohydrate or protein, characteristic of pancreatic insufficiency, may also reproduce this effect when these substances pass undigested to reach the colon.

In secretory diarrhoeas, which occur due to overstimulation of intestinal secretory capacity, severe disturbances of electrolyte balance are more common, and left untreated may be fatal. The electrolyte content of stool in those affected by secretory diarrhoea exhibits similar concentrations of sodium, potassium, and chloride to that found in plasma. In contrast, normal stool has much lower sodium concentrations, due to reabsorption in the colon. As the absorptive apparatus of the intestine is not impaired in those affected by secretory diarrhoeas, an orally administered isotonic solution containing equimolar amounts of sodium and glucose can be effectively used to replace diarrheal losses. This principal is exploited in the mechanism of oral rehydration therapy. The driving force behind the absorption of sodium and water in this situation is provided by the active transport of sodium from the intestinal baso-lateral membrane. These cells can, thereby, potentiate an electrochemical gradient which allows the inward flux of sodium coupled to organic solutes such as glucose or amino acids. In fact, the properties of the transmembrane ion transporters allow two sodium ions and two counterions (mainly chloride) to be absorbed for every glucose molecule; thus, glucose-coupled sodium transport enhances total solute and water absorption approximately fourfold.

Congestive heart failure and cirrhosis

Sodium retention is a hallmark of congestive heart failure and advanced liver cirrhosis. A unifying hypothesis for these and perhaps other oedematous states has been put forward, emphasising the role of arterial underfilling as the initial pathophysiological phenomenon. This phenomenon consists of reduced effective blood flow in the arterial system despite relative or absolute expansion of the ECF. Arterial underfilling would be caused by poor cardiac contractility and/or arteriolar vasodilatation. Arterial underfilling leads to:

(1) Reduction in renal blood flow, produced by the almost simultaneous operation of alpha- and beta-catecholamines, antidiuretic hormone, the endothelins, and angiotensin II.
(2) Activation of the tubuloglomerular feedback system, enhancing intrarenal angiotensin II release.
(3) Activation of apical sodium channels of principal cells in the cortical collecting tubule by aldosterone and antidiuretic hormone (ADH).
(4) Resistance of the inner medullary collecting ducts to the action of ANP.

In the presence of oedema and overt heart failure, sodium should be eliminated or severely reduced from feeding formulas, either enteral or parenteral. As has already been mentioned, ECF expansion – and even oedema and heart failure – may occur during aggressive refeeding of severely under-nourished patients given too much glucose, sodium, and water. Thus, refeeding should be done cautiously, using, when possible, the enteral route.

Stroke, dysphagia, and the elderly

The ability to adjust to variations in environmental conditions is characteristic of the young and healthy.

However, in the natural process of ageing, the capacity of organ systems to cope with physiological demands is reduced, and alterations in fluid and electrolyte homeostasis manifest, such that individuals may become vulnerable to adverse conditions. Furthermore, the presence of comorbidity and the intake of drugs may compound this situation, so that even small perturbations in fluid and electrolyte balance may result in significant metabolic derangement. Dehydration is one of the 10 most common reasons for hospital admission in the over-65 population, with mortality of over 50% when untreated.

As a result of ageing, there is a reduction in total body water of 10–15%. This is accounted for by the loss of lean body mass, and, analogous with the effect of starvation, results in relative expansion of the ECF. Renal function is adversely affected by the process of ageing, with reductions in both creatinine clearance and renal tubular function. As a consequence of reduced ability to concentrate the urine, the renal obligatory water loss is increased. However, as GFR is reduced, free water clearance and the ability to excrete a water load is diminished. Perilous falls in ECF osmolality can result, secondary to the administration of hypotonic solutions in this setting. To compound the problem, there is an age-related decrease in sensitivity to fluctuations in arterial volume and ECF osmolality. This, together with the regular intake of diuretics and antihypertensive medication, can precipitate dehydration.

Inadequate water intake is also a hallmark of patients with cerebrovascular accidents who suffer from swallowing difficulties. In a recent study, patients with a newly diagnosed acute stroke and dysphagia had a water intake that amounted to only 60% of the daily requirement.

In this group of patients, and more broadly speaking in the elderly with acute disease, dehydration due to poor water intake may go unnoticed due to a diminished threshold for thirst and cognitive impairment. Attention to hydration then becomes an essential part of clinical management in the elderly. In addition, since some of these patients may also be candidates for supplementary enteral feeding, attention should be paid to adequate provision of fluids to prevent dehydration due to both hypodipsia and substrate load.

3.12 Concluding remarks

Our knowledge of fluid and electrolyte balance has increased steadily over the past 50 years, although current prescribing practices indicate that this is still an area that is poorly understood. Inappropriate prescribing can cause increased morbidity, especially in patients undergoing surgery. Furthermore, knowledge of fluid and electrolyte balance is important when prescribing fluids and enteral or parenteral nutrition, and should be given the same careful consideration as other nutritional and pharmacological needs, especially in the elderly. Future studies will aim to evaluate the impact of balanced intravenous solutions and assess the value of individualised therapy and GDFT in the clinical setting.

References and further reading

Abbas SM, Hill AG. Systematic review of the literature for the use of oesophageal Doppler monitor for fluid replacement in major abdominal surgery. Anaesthesia 2008; 63: 44–51.

Allison S. Fluid, electrolytes and nutrition. Clin Med 2004; 4: 573–578.

Awad S, Allison SP, Lobo DN. The history of 0.9% saline. Clin Nutr 2008; 27: 179–88

Brandstrup B, Tonnesen H, Beier-Holgersen R, et al. Effects of intravenous fluid restriction on postoperative complications: comparison of two perioperative fluid regimens: a randomized assessor-blinded multicenter trial. Ann Surg 2003; 238: 641–648.

Chowdhury AH, Lobo DN. Fluids and gastrointestinal function. Curr Opin Clin Nutr Metab Care 2012a; 256: 18–24.

Chowdhury AH, Cox EF, Francis ST, et al. A randomized, controlled, double-blind cross-over study on the effects of 2-liter infusions of 0.9% saline and Plasma-Lyte® 148 on renal blood flow velocity and renal cortical tissue perfusion in healthy volunteers. Ann Surg 2012b; 256: 18–24.

Edelman IS, Leibman J. Anatomy of body water and electrolytes. Am J Med 1959; 27: 256–277.

Fleck A, Raines G, Hawker F, et al. Increased vascular permeability: a major cause of hypoalbuminaemia in disease and injury. Lancet 1985; 1: 781–784.

Gamble JL. Physiological information gained from studies on life raft ration. Harvey Lectures 1946; 42: 247–273.

Gil MJ, Franch G, Guirao X, et al. Response of severely malnourished patients to preoperative parenteral nutrition: a randomized clinical trial of water and sodium restriction. Nutrition 1997; 13: 26–31.

Hill GL. Body composition research: implications for the practice of clinical nutrition. JPEN J Parenter Enteral Nutr 1992; 16: 197–218.

Klahr S, Davis TA. Changes in renal function with chronic protein-calorie malnutrition. In: Nutrition and the Kidney (WE Mitch, S Klahr, eds). Boston: Little, Brown and Co., 1988, pp. 59–79.

Ljungqvist O, Jansson E, Ware J. Effect of food deprivation on survival after hemorrhage in the rat. Circ Shock 1987; 22: 251–260.

Lobo DN. Fluid, electrolytes and nutrition: physiological and clinical aspects. Proc Nutr Soc 2004; 63: 453–466.

Lobo DN. Fluid overload and surgical outcome: another piece in the jigsaw. Ann Surg 2009; 249: 186–188.

Lobo DN, Bjarnason K, Field J, et al. Changes in weight, fluid balance and serum albumin in patients referred for nutritional support. Clin Nutr 1999; 18: 197–201.

Lobo DN, Stanga Z, Aloysius MM, et al. Effect of volume loading with 1 liter intravenous infusions of 0.9% saline, 4% succinylated gelatine (Gelofusine) and 6% hydroxyethyl starch (Voluven) on blood volume and endocrine responses: a randomized, three-way crossover study in healthy volunteers. Crit Care Med 2010; 38: 464–470.

Moore FD. The effects of haemorrhage on body composition. N Engl J Med 1965; 273: 567–577.

Moore FD. Energy and the maintenance of the body cell mass. JPEN J Parenter Enteral Nutr 1980; 4: 228–260.

Powell-Tuck J, Gosling P, Lobo DN, et al. British Consensus Guidelines on Intravenous Fluid Therapy for Adult Surgical Patients (GIFTASUP). The British Association for Parenteral and Enteral Nutrition (BAPEN), 2008. Available from http://www.bapen.org.uk/pdfs/bapen_pubs/giftasup.pdf. Accessed 1 October 2011.

Rose BD, Post TW. Clinical Physiology of Acid-base and Electrolyte Disorders. New York: McGraw-Hill, 2001.

Schnuriger B, Inaba K, Wu T, et al. Crystalloids after primary colon resection and anastomosis at initial trauma laparotomy: excessive volumes are associated with anastomotic leakage. J Trauma 2011; 70: 603–610.

Schrier RW, Gurevich AK, Cadnapaphornchai MA. Pathogenesis and management of sodium and water retention in cardiac failure and cirrhosis. Semin Nephrol 2001; 21: 157–172.

Varadhan KK, Lobo DN. A meta-analysis of randomised controlled trials of intravenous fluid therapy in major elective open abdominal surgery: getting the balance right. Proc Nutr Soc 2010; 69: 488–498.

Winick M, editor. Hunger Disease. Studies by the Jewish Physicians in the Warsaw Ghetto. Current Concepts in Nutrition, Vol. 7. New York: Wiley, 1979.

4
Over-nutrition

Gema Frühbeck

Clínica Universidad de Navarra-CIBERobn, Spain

Key messages

- The World Health Organization (WHO) has declared obesity the largest global chronic health problem in adults, which by 2025 will emerge as a more serious world problem than malnutrition.
- In 2008, 1.5 billion adults, aged 20 and older, were overweight. Of these, over 200 million men and nearly 300 million women were obese. Nearly 43 million children under the age of five were overweight in 2010. Around 65% of the world's population lives in countries where overweight and obesity kills more people than underweight.
- Many factors contribute to the development of overweight and obesity, including energy intake and expenditure, genetic

factors, endocrine disorders, environmental factors, psychosocial influences, and other factors to a greater or lesser extent.
- The hazards of excess body weight have been clearly established by epidemiological and clinical studies, highlighting the need for careful diagnosis and effective treatment programmes.
- A multidimensional approach involving politicians, medical and health professionals, as well as industry, communities, and individuals is necessary to successfully tackle the obesity pandemic.
- The most effective treatment in the long term is, and will be, obesity prevention.

4.1 Introduction

Obesity was introduced into the International Classification of Diseases (ICD-9 code 278.0) in the 1950s. However, in the twenty-first century it has already reached epidemic proportions and it will be the leading cause of death and disability in this century worldwide, thus threatening to reverse many of the health gains achieved in recent decades. Surprisingly, obesity is often neglected, being frequently not even thought of as a serious, life-threatening chronic disease.

Definitions and classification

The widely used clinical term 'obesity' derives from the Latin *ob*, for 'on account of', and *esum*, meaning 'having eaten'. Strictly speaking, obesity is not defined as an excess of body weight but of body fat, to the extent that health may be adversely affected. Despite this important difference, medical criteria for the diagnosis of overweight and obesity do not rely on the measurement of adiposity. By convention set out in international guidelines, overweight and obesity are arbitrarily defined on the basis of the body mass index (BMI) or Quetelet's index (Table 4.1). The index is calculated by dividing the individual's weight (expressed in kilograms) by the square of his or her height (expressed in metres). A graded classification is valuable in diagnosing individuals, establishing meaningful comparisons of weight status within and between populations, identifying intervention priorities, and providing a firm basis for evaluating treatments and interventions. Although BMI is widely used as a simple surrogate measure of body fat and has been shown to correlate closely with adiposity, it does not provide an exact description of body composition. The principal limitation of BMI as a measure of body fat is that it does not distinguish fat mass from fat-free mass.

Table 4.1 WHO classification of overweight and obesity in adults according to body mass index (BMI). © WHO (2000).

Classification	BMI (kg/m^2)	Risk of comorbidity
Underweight	<18.5	Low[a]
Normal range	18.5–24.9	Average
Overweight	25.0–29.9	Increased
Obesity	≥30.0	
Class I	30.0–34.9	Moderate
Class II	35.0–39.9	Severe
Class III (morbid)	≥40.0	Very severe

[a]Low for the noncommunicable diseases associated with obesity, but there is increased mortality due to cancer and infectious diseases.

The classification of overweight and obesity in children and adolescents is especially complicated by their continually changing height and body composition. During these developmental periods, the changes often take place at different rates and times in diverse populations, making agreement over the diagnosis of overweight and obesity in children and adolescents difficult to establish. Paediatricians in the USA have classically used the 85th and 95th centiles of BMI for age and sex based on US nationally representative survey data as cut-off points to identify overweight and obesity. However, by choosing percentile values, any public health analyses and comparison purposes are minimised due to the fact that cut-off points vary between populations and over time. A standard definition for child overweight and obesity cut-off points for BMI based on international data and linked to the widely accepted adult cut-off points of 25 and 30 kg/m² has been established, which is more practical and allows comparisons.

The scale of the problem

The obesity epidemic rolls on, without signs of abatement (see *Public Health Nutrition* in this series). The World Health Organization (WHO) has declared obesity the largest global chronic health problem in adults, emerging as a more serious world problem than malnutrition. Throughout this chapter, the term 'malnutrition' refers to under-nutrition. In 2008, 1.5 billion adults, aged 20 and older, were overweight. Of these, over 200 million men and nearly 300 million women were obese. Approximately 65% of the world's population lives in countries where overweight and obesity kill more people than underweight. While in 1980, 6% of men and 8% of women in Britain were clinically obese, by 1998 those figures had ballooned to 17% of men and 21% of women, and by 2003 the numbers had increased to 22% of men and 24% of women (Figure 4.1). About a fifth of the population was obese and nearly two-thirds of men and over a half of women in England were either overweight or obese. In 2007, the government-commissioned Foresight report predicted that if no action were taken, 60% of men, 50% of women, and 25% of children would be obese by 2050. The extrapolation of current trends indicates that by 2015, 36% of males and 28% of females will be obese, while by 2025, these figures will rise to 47% and 36%, respectively. The growth of obesity in England reflects a worldwide trend. In 1991, 12.0% of US adults were clinically obese (defined as a BMI ≥30.0 kg/m²). By 2000, that figure had grown to 19.8%, representing a 65% increase in a decade. In 1999, an estimated 61% of US adults were overweight or obese, along with 13% of children and 14% of adolescents. In recent decades, the percentages of children and adolescents who are overweight have nearly doubled and almost trebled, respectively. Disparities in overweight and obesity prevalence exist in many segments of the population, based on race and ethnicity, gender, age, and socioeconomic status. In general, the prevalence is higher in women who are members of racial and ethnic minority populations and in those with a lower family income.

Economic impact and global burden

'Economic evaluation of healthcare' is the generic term referring to the various methods used to make the costs and benefits associated with any change in health service delivery explicit, while burden- and cost-of-illness studies estimate the absolute amount of resources used in treating a disease over a given period. Unfortunately, the consequences of overweight and obesity are more far-reaching than mere aesthetic problems (Tables 4.2 and 4.3). Excess body weight puts patients at a higher risk of heart disease, hypertension, diabetes mellitus, dyslipidaemia, stroke, osteoarthritis, sleep apnoea, certain cancers, and other serious associated diseases. The problems linked to obesity cause an estimated 18 million sick days and 30 000 deaths a year in the UK. The Foresight Committee estimated that the

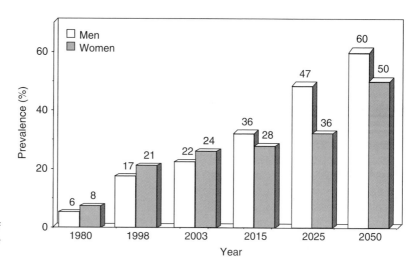

Figure 4.1 Increase in the prevalence of obesity in the UK since 1980 and the estimated figures for 2015–2050.

Table 4.2 Reported economic costs of obesity. Adapted from Caterson *et al.* (2004) © Informa Healthcare.

Country	Year	Cost		Health care
		Direct	Indirect	expenditure (%)
Netherlands	1989	US$0.5 billion		2.4
New Zealand	1991	US$208 million		>2
France	1992	US$69.7 million	US$0.69 million	4
Australia	1996	US$1.13–1.89 billion		
Canada	1997	US$1.11–4.56 billion		
Spain	1999	US$1.68 million		
USA	2000	Included in indirect	US$117 billion	6–7
UK	2003	US$0.91 billion	US$3.63 billion	>1.5

Table 4.3 Diseases used in studies of costs of obesity, and the relative risks (RR) utilised. From Caterson *et al.* (2004) © Informa Healthcare.

Frequency of use	Disease	RR range
Invariably	Type 2 diabetes mellitus	2.9–27.6
Frequently	Hypertension	2.5–4.3
	Coronary heart disease	1.7–3.5
	Gallbladder disease	1.9–10
	Cancer	1.2–1.5
Often	Dyslipidaemia	1.4–1.5
	Stroke	1.1–3.1
	Osteoarthritis	1.8
Occasionally	Gout	2.5
	Venous thrombosis	2.4

direct healthcare costs for the treatment of obesity and its consequences were between £991 and 1124 million in 2002, equating to 2.3–2.6% of NHS expenditure (McPherson *et al.*, 2007). An estimate of lost earnings attributable to obesity was £2.3–3.6 billion per year, accounting for an annual total of 45 000 lost working years. Subsequent work suggests that the total impact of obesity on employment may be as much as £10 billion (McCormack & Stone, 2007). In 2000, the total direct and indirect costs attributed to overweight and obesity amounted to US$117 billion in the US. The medical care costs of obesity in the USA are staggering, totalling about US$147 billion in 2008.

In addition to the serious life-threatening diseases associated with obesity, a range of debilitating conditions, such as osteoarthritis, respiratory difficulties, gallbladder disease, infertility, psychosocial problems, and so on, which lead to reduced quality of life and disability, are extremely costly in terms of both absence from work and use of health resources, accounting for approximately 9.4% of US healthcare expenditures (Finkelstein *et al.*, 2009). Overweight and obesity are the fifth leading risk for global deaths. At least 2.8 million adults die each year as a result of being overweight or obese. In addition, 44% of the diabetes burden, 23% of the ischaemic heart disease burden, and between 7 and 41% of certain cancer burdens are attributable to overweight and obesity. Importantly, the risk increases throughout the range of moderate and severe overweight for both men and women in all age groups.

4.2 Aetiology

Remarkable new insights into the mechanisms controlling body weight are providing an increasingly detailed framework for a better understanding of the pathogenesis underlying weight gain. Key peripheral signals have been linked to hypothalamic neuropeptide release, and the anatomic and functional networks that integrate these systems have begun to be elucidated. Obesity is a multifactorial disease influenced by both genetic and environmental factors (Figure 4.2). Since obesity has reached epidemic proportions, the epidemiological triad of host, agent, and environment can be used to consider causal factors.

The agent, by definition, is energy imbalance, where energy intake exceeds energy expenditure. This thermodynamic mismatch is determined by both genetic and environmental components.

In the epidemiological triad, features of the host affect obesity in ways that are not well understood. Some individuals appear to be more susceptible than others to weight gain. Genetic factors impinge on appetite, food choices, endocrinology, metabolism, activity, and how the body fine-tunes the balance between energy intake and expenditure. In recent years an alphabet soup of genes has been found to influence everything from food intake to how fat is stored in the body.

The third entity that facilitates an epidemic is the environment, by bringing the susceptible host and the agent together. Environmental factors include our increasingly sedentary lifestyles, as well as social and cultural values. Evidence for a genetic component to obesity is multiple and includes twin studies, adoption studies, familial aggregation, complex segregation analysis, monogenic syndromes, and gene variants that affect the obese phenotypes. Quantitating the exact genetic contribution to a predisposition to obesity has proved difficult. Great progress has been made in understanding the molecular mechanisms

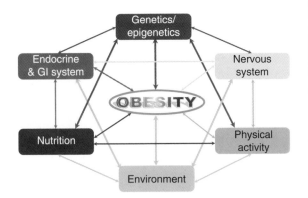

Figure 4.2 Schematic representation of the multifactorial factors influencing the development of obesity (GI: gastrointestinal).

underlying phenotypes of altered body weight, adiposity, and fat distribution.

The energy-balance equation

Energy-balance regulation is an extremely complex process, comprising multiple interacting homeostatic and behavioural pathways aimed at maintaining constant energy stores. It is now evident that body-weight control is achieved through highly integrated interactions between nutrient selection, organoleptic influences, and endocrine responses to diet, as well as being influenced by genetic and environmental factors. The brain is known to play a critical role in maintaining whole-body energy balance by regulating energy intake and expenditure in accordance with afferent and efferent signals. Regulation of body weight was once considered a simple feedback control system, in which the hypothalamus modulated food intake to compensate for fluctuations in body weight. The existing body of evidence has fostered the transition from the classic 'lipostat' to a multifactorial model, including factors emerging from several different organs.

From an evolutionary point of view, animals feed to satisfy their immediate caloric and nutritional requirements from meal to meal, but also to allow energy and nutrients to be stored in anticipation of high energy demands or seasonal food shortages. Thus, food intake control involves the integration of external environmental cues with multiple internal physiological signals, as well as external social elements and hedonic influences. An obese phenotype, which ultimately expresses a heterogeneous group of

Table 4.4 Main influences affecting the human appetite system.

Influence	Examples
Cognitive	Restraint, emotions, previous experiences, conditioned associations
Sociocultural	Religious beliefs, education, tradition, learned experiences, economy-acquisition level
Gustatory	Palatability, learned/innate preferences, food-specific satiety, nutrient-associated sensory stimuli, cephalic phase events, taste-receptor density
Neuroendocrine	Orexigenic and anorexigenic peptides, entero-insular axis, adipostatic signals, sympathetic/parasympathetic balance
Gastrointestinal	Nutrient composition, water content, energy density, digestibility, pH, osmolarity, peptidic/hormonal/neural release, stomach size, mechanical distension, emptying rate, absorption
Metabolic	Nutrient partitioning/flux, nutrient–genotype interactions, hepatic metabolism
Behavioural	Age, sex, socioeconomic status, occupation, meal patterns, physical-activity level, pathophysiology/developmental stage

conditions with multiple causes, can only occur when energy intake exceeds energy expenditure for an extended period of time. The sustained energy-balance displacement incontrovertibly leads to changes in body energy stores.

Energy intake

The amount of food consumed represents a major contributor to the control of body weight and consequently to obesity development. The biobehavioural food intake control system includes orosensory, gastrointestinal, circulating, nutritional, metabolic, and central influences, which interact to elicit facilitatory or inhibitory signals. The main food and nutrient influences affecting the human appetite system are summarised in Table 4.4. Multiple systems, ranging from elaborated cognitive influences to purely chemical signals, work at different levels to maintain a functional cascade of sequential physiological events in order to regulate hunger and satiety. Feeding patterns, including the amount, kind, and composition of food consumed, are governed by a pleiad of influences from quite diverse anthropological spheres.

With the identification of leptin, research into appetite control has progressed at a phenomenal rate (see Chapter 3 in *Nutrition and Metabolism* in this series). A complex network of synchronous, redundant, and counterbalancing peptide signals has been identified. These interactions are mainly mediated in the hypothalamus, where orexigenic and anorexigenic signals regulate feeding behaviour via effects on hunger and satiety (Table 4.5). The means by which the body strives to defend fat stores in the face of large variations in day-to-day energy intake and expenditure is a topic of paramount biomedical importance. In this sense, it can be stated that not all peptides are 'equal', which implies that the adaptive responses to weight gain and loss are critical and have evolved differentially over time based on teleological reasons. Thus, the efficiency of the peptides and systems aimed at defending the organism against starvation is more important than the anorexigenic pathways.

Progress in understanding the contribution of energy intake to the aetiology of obesity has been seriously confounded by underreporting, averaging about 30% of energy consumption in obese subjects. Whether this phenomenon takes place consciously or subconsciously has not been established. Several causes may underlie underreporting, ranging from changes in eating habits subsequent to the pressure of recording food intake to underestimation of portion size and inadequate knowledge of food composition, as well as forgetfulness. In addition, individual macronutrients are known to exert different effects on eating behaviour as a consequence of their diverse satiating ability.

Based on experiments with manipulated foods and retrospective analyses of dietary records, protein has been suggested to be the most satiating macronutrient, while fat appears to have the weakest effect, which provides support for subjects readily over-eating in response to high-fat foods. However, other factors such as energy density have also to be taken into consideration, since under conditions of isoenergetically dense diets, the high-fat hyperphagia does not occur. The role played by sensory preferences for particular food groups in association with obesity has also been addressed, but the high intersubject variability may mask any potential obese–lean differences. Initially, some epidemiological studies suggested that individuals who reported eating a greater number of small meals had a lower relative weight than those eating fewer but large meals. A review of the literature failed to find any significant association between eating frequency and obesity development.

Table 4.5 Hormones, neurotransmitters, and peptides implicated in food intake control.

Orexigenic	Anorexigenic
Agouti-related protein (AGRP)	Amylin
Beacon	Alpha-melanocyte-stimulating hormone (α-MSH)
Cerebellin 1	Bombesin
Dynorphin	Brain-derived neurotrophic factor (BDNF)
Endocannabinoids	Calcitonin-gene related peptide (CGRP)
Gamma-aminobutyric acid (GABA)	Cholecystokinin
Galanin	Ciliary neurotrophic factor (CNTF)
Glucocorticoids	Cocaine- and amphetamine-related transcript (CART)
Ghrelin	Corticotropin-releasing hormone (CRH)
Growth hormone-releasing hormone (GHRH)	Enterostatin
Insulin	Gastrin-releasing peptide (GRP)
Interleukin 1 receptor antagonist	Glucagon
Melanin-concentrating hormone (MCH)	Glucagon-like peptide 1 and 2 (GLP-1, GLP-2)
Motilin	Histamine
Neuropeptide Y (NPY)	Interleukin 1, interleukin 2
Noradrenaline (α_2 receptor)	Leptin
Opioid peptides (β-endorphin)	Neurotensin
Orexins/hypocretins	Norepinephrine (β receptor)
	Oxytocin
	Oxyntomodulin
	Peptide YY$_{3-36}$
	Pituitary adenylate cyclase-activated peptide (PACAP)
	Prolactin-releasing peptide
	Serotonin
	Somatostatin
	Thyrotropin-releasing hormone (TRH)
	Tumour necrosis factor alpha (TNFα)
	Urocortin
	Xenin

Energy expenditure

Total energy expenditure (TEE) reflects the sum of three major components: basal metabolic rate (BMR), thermogenesis, and physical activity (Figure 4.3). BMR represents 60–75% of the TEE in sedentary people; it is the energy required to maintain the basic physiological functions such as respiration, circulation, cellular homeostasis, and tissue regeneration. BMR is measured under highly standardised conditions, including determination early in the morning, with the subject at complete rest, in a thermoneutral environment, and after an overnight fast. Approximately 80% of the interindividual variance in BMR can be accounted for by age, fat-free mass, and gender. Potential mechanisms for the remaining variance can be attributed to differences in sympathetic nervous-system activity and skeletal muscle metabolism. Although this leaves some scope for subjects with a relatively low BMR to be predisposed to obesity development, BMR studies have conclusively shown

that obese individuals have an increased BMR relative to their lean counterparts.

The thermogenesis compartment comprises the heat production specifically generated for body-temperature maintenance (thermoregulatory thermogenesis), the obligatory heat loss associated with the absorption, transport, and metabolism of recently ingested food (diet-induced thermogenesis, DIT), and the heat production switched on in order to dissipate excess dietary energy as heat (adaptive thermogenesis or luxus consumption). In humans, due to the large body size and subsequent low surface area : volume ratio, thermoregulatory thermogenesis is usually of minor importance. In addition, clothing and heating have minimised the thermogenic challenge of cold stress. Until recently it was assumed that only vestigial amounts of brown adipose tissue (BAT) were present in adulthood. But since 2000, positron emission tomography (PET) studies have clearly shown that BAT is present mainly in the cervical, supraclavicular, axillary, and paravertebral

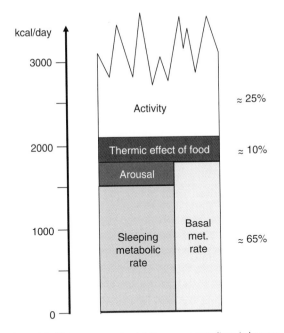

Figure 4.3 Major components of daily energy expenditure in humans (example for a 70 kg man).

to weight gain during periods of overfeeding. Under carefully controlled experimental conditions and with rigorous determination techniques, any significant role for this energy compartment in the modulation of energy balance during overfeeding has been discarded. However, evidence that the best predictor of interindividual differences in fat gain during over-eating is the so-called non-exercise activity thermogenesis (NEAT) has been provided. Besides the calorie expenditure of activities of daily living, NEAT encompasses the energy costs of all nonvolitional muscle activity, such as muscle tone, posture maintenance, and fidgeting. Interestingly, changes in NEAT have been reported to account for differences in fat storage between individuals, suggesting that as humans over-eat, activation of NEAT dissipates excess energy to preserve leanness, and that failure to activate NEAT may lead to weight gain. Since thermogenesis accounts for only a fraction of TEE (about 10%), the potential for a significant contribution in humans is relatively small, though not negligible.

The most variable component of energy expenditure is represented by physical activity, which may account for 20–50% of TEE. This consists of the sum of all gross muscular work involved in body displacement – including all minor movements – as well as in performing physical work. The ratio of TEE:BMR gives an index of the activity of an individual: the physical activity level (PAL). In humans, the freedom to undertake exercise and everyday lifestyle physical activities accounts for a further high interindividual variability in this energy fraction. Physical work can be divided into weight-independent and weight-dependent activities. Consequently, the energy cost of weight-bearing exercises is highly correlated with body mass and is therefore much higher in obese individuals. Moreover, activity can be further divided according to whether it is essentially obligatory or discretionary. In modern societies, mechanisation has replaced most manual labour. Therefore, leisure-time physical activity is gaining a dominant role in determining energy expenditure. In this respect, the general secular trend towards less-active lifestyles in affluent countries appears as the major contributor to the obesity epidemic.

Genetic factors

Although the search for genes responsible for human obesity has experienced outstanding advances, the genetic explanation for, or susceptibility to, obesity in

regions of adult humans, providing support for its potential relevance in whole-body energy homeostasis (Frühbeck *et al.*, 2009). The prevalence of active BAT in adults can be estimated only indirectly, but it is thought to be present in at least about 10% of the general population. Recent studies have detected BAT in 3.1% of the men and 7.5% of the women indicating a sexual dimorphism. Nonetheless, prevalence data vary considerably, ranging from as much as 80% in women with breast cancer to 50% in a teenage population. The amount of BAT is inversely correlated with BMI, especially in older people. Furthermore, the probability of detecting active BAT regions is inversely associated with increasing age, suggesting an age-related decline in thermogenesis and energy expenditure. BAT activity is acutely enhanced by cold exposure and stimulated by the sympathetic nervous system. However, it should be borne in mind that statistical association does not imply causality, especially in such a multifactorial biological process as energy-balance regulation. The DIT, also termed postprandial thermogenesis, is mostly obligatory, but does also contain a so-called 'facultative' fraction, which is non-obligatory and is stimulated by the sympathetic nervous activity.

The capacity for facultative thermogenesis has been suggested to explain the differential propensity

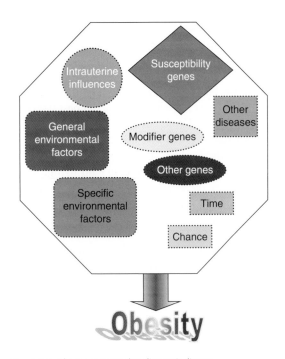

Figure 4.4 Obesity as a complex oligogenic disease.

the vast majority of patients has not been identified. In some rare cases of severe childhood-onset obesity, single gene defects have been accounted for. Further evidence for a genetic component to obesity is derived from twin studies, adoption studies, familial aggregation, complex segregation analysis, monogenic syndromes, and gene variants that affect the obese phenotypes. Quantitating the exact genetic contribution to a predisposition to obesity has proved difficult. Great progress has been made in understanding the molecular mechanisms underlying phenotypes of altered body weight, adiposity, and fat distribution by creating transgenic animal models. A role of utmost importance for genetic factors in body-weight regulation seems difficult to reconcile with the burgeoning of human obesity in the past decades. Available evidence supports the notion that obesity is an oligenic disease, whose expression can be modulated by numerous polygenic modifier genes interacting with each other and with environmental factors such as food choices, physical activity, and smoking (Figure 4.4).

Genetic epidemiology

Genetic epidemiology studies are useful for addressing specific questions pertaining to the extent of familial

aggregation in obesity, the relative contribution of nongenetic versus genetic factors, paternal versus maternal transmission, the contribution of shared genetic and environmental factors to covariation among phenotypes, and so on. Monozygotic (MZ) twins share 100% of their genes, while dizygotic (DZ) twins twins share on average half of them. Therefore, twin studies allow for separation of the genetic component of variance. Nonetheless, twins may also share common environmental influences, thus masking the real genetic component. Heritability estimates for BMI derived from twin studies typically cluster between 50 and 80%. The correlations of MZ twins reared apart provide a direct estimate of the genetic effect, given that members of the same pair were not placed in similar environments, that behavioural characteristics were different, and that intrauterine factors did not affect long-term variation in BMI. The heritability of BMI under these circumstances would be in the range of 40–70%.

Adoption studies represent a useful tool for quantifying the contribution of common environmental effects as the adoptive parents and their offspring (and adopted siblings) are exposed to the same environmental sources of variation, while the adoptees and biological parents share only genetic sources of variance. It has to be taken into consideration, however, that selective and late placement in the adoptive home may result in inflated common environmental estimates (translating to reduced heritability estimates) if the placement is based in part on genetic similarity between the biological and adoptive parents. Heritability estimates for the BMI tend to cluster around 30%, with all the remaining variance attributable to nonshared individual environmental factors.

Comparison of resemblance in pairs of spouses, parents, children, brothers, and sisters, including sometimes MZ and DZ twins, for body weight, BMI, and selected skinfold thicknesses, has been approached in family studies. As would be expected, the highest familial correlation appears among MZ twins (0.73), while the lowest is among spouses (0.13). In an intermediate position are the parent–offspring, sibling, and DZ twin correlations, with 0.22, 0.28, and 0.27, respectively. In the Quebec Family Study, based on 1698 members and 409 families, and including nine types of relatives by descent or adoption, a total transmissible variance across generations for BMI of about 35%, but a genetic effect of only 5%, was observed. It can be concluded that the heritability of obesity phenotypes is highest with twin studies, intermediate with nuclear family data, and lowest when derived from adoption data. When several different types of relatives are used jointly in the same design, the heritability estimates typically cluster around 25–40% of the age- and gender-adjusted phenotype variance. In addition, they always tend to be slightly higher for fat-distribution phenotypes than for overall body fat, reaching a value of about 50% for abdominal visceral fat.

In segregation analysis, the phenotype is assumed to be influenced by the independent and additive contributions from the major gene effect, a multifactorial background due to polygenes, and a unique environmental component (residual). An overview of the segregation analysis studies for obesity phenotypes provides evidence for the segregation of a recessive locus with a frequency of about 0.2 and accounting for 35–45% of the variance, with a multifactorial component accounting for 40–45% of the variance. Taken together, the several different existing segregation studies quite consistently indicate that body fat and abdominal visceral fat are influenced by the segregation of a recessive locus, explaining up to about 65% of the variance, in addition to a multifactorial component, accounting for 20–40% of the residual variance. These observations provide evidence for the existence of a subset of obese families in which some genes appear to be more important than others in the genetic aetiology of obesity.

Another interesting topic is the genetic covariation between obesity and comorbidities. Multivariate genetic studies try to address whether or not, and to what extent, the associations between overweight and its associated comorbidities share common genetic and/or environmental aetiologies. In this regard, the Quebec Family Study examined the hypothesis of a shared genetic basis between measures of body fat and other traits of the metabolic syndrome, showing that adiposity and glucose and insulin concentrations are influenced by specific genetic and environmental factors. Furthermore, shared genetic and environmental factors were shown to contribute to the common variance ranging from 5 to 25% between indicators of body fat and insulin within individuals. The obtained results illustrated that there is a shared genetic basis between the two traits, with a bivariate heritability estimate of about 10%. Other studies have investigated the cross-trait familial resemblance between measures of body fat and cardiovascular elements (blood pressure, cholesterol, triglycerides, waist-to-hip ratio, etc.).

In summary, the multivariate genetic studies strongly support the presence of familial aggregation in the clustering of obesity and most of its comorbidities, with family studies showing a common familial basis for the covariation between insulin and body fat, adiposity distribution, blood pressure, lipidaemia, and high-density lipoprotein (HDL) fractions, as well as HDL particle size. Nevertheless, the shared genetic variance between body-fat phenotypes and circulating concentrations of cholesterol and lipoproteins may be lower than for other manifestations of the metabolic syndrome.

Molecular epidemiology

The identification of genes and mutations predisposing to obesity has been principally based on linkage and association studies with candidate genes. Both strategies rely on the principle of co-inheritance of adjacent DNA markers. Linkage studies analyse the cosegregation between a marker locus and a trait within families, whereas association studies test in the population for the cooccurrence of an allele at a marker locus and a trait in unrelated individuals. Candidate genes can be selected on the basis of several approaches:

- Observed influence of the trait in animal models – candidate genes by mutation.
- Known chromosomal locations physiologically or metabolically relevant for the obesity phenotype – functional candidate genes.
- Position in a region of the genome – positional candidate genes, near a Mendelian obesity syndrome, within a quantitative trait locus (QTL) homologous to a locus linked to obesity in animal models or identified through human genome-wide scans.

Single gene-mutation mouse models

So far, a small number of single genes with spontaneous mutations have been observed to be responsible for mouse models of obesity. These mutations are listed in Table 4.6. Most human linkage and association studies of the cloned genes from obesity mouse

Mutation	Gene product	Genetic effect	Chromosome Mouse	Human
Obese (*ob*)	Leptin	Recessive	6 (10.5)	7q31.1
Diabetes (*db*)	Leptin receptor	Recessive	4 (46.7)	1p31
Agouti yellow (*A^y*)	Agouti-signaling peptide	Dominant	2 (89.0)	20q11.2
Fat (*fat*)	Carboxypeptidase E	Recessive	8 (32.6)	4q32
Tubby (*tub*)	Insulin-signaling protein	Recessive	7 (51.5)	11p15.5
Mahogany (*mg*)	Attractin	Recessive	2 (73.9)	20p13

Table 4.6 Single-gene mutations of mouse models of obesity and their corresponding chromosomal regions in the human genome.

models have yielded negative results, with only a small number of cases of human obesity related to the specific mutations mentioned. Nevertheless, these candidate genes have been extremely useful in providing more insight into the molecular basis of human body-weight control. This is extraordinarily evident in the case of leptin, and how it has contributed to the unravelling of new pathways in the regulation of food intake and energy balance.

Functional candidate genes

Potentially, candidate genes can be defined on the basis of an impact on body mass, adiposity, fat distribution, food intake, satiety signals, energy expenditure, diet-induced thermogenesis, physical activity, nutrient partitioning, and comorbidities, among other things. The last update of the human obesity gene map was published in 2006. It reports the number of genes and DNA sequence variations known to be associated and/or linked with obesity-related phenotypes, together with the exact chromosomal locations of the genes (Rankinen *et al.*, 2006). As of October 2005, 176 human obesity cases due to single-gene mutations in 11 different genes had been reported and 50 loci related to Mendelian syndromes relevant to human obesity had been mapped to a genomic region, and causal genes or strong candidates have been identified for most of these syndromes. There are 244 genes that, when mutated or expressed as transgenes in a mouse, result in phenotypes that affect body weight and adiposity. The number of human obesity QTLs derived from genome scans continues to grow, with 253 QTLs for obesity-related phenotypes from 61 genome-wide scans. A total of 52 genomic regions harbour QTLs supported by two or more studies. The number of studies reporting associations between DNA sequence variation in specific genes and obesity phenotypes has also increased

considerably, with 426 findings of positive associations with 127 candidate genes. A promising observation is that 22 genes are each supported by at least five positive studies. Among them, those showing replications in 10 studies or more include *PPARG*, *ADRB3*, *ADRB2*, *LEPR*, *GNB3*, *UCP3*, *ADIPOQ*, *LEP*, *UCP2*, *HTR2C*, *NR3C1*, and *UCP1*. It is worth noting that the obesity gene map shows putative loci on all chromosomes except Y. Unfortunately, the Web site devoted to the Human Obesity Map is no longer available.

Positional candidate genes

Positional candidate genes of obesity are considered those whose position in the human genome maps to a chromosomal region containing genes or loci that could influence obesity. Undoubtedly, Mendelian syndromes of obesity represent a good example of positional candidate genes. Although it has been observed that overweight and obesity run in families, most cases do not segregate in families according to a clear pattern of Mendelian inheritance. Nonetheless, some rare Mendelian disorders with obesity as a clinical feature have been described; these are summarised in Table 4.7. Prader–Willi syndrome is the most common of the listed disorders, with an estimated prevalence of 1 in 25 000. For many of the listed syndromes, the specific genetic or molecular defect remains unknown.

Most of the disorders listed share some other clinical features in addition to obesity, such as mental retardation, delayed growth and maturation, hypogonadism, or dysmorphic characteristics such as facies and those affecting the limbs, making them difficult to distinguish and sometimes leading to misclassifications. In this sense, the Laurence–Moon and the Bardet–Biedl syndromes have long been considered a single entity (Laurence–Moon–Bardet–Biedl syndrome) because of the presence of mental retardation,

Table 4.7 Disorders with Mendelian inheritance in humans which have obesity as a clinical feature. NA, not available.

Inheritance	Disorder	Mapping
Autosomal dominant	Achondroplasia	4p16.3
	Adiposis dolorosa (Dercum disease)	NA
	Albright hereditary osteodystrophy	
	AHO	20q13.3
	AHO2	15q11–q13
	Posterior polymorphous corneal dystrophy	20p11.2
	Morgani–Stewart–Morel syndrome	NA
	Momo syndrome	NA
	Prader–Willi syndrome	15q11.2–q12
	Angelman syndrome	15q11.2
	Ulnar-mammary Schnizel syndrome	12q24.1
	Familial partial lipodystrophy	
	type 2	1q22
	type 3	3p25
	type 4	15q26
	Insulin-resistance syndrome (Rabson–Mendenhall syndrome)	19p13.3–p13.2
	Thyroid hormone-resistance syndrome	3p24.2
	Polycystic ovarian syndrome (PCOS1)	19p13.2
Autosomal recessive	Alström syndrome	2p13
	Bardet–Biedl syndrome	
	BBS1	11q13
	BBS2	16q21
	BBS3	3q11.2
	BBS4	15q22.3–23
	BBS5	2q31.1
	BBS6	20p12
	BBS7	4q27
	BBS8	14q31.3
	BBS9	7p14
	BBS10	12q21.2
	BBS11	9q33.1
	BBS12	4q27
	BBS13	17q22
	BBS14	12q21.32
	BBS15	2p15
	Berardinelli–Seip congenital lipodystrophy	
	type 1	9q34
	type 2	11q13
	type 3	7q31.1
	type 4	17q21.2
	Biemond syndrome	NA
	Cohen syndrome	8q22.2
	Carbohydrate-deficient glycoprotein syndrome t la	16p13
	Fanconi–Bickel syndrome	3q26.1–26.2
	Cushing disease	NA
	Macrosomia adiposa congenita	NA
	Pickwickian syndrome	NA
	Urban–Rogers–Meyer syndrome	NA
	Short stature–obesity syndrome	NA
	Summitt syndrome	NA
X-linked	Börjeson–Forssman–Lehman syndrome	Xq26.3
	Choroideremia with deafness and obesity	Xq21.1
	Mehmo syndrome	Xp22.13–p21.1
	Chudley-McCullough syndrome	NA
	Wilson–Turner syndrome	Xp21.1–q22
	Simpson–Golabi–Behmel syndrome	
	SGBS1	Xq26.1
	SGBS2	Xp22

hypogenitalism, and pigmentary retinopathy in both. However, the Laurence–Moon syndrome cannot be considered an obesity syndrome, since obesity is not present in all cases, while it is a characteristic feature of the Bardet–Biedl syndrome. Similarly, the Carpenter syndrome resembles the Summitt syndrome, but obesity is only developed in older patients in the former.

Furthermore, positional candidate genes of obesity can be identified from genomic scans with a set of evenly spaced genetic markers covering the entire genome. Box 4.1 lists the first nine relevant genome-wide scans of obesity carried out, while Table 4.8 shows the genomic regions with obesity QTLs identified in at least two studies. QTLs represent regions of the genome containing markers that have shown significant evidence of linkage with obesity phenotypes. More recently, in genome-wide association scans for obesity-related traits performed in very large populations, FTO (fat mass and obesity-associated protein) and MC4R (melanocortin 4 receptor) came out as the most robust and frequent loci associated with increased BMI in humans. While rare MC4R mutations are the most common cause of monogenic forms of extreme, early-onset obesity, growing evidence shows that common MC4R variants contribute to obesity in the general population (Loos, 2011). A subsequent search in a meta-analysis of 15 genome-wide association studies identified six additional loci: TMEM18, KCTD15, GNPDA2, SH2B1, MTCH2, and NEGR1 (Willer *et al.*, 2009). Several of the likely causal genes are highly expressed or are known to act in the central nervous system (CNS), emphasising, as in rare monogenic forms of obesity, the role of the CNS in predisposition to obesity. A further recent study confirmed 14 known obesity susceptibility loci and identified further new loci associated with BMI, one of which includes a copy number variant near GPRC5B. As in previous analyses, some loci (at MC4R, POMC, SH2B1, and BDNF) map near key hypothalamic regulators of energy balance, and one of these loci is near GIPR, an incretin receptor (Speliotes *et al.*, 2010). Note that the most frequent loci associated with BMI have actually shown small size effects of the implicated genes. Furthermore, physical activity is able to counterbalance the genetic predisposition to obesity (Li *et al.*, 2010), thereby further attenuating the true impact of genetics.

Box 4.1 First relevant studies to perform genome-wide scans of obesity

- Pima Family Study (PFS)
- Quebec Family Study (QFS)
- San Antonio Family Heart Study (SAFHS)
- Paris-Lille French Study (PLFS)
- University of Pennsylvania Family Study (UPFS)
- Finnish Family Study (FFS)
- TOPS (Take Off Pounds Sensibly) Family Study
- HERITAGE Family Study
- Old Order Amish Population (OOAP)

Table 4.8 Genomic regions with obesity quantitative trait loci (QTLs) found in at least two of the studies in Box 4.1.

Gene	Evidence in
1p11–31	PFS, QFS
2p21	PLFS, SAFHS
7q31	OOAP, QFS
8q11–23	HERITAGE, SAFHS
9q22–34	HERITAGE, QFS
10p12–15	HERITAGE, OOAP, PLFS
14q11–31	HERITAGE, OOAP
17q11–21	QFS, SAFHS
18q12–21	PFS, FFS, QFS
20q11–13	PFS, UPFS

Although the ethnic groups, sampling strategies, densities of markers, phenotypes selected, and analytical strategies vary across the different studies, the information obtained suggests that there are some common genes and sequence variants involved in the genetic predisposition to obesity across a variety of populations and ethnic groups. Moreover, it appears that the predisposition to obesity might also be influenced by other genes and alleles whose prevalences and effect sizes vary from population to population.

The genetic and molecular epidemiology studies carried out in recent decades have considerably enhanced our understanding of the genetic factors contributing to the development of obesity and involved in shaping interindividual differences not only in body weight and adiposity, but in susceptibility to response to energy-balance challenges and the development of several obesity-associated comorbidities. Linkage and association studies are underway in various populations, aimed at identifying these genes, analysing a variety of obesity subphenotypes, and exploring gene–gene/gene–nutrient/gene–environment interactions. In addition, new technological aids – as embodied by the application of the whole array of '-omics' techniques – will further contribute to broaden our knowledge in this complex field.

Endocrine disorders

While genetic factors cause obesity mainly through endocrine mechanisms, most endocrinological changes taking place in obese patients are due to obesity itself. Primary endocrine causes of obesity encompass hypothalamic structural lesions due to tumours (craniopharyngioma, pituitary macroadenoma with suprasellar extension) as well as other space-occupying lesions produced by trauma, infiltration, inflammation, or iatrogenic damage through surgery or radiotherapy. Panhypopituitarism, growth hormone (GH) deficiency, and hypogonadism represent further contributing factors of primary endocrine obesity. Among the recently described monogenetic syndromes of obesity with hypothalamic dysfunction, the mutations in leptin, leptin receptor, pro-opiomelanocortin, pro-hormone convertase 1, and melanocortin-4 receptor (MC4R) need to be mentioned. These are extremely rare syndromes in everyday clinical practice, except for the MC4R mutation, which has been reported to appear in approximately 4% of morbidly obese patients.

Endocrinopathies

Contrary to common belief, primary endocrine disorders are not the underlying cause in most cases of human obesity. However, a number of known endocrinopathies causally associated with obesity in their clinical presentation should be taken into consideration. The diagnostic process should explore the potential presence of adrenocortical, thyroid, ovarian, and pancreatic diseases. The hypercortisolemia characteristic of Cushing's syndrome (due to primary adrenal disease, increased pituitary stimulation, or ectopically secreted adrenocorticotropic hormone (ACTH)) is accompanied by an enlarged visceral adipose tissue depot as well as all the features of the metabolic syndrome. Hypothyroidism may lead to weight gain in about 60% of patients. Since the prevalences of hypothyroidism and obesity are about 4 and

15%, respectively, it is feasible that both conditions will coexist in some patients.

The exact mechanisms linking polycystic ovary syndrome (PCOS) with obesity have not been completely established. The hyperandrogenism with chronic anovulation is not always accompanied by increased body weight, while the insulin resistance is universal and independent of the effect of obesity. Pancreatic insulin-secreting tumours are extremely rare (with an approximate incidence of 1 in 1 000 000), with the spontaneous hyperinsulinism producing recurrent hypoglycaemia leading to hyperphagia and subsequent weight gain.

Endocrine changes as a consequence of obesity

Adipose tissue has been shown to release a number of hormones, cytokines, and factors, collectively termed 'adipokines', such as tumour necrosis factor alpha (TNFα), interleukin 6 (IL-6), leptin, resistin, and adiponectin, with known effects on insulin secretion and/or action. Overweight and obesity are characterised by hyperinsulinaemia and increased insulin response to an oral glucose load. Hepatic insulin extraction is decreased in obesity, particularly central obesity, contributing further to insulin resistance and finally leading to type 2 diabetes mellitus. Obese individuals display elevated plasma fatty acid concentrations, which impair insulin-stimulated skeletal muscle glucose uptake and oxidation, as well as insulin-mediated hepatic glucose output suppression. The main disturbances of the principal endocrinological axes associated with obesity are summarised in Table 4.9, while Figure 4.5 illustrates the endocrine consequences of increased adiposity.

The dysregulation of the hypothalamic–pituitary axis (HPA) in obesity is characterised by centrally driven altered ACTH secretory dynamics and hyperresponsiveness, together with a peripheral elevation of cortisol production and local response at the adipocyte level. The association of increased activity of the HPA with central obesity is based on the effect of elevated cortisolemia on visceral adipose tissue, which exhibits a high density of glucocorticoid receptors. Elevated receptor binding together with low circulating binding globulins may lead to an accelerated clearance of cortisol. Increased expression of 11-β-hydroxysteroid dehydrogenase in visceral adipocytes may further contribute to exaggerated local cortisol production, thereby leading to central obesity.

Table 4.9 Disturbances in the main hormonal axes in obesity. ACTH, adrenocorticotropic hormone; GH, growth hormone; GHBP, growth hormone-binding protein; IGFBP, insulin-like growth factor-binding protein; LH, luteinizing hormone; SHBG, sex hormone-binding globulin; PCOS, polycystic ovary syndrome.

Axis/circumstance	Finding
Hypothalamic–pituitary–adrenal	Normal plasma and urinary cortisol concentrations
	Normal 24-hour ACTH/cortisol levels
	Increased cortisol production and breakdown
	Decreased daytime cortisol changes and reduced morning peaks
	Increased ACTH pulse frequency + decreased pulse amplitude
	Impaired cortisol suppression after dexamethasone challenge
	Increased stress-induced ACTH secretion
	Elevated adrenal androgen production
Growth hormone–insulin-like growth factor 1	Decreased GH concentrations, reduced pituitary secretion
	Elevated GHBP release
	Decreased IGFBP-1 and IGFBP-3
	Blunted response to stimuli
Hypothalamic–pituitary–gonadal	Decreased total and free testosterone
In men	Reduced C19 steroids
	Elevated oestrogen production
	Potential aromatase activity alteration
	Decreased LH secretion
	Reduced SHBG levels
In women	Increased free testosterone fraction
	Elevated oestrogen production
	Normal gonadotropin secretion
	Reduced SHBG synthesis and levels
	Elevated SHBG-bound and nonbound androgen production
With PCOS	Elevated adrenal androgen secretion
	Increased ovarian testosterone release
	Elevated oestrone/oestradiol ratio
	Increased androstendione aromatisation
	Elevated free steroid levels
	Reduced SHBG
	Decreased IGFBP-1
	Insulin resistance, metabolic syndrome

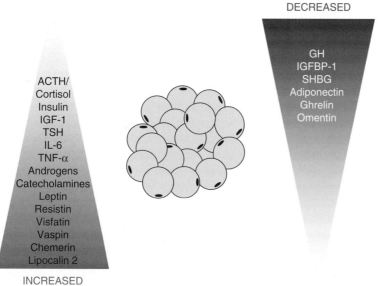

Figure 4.5 Main endocrine changes associated with increased adiposity.

In women, increased body fat is associated with hyperandrogenism and ovulatory dysfunction, often leading to infertility. Circulating testosterone and androstenedione levels are usually increased in obese women, whereas sex hormone-binding globulin (SHBG) concentrations are decreased, with an elevated oestrone/oestradiol plasmatic ratio. The low SHBG activity facilitates accelerated testosterone clearance rates, resulting in an elevated proportion of unbound testosterone available for hepatic extraction and clearance. In obese men, a decrease in circulating levels of total and free testosterone and SHBG is observed.

The hypothalamic–pituitary–thyroid axis (HPT) exerts a relevant role on energy homeostasis, as evidenced by adaptive changes taking place during the course of overfeeding and fasting periods. Despite the observation of normal free thyroid hormone concentrations in obese adults, other studies have suggested a central upregulation based on increased TSH and decreased prolactin responses to TRH. While overfeeding increases total thyroid hormone concentrations and decreases reverse T3 levels, fasting has been shown to be accompanied by low free T3 and T4 concentrations in obese individuals. The changes in the pituitary–thyroid axis involve the action of leptin in the arcuate nucleus on neuropeptide Y (NPY) and pro-opiomelanocortin (POMC)-expressing neurones.

The alterations present in the growth hormone/insulin-like growth factor (GH/IGF) axis of obese subjects include a nutrient- and neuroendocrine-induced inhibition of secretion as well as increased binding and clearance, which lead to decreased GH concentrations. Hyposecretion of GH depends more on pulse amplitude decrease than on reduced pulse frequency. Elevated concentrations of GH-binding protein further contribute to the low GH levels observed in obesity. The increased circulating free fatty acids (FFAs) present in obese individuals downregulate pituitary GH secretion, while a dysregulated hypothalamic glucose sensing with a blunted inhibitory effect of glucose on GH secretion takes place in obesity.

Given the suppressing effect of insulin on GH secretion, the hyperinsulinaemia characteristic of obesity further contributes to decreases in its secretion. Elevated IGF-1 resulting from adipose mass enlargement contributes to GH hyposecretion via a negative feedback on pituitary cells. Recently, the decreased ghrelin concentrations observed in obesity have also been suggested as a potential mechanism of reduced GH secretion.

Environmental factors

Recent trends indicate that the primary causes of obesity lie in environmental or behavioural changes, since the escalating rates of obesity are ocurring in a relatively constant gene pool and, hence, against a constant metabolic background. In their elegant study, Prentice and Jebb (1995) clearly showed that in the previous decades average recorded energy and fat intakes in Britain had declined substantially, so that at the population level energy intakes had fallen, while obesity rates experienced a continuous escalation.

The paradox of increasing obesity in the face of decreasing food intake can only be explained if levels of energy expenditure have declined faster than energy intake, thus leading to an overconsumption of energy relative to a greatly reduced requirement. The implication is that levels of physical activity, and hence energy needs, have declined even faster than intake. The development and use of new forms of technology that affect everything from global warming to housing to transport, as well as clothing, communications, and an increasingly larger scope of other factors, has led to a postindustrial society in which lower energy expenditure by humans through improved insulation and automatisation causes less energy to be spent in human activities.

For many people today, leisure-time pursuits are dominated by TV viewing and other inactive pastimes. Proxy measures of physical inactivity such as car ownership and TV viewing have rocketed. The rapid rise in childhood obesity has been mirrored by an explosion of nonactive leisure pursuits for children, such as computers and video games. Current evidence suggests that modern inactive lifestyles are important determinants in the aetiology of obesity, possibly representing the dominant factor.

Due to the fact that obesity is intricately bound up with an individual's lifestyle, a number of public-sector agencies play a potentially significant role in reshaping what can be called an 'obesogenic' environment (Figure 4.6), in which sedentarism and cheap, high-fat foods dominate over active leisure-time

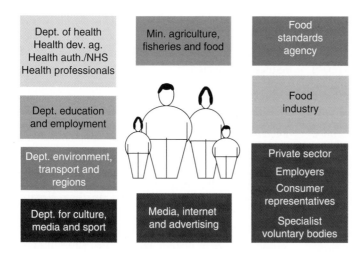

Figure 4.6 Multifaceted influences and institutions in the UK impinging on the family and the individual with a potential impact on reversing the current obesogenic environment.

occupations and healthy food choices. However, successful efforts must focus not only on individuals, but on group, institutional, and community influences, as well as on public policy. A multidimensional approach understands that individual changes can only occur in a supportive environment with accessible and healthy food choices, opportunities for engaging in regular physical activity, and access to adequate medical treatment. The environment has to be considered as encompassing not just the physical world, such as the layout of cities, but also economic and social organisation and cultural values. In this sense, public health would benefit from going beyond a narrowly mechanistic focus on energy intake and physical activity and examining the economic, social, and cultural context more broadly.

Clinical medicine and public health agencies have to face preventing obesity with new partners, including food marketers and manufacturers, public and private healthcare purchasers, large employers, transportation agencies, urban planners, and real-estate developers. All of these will play a key role in shaping and supporting social and environmental policies which can help people in general and children in particular improve their diet and become more physically active.

Psychosocial influences

Obesity is a dynamic, multidimensional biosocial phenomenon exerting a complex synergistic interaction between pathophysiology and the social world. For this reason, excess body weight has to be studied within its particular cultural and historical circum-

stances. The main social characteristics known to be associated with body-weight regulation include sex, age, race, education level, type of occupation, employment status, income, marital status, household size, parenthood, residential density, and geographical region. In addition, psychological factors focusing on the association between over-nutrition and behavioural, cognitive, and emotional processes, which may be under genetic or environmental influence, have to be taken into consideration. Large-scale comparative studies using objective measures of personality or psychiatric disorder are necessary to provide a scientific basis for the relation between emotional disorders and obesity. In general, community studies fail to find a higher prevalence of psychiatric disorders among obese patients compared with normal-weight individuals. However, some disorders – in particular depression and anxiety – do appear to be overrepresented among a subset of obese adults who also report binge-eating.

The psychosomatic model of obesity proposes that certain personality characteristics or types accompanied by higher-than-normal levels of emotional distress and lower self-esteem are linked to the development of obesity. Although this may be the case among specific subgroups, such as severely obese patients and obese binge-eaters, no clear-cut evidence of the association of any particular personality type with a higher risk of obesity has been established. Nevertheless, personality and emotional distress may play an important role in the response to treatment, especially in failure to comply with dietary indications. The role of dietary restraint in the understanding of obesity suggests that in susceptible subjects it may precipitate eating disorders, while in other individuals it may represent an effective strategy for body-weight regulation. The psychobiological model suggests that obese individuals are particularly responsive to external food cues or have a diminished responsiveness to internally generated satiety cues.

Community studies have identified a prevalence of binge-eating disorder as high as 2.5% in the general population, reaching about 20–30% rates among obese patients. Emotional eating resulting from arousal is caused by disinhibition of restraint and represents a less-severe form of binge-eating. Food addictions, especially craving for specific items or macronutrients such as chocolate or carbohydrates, suggest that self-control might be impaired because of biologically based drives for intake. Volitional control of food intake may be difficult for some individuals because hunger is a powerful drive, leading to food-seeking and consumption. However, specific experimental evidence to support the addiction theory is required in order to exclude conditioned effects. In addition, food consumption implies a reward experience, which has also to be taken into account. Cognitive-behaviour specialists have recognised the beneficial effect of decreasing body-image dissatisfaction among obese individuals in order to reduce distress and improve treatment.

Miscellaneous causes

Several different causes of either physiological, sociological, behavioural, pharmacological, or pathological nature, covering a broad spectrum of human conditions, are able to impact on the complex mechanisms implicated in energy homeostasis. Viruses have been suspected of being involved in obesity in humans. Whether this represents an important mechanism for the induction of obesity remains, as yet, unclear.

Under normal circumstances in developed countries, mean gestational weight gain in normal-weight, healthy, well-nourished women with uncomplicated pregnancies ranges from 11 to 16 kg, with approximately 25% of the increase being attributable to fat deposition in maternal adipose tissue. Reports showing a net increase in BMI with successive pregnancies provide evidence for a positive correlation between raising body weight and parity. Changes derived from lactation, dietary habits, and PALs related to child-rearing rather than to child-bearing may underlie the excess weight gain associated with parity. Confounding variables that need to be taken into consideration when studying the relation between parity and weight gain include age, education, initial body weight, marital status, health status, smoking, drinking habits, and dieting.

Pregnancy does not lead to obesity in the majority of women; most regain their pre-pregnant weight within around 12 months after delivery. Nevertheless, about 10–15% of women weigh at least 5 kg more after pregnancy compared with their pre-conception body weight. Risk factors for maternal obesity development include those associated with the period of pregnancy itself (weight gain and smoking cessation during pregnancy), factors common to both the pregnancy and postpartum periods (changes in body image, energy intake, and eating patterns; dieting or attitudes towards weight gain), as well as elements specific to the postpartum period (breastfeeding and psychosocial factors, such as stress, self-esteem, and social support).

Middle-aged and older smokers have been shown to weigh on average around 3–4 kg less than non-smokers of a similar age. In contrast, among adolescents and young adults weight differences are small or nonexistent, with smoking initiation not evidencing an association with weight loss. However, a number of large prospective studies have observed that smoking cessation is accompanied by a weight gain of about 2–4 kg, which is more evident in women, younger people, black people, people of lower prior weight, and heavy smokers. In general, approximately 20% of quitters experience a postcessation weight gain of about 10 kg. An increase in energy intake together with the loss of the potentially acute metabolic-enhancing actions attributed to nicotine may contribute to a shift in the balance equation towards weight gain. Undoubtedly, the benefits of quitting smoking outweigh the detrimental effects associated with weight gain and, therefore, smoking cessation attempts should not be discouraged.

The incidence of weight gain during treatment with several different frequently prescribed drug groups (Table 4.10) has been clearly established. Among antidepressant medications, the tricyclic drugs are effective for normal-mood restoration, but their use is accompanied by a noticeable weight gain, which may sometimes affect medication compliance.

Table 4.10 Drugs commonly associated with weight gain.

Pharmacological group	Drugs
Adrenergic antagonists	Alpha- and beta-blockers
Anticonvulsants	Valproate, carbamazepine, vigabatrin
Antidepressants	Amitriptilin, imipramine, doxepine, fenelzine, amoxapine, desipramine, trazadone, tranilcipromine, lithium
Antidiabetics	Insulin preparations, sulphonylurea agents, glitazones, tiazolidinediones
Antimigraine drugs	Flunarizine, pizotifen
Antipsychotics	Chlorpromazine, chlordiazepoxide, thioridazine, trifluoperazine, mesoridazine, promazine, mepazine, perphenazine, prochlorperazine, loxapine, haloperidol, thiothixene, fluphenazine, clozapine, olanzapine, risperidone, quetiapine, sertindole
Antiserotoninergics	Cyproheptadine, sanomigran, loratadine, astemizole
Steroids	Glucocorticoids, estrogens (at pharmacological doses), megestrol acetate, tamoxifen
Others	Some antineoplastic agents and immunosuppressants

The mechanisms of action by which tricyclics promote weight gain have not been completely disentangled, but they certainly reflect changes in energy balance due to a decrease in energy expenditure related to a reduced sympathetic nervous activity and, to a smaller extent, an increase in caloric intake.

The serotonin-specific reuptake inhibitors represent an alternative antidepressant treatment option which usually does not have the side effect of excessive weight gain, due to the lack of influence in increasing appetite, and at the same time exerts a potential enhancement of resting energy expenditure. Weight gain has been reported in relation to the use of older monoamine oxidase inhibitors; however, with the newer generation of drugs, this side effect appears to be less important. Lithium treatment is commonly followed by weight gain, especially in already overweight patients, related to increased food and fluid intake, as well as a hypothyroidism-related decreased energy expenditure.

Antipsychotics are known to promote weight gain during prolonged treatment. The effect is more evident among the conventional drugs than among the novel antipsychotics. An increased energy intake and a reduction in physical activity have been proposed to be the apparent mechanisms of this medication-induced weight increase. A commonly described side effect of epilepsy and mania treatment includes weight gain. This effect can be especially pronounced in susceptible subjects, with an increase of up to 15 kg over a few months due to a marked influence on food intake.

Anxiolytics, such as benzodiazepine and its derivatives, are not likely to produce a significant weight change in clinical practice, although an increase in body weight has been observed in short-term administration in rodents due to an effect on dopamine D2 receptors or gamma-aminobutyric acid neurons, whereas no influence in long-term experiments has been shown.

The combined antihistaminergic and serotoninergic effects of cyproheptadine and pizotifen probably lead to early but rather modest weight gain, attributable to an increase in appetite. The nonsedating antihistaminergic compounds loratadine and astemizole induce weight gain too, but to a smaller degree than the older drugs. The appetite-inducing effect of these compounds has been tried in patients with anorexia nervosa and cancer cachexia, but without successful results. Flunarizine, a calcium antagonist applied in migraine prophylaxis, promotes a dose-dependent increase in body weight of up to 4 kg during the first months of treatment by stimulating food intake. The use of nonspecific beta-blockers has been associated with a modest but sustained weight gain due to a decrease in energy expenditure, including facultative thermogenesis.

Intensive insulin therapy for the treatment of either type 1 or type 2 diabetes mellitus has been shown to promote weight gain attributable to reduced glucosuria and decreased energy expenditure due to the reversal of the catabolic metabolism. Metformin treatment for obese type 2 patients was not accompanied by significant changes in body weight compared with the conventional control group, while a more favourable outcome as regards diabetes complications and mortality was evident. Glitazones have been also reported to be associated with a modest though significant weight gain.

A common adverse effect of long-term glucocorticoid therapy is weight gain, which clearly has an impact on body fat distribution by predominantly increasing the abdominal fat depot as well as inducing insulin resistance. The underlying mechanism of action seems to be related to centrally mediated effects which increase NPY activity and a pronounced decrease in uncoupling proteins expression. Women using oral contraceptives often find that they gain weight, while postmenopausal women also report an impact on body weight control following hormone replacement therapy. High to moderate doses of megestrol acetate produce an increase in appetite and, consequently, in body weight, while tamoxifen, a partial oestrogen receptor antagonist, also induces weight gain. Some other nonhormonal antineoplastic drugs, such as cyclophosphamide and fluorouracil, have been associated with weight increase through an unknown mechanism.

4.3 Clinical presentation

The hazards of excess body weight have been clearly established by epidemiological and clinical studies. Although obesity can be easily identified and several different assessment methods are available (Table 4.11), patients who are mildly or moderately overweight may be overlooked. In this context, studies have shown that about 25% of overweight patients were thought to be of normal weight by their primary care physicians. It is worrisome that obesity itself is being underestimated by healthcare professionals. In spite of the high prevalence of this chronic, life-threatening disease, it is documented by physicians only in a small proportion of patients, indicating it is considerably underreported in medical records.

Similarly, a retrospective analysis has observed an apparently low rate of obesity in hospital outpatient departments treating obesity-related conditions (4% cardiology, 5% rheumatology, and 3% orthopedics) when compared to the true prevalence (30% cardiology, 20% rheumatology, and 25% orthopedics). The large disparity between apparent and true prevalence clearly shows that opportunities for obesity diagnosis and treatment are being missed.

Body composition

BMI is an accepted index by which to define differing levels of overweight and obesity, and clinical protocols can easily be adapted to record weight, height, and the resulting BMI calculation. However, obesity is defined by an excess body fat, not simply by an increased body

Table 4.11 Methods for the assessment of overweight and obesity.

Measurement	Methods
Energy intake	24-hour dietary recall
	72-hour dietary recall
	Food-frequency questionnaire
	Macronutrient-composition record
Energy expenditure	Indirect calorimetry
	Physical activity-level questionnaire
	Movement detector
	Heart-rate monitoring
	Doubly labelled water
Body composition	Body mass index (BMI)
	Skinfold thickness
	Bioelectrical impedance
	Near-infrared interactance
	Dual-energy X-ray absorptiometry (DXA)
	Air-displacement plethysmography (BOD-POD)
	Underwater weighing
	Isotope dilution
Regional fat distribution	Waist circumference, waist-to-hip ratio
	Computerized axial tomography
	Ultrasound
	Magnetic resonance imaging

weight relative to height. The normal range is 10–20% body fat for males and around 20–30% for females. Overweight is considered with a body fat value between 20 and 25% for males, while for females the body fat ranges from 30 to 35%. The exact values by which to classify a man or woman as morbidly obese according to body fat content have not been clearly established, but obesity might be considered for a body fat ≥40% for males and ≥50% for females. It is well known that neither body weight nor BMI provides an exact description of body composition. Therefore, a further step needs to be taken, by drawing attention not only to weight but to body composition itself (see Chapter 2 in *Introduction to Human Nutrition* in this series). The principal limitation of the BMI as a measure of body fat is that it does not distinguish fat mass from fat-free mass. Furthermore, when lifestyle interventions are introduced, measured body fat and BMI can travel in opposite directions. When patients follow a calorie-restricted diet only, body fat may increase despite the weight lost if the majority of the decrease is at the expense of lean body mass. In contrast, an increase in physical activity accompanied by a decrease in energy intake may lead to an increase in total body weight due to the fact that

Method	Practicality	Accuracy	Sensitivity to change	Cost
Skinfold thickness	++++	++	+	$
Circumference	++++	++	+	$
Body mass index (BMI)	+++++	+	++	–
Bioelectrical impedance	+++	+	++	$
Near-infrared interactance	+++	+	+	$
Total body electrical conductivity	+++	+	+	$
Underwater weighing	+	+++++	++++	$$$$$
DXA	++	+++	++	$$$$
Potassium-40 counting	+	+++	+	$$$$$
Computerised tomography	++	+++++	++++	$$$$$
Magnetic resonance imaging	++	+++++	++++	$$$$$
BOD-POD	+++	+++++	++++	$$$
Multicompartment models	+	++++	++	$$$

Table 4.12 Characteristics of body-fat estimation methods applied to obesity. DXA, dual-energy X-ray absorptiometry; BOD-POD, air-displacement plethysmography.

the reduced total fat is masked by the incremented lean body mass, resulting in a satisfactory and clinically relevant change in percentage fat and hence obesity-associated risk factors. It is therefore important to measure the body compartment that actually creates the health risks, namely body fat. This challenge, together with the effect of therapeutic interventions on adiposity distribution, has relevant implications for clinical practice and research.

In the context of tissue, total body weight can be divided into adipose tissue, skeletal muscle, skeleton, and the remaining organs and viscera. The classical methods of body-composition estimation are based on a two-compartment model, in which the body is divided into fat and fat-free mass, the latter including water, protein, glycogen, and mineral. This model assumes that the densities of adipose and lean tissue are constant, namely 0.9 and 1.1 kg/l, respectively. Table 4.12 summarises the characteristics of the currently available methods for the estimation of body fat. The selection of the most appropriate method varies according to the specific circumstances and aims (cross-sectional versus longitudinal assessment, clinical versus laboratory studies, special sub-populations, etc.). Simple and cheap anthropometric methods are useful for epidemiological surveys of large populations, while more sophisticated and expensive techniques are reserved for research studies aimed at gaining insight into the pathophysiological basis underlying body-weight homeostasis.

Further relevant issues to take into consideration are the cost, facilities, and time associated with the use of each of the methods, as well as the need for cooperation from the subjects and expertise in the staff. One of the difficulties in evaluating *in vivo* body-composition methods is the lack of a true optimal technique. Body-composition techniques are frequently compared using correlation analysis. This provides only partial information, since methods may show a good relationship with each other but may not always agree or be equally inaccurate. Therefore, it is of utmost importance to validate the data obtained against a reference method and also in a similar population. This is especially true in overweight and obese individuals in whom body-fat loss is being monitored.

Up-to-date underwater weighing is considered the traditional 'gold standard', but is impractical for widespread application at the clinical level. Air-displacement plethysmography (BOD-POD) has been reported to agree closely with the reference hydrodensitometry underwater weighing method, showing that the plethysmographic technique predicts fat mass and fat-free mass more accurately than dual-energy X-ray absorptiometry (DXA) and bioelectrical impedance.

Fat distribution

Regional distribution of body fat is known to be an important indicator for metabolic and cardiovascular alterations, providing an explanation for an inconstant correlation between BMI and these disturbances in some individuals. The observation that the topographic distribution of adipose tissue is relevant to understanding the relation of obesity to

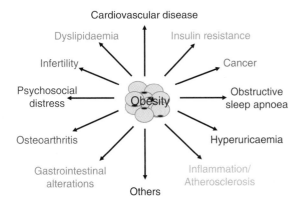

Figure 4.7 Main comorbidities associated with obesity.

disturbances in glucose and lipid metabolism was formulated before the 1950s. Since then, numerous prospective studies have revealed that compared with 'gynoid or female-type obesity', with a predominantly lower-body, gluteofemoral, or peripheral fat deposition, 'android or male-type obesity' (also termed 'central' or 'abdominal' obesity), characterised by an increased fat in the upper body, correlates more often with an elevated mortality and risk for the development of diabetes mellitus type 2, dyslipidaemia, hypertension, and atherosclerosis.

The waist-to-hip circumference ratio (WHR) represents a simple, convenient, and useful anthropometric measurement for the estimation of the proportion of abdominal or upper-body fat. However, the WHR does not distinguish between accumulations of deep (i.e. visceral) and subcutaneous abdominal fat. In this sense, imaging techniques, especially computed tomography and magnetic resonance, allow the topographical differentiation of the fat depots, showing that the detrimental metabolic and cardiovascular influences of abdominal obesity are mediated by the intra-abdominal fat accumulation.

Comorbidities

Obesity has been reported to cause or exacerbate a large number of health problems (Figure 4.7), which are known to impact on both life expectancy and quality of life. The associations between increased body weight and the main systemic comorbidities extending across most major medical specialities are summarised in Table 4.13. Obesity is accompanied by important pathophysiological alterations as a

Table 4.13 Association of systemic comorbidities with overweight and obesity. FRC, functional residual capacity; FVC, forced vital capacity; TLC, total lung capacity.

System	Pathology/effect
Metabolic	Hyperinsulinism, hyperglycaemia
	Insulin resistance, type 2 diabetes mellitus
	Dyslipidaemia
	Hyperuricaemia, gout
	Syndrome X
Cardiovascular	Hypertension
	Left-ventricular hypertrophy, congestive heart failure
	Arrhythmias, sudden death
	Cerebrovascular disease, stroke
	Endothelial dysfunction
	Low-grade chronic inflammation
	Increased sympathetic activity
Haematologic	Impaired fibrinolysis
	Procoagulant state
	Hyperviscosity
	Atherothrombosis, thrombophlebitis
Endocrine	Hirsutism
	Elevated adrenocortical activity
	Disturbances in circulating sex steroids and binding globulins
	Infertility
	Polycystic ovary syndrome
	Breast cancer
Gastrointestinal	Hiatus hernia
	Gastroesophagic reflux
	Gallstone formation, gallbladder hypomotility and stasis
	Gallbladder carcinoma
	Steatosis, cirrhosis
	Colorectal cancer
Respiratory	Restrictive ventilatory pattern, decreased FRC, FVC, and TLC
	Dyspnoea/shortness of breath in exercise and/or at rest
	Obesity hypoventilation syndrome
	Obstructive sleep apnoea
Renal	Proteinuria, albuminuria
	Enhanced sodium retention
	Renin–angiotensin–aldosterone-system stimulation
	Disturbed Na/K ATPase activity, Na/K cotransport
Genitourinary	Incontinence
	Prostate/endometrial/ovarian cancer
Locomotor	Nerve entrapment
	Low-back pain, joint damage
	Osteoarthritis
Dermatologic	Increased sweating
	Oppositional intertrigo
	Wound dehiscence
	Lymphoedema
	Acanthosis nigricans

consequence of metabolic and/or mechanical effects associated with excess body weight, such as type 2 diabetes mellitus, dyslipidaemia, cardiovascular disease, hypertension, stroke, gallbladder disease, infertility, respiratory difficulties, sleep apnoea, certain forms of cancer, osteoarthritis, and psychosocial problems, which lead to reduced quality of life, decreased life expectancy, and increased mortality (Williams & Frühbeck, 2009). The comorbidities which directly cause mortality are cancer and cardiovascular disease (see *Public Health Nutrition*).

In a recent large prospective cohort study, high BMI values were shown to be associated with increased mortality from cancer for overweight individuals. The underlying biological mechanisms that have been regularly invoked to explain the association between adiposity and cancer involve mainly steroid hormones and the insulin-like growth-factor system. However, recent evidence provided by an extensive study reports an increase in all-cancer mortality, suggesting the contribution of further adipocyte-related factors to mutagenesis.

In response to the emerging body of scientific medical data linking excess adiposity to coronary heart disease (CHD), the American Heart Association reclassified obesity as a major, modifiable risk factor for CHD in 1998. The pathophysiological relevance of adipocyte-derived molecules resides in the participation of some of these factors beyond body-weight control in vascular homeostasis through effects on blood pressure, fibrinolysis, coagulation, angiogenesis, insulin sensitivity, proliferation, apoptosis, and immunity, among other things. In this respect, adipokines have been shown to be implicated either directly or indirectly in the regulation of several processes that regulate the development of inflammation, atherogenesis, hypertension, insulin resistance, and vascular remodelling. Cardiovascular disorders weaken the heart and tire the patient, thus leading to inactivity and weight gain. Similarly, cardiovascular-related target-organ damage alters endothelial, vascular, and renal functions, thereby worsening hypertension. In addition, obesity *per se* can lead to hypertension, thus completing a 'vicious triangle', which perpetuates the phenomenon.

Cardiac alterations in obese patients reflect an integrated response to multiple haemodynamic, structural, functional, biochemical, metabolic, and endocrine derangements. An elevated BMI results in an increase in blood volume, as well as in sympathetic activity. In addition to increased blood pressure, obese individuals show elevated viscosity and risk factors, such as fibrinogen, plasminogen activator inhibitor type 1 (PAI-1), C-reactive protein, and so on, which alter the rheological properties, adding further to the pressure load of the heart. Thus, pressure and volume load increase simultaneously. Consequently, structural changes to the heart take place. Cardiac mass and geometry alterations lead to left-ventricular (LV) hypertrophy. LV wall thickness and myocardial remodelling result in a progressive impairment in LV filling, and thus a high risk of diastolic dysfunction. Alterations in systolic function may also become evident. In particular, long-standing obesity may result in a decrease in mid-wall fibre shortening and ejection fraction.

In addition to heart failure, arrhythmias take place, particularly ventricular ectopic beats in relation to a concentric pattern of LVH and atrial fibrillation due to atrial enlargement. In synergy, these maladaptive changes increase the risk of cardiovascular death.

Other conditions, such as type 2 diabetes, syndrome X, dyslipidaemia, atherothrombosis, hypertension, and pulmonary alterations, are responsible for the direct morbidity related to obesity, and at the same time contribute indirectly to mortality. Osteoarthritis, gallstone formation, gastrointestinal alterations, and psychosocial problems, on the other hand, represent disturbances more likely to cause morbidity than mortality. Since these topics are extensively reviewed in *Public Health Nutrition* as well as in Chapter 6 of this volume, the reader is referred to these places for more detailed information.

4.4 Clinical assessment

Given the escalating prevalence rates, obesity will be the leading cause of death and disability worldwide in the twenty-first century. The rapid increase of obesity to epidemic proportions collides with a scenario where, paradoxically, preoccupation with body weight, fitness, and diet pervades today's society in the developed world. The hazards of excess body weight have been clearly established by epidemiological and clinical studies, highlighting the need for programmes for early competent diagnosis, treatment, and prevention. Interestingly, obesity has until recently not featured strongly in medical training, with medical school curricula not even addressing obesity as a disease. Moreover, it has been reported that health professionals hold negative views of overweight and obese patients. Negative attitudes have been observed in medical students, qualified practitioners, nurses, and dietitians, and may lead to beliefs about the usefulness of intervention, thus representing a barrier to good practice.

A thorough clinical evaluation of the overweight or obese patient includes a medical history and physical examination, with the review-of-systems section specifically addressing the identification of the aetiological factors mentioned above, as well as providing particular emphasis on the assessment of risk factors and the presence of comorbidities (see Table 4.13). The history should focus on the age of onset of obesity, minimum body weight in adulthood, special events related to weight gain and loss (in women: menstrual history, pregnancies, age at menopause), previous weight-loss attempts, treatment modalities, outcomes, and complications. A dietetic history, including usual eating pattern, current PAL (type and regularity), habitual lifestyle, and the family and social constellation of the patient, should be obtained. Smoking history and alcohol and substance abuse also need to be asked about.

It is also important to get a clear picture of the nutritional knowledge of the patient, since this will determine whether a basic or a more sophisticated level of nutrition education will be applied in the sessions. As described earlier, several different medications are known to promote weight gain, and these should be recorded and, if possible, changed to plausible alternatives with a lower impact on body weight. With the current high prevalence rates of obesity, easily obtained nonprescription weight-loss products are an appealing alternative, and their use is on the rise. Because over-the-counter weight-control products, cold remedies, and dietary supplements are generally regarded as safe by the general population, many patients do not inform their physicians about the use of these products. However, due to the possibility of herb–drug and drug–drug interactions, physicians should ask their patients about the use of nonprescription weight-loss products as well as other supplements.

It is noteworthy that individuals with uncontrolled or undiagnosed diabetes, hypertension, heart disease, and other weight-related health conditions may be frequent users of nonprescription weight-loss products. In this group of patients, the use of the mentioned nonprescription products in general, and of ephedra and ephedrine in particular, may result in especially adverse effects.

Height and weight should be determined and BMI calculated. Waist circumference, WHR, and neck circumference should be measured with a tape. Depending upon the availability of resources, the physician should try to get information on body composition and fat distribution. Blood pressure should be checked with an appropriately sized cuff. Any evidence of cardiac and pulmonary alterations, as well as signs of hyperlipidaemia, thyroid disease, and other endocrinopathies, should be investigated. The clinician should search for all of the aforementioned obesity-associated complications. Signs and symptoms of these conditions may have been overlooked by the patient and not related to obesity itself, and, therefore, should be carefully screened by the physician.

The third part of the clinical evaluation encompasses the laboratory tests, which are relevant for risk assessment and decision-making. These include fasting plasma glucose (if necessary, impaired glucose tolerance or type 2 diabetes is confirmed by a 2-hour value after an oral glucose tolerance test; in already diagnosed diabetic patients, glycated haemoglobin HbA1c is determined), lipid profile (cholesterol-total, low-density lipoproteins (LDLs), HDLs, and triglycerides), basal insulin (using several insulin-sensitivity/insulin-resistance indices, if possible), liver function tests for steatohepatitis, thyroid-stimulating hormone (TSH) to discount a potential hypothyroidism, and prostate-specific antigen (PSA) in men as a screening test for prostate cancer. In some specialised centres, analysis of known cardiovascular risk factors such as fibrinogen, homocysteine, C-reactive protein, and PAI-1 are also carried out.

According to the outcome of the medical history and physical examination, a number of complementary explorations may be indicated, such as an ophthalmic evaluation in diabetes or sustained hypertension, referral to the cardiologist for a potential echocardiogram, a polysomnographic study in heavy snorers, sleep apnoea, nighttime awakening, daytime fatigue with episodes of sleepiness and/or morning headaches, mammography and gynaecological screening tests, evaluation of gastroesophageal reflux/hiatus hernia in patients complaining about

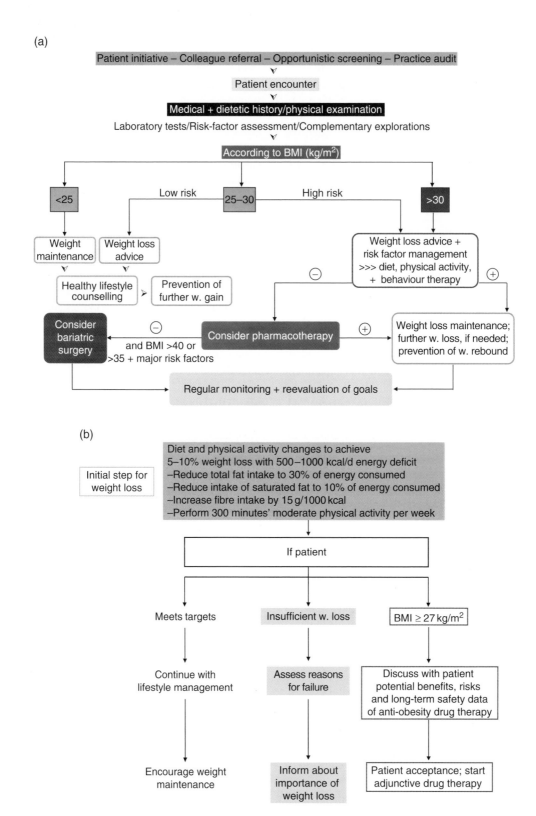

Figure 4.8 Algorithms developed to identify and manage overweight and obesity: (a) global screening for treatment selection; (b) initial steps for weight-loss therapy; (c) regular follow-up on treatment progress; (d) special considerations for instauration of pharmacotherapy.

(c)

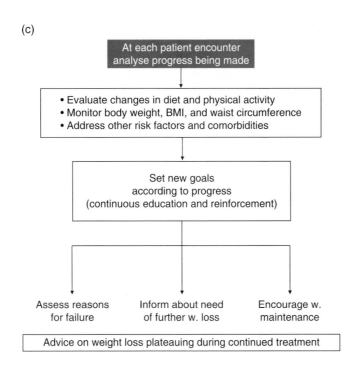

At each patient encounter
analyse progress being made

• Evaluate changes in diet and physical activity
• Monitor body weight, BMI, and waist circumference
• Address other risk factors and comorbidities

Set new goals
according to progress
(continuous education and reinforcement)

Assess reasons
for failure

Inform about need
of further w. loss

Encourage w.
maintenance

Advice on weight loss plateauing during continued treatment

(d)

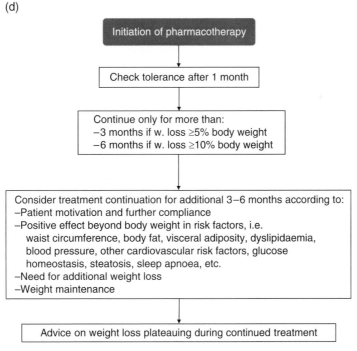

Initiation of pharmacotherapy

Check tolerance after 1 month

Continue only for more than:
−3 months if w. loss ≥5% body weight
−6 months if w. loss ≥10% body weight

Consider treatment continuation for additional 3−6 months according to:
−Patient motivation and further compliance
−Positive effect beyond body weight in risk factors, i.e.
   waist circumference, body fat, visceral adiposity, dyslipidaemia,
   blood pressure, other cardiovascular risk factors, glucose
   homeostasis, steatosis, sleep apnoea, etc.
−Need for additional weight loss
−Weight maintenance

Advice on weight loss plateauing during continued treatment

Figure 4.8   *(Continued)*

indigestion, or an ultrasound of the gallbladder in case of abdominal pain.

Several different algorithms have been outlined to help in identifying and managing these complicated patients (Figure 4.8). Most of them are based on BMI assessment and quantification of additional comorbidities and aim at applying the most appropriate treatment options for both weight and risk-factor management. Before starting any treatment, both patient and physician should have realistic expectations. It may be useful to instruct patients about what can be considered a successful outcome and the timescale needed to reach it. Once the original therapeutic goal has been achieved, it is also important to provide weight-maintenance programmes and continuous follow-up, since obesity has to be considered a chronic disease.

4.5 Treatment approaches

Obesity is a particularly challenging medical condition to treat, and goes beyond the mere cosmetic problem. It is evident that obesity requires a coordination of care from multiple healthcare providers, with a multidisciplinary group with varied expertise working together as a team to assist patient care. There are three recognised approaches to the treatment of the complex aetiology and multifactorial nature of obesity: lifestyle changes, pharmacotherapy, and bariatric surgery, which should be applied either alone or in combination according to the characteristics of the patients.

General principles

The foundation of any effective strategies for successfully tackling excess body weight is information. As described in this chapter, weight gain is the consequence of many interacting processes. As for any disease with a multifactorial aetiology, there are many different approaches to its management, which are more or less effective for different individiuals. Any intervention which achieves a negative energy balance over an extended period of time will result in weight loss. For this reason, it is important to inform patients about the rationale and beneficial effects of the different recommendations and treatment strategies.

Lifestyle changes

The most successful weight-reduction programmes are those that combine diet with exercise within a matrix of behaviour modification. The main modifiable factors affecting energy balance are dietary energy intake and energy expended through physical activity. Treatment of obesity is most successful if realistic goals are set, a balanced diet is stressed, and a safe rate of weight loss per week is achieved through a combination of moderate caloric intake reduction (diet) and increased energy expenditure (physical activity).

Dietary management

It is worth remembering that the word 'diet' originally comes from the Greek *diaita*, meaning 'manner of living', and it is truly this that the obese patient must change. Fad diets promising a quick fix should be avoided. Unlike drugs, which must go through stringent clinical testing before they are licensed, fad diets can be promoted without being put on a trial. Diets with altered levels of protein, carbohydrate, or fat are very popular with the dieting public, which is desperate to find 'new' strategies for successful weight loss and maintenance.

The Nutrition Committee of the American Heart Association has published a statement for healthcare professionals analysing the frequently followed high-protein diets. The Science Advisory concludes that high-protein diets are low-calorie diets, even though none is advertised as such. In obese individuals, the macronutrient composition of the diet has little effect on the rate or magnitude of weight loss unless nutrient composition influences caloric intake. The amount of protein recommended in high-protein diet regimens exceeds established requirements and may impose significant health risks. Animal proteins, rather than plant-based ones, are generally advocated, leading to increased intake of purines and saturated fat, ultimately resulting in raised uric acid and LDL cholesterol concentrations, elevating the risk of gout and cardiovascular disease in susceptible individuals. Due to the omission of certain foods, and sometimes entire food groups, the diets are deficient in fibre and carbohydrates, as well as some vitamins, minerals, and protective phytochemicals, with detrimental effects on cancer development and osteoporosis.

High-protein, high-fat diets induce ketosis and are initially attractive because they promote a quick weight loss attributable to water loss and glycogen depletion, which engenders a false sense of accomplishment. If the imbalance is maintained, loss of appetite associated with ketosis results in lower total caloric intake, potentially leading to muscle breakdown and, consequently, increased per cent body fat. It is concluded that high-protein diets are not recommended because they restrict healthful foods that provide essential nutrients, leading to potential cardiac, renal, skeletal muscle, bone, and liver abnormalities.

Similarly, the promotion of the eating of certain foods in a specific order, at concrete times, or in purposeful combinations has no nutritional–medical basis.

Physical activity

Together with energy intake, the other main modifiable factor affecting the energy-balance equation is energy expended through physical activity. The addition of exercise to a diet programme is important because it determines the composition of weight loss. Two meta-analyses pooling data from 74 published trials have found that exercise is able to attenuate fat-free mass loss. Interestingly, it has been shown that in previously sedentary people, a lifestyle physical-activity intervention is as effective as and has similar effects to a structured exercise programme in improving physical activity itself, cardiorespiratory fitness, systolic and diastolic blood pressure, and insulin sensitivity, serum triglycerides, and total cholesterol concentrations. Moreover, physical activity has been shown to be of utmost importance for long-term weight management. Therefore, patients should be urged to cut down on sedentary activities while increasing everyday lifestyle activities. In fact, less than one-third of the general population meets the recommendation to engage in at least 30 minutes of moderate physical activity 5 days per week, while 40% of adults engage in no leisure-time physical activity at all.

Pharmacotherapy

In comparison with other diseases, at present there is a paucity of drug-therapy options for obesity, influenced by a history of past failures in trying to overcome the regulatory requisites of safety and efficacy that are defined for an acceptable weight-loss product. Since effective pharmacotherapy for obesity is likely to require long-term application, it is essential to weigh potential risks, side effects, and costs against benefits. No prospective randomised controlled trials have evaluated the efficacy of currently approved anti-obesity drugs for longer than 2 years. Treatment discontinuation should be considered in nonresponders after an unsuccessful 1-month period.

Currently, only one product is available on the market as an anti-obesity drug: namely orlistat, a lipase inhibitor which works peripherally in the digestive tract to prevent breakdown, and hence absorption, of approximately 30% of dietary fat. The standard dose of 120 mg three times daily, taken with the main meals, has been evaluated in seven prospective randomised controlled trials, showing that at 1 year about twice as many patients treated with orlistat lost 10% or more of their initial body weight as those in the placebo group, while one-third more patients taking orlistat lost 5% or more of their initial body weight compared with placebo-treated individuals. Successful weight loss was more difficult to achieve in patients with associated risk factors like CHD and type 2 diabetes mellitus. Recently, orlistat has become available as an over-the-counter product at the lower dose of 60 mg per tablet.

Volunteers enrolled in a trial conducted within a primary care setting with no dietitian or behaviour modification counselling were less successful in achieving weight loss. Four trials included a second-year extension of the 1-year studies, with the aim of preventing weight regain, rather than inducing further weight loss.

Due to its mechanism of action, orlistat may be associated with unpleasant side effects, including the production of oily stools, abdominal pain, flatulence, faecal urgency, and incontinence when ingested with high-fat diets. In 1- and 2-year trials, about 70–80% of volunteers treated with orlistat experienced one or more gastrointestinal events, compared with approximately 50–60% of subjects treated with placebo. Gastrointestinal side effects usually occurred within the first month and were of mild to moderate intensity. About 4% of orlistat-treated subjects versus 1% of placebo-treated subjects withdrew from the study because of gastrointestinal complaints.

Many of the gastrointestinal side effects of orlistat can be prevented by concomitant therapy with a gel-forming fibre (psyllium mucilloid). Inhibition of fat digestion prevents fatty acid release into the lumen, which is needed to stimulate cholecystokinin secretion and gallbladder contraction, thus laying the base for an increased risk of gallstone formation by orlistat. However, orlistat administered with meals of varying fat content reportedly did not reduce gallbladder motility, and no evidence of increased gallstone formation has been observed in any trial. In addition, the increased delivery of fat to the colon has raised concern over a potential increased risk of colon cancer. However, orlistat administration in volunteers has been shown not to increase colonocyte proliferation, and no increased incidence of colon cancer in the different clinical trials has been noticed.

Long-term orlistat treatment can affect the homeostasis of fat-soluble vitamin. It has been observed that concentrations of vitamins D, E, and beta-carotene decreased below normal limits in around 5% more orlistat- than placebo-treated volunteers, which normalised rapidly with vitamin supplementation. Therefore, it is recommended that all patients treated with orlistat should be given a daily multivitamin supplement that is taken at a time when orlistat is not being ingested.

It is important to bear in mind that orlistat may interfere with the absorption of lipophilic drugs when they are taken simultaneously. A few cases of subtherapeutic circulating concentrations of cyclosporine in organ-transplant recipients starting orlistat treatment for obesity have been reported. Orlistat should not be taken for at least 2 hours before or after ingestion of lipophilic drugs, and circulating drug concentrations should be followed to ensure appropriate dosing, if needed. Pharmacokinetic studies suggest that orlistat does not interfere with absorption of selected drugs with a narrow therapeutic index, such as warfarin, digoxin, and phenytoin, or of other products that are likely to be taken simultaneously with the lipase inhibitor, such as glyburide, oral contraceptives, furosemide, captopril, nifedipine, atenolol, and alcohol.

Sibutramine, a mixed serotonin–noradrenaline reuptake blocker which causes increased levels of neurotransmitters, which also caused a decrease in food intake, used to be available for the pharmacological treatment of obesity. However, the US Food and Drugs Administration (FDA), as well as the European Medicines Agency (EMA), decided to withdraw sibutramine in 2010 because of safety concerns based on data derived from the SCOUT (Sibutramine Cardiovascular Outcome Trial) study, which found that the drug increased morbidity from cardiovascular disease. The SCOUT study was initially aimed at proving that the anti-obesity drug could reduce cardiovascular risk. Therefore, the patient group included patients with an already increased cardiovascular risk profile, where the potential beneficial effects of sibutramine could not be shown.

The inhibition of the reuptake of noradrenaline had, on one hand, the added effect of increasing resting energy expenditure, and on the other, side effects related to increased heart rate and blood pressure. Sibutramine treatment at doses between 1 and 30 mg per day for 6 months has shown a dose-dependent weight-loss effect, amounting to 0.9 and 7.7% of initial body weight for placebo and 30 mg/day, respectively. The recommended starting dose was 10 mg/day, which could be increased by 5 mg if needed.

The efficacy of sibutramine therapy in producing and maintaining weight loss was evaluated in two prospective 1-year randomised controlled trials. Interestingly, it was shown that weight loss was equivalent in intermittent (15 mg/day during weeks 1–12, 19–30, and 37–48) and continuous sibutramine treatment. Evaluation of sibutramine therapy in long-term weight management after an already-achieved weight loss showed that approximately 43% of sibutramine-treated and 16% of placebo-treated volunteers maintained 80% or more of their original weight loss.

Mild and usually transient side effects associated with sibutramine were dry mouth, headache, constipation, and insomnia. More importantly, sibutramine was reported to cause a dose-related increase in heart rate and blood pressure. On average, an increase of 2–4 mmHg systolic and diastolic blood pressure, accompanied by an elevation of 4–6 beats/min, was observed at a dose of 10–15 mg/day. However, some patients suffered much larger increases in both heart rate and blood pressure, requiring dose reduction or treatment discontinuation, which led to the inclusion of hypertension and other cardiovascular risk factors as a contraindication for its use. Therefore, in the originally commercialised prescription, sibutramine therapy was contraindicated in patients with poorly controlled hypertension, while the risk of adverse effects was not increased in patients with controlled hypertension compared with normotensive volunteers. For this reason, the FDA and EMA withdrawal due to a side-effect that was already stated as a contraindication proved somewhat surprising.

Recently, the Italian regulatory authorities have suspended the sale of sibutramine after reports of serious cardiac alterations, including two deaths, in patients taking the product. Authorities in England, Germany, and France have not suspended sales of sibutramine but are reviewing the evidence.

Pharmacological treatment of obesity is currently approved in adults with a BMI above $30 \, kg/m^2$, or above $27 \, kg/m^2$ with comorbidities. Surprisingly, between 1996 and 1998 only about 10% of women and 3% of men with a BMI of $30 \, kg/m^2$ reported using prescription weight-loss medication. With the high prevalence rates of obesity, nonprescription product use is on the increase. Easily obtained nonprescription weight-loss products are appealing. From 1996 to 1998, in a multi-state survey with a population-based sample of 14 679 adults, 7% reported overall nonprescription weight-loss product use, 2% declared phenylpropanolamine (PPA) use, and 1% reported ephedra consumption. In addition, among prescription weight-loss product users, 33.8% also took nonprescription agents.

PPA, the main ingredient in the over-the-counter weight-loss aids reported in the study, is a synthetic ephedrine alkaloid with stimulant properties that reduce appetite. Case reports of adverse cerebrovascular and cardiac events and a study showing an increased risk of stroke resulted in the voluntary withdrawal of all over-the-counter PPA products from the market in November 2000. Dietary supplements are generally regarded as safe and are regulated as foods rather than drugs. In addition, there can be a discrepancy between the actual composition or potency of a product and the specifications on the label. In this sense, 55% of ephedra supplements tested failed to list the ephedrine alkaloid content on the label, or else had more than a 20% difference between the actual amount and the amount listed on the label.

Unfortunately, 'nontraditional' or 'alternative' treatments are extremely popular and widely used. There is no clear support by existing data in the peer-reviewed literature concerning their efficacy and safety. Of 18 methods/products advocated as potential anti-obesity/fat-reducing agents, none was convincingly demonstrated to be safe and effective in two or more peer-reviewed publications of randomised double-blind placebo-controlled trials conducted by at least two independent laboratories.

Bariatric surgery

'Bariatric' is a term derived from the Greek words for 'weight' and 'treatment'. Bariatric surgical procedures are major gastrointestinal operations that (a) seal off most of the stomach to reduce the amount of food one can eat, and (b) rearrange the small intestine to reduce the calories the bodies can absorb. There are several different types of bariatric weight-loss surgical procedure, but they are known collectively as 'bariatric surgery'.

Bariatric surgery should be considered for morbidly obese (BMI above $40 \, kg/m^2$, or over $35 \, kg/m^2$ with comorbidities), well-informed, and motivated patients with previous failure in conventional treatment who fulfil the established selection criteria and in whom the operative risks are acceptable. Candidates for surgical procedures should be selected carefully after evaluation by a comprehensive, multidisciplinary team with medical, surgical, nutritional, and psychiatric expertise, working in a clinical setting with adequate support for all aspects of management and assessment, and providing both preoperative and postoperative counselling and support. In this context, it is important to bear in mind that effectiveness of surgery does not necessarily need to be based on body weight alone but may focus on beneficial effects on obesity-associated diseases.

The aim of surgery is to produce a dramatic decrease in energy intake, which can be achieved by triggering an early and enhanced satiety sensation, reducing hunger signals, and bypassing relevant parts of the gastrointestinal system, thereby allowing rapid transit via the digestive tract and a subsequent partial malabsorption resulting from undigested food quickly being shunted into the large intestine.

According to the underlying mechanism of action, bariatric procedures can be classified into restrictive, malabsorptive, and mixed techniques. Restrictive procedures increase oesophageal and gastric distension, producing an early satiety sensation. The placement of an adjustable gastric band represents a purely restrictive procedure, producing a small gastric pouch and a narrow passage into the remainder of the stomach. The partitioning of the stomach into two parts (either vertically or horizontally), producing a slow emptying into the digestive tract, is known as gastroplasty. Sleeve gastrectomy has emerged as a relatively easy-to-perform restrictive surgery in its different forms of application, either as a primary, staged, or revisional operation, due to the relative simplicity and safety of performing a vertical gastrectomy along the greater curvature of the stomach. Malabsorptive techniques involve bypassing large parts of the absorptive gastrointestinal tract. Exclusively malabsorptive procedures like the jejuno-ileal bypass are no longer performed and have been replaced by mixed techniques combining restriction and malabsorption.

The proximal Roux-en-Y gastric bypass is one of the most frequently applied mixed techniques. It leaves a small stomach pouch near the oesophago-gastric junction, which excludes the major curvature, and bypasses most of the stomach and duodenum. Like the gastric bypass, the biliopancreatic diversion is also a mixed intervention. However, the latter technique consists in a subtotal horizontal gastrectomy, leaving on average a 200 ml upper-gastric remnant, and involves a more extensive malabsorptive element, as the gastric pouch is connected to the final segment of the intestine, completely bypassing the duodenum and jejunum.

Traditionally, gastric surgery was carried out as an open procedure, but today all techniques can be performed via laparoscopy. The results from initial large series and a randomised controlled trial show that weight loss is the same with the open versus the laparoscopic approach. However, laparoscopic access for bariatric surgery has proved to reduce postoperative pain, recovery time, and perioperative complications.

Complications related to bariatric surgery include early haemorrhage problems, gastrointestinal leakage leading to peritonitis, splenic laceration with potential need for splenectomy, subphrenic abscesses, wound infection, wound seromas, pulmonary embolism, and late complications derived from stomal stenosis, marginal ulcers, staple-line disruption, dilation of the bypassed stomach, internal hernias, torsion of the intestinal limb, closed-loop obstruction, cholelithiasis, vomiting, dumping syndrome, and specific nutrient deficiencies.

Impaired absorption and decreased intake are responsible for the appearance of certain nutrient deficiencies, especially of iron, calcium, folic acid, and vitamin B_{12}. Nonetheless, these deficiencies can be easily prevented by starting prophylactic vitamin and mineral supplementation after surgery. The perioperative mortality rate after open obesity surgery, taking into account studies including large numbers of patients, is usually less than 1.5%. Approximately 75% of deaths are caused by anastomotic leaks and peritonitis, while 25% are due to pulmonary embolism. Recent series evaluating laparoscopic gastric bypass alone establish the perioperative mortality around 1% and the risk of early postoperative complications about 10%.

The clinical effectiveness of bariatric surgery has been compared with conventional therapy and with different types of surgery in 17 randomised clinical trials and one nonrandomised clinical trial. Comparing horizontal gastroplasty with a very low-calorie diet, no significant difference in weight loss at 12 months was observed (23 vs. 18 kg), although at 24 months patients undergoing gastroplasty had lost significantly more weight (32 vs. 9 kg), with about 58% of gastroplasty patients exhibiting less than 40% overweight compared with only 7% of nonsurgical patients. In the Danish Obesity Project trial, comparing jejunoileostomy with medical management, surgically treated patients had also lost significantly more weight at 2 years (42.9 vs. 5.9 kg). In the Swedish Obese Subjects (SOS) cohort study (the most extensive study in terms of sample size and years of follow-up performed so far) comparing bariatric surgery (vertical banded gastroplasty, gastric banding, and gastric bypass, $n = 1210$) with conventional treatment ($n = 1099$), patients treated surgically had lost significantly more weight after 2 years than conventionally managed obese subjects (23 vs. 0% weight loss). All patients treated surgically exhibited significant improvements in all health-related quality-of-life measures at 2 years compared with patients on conventional treatment. At 8 years, patients in the surgical group had a 16.3% weight loss, compared with a 0.9% weight gain in the conventional-treatment group.

Among the three different bariatric-surgery procedures, the gastric bypass-group patients had a lower weight at 8 years than gastroplasty and gastric-banding patients. Moreover, in the SOS study, beneficial effects of surgical treatment over 10 years have been observed with respect to body weight, diabetes, triglycerides, HDL-cholesterol, uric acid, and quality of life, but not necessarily with total cholesterol or blood pressure.

Four prospective, randomised trials comparing vertical-banded gastroplasty with gastric bypass have further shown that weight loss was greater with the latter, with an average loss of excess weight of 42 versus 68% at 1 year, and about 35 versus 62% after a 3-year follow-up period. Moreover, average weight loss after gastric bypass has reportedly been maintained up to 14 years after surgery.

The majority of surgeons contend that gastric bypass is the bariatric procedure of choice for most patients with severe obesity. Although it is a technically complex operation, needing experienced professionals, the physical, psychological, and social benefits outweigh the low perioperative risk. High-risk morbidly obese patients with multiple comorbidities may in particular benefit from a less-invasive approach, because they are more vulnerable to cardiopulmonary and wound-related complications.

Recently, a bariatric-surgery algorithm taking into consideration variables of BMI, age, gender, race, body habitus, comorbidities, and outcomes provided a logical framework for the selection of the appropriate bariatric operation for each patient. It has to be stressed that gastrointestinal surgery is an effective last-resort remedy in morbidly obese patients with previous failure in conventional treatment. A weight loss of 50–70% of excess body weight has been reported with surgical treatment. More importantly, long-term weight loss has been shown to extend to 10 years and longer. The importance of carefully reviewing patients' treatment expectations and setting realistic goals should be underscored, since many patients who seek bariatric surgery often have unrealistically high weight-loss expectations. Assessment of the efficacy of gastric surgery requires evaluation beyond weight-loss variables alone.

The long-term benefits of bariatric surgery are more fully characterised by its ability to reduce or eliminate comorbid diseases and their associated morbidity and mortality. Significant improvements in diabetes and hypertension, as well as in pulmonary function, cardiovascular risk factors, osteoarthritis, reproductive performance, self-esteem, sick leave, and quality of life, among other factors, have been extensively reported. In any case, after gastrointestinal surgery, patients have to undergo lifelong medical follow-up and surveillance.

Gradually, more insurers are beginning to cover bariatric operations, recognising that this kind of surgery can have powerful medical benefits, saving money in the long run. Surgical therapy in patients with morbid obesity is significantly more effective at producing and maintaining weight loss than medical and psychosocial approaches, and, hence, more convenient from a cost-effectiveness, cost-utility, and cost–benefit-analysis perspective. However, contrary to what would be expected given existing evidence of weight loss and impact on obesity-related comorbidities, bariatric surgery is underutilised, with only a small fraction of eligible patients being referred to the specialist. Given the favourable long-term outcomes of surgery for the treatment of morbid obesity and the current underprovision of services and skills to support bariatric surgery via laparoscopy, detailed implementation strategies to mainstream this surgical approach in carefully selected patients should be considered by health systems.

Other options

Since morbid obesity is not showing signs of abatement and gastroplasty and gastric bypasses represent ablative, irreversible surgical procedures, new minimally invasive and reversible approaches are constantly being sought.

Intragastric balloon

Intragastric balloon (IGB) therapy is a nonsurgical attempt to induce early satiety by placing a silicone elastic balloon with a self-sealing radio-opaque valve into the body of the stomach endoscopically, under sedation. After placement, the device is inflated under direct vision. The IGB should be viewed as a temporary treatment option that achieves moderate weight loss (around 15 kg). It is rarely successful if not associated with dieting and behaviour modification. Peptic ulceration or a large hiatus hernia preclude insertion of the balloon. Major complications of this procedure include balloon displacement, resulting in intestinal obstruction, and balloon deflation at around 3–4 months. A 5% risk of laparotomy for major complications associated with the balloon and a 1.4% conversion rate for gastric banding have been observed.

In the early days, commercial suppliers recommended a 3-month limit for balloon placement. At the end of 1999, new designs prompted a recommendation by the manufacturers of balloon placements of up to 6 months. Ulcer prophylaxis with a proton-pump inhibitor for the duration of IGB therapy has proved useful in avoiding peptidic ulceration and gastrointestinal bleeding. Strict and regular follow-up, together with removal of the device at between 3 and 6 months is essential to avoiding potentially serious complications. The utility of the IGB has been advocated in relation to desirable BMI reduction and, hence, operative risk reduction before embarking on definitive bariatric surgery. However, to date no evidence for this application has been provided by studies especially designed for this purpose.

Gastric pacing

Gastric pacing represents a novel potential therapy for the treatment of obesity. It showed promising results in experimental animal models. Preliminary effects of the application of an implantable gastric stimulator in 24 morbidly obese patients included a significant weight loss of an average $4.7 \, \text{kg/m}^2$ reduction over 9 months, due to an increased satiety conducive to a reduced food intake. The electrical-stimulator system is composed of a bipolar electro-catheter (the gastric lead), which is tunneled intramuscularly at the lesser curve of the anterior gastric wall (upper third of the antrum), and a gastric pacemaker (a microcircuit with a battery), connected to the lead and located outside the abdomen. The electrical-stimulator system can be implanted either laparoscopically or using open surgery under general anaesthesia. Intraoperative fibreoptic flexible endogastroscopy is usually performed to ensure that the mucosa has not been damaged during electrode implantation, as well as to warrant that no intracavity penetration has taken place. After placement of the lead, the gastric pacer is located in a subcutaneous pocket created in the anterior abdominal wall.

In a recent study, gastric pacing has been reported to elicit a 20% excess weight loss after 6 months, accompanied by a decrease in plasma concentrations of cholecystokinin (CCK), somatostatin, glucagon-like peptide 1 (GLP-1), and leptin. The safety and efficacy of gastric pacing is being evaluated in clinical trials in many countries, and an analysis of long-term effects is still required.

4.6 Prevention

The relevance of obesity prevention is evident not only for health professionals but also for politicians, given the far-reaching medical, social, and economic consequences of having to deal with the ill consequences and difficulties associated with its management. To some extent, past and recent prevention efforts may have been inhibited by a number of external factors, ranging from the lack of acceptance of obesity as a serious health problem to the commercial interests of the food industry in continuing with a blossoming market.

Childhood obesity

Obesity prevention in children is a key factor in urging a strong response to the current epidemic. General practitioners and paediatricians, therefore, need to provide a much more prevention-orientated, systematic, and vigorous weight-loss approach. Health professionals should be especially alert in early identification of overweight and obese children, at the same time as being less complacent and more active in starting their treatment. Not surprisingly, obesity in childhood is associated with many of the same diseases observed in adults, such as hypertension, sleep-disordered breathing, dyslipidaemia, and insulin resistance, and is also accompanied by social stigmatisation.

The rapid rise in childhood obesity has been mirrored by an explosion of nonactive leisure pursuits for children, such as computers and video games. Television-watching represents the principal source of inactivity for most children in developed countries, and has been linked to the prevalence of obesity. Substantial declines in physical activity have been reported to occur during adolescence in girls, and have been shown to be associated with higher BMI. Public-health approaches in schools should extend beyond education to include the physical and social environment, together with school policy and links to family and community. Age-appropriate and culturally sensitive instruction develops the knowledge, attitudes, and behaviours needed to adopt healthy lifestyle changes. Increased general activity and play appear to be more effective than competitive sport and structured exercise. Adherence may be

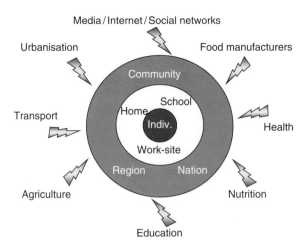

Media / Internet / Social networks

Urbanisation

Food manufacturers

Community

Transport

Home

School

Indiv.

Health

Work-site

Region

Nation

Agriculture

Nutrition

Education

Figure 4.9 Multidimensional approach to target the obesity epidemic.

improved by making the activity enjoyable, increasing the choice over type and level of activity, and providing positive reinforcement of even small achievements.

Initiatives in key settings

To halt the drift from healthy weight into overweight and obesity, diverse initiatives have identified activities and interventions in five key settings: families and communities, schools, healthcare, media and communications, and worksites. Individual behavioural change obviously lies at the core of all strategies to reduce excess body weight. Clinical medicine and public health agencies have to face preventing obesity at multiple levels with new partners, including food marketers and manufacturers, agricultural, nutritional, and educational authorities, public and private healthcare purchasers, mass media, the Internet and social networks, opinion leaders, large employers, transportation agencies, urban planners, and real-estate developers (Figure 4.9). All public- and private-sector stakeholders with the potential to influence lifestyle and body weight will play a key role in shaping and supporting social and environmental policies that can help citizens improve their diet and become physically active.

Additionally, physicians play a key role in the correct diagnosis and management of overweight and obesity, and have a particular need to focus on children and adolescents, whose excess weight and sedentary lifestyle will form the basis for a lifetime of preventable morbidity and increased premature mortality.

4.7 Concluding remarks

We are currently facing a paradoxical situation in which high prevalence rates of obesity and overweight collide with a scenario where clear opportunities for diagnosis and effective treatment are being missed. Information forms the foundation of the development of evidence-based strategies to successfully tackle the obesity epidemic. Physiological and genetic studies are improving our understanding of the complex mechanisms controlling appetite and energy expenditure. Overweight and obesity can no longer be viewed as strictly a personal matter; it is everybody's responsibility, since health problems resulting from this disease are threatening health gains achieved worldwide.

The hazards of excess body weight have been clearly established by epidemiological and clinical studies, highlighting the need for careful diagnosis and effective treatment programmes. Overweight and obesity are serious health issues that will only worsen without thoughtful and evidence-based interventions. Numerous weight-loss strategies have been proposed over recent years, making the task of obesity management-evaluation daunting.

Undoubtedly, in order to tackle the obesity epidemic, it is important to persuade politicians, medical and health professionals, industry, communities, and individuals to take up the fight. It is important to bear in mind that actions to reduce overweight and obesity will fail without a multidimensional approach. Moreover, special attention should be paid to the role played by physicians. Lack of motivation to work with overweight and obese patients due to negative perceptions of the efficacy of treatments or of adherence to treatment may be an important barrier to successfully implementing interventions in the healthcare setting. According to the particular characteristics of the patient, either lifestyle changes, pharmacotherapy, surgery, or a combination should be applied. In morbidly obese patients refractory to diet and drug therapy, a substantial and sustained weight loss after bariatric surgery is obtained. However, the most effective treatment in the long term is, and will be, obesity prevention.

Acknowledgements

This work was supported by CIBER Fisiopatología de la Obesidad y Nutrición (CIBERobn) and Fondo de Investigaciones Sanitarias (FIS PS0902330), both from the Spanish Instituto de Salud Carlos III.

References and further reading

The information in this chapter has been obtained from existing textbooks and PubMed searches of obesity-related topics, as well as from the Web sites of the most relevant international health institutions, such as the World Health Organization (WHO), the British National Health Service (NHS) and National Institute of Clinical Excellence (NICE), and the US National Institutes of Health (NIH), which have convened expert panels to carry out comprehensive and critical evaluations of multiple clinical trials in an effort to establish evidence-based guidelines.

Caterson ID, Franklin J, Colditz GA. Economic costs of obesity. In: Handbook of Obesity. Etiology and Pathophysiology, 2nd edn (GA Bray, C Bouchard, eds). New York: Marcel Dekker, 2004, pp. 149–156.

Finkelstein EA, Trogdon JG, Cohen JW, Dietz W. Annual medical spending attributable to obesity: payer- and service-specific estimates. Health Affairs 2009; 28(5): w822–w831.

Frühbeck G, Becerril S, Sáinz N, Garrastachu P, García-Velloso MJ. BAT: a new target for human obesity. Trends Pharmacol Sci 2009; 30(8): 387–396.

Li S, Zhao JH, Luan J, Ekelund U, Luben RN, Khaw KT, Wareham NJ, Loos RJ. Physical activity attenuates the genetic predisposition to obesity in 20 000 men and women from EPIC-Norfolk prospective population study. PLoS Med 2010; 7(8). pii: e1000332.

Loos RJ. The genetic epidemiology of melanocortin 4 receptor variants. Eur J Pharmacol 2011; 660(1): 156–164.

McCormack B, Stone I. Economic costs of obesity and the case for government intervention. Obesity Rev 2007; 8(s1): 161–164.

McPherson K, Marsh T, Brown M. 2007. Modelling Future Trends in Obesity and the Impact on Health. Foresight Tackling Obesities: Future Choices. Available from http://www.foresight.gov.uk.

Prentice AM, Jebb SA. Obesity in Britain: gluttony or sloth? BMJ 1995; 311: 437–439.

Rankinen T, Zuberi A, Chagnon YC, Weisnagel SJ, Argyropoulos G, Walts B, Pérusse L, Bouchard C. The human obesity gene map: the 2005 update. Obesity (Silver Spring) 2006; 14(4): 529–644.

Speliotes EK, Willer CJ, Berndt SI, Monda KL, Thorleifsson G, Jackson AU, et al. Association analyses of 249 796 individuals reveal 18 new loci associated with body mass index. Nat Genet 2010; 42(11): 937–948.

WHO. Obesity: preventing and managing the global epidemic. Report of a WHO consultation. WHO Technical Report Series 894. Geneva: World Health Organization, 2000.

Willer CJ, Speliotes EK, Loos RJ, Li S, Lindgren CM, Heid IM, et al. Six new loci associated with body mass index highlight a neuronal influence on body weight regulation. Nat Genet 2009; 41(1): 25–34.

Williams G, Frühbeck G, editors. Obesity: Science to Practice. Chichester: Wiley-Blackwell, 2009.

Web sites of interest

Catalog of published genome-wide association studies. http://www.genome.gov/26525384.

Economic costs of obesity. http://www.cdc.gov/obesity/causes/economics.html.

FORESIGHT report: Tackling Obesities: Future Choices. http://webarchive.nationalarchives.gov.uk/+/http://www.bis.gov.uk/foresight/our-work/projects/current-projects/tackling-obesities.

International Association for the Study of Obesity. http://www.iaso.org/.

International Obesity Task Force. http://www.iaso.org/iotf/.

National Heart, Lung, and Blood Institute (NHLBI) of the NIH. What are overweight and obesity? http://www.nhlbi.nih.gov/health/health-topics/topics/obe/.

National Human Genome Research Institute: Hindorff LA, Junkins HA, Hall PN, Mehta JP, Manolio TA. A Catalog of Published Genome-wide Association Studies. http://www.genome.gov/gwastudies.

NICE. Guidance on surgery for morbid obesity. http://www.dh.gov.uk/en/Publichealth/Obesity/index.htm.

UK obesity statistics. http://www.annecollins.com/obesity/uk-obesity-statistics.htm.

WHO global infobase. https://apps.who.int/infobase/.

WHO on obesity. http://www.who.int/topics/obesity/en/; http://www.who.int/mediacentre/factsheets/fs311/en/index.html.

5
Under-nutrition

Anura V Kurpad[1] and Isabelle Aeberli[2]

[1]St John's Research Institute, Bangalore, India
[2]St John's Research Institute, Bangalore, India and ETH Zurich, Zurich, Switzerland

Key messages

- Acute under-nutrition is suspected when an involuntary weight loss of greater than 10% of the body weight occurs over a 3–6-month period.
- Chronic under-nutrition is similar to chronic energy deficiency; this is characterised by a low body mass index (BMI) in weight-stable individuals.
- Under-nutrition that is uncomplicated by disease is associated with several nutrient-saving and homeostatic responses.
- When disease and under-nutrition coexist, the adaptive nutrient-saving responses are generally reversed, such that the depletion of body nutrient stores and tissue is accelerated.
- Nutritional screening is a rapid generic procedure, often undertaken by nonspecialist health professionals to identify individuals

- at risk of under-nutrition. Nutritional assessment is a more in-depth evaluation of nutritional status, which is normally undertaken by a specialist in nutrition, such as a dietician, and is specific to the disease and the patient.
- The assessment of under-nutrition can be made in the clinic using simple clinical techniques. More complex techniques for measuring depletion and body composition or function are also available.
- Nutritional support in under-nutrition should be tailored to the clinical situation; in any case, a modest and balanced diet should be instituted as soon as possible. Monitoring the nutritional support given is essential for a successful outcome.
- There are dangers associated with aggressive and unbalanced diet administration.

5.1 Introduction

'Under-nutrition' is often used as a generic term to describe a variety of nutrient deficiencies. The common way to think of under-nutrition is in terms of body weight; this has often led to the terms 'underweight' and 'under-nourished' being used interchangeably. Under-nutrition is caused by a less-than-adequate intake of nutrients, most of which are related to the energy intake. In adults, this has led to the term 'energy deficiency', with a further subclassification into acute – which is sudden, and associated with a declining body weight – and chronic – which occurs over a long period of time, such that the body weight over the preceding few months may be low, but stable.

The definition of under-nutrition in a clinical setting needs to highlight the differences between cachexia, sarcopenia, and under- or malnutrition.

There is much debate regarding the definitions of these conditions, and it may be reasonable to think that cachexia and sarcopenia are part of the syndromes of under-nutrition. Cachexia is a catabolic condition caused by disease-related inflammatory activity and negative nutrient balance due to anorexia and/or a decreased absorption of nutrients. In that sense, although this is a catabolic condition, inflammation is the key feature, and muscle or the fat-free mass (FFM), as well as fat mass (FM), decreases in size. The diagnosis of cachexia rests principally on a loss of body weight. In sarcopenia, however, which is now recognised as a multifactorial geriatric syndrome, there is primarily a loss of muscle tissue, as well as decline in muscle strength as a result of ageing and physical inactivity, along with the general wear and tear of the normal life course; therefore, the tissue loss occurs primarily in the FFM. The diagnosis of sarcopenia is

Clinical Nutrition, Second Edition. Edited by Marinos Elia, Olle Ljungqvist, Rebecca J Stratton and Susan A Lanham-New.

thus dependent on an assessment of muscle mass as well as of muscle function. It may not need to be accompanied by a negative nutrient balance, although this can occur when sarcopenia happens in old age. While under-nutrition may be regarded as the inadequate consumption and absorption of nutrients, along with a possible increased loss of these nutrients from the body, cachexia is a multifactorial syndrome characterised by severe body-weight, fat, and muscle loss and increased protein catabolism due to underlying disease. It is rare to see pure under-nutrition in adult patients, and most often a combination of cachexia and under-nutrition occurs.

There are several factors that predispose to the occurrence of under-nutrition within a care setting; these include a very young or advanced age, apathy and depression leading to a decreased intake, and the simple inability to eat food. Equally, carers may fail to recognise the need for nutrition in a timely manner.

The consequences of under-nutrition can be physical, psychological, or behavioural. Examples of these are shown in Table 5.1. On a physical level, a loss of muscle and FM, reduced respiratory muscle and cardiac function, and atrophy of visceral organs occurs. At a psychological level, under-nutrition can be associated with fatigue and apathy, which in turn impact on food intake and can worsen the nutritional status. On a behavioural level, under-nutrition is also associated with an increased length of hospital stay, and such patients are more prone to experiencing complications.

Table 5.1 Some of the functional consequences of under-nutrition.

Physical	Muscle strength and fatigue
	Hypothermia
	Reduced respiratory muscle function and reduced cough pressure, predisposing to chest infections
	Immobility, predisposing to venous thrombosis and embolism
	Impaired immune function
	Reduced wound-healing
	Reduced final height in women, leading to small pelvic size and small-birth-weight infants
Psychological and behavioural	Depression
	Anxiety
	Reduced will to recover
	Self-neglect
	Poor bonding with mother and child
	Loss of libido

It has now been proposed that an aetiology-based terminology be used for the diagnosis of under-nutrition in adults in clinical settings, which gives recognition to the interacting effect of inflammation on nutritional status. Therefore, when there is chronic starvation without inflammation, the term 'starvation-related malnutrition' is used. An example of this condition is anorexia nervosa. When chronic inflammation is present, the term 'chronic disease-related malnutrition' is used. Examples of this condition include organ failure and sarcopenic obesity. When acute inflammation is present, the term 'acute disease-related malnutrition' is used. Examples include major infections, burns, and trauma.

5.2 Pathophysiology of under-nutrition

Body composition

Body-weight loss on starvation is initially rapid (up to 5 kg over a few days), due to the emptying of glycogen reserves, the utilisation of body protein, and the accompanying water loss. The later loss of body tissue that accompanies negative energy balance primarily comprises fat, although varying amounts of lean tissue are lost as well. This is demonstrated in a classic study on the effect of long-term semi starvation on healthy men by Keys *et al.* (1950). During their 6-month semi-starvation study, the lean-tissue loss observed in the subjects represented about half of the total weight loss. Although physical activity would be expected to maintain muscle mass in such a situation, it is clear that lean tissue is also catabolised to provide energy in the face of large energy deficits. The composition of weight loss is dependent on different conditions under which the negative energy balance is imposed: in healthy, normal young men, the weight loss is composed of fat and FFM, while in obese individuals, it may be primarily FM.

Energy metabolism

Accompanying the changes in body composition during acute negative energy balance are adaptive changes in energy expenditure. These changes can occur in one or more of: the basal metabolic rate (BMR), thermogenesis (the production of heat by the body in response to various stimuli), and physical activity (Figure 5.1).

Reductions in the BMR are partly mediated through weight loss itself, in which metabolically demanding tissues of the body are reduced in size, and partly through reductions in the metabolic activity of these tissues. In the semi-starvation study referred to before, the subjects' BMR decreased by about 25% when expressed per kilogram of their FFM (or metabolically active tissue). This decline was most rapid in the first 2 weeks, indicating that the reduced metabolic activity of the fat-free tissue occurred quickly in response to energy deficiency.

The factors underlying the decrease in the activity of the FFM include reduced activity of the sympathetic nervous system – which is a part of the autonomic nervous system and which partly drives the heat-producing activity of the FFM – as well as altered peripheral thyroid metabolism, lowered insulin secretion, and substrate utilisation designed to maintain glucose production and maximise fat usage. Leptin is a hormone that plays a key role in regulating energy intake and energy expenditure. It is expressed in adipose tissue (the *ob* gene product) and, once secreted into the circulation, acts at the hypothalamic level to inhibit appetite. It therefore forms a link between the FM, energy intake, and expenditure, acting as a lipostatic mechanism through modulation of satiety and the activity of the sympathetic nervous system. Leptin levels are low in anorexia nervosa, suggesting that leptin may be important in under-nourished, low-FM states as a potential modulator of the energy-sparing response to energy deficiency. An additional modulator of the

response to underfeeding is the genetic makeup of the individual. In an interesting study on monozygotic twin pairs, body weight and compositional change were studied after 93 days of negative energy balance induced by increased exercise with constant dietary intake. The within-pair variation was much less than the between-pair variation for loss of weight, body fat, visceral fat, and respiratory exchange ratio during exercise (see Figure 5.2 for weight change), showing that subjects with the same genotype were more alike in responses than subjects with different genotypes.

On the other hand, there are also findings of an increased BMR per kilogram body weight in a number of clinical studies arising from energy deficiency. These conflicting findings may be due to factors including whether or not the patient was in a state of recovery, and methodological errors during the conduct of BMR measurement. The increased BMR could also be due to the stress imposed by illness in clinical situations (see later in this chapter).

Even though thermogenesis only accounts for a small part of overall energy expenditure, changes which occur as a result of total or semi-starvation can add to the decreased energy expenditure observed in this condition. Compared to the dramatic fall in

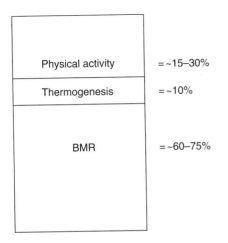

Figure 5.1 Components of total 24-hour energy expenditure.

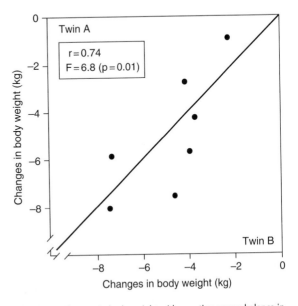

Figure 5.2 Changes in body weight with negative energy balance in seven pairs of twins. Twin A on the ordinate, twin B on the abscissa. Reprinted from Bouchard *et al.* (1994), with permission of Nature Publishing Group.

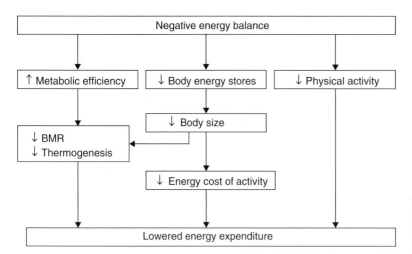

Figure 5.3 Interaction between factors leading to lowered energy expenditure as a result of negative energy balance. BMR, basal metabolic rate.

BMR during acute energy deficiency, the influence of thermogenesis is much less pronounced and less consistent, but still measureable. For example, in elderly, under-nourished women admitted into hospital with fractured femurs, the thermogenic response to a cold stimulus was diminished.

Even with otherwise healthy individuals, semi-starvation or starvation leads to a reduction in physical activity. From the behavioural viewpoint, the imposition of an acute energy deficiency also causes apathy, with a marked reduction in spontaneous activity. A decrease in food intake results in a change in selection of discretionary activity patterns, such that lower-activity discretionary patterns are selected. These behavioural changes are obviously designed to maximise the chances of survival under conditions of acute energy deficiency.

Overall, therefore, it appears that energy deficiency is associated with body-weight loss, along with changes in body composition and a reduction in BMR and physical activity. Figure 5.3 shows how these factors interact with each other to attain lower energy expenditure when an acute negative energy balance exists.

If the lowered energy expenditure is adequate to compensate for the decreased energy intake that caused the negative energy balance, and allows for a new neutral energy balance to be achieved, the person can survive, albeit at a lower plane of nutrition. This leads to a chronic energy deficiency (CED), discussed in Section 5.4. If a homeostatic response is not possible, due to a severe energy deficit, body energy and muscle stores continue to be lost until a lethal weight loss occurs, usually when body weight or FFM has fallen to about half its original value.

Protein metabolism

When nitrogen (protein) intake is reduced, the nitrogen output also decreases, although this can take some days to occur. In subjects who are put on low-protein diets, some 7–14 days may be required for the N output to stabilise at a new lower level (Figure 5.4). This is important when assessing N balance, particularly over a short time period, since the previous N intake influences the amount of N output.

This adaptation spares body protein and preserves essential functions in the body; since the protein loss never reaches zero, there will be losses of protein from the body, primarily from the skeletal muscle mass. In more chronic under-nutrition (but not starvation), the relatively greater loss of muscle mass leads to an increase in the viscera-to-skeletal muscle mass ratio of the FFM. An important point is that when the protein intake is acutely reduced, there is a transient loss of N over a period of days. This has been attributed to a 'labile' pool of body protein, which contracts when protein intake is reduced (and, conversely, expands when protein intake is increased), but the identity of this pool of body protein has not been established in humans.

The adaptive reduction in N output during protein deprivation can be mediated though a decrease in amino acid oxidation, reduced formation of ammonia in the kidney, or reduced formation of glucose (gluconeogenesis) in the liver. Glucose is primarily

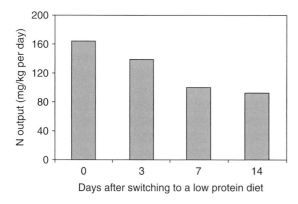

Figure 5.4 Rate of change in nitrogen (N) excretion after changing from a high to a low protein intake. Data from Quevedo *et al.* (1994) © The Biochemical Society.

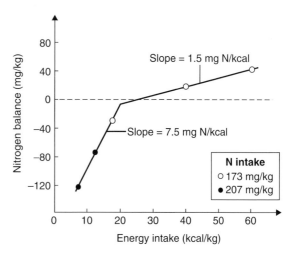

Figure 5.5 Relationship between N balance and energy intake. From Elwyn DH. Nutritional requirements of adult surgical patients. Crit Care Med 1980; 8: 9–20. Copyright © Wolters Kluwer Health.

needed by organs such as the brain. This need is met in conditions of starvation by proteolysis. Although ketoacids, which derive from fat, become important fuels for the brain as starvation progresses, they do not eliminate brain glucose requirements. Increasing the energy intake will improve N balance, just as increasing the N intake would, and when both N and energy are provided at their minimum requirement level, the N balance is expected to be zero. Thus, energy can be said to have a protein-sparing effect in the submaintenance range of protein intakes. The effect of N and energy intake on N balance is interdependent and complex. The level of N intake determines the change in N balance that can be achieved with an increase in energy intake. On the other hand, the effect of energy intake on N balance depends on the intake range within which alterations in energy intake occur, and a value of 7.5 mg N/kcal has been reported for submaintenance energy intakes of up to about 15 kcal/kg (Figure 5.5). About one-third of the variation in N balance can be attributed to variations in energy intake relative to the requirement, and 1–1.5 mg N/kg body weight is gained (or spared) per extra 1 kcal/kg body weight of energy intake at maintenance levels of intake. This has led to the suggestion that in under-nutrition, the high slope of the N balance-to-energy intake relationship is due to replenishment or maintenance of the body cell mass, while at high energy intakes, the N retained may be needed to support the extra energy retained as fat.

The type of energy source (carbohydrate or fat) is also important in determining the influence of energy on N balance. In the submaintenance range of

protein intakes, it has been shown that carbohydrate is more effective than fat, perhaps because of the greater insulinogenic influence of carbohydrate. At maintenance intakes, as well as in the clinical setting, both carbohydrate and fat have been found to be equally effective, although some studies suggest that a fat/glucose regimen is better than a glucose-alone regimen. The message from these observations is that energy spares protein, and 100–150 g of glucose per day has been described to be effective in reducing urea N excretion by about half.

Measurements of the rate of protein turnover show that it changes little, if at all, with moderate reductions in protein intake, although with severe protein deficiency there is a reduction in whole-body protein turnover. Whole-body protein synthesis does not appear to change with feeding, and changes in proteolysis appear to mediate most of the acute regulatory changes associated with feeding and fasting. While whole-body protein synthesis rates are relatively unchanged, there may be differences in tissue-specific protein synthesis rates. In rats given a low protein intake, rates of protein synthesis are reduced in the muscle, but increased in the liver. The rate of synthesis of albumin is also decreased with a low protein intake; however, this is followed by a decrease in the rate of catabolism as well after a few days. In addition, there is a transfer of albumin from the extravascular to the intravascular pool, preserving serum albumin concentrations. Similarly, a relatively low protein intake does not change the concentrations of other liver secretory proteins such as retinol-binding protein and transferrin.

There are other nutrients that are important in the maintenance of the FFM. Intracellular constituents such as potassium and phosphorus are important in maintaining a positive N balance when a diet adequate in protein and energy is given to malnourished patients. Diets lacking in potassium or phosphorus lead to negative N balances even when all other nutrients are adequate, while a lack of sodium reduces the extent of the observed positive N balance in malnourished patients receiving an otherwise adequate diet.

Hormonal mediators

During starvation, the maintenance of blood glucose levels is paramount for the organism. Thus, starvation is associated with a decrease in the hypoglycaemic hormone insulin and an increase in counter-regulatory hormones that aim to increase glucose, including glucagon, which promotes hepatic glucose production. The lowered insulin concentrations also allow for a reduced peripheral utilisation of glucose and an increased mobilisation of fat. Thus, fatty acids become an important oxidative fuel for peripheral tissues during starvation. Thyroid hormone levels also show changes, in that the active form of the hormone (T_3) is reduced, while the inactive form (reverse T_3) is increased in the serum. The activity of the sympathetic nervous system is also reduced, as are serum concentrations of catecholamines. The implication of a decrease in these hormones in nutritional terms is that energy expenditure decreases, thus reducing the magnitude of the negative energy balance.

Immune function in under-nutrition

The immune system depends on cellular and secretory activities, which require nutrients in much the same way as other processes in the body. Severe protein-calorie malnutrition causes a decline in immune function, in terms of lymphocyte number, cell-mediated immunity, antibodies, and phagocytosis, and therefore an increase in infective morbidity. The levels of other immune mediators, including most complement factors (complement is an important mediator of inflammation activated by antibodies)

are also decreased in protein–energy malnutrition. The decreased immunocompetence seen with under-nutrition is a type of acquired immunodeficiency, and several adverse clinical effects, such as opportunistic infections, marked depression of the delayed cutaneous hypersensitivity response, and increased frequency of septicaemia, occur. A low protein intake on its own also results in a decline in both cell-mediated and antibody-based immunity.

Although single nutrient deficiencies are rare in humans, experimental evidence is available for the importance of several nutrients, such as vitamins (vitamins A, C, and E, pyridoxine, folate), and minerals, such as zinc, iron, copper, and selenium. Some amino acids, such as arginine and glutamine, and other nutrients, like n-3 polyunsaturated fatty acids, are important for specific immune functions, including T-cell immunity, and may be beneficial in wound-healing and resistance to infections and tumourigenesis as well.

5.3 Pathophysiology of under-nutrition complicated by stress

The coexistence of under-nutrition and the stress of an injury or infection will lead to a potentiation of the rate at which nutritional depletion occurs. This is illustrated in Figure 5.6, where a reduction in body weight occurs much faster if starvation is associated with injury or infection.

Energy metabolism

During injury or infection, there is an increase in BMR, and this increase is dependent on the severity of the injury. Thus the BMR may even double with burns of more than 40% of the body surface, whereas it may only increase by about 25% in patients with long bone fractures, and even less after surgery (Figure 5.7). If there is fever associated with the injury, the metabolic rate will increase concomitantly. However, this does not necessarily mean that the energy requirements of a patient are raised dramatically. In sick patients who are likely to be in bed, the increase in BMR due to the stress imposed by the disease may be offset by the decrease in physical activity, such that the total daily energy expenditure may not change by much.

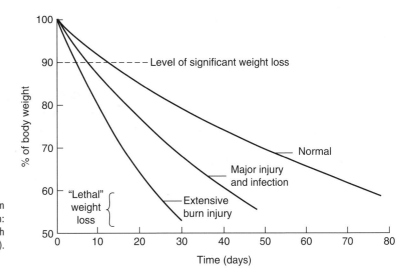

Figure 5.6 Effect of infection and injury on weight loss. Souba WW & Wilmore DW. In: Modern Nutrition in Health and Disease, 9th ed (Shils M, Olson J, Shike M & Ross A, eds). Lippincott Williams & Wilkins, 1999.

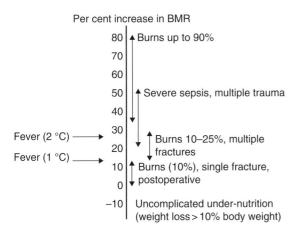

Figure 5.7 The effect of disease and malnutrition on the basal metabolic rate (BMR). Modified from Elia (1991).

Protein metabolism

With injury, nitrogen loss also occurs, and this may be extensive enough to lead to muscle wasting and muscle weakness. The amount of N lost varies depending on the severity of injury, but in general there is always an increased N loss. This contrasts with the picture of reduced N losses due to adaptation to low protein intake shown in Figure 5.4. There is an increase in protein synthesis rates, associated with an even greater increase in protein breakdown rates, leading to net N loss. The prior nutritional status of

the patient is important in determining their muscle mass, and possibly the amount of N that is lost from their muscle after injury. The amino acids that are released from the muscle in response to injury do not match the composition of the muscle that is broken down, and alanine and glutamine represent about 60% of the amino acids released from muscle after injury. While the kidney takes up glutamine for ammonia generation and the gut takes it up as an oxidative fuel, the liver takes up alanine for glucose synthesis. In addition, the outflow of amino acids from muscle also serves to fuel the acute-phase protein synthesis in the liver. In an under-nourished or starved patient, this loss will be magnified because of an inability to replenish the protein breakdown required to fuel these processes. A depleted muscle can then no longer provide enough substrates to allow the splanchnic organs to maintain intestinal integrity and to maintain a high immunocompetence, thereby creating a vicious cycle. It is not known how fast depleted muscle can be restored in under-nourished patients, and it is likely that depleted muscle will be restored back to normal only very slowly, depending on activity and exercise during rehabilitation.

Hormonal mediators

There are several hormonal and cytokine mediators of the catabolic response to injury. Elevated levels of catecholamines and cortisol are characteristic, in contrast to what is seen in uncomplicated starvation, and promote an increased energy expenditure, nitrogen loss, and glucose production, along with the mobilisation of free fatty acids. Insulin levels are reduced in the early response to injury, but are raised later in the course of the injury response as insulin resistance appears, probably mediated by cortisol and catecholamines. Glucagon levels are also increased, to facilitate glucose production. Proinflammatory cytokines such as tumour necrosis factor alpha (TNFα), interleukin-1 (IL-1), and interleukin-6 (IL-6) are also important in stimulating acute-phase protein synthesis (which is in turn fuelled by amino acids from muscle), increased loss of muscle protein, increased lipolysis, and fever, leading to an increased energy expenditure.

If the increased metabolic response continues along with under-nutrition, it results in cachexia, which is characterised by extreme weight loss, tissue-wasting, and anorexia. The latter contributes in turn to the wasting in a vicious cycle. Cachexia can occur in chronic illnesses, cancers, and AIDS.

5.4 Chronic under-nutrition

Chronic under-nutrition (or CED) is a weight-stable condition found in the presence of lower-than-normal energy intakes. This state is achieved by the presence of low body weight and fat stores, but the individual's health is normal and body physiological function is not compromised to the extent that the individual is unable to lead an economically productive life. While this condition exists to a very small extent in developed countries, between 25 and 50% of adults from developing countries can be described as having CED.

The consequence of an inadequate energy intake during the childhood and adolescence of an individual is a reduced body size and a low body mass index (BMI). There is also stunting, due to the presence of low energy intakes and concomitant repeated infections in childhood and adolescence. Both the body fat and the FFM are decreased when compared to normally-nourished individuals. Within the FFM, relatively more muscle is lost, which means that the viscera-to-muscle ratio is increased. It is important to note that in individuals with chronic under-nutrition, the BMR expressed per kilogram body weight or

FFM may not be decreased as it is in individuals with acute under-nutrition. When the relationship between BMR and body weight is examined, it shows a line with a positive slope; when this line is extended back to a zero body weight, the BMR does not drop to zero as one would expect with a simple ratio relationship, but has a positive intercept on the y-axis. Therefore, a simple expression of the BMR per kilogram body weight may not be the best way to look for differences in BMR between normal and under-nourished individuals. However, there may also be a physiological explanation for the conflicting findings of an increase in the BMR per kilogram body weight or FFM, which can partly be explained by the relatively higher contribution of the viscera to the metabolic rate. Similarly, these individuals have an increase in their rate of protein turnover expressed per kilogram body weight, and although the relation between protein turnover and body weight will also have a positive y-intercept, a physiological explanation for the higher protein turnover is the relative loss of slow-turnover tissues such as muscle, compared to the preservation of the more rapid-turnover proteins of the viscera.

Chronic marginal malnutrition is also associated with reduced grip strength, and studies have shown that adults with CED have lower hand grip strengths, both in absolute terms and when corrected for forearm muscle area, than well-nourished subjects. In addition, it has been found that CED subjects fatigue faster when subjected to standard laboratory isotonic and isometric exercise protocols than their well-nourished counterparts, although some studies could not find any differences in endurance between under-nourished and normal individuals. Taken together, individuals with CED have reduced skeletal muscle performance, which is largely explained by the reduction in muscle mass, but may also be partly due to functional changes in skeletal muscle.

5.5 Under-nutrition in the elderly

There is an increase in the number of elderly in most populations today due to a longer life expectancy, but few data exist on the effects of under-nutrition on such individuals in the long term, or on chronically energy-deficient elderly subjects. The total daily energy expenditure of elderly individuals reduces with progressive age, by about 95 kcal/day/decade. A reduction in BMR and physical activity largely accounts for this change, along with smaller changes in thermogenesis. The elderly also lose muscle mass, in a process called sarcopenia, which is associated with a reduction in skeletal muscle strength. The reduction in skeletal muscle mass has been linked at least in part to suboptimal intakes of protein and the availability of amino acids. In elderly women, consumption of energy-adequate but protein-deficient diets resulted in significant decreases in adductor pollicis function, while in supplemented elderly people on a resistance-exercise schedule, muscle mass increased. Ageing is also associated with a decline in immune function, which compounds the problem in a clinical situation; an adequate nutritional intake can modify this decline in immunity.

A 3-week underfeeding trial of elderly subjects, by about 3.4 MJ/day, showed that they reduced their resting and total energy expenditure by the same degree as normal young subjects subjected to an energy restriction of similar magnitude. The decline in resting energy expenditure was greater than what would have been expected from the weight loss alone, as is expected in acute under-nutrition, but this decline was smaller than that observed in the younger adults. A longer-term study of underfeeding by about 3.7 MJ/day for 6 weeks showed that the older individuals lost greater amounts of weight than their younger counterparts and reported a significantly lower frequency of hunger during underfeeding. When they were followed up over a period of 6 months of normal unrestricted feeding, they did not regain their lost weight. It is thought that ageing is associated with a significant impairment in the control of food intake in response to prior changes in energy intake.

Hospitalised elderly patients have a high prevalence of malnutrition, with adverse outcomes related to complications, mortality, and length of stay in hospital. These patients need to be identified, as nutritional support can improve their clinical outcome. Nutritional support also has beneficial effects on the readmission rate into hospital and the ability of elderly patients to be maintained at home, although the regaining of depleted muscle mass seems unlikely. There is a case for adequate nutrition being given to elderly patients; a study on malnourished elderly patients with hip fractures showed that their ability to walk after surgery was improved after nutritional support; however, strong evidence is still unavailable for many other outcomes in these patients, particularly on morbidity and mortality.

5.6 Severe acute malnutrition in children

Severe acute malnutrition (SAM) is still a problem in young children in many parts of the developing world, and is associated with a high mortality rate. It has been estimated that some 20 million children are affected by SAM, mainly in South Asia and sub-Saharan Africa. This type of severe malnutrition requires targeted care, and is diagnosed when the weight-for-height 'z' scores (WHZ) are less than or equal to -3, when there is severe visible wasting, or when there is symmetrical oedema (oedematous malnutrition, kwashiorkor). While it may be difficult to rapidly survey many children for their weight and height, a simpler method is to measure the mid-upper arm circumference (MUAC), using either a tape or simple ready-made plastic strips. An MUAC of less than 110 mm in children aged 6–59 months is indicative of SAM. While the mortality rate can be high in these children, it can be reduced when the guidelines for management are followed. A proportion of under-5 children with SAM require management in a clinical facility because of medical complications, but the majority can be nutritionally cared for through a community or home-based care approach.

Children with SAM need to be free from medical complications and therefore need to be treated for any dehydration or infections before they receive the therapeutic food, which is safe, soft, easily ingested, and palatable, and has a high energy content and vitamins and minerals. Severely malnourished children cannot tolerate normal amounts of protein and sodium, or high amounts of fat (which may be used in a diet designed to encourage catch-up growth), and therefore may need a less intensive diet as a starter formula until they are metabolically stable. Ready-to-use therapeutic foods (RUTFs) are now used to encourage catch-up growth; these formulas have a low water content and are therefore less susceptible to spoiling in harsh field conditions. It is important to remember that breast-fed children should always get breast milk before they are given the therapeutic food, and also on demand. Typically, children need to be fed this food for about 6–8 weeks before they return to their habitual diets, and since this is a therapeutic food, it needs to be given under some supervision.

5.7 Assessment of under-nutrition

A distinction should be made between nutritional screening and nutritional assessment. The first is a rapid generic procedure, often undertaken by non-specialist health professionals, to identify individuals at risk of under-nutrition. Nutritional assessment is an in-depth evaluation of nutritional status, which is normally undertaken by a specialist in nutrition, such as a dietitian, and is specific to the disease and patient.

The assessment of under-nutrition has to be viewed from two perspectives: from a nutritional and physiological perspective, one would like to know the consequences of under-nutrition on body composition and function; from the clinical perspective, one would like to know the predictive value of the assessment, particularly in judging what the clinical outcome will be. In addition, the clinical perspective also places value on those assessments that provide an early diagnosis of under-nutrition, so that nutritional support can be started promptly. It would seem to be ideal to have a single test or index that can provide a specific and sensitive nutritional assessment, as well as predictive information on the clinical outcome. In practice, this is not so, and simple clinical assessments of the nutritional state have proved as useful as complex sophisticated tests in defining the nutritional status for clinically useful purposes. A good nutritional assessment is also important in deciding the nutrient requirements of the individual (see Chapter 2).

5.8 Treatment

The aim of treatment of under-nutrition in the clinical setting is twofold: there is a need to prevent under-nutrition from progressing (to prevent weight loss and maintain body weight) and to provide nutrients so that nutritional repletion (weight gain) can occur; equally, the provision of nutrients to sick under-nourished patients is unlikely to be effective in terms of clinical outcome in the presence of sepsis and altered metabolism – such as insulin resistance and cytokine-mediated events – unless the underlying pathology is addressed. The first step is to assess the nutritional requirements of the patient. Decisions can then be made on how to deliver nutrients to them.

Assessment of energy and protein requirements

The assessment of the energy requirement in an under-nourished patient is based on the energy expenditure. As Figure 5.1 shows, the major component of the energy expenditure is the BMR, which can be either measured by indirect calorimetry or predicted by equations that use easily measurable parameters such as the body weight, height, and age of the patient. The actual measurement of the BMR requires several conditions to be met, including a state of fast, complete rest when awake, and the thermoneutrality of the environment. These conditions are unlikely to be met in the clinical state, and a measurement of the metabolic rate under these conditions can at most be called a 'resting metabolic rate' (RMR). The prediction of BMR can be made through the use of age- and gender-based predictive equations, which are recommended by the UN's Food and Agriculture Organization (FAO), the World Health Organization (WHO), and the United Nations University (UNU) (FAO/WHO/UNU, 2004).

A single equation that incorporates weight, height, and age for each gender is the Harris–Benedict equation. This states that energy requirement (kcal/day) can be calculated by:

$$\text{Men: } 66.4730 + (13.7516 \times W) + (5.0033 \times H)$$
$$- (6.7550 \times A)$$
$$\text{Woman: } 655.0955 + (9.5634 \times W) + (1.8496 \times H)$$
$$- (4.6756 \times A)$$

where W is weight in kg, H is height in cm, and A is age in years.

Some error would be expected with the use of these equations, of the order of 10–20%. If there is a coexisting illness, this will cause the BMR to be increased, and an appropriate stress factor for the illness will have to be multiplied into the BMR. For

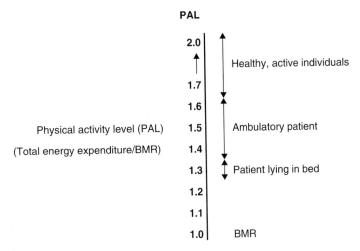

PAL

2.0
↑
1.7   Healthy, active individuals
1.6
1.5   Ambulatory patient
1.4
1.3   Patient lying in bed
1.2
1.1
1.0   BMR

Figure 5.8 Physical-activity levels (PALs). This factor is multiplied into the basal metabolic rate (BMR) to obtain total energy expenditure.

instance, if the measured BMR is 1200 kcal/day, and the stress factor related to the illness is 1.3, the BMR becomes $1400 \times 1.3 = 1560$ kcal/day.

Once the BMR is known, the total energy expenditure can be obtained by the use of factors representing the other components that are multiples of the BMR. In general, since the other major component of energy expenditure is the physical activity, only this needs to be taken into consideration for practical purposes. The physical-activity factor depends on whether the patient is confined to bed or moving around. The total energy expenditure based on the activity ranges from about 1.3 to 1.5 times the BMR (Figure 5.8).

The decrease in physical activity during illness usually offsets any increase in the BMR due to stress, and overall it is usually never necessary to provide any more than a modest energy intake. The use of hyper-alimentation or the feeding of large amounts of energy to sick patients has no evidence to support its use.

The requirement for protein is to some extent dependent on the energy provided, but it must be met in under-nourished patients. As stated above, the energy requirement is usually not increased, and simply providing an excess of energy will not promote a positive N balance if the protein intake is less than adequate. The normal protein intake that is considered safe, in the sense that it meets the requirements of 95% of the healthy population, is 0.83 g/kg/day. This protein also needs to deliver essential amino acids in amounts that are adequate. Recent data (which are still a matter of debate) on essential amino

acid requirements indicate that these are higher than was earlier thought, and require the inclusion of good-quality protein in the diet. Thus, proteins from cereals given alone are likely to be limited in lysine, and appropriate complementary foods, such as legumes or animal protein sources, should also be provided in the diet. When protein accretion is the goal of nutritional therapy (although this will not occur by increasing protein intake only), the protein intake will have to be raised to about 1.5 g/kg/day, but ideally should not exceed 2 g/kg/day, since the kidney and liver may have a diminished ability to tolerate a high amino acid load. Expressed as a percentage of the energy given, the energy from protein intake should be about 15%.

Even though they are very important, protein intake should not consist of essential amino acids only. Also, the nonessential amino acids are now recognised to have important roles in maintaining functions of the body, such as those involved in defence, movement, and absorption of nutrients. These include skeletal muscle, immune, and intestinal functions, which are particularly important during stress (Table 5.2). Given the recent data on essential amino acid requirements, the non-essential amino acids would constitute about 70% of the total daily amino acid intake. In disease states, certain amino acids may become essential, and this is called conditional essentiality. Glutamine is an example of a conditionally essential amino acid, and acts as the preferred respiratory fuel for lymphocytes, hepatocytes, and intestinal mucosal cells. Low concentrations of

Table 5.2 Nonessential amino acids in maintenance functions of the body. Glu, glutamate; Asp, asparate; Gly, glycine; Cys, cysteine; Arg, arginine; Gln, glutamine. Modified from J Nutr (2000; 130: 1835S-1840S), American Society for Nutrition.

System	Function	Product	Precursor
Intestine	Energy	ATP	Glu/Asp/Gln
	Growth	Nucleic acids	Gln/Asp/Gly
	Protection	Glutathione	Cys/Glu/Gly
		Nitric oxide	Arg
Muscle	Energy	Creatine	Gly/Arg
Nervous	Transmitters	Glutaminergic	Glu
		Glycinergic	Gly
		Nitric oxide	Arg
Immune	Peroxidative	Glutathione	Cys/Glu/Gly
	Lymphocytes		Glu/Arg/Asp
Cardiovascular	Blood-pressure regulation	Nitric oxide	Arg

Table 5.3 Clinical manifestations of micronutrient deficiencies.

Micronutrient	Symptom/sign
1. Thiamine (B_1)	Beriberi
	Wernicke's encephalopathy
2. Riboflavin (B_2)	Glossitis, cheilosis
3. Pyridoxine (B_6)	Dermatitis, neuropathy
4. Niacin[a]	Pellagra
5. Folic acid	Megaloblastic anaemia
6. Cobalamine (B_{12})	Megaloblastic anaemia, glossitis, diarrhoea, neuromyopathy
7. Ascorbic acid (C)	Scurvy
8. Vitamin A	Xerophthalmia, night blindness, infections
9. Vitamin D	Osteomalacia
10. Vitamin K	Clotting abnormalities
11. Iron	Anaemia
12. Zinc	Rashes, anorexia, growth retardation, alopecia
13. Iodine	Hypothyroidism
14. Calcium	Rickets, osteoporosis
15. Selenium	Cardiomyopathy, myositis
16. Copper	Anaemia, neutropaenia, infections

[a]Niacin equivalents.

glutamine in plasma reflect reduced stores in muscle, and this reduced availability of glutamine in the catabolic state seems to correlate with increased morbidity and mortality. Adding glutamine to the nutrition of clinical patients, either in enteral or parenteral feeds, may reduce morbidity, and several clinical trials have evaluated the efficacy and feasibility of the use of glutamine supplementation. Similarly, arginine may limit immune function and thus be conditionally essential; nutrition that is enhanced in specific nutrients designed to boost immunity is called immunonutrition. Critically ill patients fed a high-protein diet enriched with arginine, fibre, and antioxidants had a significantly lower catheter-related sepsis rate, although there were no differences in mortality or length of hospital stay. The response of under-nourished patients to such immunonutrition is dependent on their prior level of antioxidants and perhaps their genotype.

Requirements for other nutrients

The provision of adequate energy and protein to the patient must be accompanied by other nutrients such as micronutrients and electrolytes. When tissue depletion occurs in under-nutrition, fluid and electrolyte shifts occur, which on feeding the patient can cause problems (discussed in Section 5.9). As stated earlier, diets that are lacking in potassium or phosphorus lead to negative nitrogen balances even when all other nutrients, like energy and protein, are

adequate, while a diet lacking in sodium can reduce the extent of a positive nitrogen balance in malnourished patients receiving an otherwise adequate diet. Similarly, micronutrient deficiencies can interfere with refeeding of under-nourished patients. Body zinc concentrations fall when malnourished patients are fed, and energy supplements to children with protein-energy malnutrition are not effective in the absence of zinc. Further, zinc is also an important micronutrient in diarrhoea and surgical stress. Iron and folic acid are important micronutrients in anaemic patients. In general, a diet lacking in any of the vitamins or minerals will lead to one deficiency symptom or another, even if energy and protein supply are adequate, and will thus interfere with the recovery of the under-nourished patient. Table 5.3 gives the symptoms and signs caused by a deficiency of vitamins and minerals in the body. Overall, it is very important to provide a diet that is balanced in all nutrients. Unbalanced nutrient intakes can often occur in situations where artificial feeding is instituted by the use of elemental mixtures or where energy supplements are given without attention to protein and micronutrients. Specifically, in disease, where requirements for vitamins and minerals are likely to be increased, the risk of deficiencies is elevated.

5.9 Potential problems with nutritional supplementation in under-nutrition

Several complications are possible when delivering nutrients to patients. These range from problems related to aggressive- and over-feeding (discussed later) to those associated specifically with enteral and parenteral nutrition. Gastric retention and the hazard of aspiration of the gastric contents is a complication of enteral feeding. A slow rate of administration of calories is important, as is the evaluation of the food residue in the stomach, particularly in the early stage of feeding. In order to avoid this problem, nasoenteral tubes are used. Another problem linked to enteral feeds is diarrhoea, with associated cramps and nausea. Important reasons for this may be bacterial contamination of feeds or a rapid rate of infusion of the feed. Electrolyte disturbances arising secondary to the diarrhoea should also be investigated.

When total parenteral nutrition (TPN) is given, it is through a central vein, and there are several technical problems that arise with insertion of the catheter. In order to avoid catheter sepsis and other serious complications, it is important to adhere to the guidelines for catheter care. Even with a well-placed and -maintained catheter, metabolic complications can occur. Hyperglycaemia may be the result of the administration of glucose at a faster rate than its utilisation by the body. In addition, illness by itself can also decrease the body's ability to utilise glucose. Other metabolic complications related to electrolyte disturbances are also common, and are discussed later. The metabolic complications of overfeeding can be curtailed by identifying patients at risk, providing adequate assessment, coordinating interdisciplinary care plans, and delivering timely and appropriate monitoring and intervention.

Monitoring the nutritional support given is essential to maintaining metabolic stability and promoting recovery. Complications should be documented, and interventions and the outcomes of clinical care evaluated on a regular basis in order to assess the appropriateness of the nutritional support that is given.

Refeeding syndrome

The refeeding syndrome can occur in patients who are starved or severely under-nourished upon the aggressive reinstitution of adequate nutrition. As soon as depleted patients are given energy and protein supplements, insulin secretion is stimulated, resulting in N retention, with increased cellular protein synthesis, and glycogen storage. There is also an enhanced cellular uptake of glucose, phosphorus, and other minerals such as potassium and magnesium. As a result of these shifts, water and electrolyte disturbances can occur, usually within 4 days of initiating refeeding. The occurrence of low serum phosphate levels, along with low serum potassium and magnesium levels, is particularly important in this context, leading to cardiac arrhythmias or failure, and even death. On the other hand, an expanded extracellular and circulatory volume as a result of fluids administered during refeeding can stress the depleted cardiac muscle in such patients.

Thus it is important to be aware of the refeeding syndrome when starting nutritional therapy for the under-nourished patient. Energy and protein feeding, and the restoration of circulatory volume, should be instituted slowly, with energy intake remaining at only 50–70% of requirements for the first few days. Electrolytes, particularly phosphorus, potassium, and magnesium, should be monitored for abnormalities, especially in the first week. It is also worth administering vitamins routinely and restricting sodium intake. The axiom, 'A little nutrition support is good, too much is lethal,' is apt in this situation, and the goals for nutritional support should be instituted accordingly. In the short term, it is unlikely that protein accretion will take place to a clinically observable extent; what is more important is that previously lost function, such as muscle strength, can be recovered. Overfeeding with energy in an attempt to make the patient gain weight will only result in fat deposition (discussed later) and eventually in clinical complications.

Nutritional supplementation in chronic under-nutrition

It is well known that the refeeding of semistarved individuals leads to an increase in body weight, particularly fat, as described by Keys *et al.* (1950). Studies on energy repletion (with low-protein supplements) of individuals with a low BMI for about 6 weeks showed that the body weight increased, but also that a large part of the weight gained was fat. This pattern of weight gain was altered when these individuals were given extra protein repletion in addition to their energy-replete diets, where an increase in protein intake to about 2 g/kg/day (compared to about 0.6 g/kg/day in their habitual diets) in addition to the increased energy intake led to an increase in the FFM, in terms of both muscle and visceral mass. While body fat continued to increase, its rate of increase relative to the body-weight change was slower. This suggests that a healthier pattern of weight gain can be achieved by paying attention to protein intake. Significant improvements in VO_2 max after protein and energy feeding has also been observed, due to an improvement in muscle mass, but this is not observed with energy supplementation alone. It is also important that an appropriate level of physical activity is followed, in order to regain muscle mass.

The potential for an increase in fat stores on refeeding raises important public-health issues related to the epidemic of type 2 diabetes and coronary heart disease (CHD) in transitioning populations in developing countries. Asians and Mexican Americans seem to have a higher amount of body fat at a given BMI, and it is thought that insulin resistance is related to circulating concentrations of the proinflammatory cytokines secreted by adipose tissue, such as TNFα, and, in conditions where there is a higher possibility of subclinical infections, this may be a significant factor in the development of insulin resistance. A common thread that runs through these observations is the role of accumulated body fat in general, which points to a dual problem, particularly in developing countries: while CED will remain a major public health problem, economic growth and development may lead to an equally large burden of chronic disease. Appropriate preventative measures that avoid excessive nutrient intake, as well as the aggressive promotion of healthier lifestyles, will be needed.

5.10 Prevention

It is relatively common for patients who are admitted into hospital to become under-nourished. There are several reasons why under-nutrition can occur: it could be due to a reduced food intake or to increased requirements for nutrients. The questions that need to be asked are whether under-nutrition affects patients' clinical outcome, and therefore, should it be treated?

Further, does treating malnutrition have a beneficial effect on the clinical outcome? There is little doubt that under-nutrition affects the clinical outcome in terms of recovery, lower morbidity, hospital stay, and even quality of life in under-nourished patients, and therefore there is little doubt that it should be treated. A further question is how much a lack of feeding can be tolerated without ill effect, in both normally-nourished and under-nourished patients. For the latter group, it seems clear that feeding should be instituted as quickly as possible, building up rapidly to full-strength feeding. In normally-nourished patients, it appears that a week of low nutrient intake can be tolerated without ill effect; this can happen, for instance, during the course of elective surgery. However, it should be reiterated that it is best to feed patients as soon as it is possible to do so.

The beneficial effect of nutritional support in patients is more difficult to establish, given that studies are done over short periods of time in heterogeneous patient populations with different treatment regimens. For many diseases complicated by malnutrition, strong data are still lacking in terms of the beneficial effect of nutritional support on disease outcome, due to the many confounders that exist when such clinical trials are done. This task becomes even more difficult with seriously ill patients. However, there is evidence available to suggest that nutritional intervention in under-nourished patients is beneficial in changing their clinical outcome. Studies on perioperative nutritional support have shown benefits in terms of post-operative outcomes, and malnourished patients with fractured hips have also been demonstrated to recover their post-operative ability to walk sooner when they are given nutritional support. The clear course to follow clinically is to institute nutritional support promptly, in a moderate and balanced manner, after an assessment to define what the goals of nutrition are, and to follow this up with careful monitoring of the patient to prevent complications.

5.11 Concluding remarks

What is the future for the problem of under-nutrition? A challenge that still exists is to be able to diagnose the functional consequences of under-nutrition at an early stage, with a reasonable specificity. For example, while tests for muscle functions exist, there is a need to assess other functional parameters, such as cognition and gut and immune function. These tests also need to be validated for their specificity, given that there is so much variability in function.

Several functional nutritional supplements are available, based on physiological evidence for the requirement of specific nutrients in specific situations. A novel method for the delivery of nutrients such as glutamine, through the use of dipeptides, is another area of development. However, the administration of individual specific nutrient substrates (arginine, glutamine, different types of triglycerides and short-chain fatty acids) has the potential to produce a variety of metabolic responses, which could be both beneficial and harmful. These effects depend on the type and quantity of substance infused, the quality of methodology in the study, and the disease and clinical condition of the patient. For example, immunonutrition with arginine, glutamine, nucleotides, or ω-3 fatty acids either alone or in combination is said to decrease infectious complication rates. However, it has also been suggested that severe systemic inflammation might even be intensified by arginine and unsaturated fatty acids, through their direct effect on cellular defence and the inflammatory response; therefore, caution should be exercised when using immune-enhancing substrates that might actually aggravate systemic inflammation. The same reasoning is true for those substances, such as growth hormone and IGF-1, that are being evaluated for their effects in improving protein accretion and the immune response of the body. While the development of new substrates, modulators, and pharmaconutrition is likely to improve the outcome for many patients, overall, for a clinical benefit, one must differentiate between information about the effects of individual substrates on the metabolic response to illness and information on clinical outcomes, particularly in the long term. Another issue of importance is the need for information that will define the cost-efficacy of artificial nutrition across a broad spectrum of clinical practice.

More studies are required to evaluate the interaction between those parts of an individual's genotype relevant to the response to injury/infection, nutrients, and prior nutritional status. It can be anticipated that an optimal mixture of glucose, fat, and protein, along with specific nutrients and modulators (to create something like a dream diet), will prove beneficial for specific conditions, but it is prudent to evaluate these in terms of specific beneficial and adverse clinical outcomes, since, with many novel nutrients, there is perhaps a danger of creating specialised fads in the place of specialised foods.

Nutritional support for the under-nourished has the possibility of adverse effects. This is well-documented clinically and in acute under-nutrition. The effect of nutritional supplementation in under-nutrition needs to be evaluated for its potential long-term adverse effects, since it seems likely that a large part of the weight gain will be fat.

References and further reading

Akner G, Cederholm T. Treatment of protein–energy malnutrition in chronic nonmalignant disorders. Am J Clin Nutr 2001; 74: 6–24.

Bouchard C, Tremblay A, Despres JP, Theriault G, Nadeau A, Lupien PJ, Moorjani S, Prudhomme D, Fournier G. The response to exercise with constant energy intake in identical twins. Obes Res 1994; 2: 400–410.

Detsky AA, McLaughlin JR, Baker JP, Johnston N, Whittaker S, Mendelson RA, Jeejeebhoy KN. What is subjective global assessment of nutritional status? JPEN 1987; 11: 8–13.

Elia M. Organ and tissue contribution to metabolic rate. In: Energy Metabolism. Tissue determinants and cellular corollaries (JH Kinney, H Tucker, eds). New York: Raven Press, 1991, pp. 61–80.

Elwyn DH. Nutritional requirements of adult surgical patients. Crit Care Med 1980; 8: 9–20.

FAO/WHO/UNU. Human Energy Requirements. Report of a joint FAO/WHO/UNU consultation. Food and Nutrition Technical Report Series 1. Rome: FAO, 2004.

Gonzalez-Gross M, Marcos A, Pietrzik K. Nutrition and cognitive impairment in the elderly. Br J Nutr 2001; 86: 313–321.

Grimble RF. Nutritional modulation of immune function. Proc Nutr Soc 2001; 60: 389–397.

Heymsfield SB, Wang Z, Baumgartner RN, Ross R. Human body composition: advances in models and methods. Ann Rev Nutr 1997; 17: 527–558. Available from http://www.who.int/nutrition/publications/severemalnutrition/9789241598163_eng.pdf.

Jensen GL, McGee M, Binkley J. Nutrition in the elderly. Gastroenterol Clin North Am 2001; 30: 313–334.

Jensen GL, Mirtallo J, Compher C, Dhaliwal R, Forbes A, Grijalba RF, Hardy G, Kondrup J, Labadarios D, Nyulasi I, Castillo Pineda JC, Waitzberg D. Adult starvation and disease-related malnutrition: a proposal for etiology-based diagnosis in the clinical practice setting from the International Consensus Guideline Committee. JPEN 2010; 34: 156–159.

Keys A, Brozek J, Henschel A, Mickelson O, Taylor HL. The biology of human starvation. St Paul, MN: University of Minnesota Press, 1950.

Millward DJ, Layman DK, Tomé D, Schaafsma G. Protein quality assessment: impact of expanding understanding of protein and amino acid needs for optimal health. Am J Clin Nutr 2008; 87: 1576S–1581S.

NIH Technology Assessment Conference Statement. Bioelectrical impedance analysis in body composition measurement. 1994.

Quevedo MR, Price GM, Halliday D, Pacy PJ, Millward DJ. Nitrogen homoeostasis in man: diurnal changes in nitrogen excretion, leucine oxidation and whole body leucine kinetics during a reduction from a high to a moderate protein intake. Clin Sci 1994; 86: 185–193.

Reeds J. Dispensable and indispensable amino acids for humans. J Nutr 2000; 130(7): 1835S–1840S.

National Advisory Group on Standards and Practice Guidelines for Parenteral Nutrition. Safe practices for parenteral nutrition formulations. JPEN 1998; 22: 15–19.

Soeters PB, Reijven PLM, van der Schueren MAE, Schols JMGA, Halfens RJG, Meijers JMM, van Gemert WG. A rational approach to nutritional assessment. Clin Nutr 2008; 27: 706–716.

Waterlow JC. Metabolic adaptation to low intakes of energy and protein. Ann Rev Nutr 1986; 6: 495–526.

WHO. Community based management of severe acute malnutrition. A Joint Statement by the World Health Organization, the World Food Programme, the United Nations System Standing Committee on Nutrition and the United Nations Children's Fund. Available from http://www.who.int/nutrition/topics/Statement_community_based_man_sev_acute_mal_eng.pdf. Accessed 17 September 2001.

WHO. WHO child growth standards and the identification of severe acute malnutrition in infants and children. A Joint Statement by the World Health Organization and the United Nations Children's Fund.

WHO/FAO/UNU Expert Consultation. Protein and Amino Acid Requirements in Human Nutrition. Technical Report No 935. Geneva: World Health Organization, 2007.

6
Metabolic Disorders

Luc Tappy[1] and Jean-Marc Schwarz[2]

[1]University of Lausanne, Switzerland
[2]Touro University, California USA

Key messages

- The prevalence of noncommunicable diseases such as obesity, diabetes, dyslipidaemia, cardiovascular diseases, nonalcoholic fatty liver disease (NAFLD), and cancer has increased substantially in European and North American populations.
- A similar trend is now being observed in many countries within Africa and South-East Asia, and also in China, which appears to be related to improvements in average income and industrialisation/urbanisation.
- Morbidity is positively correlated with body mass index (BMI), even within the normal range of 20–25 kg/m². The hypothesis that a low energy intake is associated with an increased lifespan is supported by animal studies.
- Energy restriction is associated with increased lifespan and lower morbidity in animal models and in humans. Proposed mecha-

- nisms are decreased oxidative stress, improved DNA repair, and lower lipotoxicity due to sirtuins activation.
- The concomitant occurrence of visceral obesity, impaired glucose tolerance or type 2 diabetes, hypertension, and dyslipidaemia is known as the 'metabolic syndrome'. Insulin resistance and an excess of visceral fat appear to play a pathogenic role in each of these conditions.
- These metabolic disorders, or diseases of affluence, can be attributed not only to dietary factors but also to decreased physical activity and other environmental factors. It is also likely that the genetic background of individuals plays an important role.

6.1 Introduction

The average life expectancy of European and North American populations increased drastically during the second half of the twentieth century. This is essentially attributable to a marked reduction of the mortality associated with infectious diseases. In contrast, the prevalence and mortality associated with noncommunicable diseases, such as cardiovascular diseases, cancer, diabetes, and obesity, have increased substantially. A similar trend is currently evident in many countries within Africa and South-East Asia, and also in China, which appears to be related to improvements in average income and industrialisation/urbanisation. This epidemiological evolution suggests that the development of these diseases is strongly dependent on the way of life of affluent societies. This

may stop or even reverse the trend of increased life expectancy in some countries, because of the years of life lost by individuals as a result of obesity.

The wealth of a nation impacts indisputably on the way of life of its population. As a result of industrialisation, individuals switch from physically active, rural occupations to more sedentary factory and office jobs. The higher income associated with these jobs also promotes the use of automated housework devices, cars, and so on, which leads to a substantial reduction in physical-activity levels. Simultaneously, the mode of feeding and the types of macronutrient consumed are altered as a consequence of urban living. This includes changes in market food availability and increases in consumption of fast food and meals in restaurants. The urban feeding pattern is associated with an increased consumption of processed

Clinical Nutrition, Second Edition. Edited by Marinos Elia, Olle Ljungqvist, Rebecca J Stratton and Susan A Lanham-New.
© 2013 The Nutrition Society. Published 2013 by Blackwell Publishing Ltd.

foods with a higher proportion of fat and sugar when compared with traditional, rural diets containing high-fibre/high-complex carbohydrate foods. These changes in lifestyle are thought to be involved in the pathogenesis of nontransmissible diseases. For example, obesity has dramatically increased over the past century. While rare at the beginning of the twentieth century, it now affects 20–50% of European and North American populations. The marked increase in childhood obesity over the past two or three decades, together with the growing occurrence of type 2 diabetes mellitus in children and young adults, is of particular concern.

The development of obesity stems from an imbalance between energy intake and energy expenditure. There is evidence that energy density, portion size, and the frequency of eating/drinking occasions are contributing to a significant increase in the amount of food calories consumed per capita. From 1977 to 2006, calorie consumption is estimated to have increased by 570 kcal/day in the USA. Other studies clearly indicate that the amount of energy expended through physical activity has dropped during this period. Based on measurements of energy fluxes, it appears that a high energy intake and a low energy expenditure both play a role in the development of obesity.

In addition to nutritional changes and alterations in physical activity, other factors also affect the pattern of diseases in affluent societies. For instance, there is an important increase in the consumption of alcohol and other addictive substances which can be viewed as a consequence of affluence. Chapter 4 deals with over-nutrition; this chapter will essentially focus on the effects of caloric intake on health and its role in the pathogenesis of metabolic disorders (obesity-related metabolic alterations, type 2 diabetes, and hypertension). In addition, the effects of alcohol as a source of calories will be considered.

6.2 Energy intake, health and longevity

In order for individuals to maintain a constant body composition, energy intake must be balanced with energy expenditure. Resting energy expenditure is proportional to body mass (or more specifically, to lean body mass) and hence is increased in obese patients. As a consequence, at similar physical-activity levels, weight-stable obese patients have higher energy requirements and energy intakes in comparison to nonobese individuals. This has to be compensated by an increased food intake in order to maintain a higher body weight over time.

Excessive body weight, together with a high total energy intake, clearly has deleterious effects on health. This is illustrated by the very significant association between body mass index (BMI), an index of adiposity, and morbidity for various diseases. At the other end of the spectrum, an insufficient energy intake will lead to weight loss, which can be associated with muscle and organ wasting, immune dysfunction, and hence adverse health outcomes. Between these two extremes of obesity and underweight, there is however a full range of energy intakes which allow the maintenance of an individual BMI between 19 and 25 kg/m². This wide variation illustrates that a normal body weight and food intake are not easily defined. It appears, however, that morbidity is positively correlated with BMI even within the normal range of 19–25 kg/m² and that the Asian population may have an increased risk at a lower BMI threshold.

The hypothesis that a low energy intake (but above the starvation threshold) is associated with an increased lifespan is supported by animal studies. In protozoans, insects, rodents, and non-human primates, energy restriction reduces the incidence of diseases and extends lifespan. This suggests that the level of energy intake and/or metabolic factors modulates the ageing process. Several hypotheses can be proposed to explain these effects of caloric restriction. A low energy intake reduces body weight and the weight of most individual organs (with the exception of the brain). In some studies, energy restriction lowers the rate of oxygen consumption per kilogram of lean body weight, indicating that tissue metabolism is reduced. In relation with this lowering of tissue metabolic rate, energy restriction decreases the synthesis of reactive oxygen species, and hence the oxidative stress imposed on the organism. The reactive oxygen species generated during oxidative stress cause enzyme deactivations, induce DNA mutations, or alter cell membranes (Figure 6.1).

Energy restriction may also result in a reduction in plasma glucose and insulin concentrations, and an improved insulin sensitivity. In this context, it is of

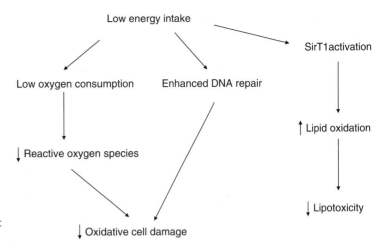

Figure 6.1 Putative mechanisms linking caloric intake with longevity.

interest that a gene associated with longevity in *Caenorhabditis elegans* belongs to the family of the insulin receptor gene. Energy restriction has also been shown to be associated with the induction of DNA repair systems. Ageing and energy restriction have opposite effects on tissue gene expression: ageing is associated with an increased expression of genes involved in the stress response in the skeletal muscle of mice, including acute-phase proteins, inflammatory mediators, and inducible DNA repair systems; energy restriction has the opposite effect, which suggests that there is induction of a stress response as a result of damaged proteins during ageing. This response may be secondary to a decrease in cellular systems involved in turnover of cellular constituents. Energy restriction, by increasing the expression of genes coding for biosynthetic processes, may attenuate the effects of ageing. It appears that a family of intracellular proteins, sirtuins, is involved in the adaptation of gene expression to calorie restriction. Sirtuins are a class of proteins that possess histone deacetylase or mono-ribosyltransferase activity, and they have been shown to be involved metabolic adaptations to stress, ageing, and energy deficiency. Sirtuin activation induced by energy deficiency leads to an activation of genes involved in lipid oxidation. Mice submitted to a severe energy restriction maintain constant energy expenditure and increase their physical activity, but these effects are abolished in mice lacking SirT1, a member of the sirtuin family. Energy restriction also failed to increase the lifespan of these sirtuin-deficient mice. Resveratrol, a natural plant phenol,

activates sirtuins, but its effects on lifespan in animal models are still under investigation.

6.3 The metabolic syndrome

Obesity, impaired glucose tolerance or type 2 diabetes, hypertension, dyslipidaemia, and nonalcoholic fatty liver disease (NAFLD) are diseases of major importance in Western societies (Box 6.1). Nutritional imbalances and, more specifically, excess calorie intake play a recognised role in the pathogenesis of each of these conditions. Furthermore, these metabolic diseases often appear together, with two or more of them being present in the same individual. The concomitant occurrence of these alterations has therefore been renamed the 'metabolic syndrome'. Additional features of the syndrome are hyperuricaemia, impaired fibrinolysis secondary to high plasminogen-activator inhibitor concentrations in blood, and ectopic lipid deposition in liver cells (NAFLD) and muscle.

The concomitant occurrence of obesity, hypertension, dyslipidaemia, and impaired glucose tolerance/diabetes has led to the search for a common factor of origin. Insulin resistance and hyperinsulinaemia are frequently observed in association with all the above abnormalities, and may represent a common pathogenic link. The presence of excess intra-abdominal fat and mesenteric fat depots is also closely associated with individual features of the metabolic syndrome. Furthermore, for any given body fat content, fat distribution in the visceral rather than subcutaneous

> ### Box 6.1 The metabolic syndrome: WHO criteria
>
> Main features:
>
> - type 2 diabetes/impaired glucose tolerance/insulin resistance;
> - and at least two of the following:
>   - visceral obesity;
>   - dyslipidaemia (high LDL cholesterol, low HDL cholesterol, high triglycerides);
>   - hypertension;
>   - hyperuricaemia;
>   - high fibrinogen microalbuminuria;
>   - NAFLD.
>
> Associated with hyperinsulinaemia/insulin resistance.

compartment is more closely associated with insulin resistance. Central, visceral obesity may therefore be a common feature linking all constituents of the metabolic syndrome. The mechanisms responsible for preferential deposition of visceral fat in some predisposed individuals are not yet fully understood. Males appear to be at higher risk than females, indicating a role of sex hormones; glucocorticoids and exposure to stress are known to favour visceral fat deposition. However, additional genetic or nutritional factors are also likely to be involved.

6.4 Pathophysiology of insulin resistance

Insulin exerts several different actions at the level of various tissues. Regulation of glucose metabolism is a major action of insulin. In skeletal muscle, adipose tissue, fibroblasts, and several other tissues, insulin increases glucose uptake, oxidation, and storage. These effects are largely secondary to the effect of insulin on specific proteins involved in the facilitated diffusion of glucose from the interstitial space into the cells. In tissues where glucose metabolism is not dependent on insulin concentrations, cells constitutively express glucose-transporter protein isoforms (e.g. GLUT1, GLUT3) on the cell surface. The permanent presence of these proteins on the cell membrane ensures a continuous entry of glucose into the cells. Insulin-sensitive tissues (skeletal muscle, adipose tissue, etc.) express a specific isoform of glucose transporter, GLUT4. GLUT4 has the special feature in that it can be essentially sequestrated into the cells

when insulin receptors are not occupied by insulin. When the insulin concentration increases (for example, after a carbohydrate meal), stimulation of insulin receptors on the surface of the cells triggers the rapid migration of GLUT4 from intracellular stores to the plasma membrane. This allows a rapid, several-fold increase in the number of glucose transporters present at the cell surface, and hence the entry of glucose into the cell.

In addition, insulin activates or inhibits several key intracellular enzymes involved in glucose, fat, and amino acid metabolism. At the level of liver cells, it inhibits glucose production. Some of these effects are due to the interaction of insulin with insulin receptors at the target cell surface and activation of complex intracellular transduction mechanisms. A substantial number of these actions on glucose metabolism can be attributed, however, to indirect effects of insulin (i.e. actions exerted on other cell types, which in turn regulate glucose metabolism in distinct cells). Thus, the decrease in free fatty acids produced by insulin contributes substantially to an increased glucose oxidation in skeletal muscle and an inhibition of glucose production in the liver.

Insulin also regulates lipid metabolism. In adipose tissue, it inhibits lipolysis and free fatty acid release. In skeletal muscle, it decreases lipid oxidation by inhibiting the transport of acyl CoA into the mitochondria. In hepatocytes, it suppresses ketogenesis. Insulin also exerts regulatory effects on protein metabolism by stimulating whole-body protein synthesis and inhibiting protein breakdown. In addition to its metabolic actions, insulin also affects a number of other processes: it stimulates Na reabsorption by the kidney, decreases K^+ concentrations through an activation of Na/K ATPase, produces vasodilation in skeletal muscle, increases the sympathetic nervous system activity, and exerts growth-promoting effects.

Insulin affects these different processes with various levels of effectiveness (Figure 6.2). Inhibition of lipolysis and the production of ketone bodies are already half-maximal at insulin concentrations about twice basal values. Stimulations of vasodilation and sympathetic nerve activity are also attained at low insulin concentrations. In contrast, half-maximal stimulation of glucose transport and oxidation requires higher insulin concentrations (about 10–20 times basal concentrations).

Sensitivity to insulin of various processes

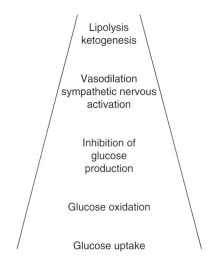

Figure 6.2 Insulin concentrations required to half-maximally affect various metabolic steps. This illustrates the differential insulin sensitivity of various tissues.

6.5 Insulin resistance

Insulin resistance corresponds to blunted insulin actions in the presence of normal or increased insulin concentrations. Insulin resistance often refers to a decreased stimulation of glucose metabolism in response to a given concentration of insulin. It can be documented *in vitro* (decreased insulin-induced glucose transport on isolated cell preparation) or *in vivo* (decreased whole-body glucose utilisation in response to insulin infusion). Insulin resistance has been reported in various clinical conditions: obesity and type 2 diabetes mellitus, dyslipidaemia, essential hypertension, and many others. Even in healthy individuals, a wide range of insulin sensitivity is observed, and a substantial portion of the normal population can be considered 'insulin resistant'. Several factors may be involved in insulin resistance (Box 6.2). Body visceral fat mass is a strong determinant of insulin sensitivity; obese patients with central, visceral obesity generally have a substantial decrease in insulin responsiveness.

In healthy individuals, insulin sensitivity is a familial trait, which suggests that (as-yet-unidentified) genetic factors are involved. Ethnic factors (possibly partly linked to genetics) are also involved: obese black African, Asian and Hispanic Americans tend to

have a more severe insulin resistance than Caucasians of a comparable BMI. Dietary factors are also involved; excess energy intake leads to obesity and insulin resistance. In addition, high-fat diets or high-fructose diets can lead to the development of insulin resistance in rodents and/or humans. In population studies, many reports indicate a relationship between total sugar intake (and/or intake of beverages sweetened with sucrose or high-fructose corn syrup) and obesity, diabetes, dyslipidaemia, and cardiovascular risk factors. Finally, physical fitness and habitual physical activity are important factors which modulate insulin sensitivity. Physical training clearly improves the action of insulin, although the multiple possible mechanisms are not yet fully understood. A lower body fat mass, an increased skeletal muscle mass, and alterations of muscle oxidative enzymes induced by training may all be involved.

Insulin resistance appears to affect specific insulin-sensitive pathways but leave other pathways unaffected. Thus, it has been shown that insulin-mediated glucose utilisation is impaired in obese patients, while the antilipolytic effects of insulin (decreased lipolysis per unit fat mass) remain modestly affected. Similarly, stimulation of kidney Na reabsorption and possibly of sympathetic nervous system activity may not be impaired. Since regulatory feedback mechanisms lead to an increased insulin secretion and development of hyperinsulinaemia in insulin-resistant individuals, this differential tissue insulin resistance may lead to overstimulation of some insulin-sensitive processes by hyperinsulinaemia. For example, this may account for the increased muscle sympathetic nerve activity and kidney Na reabsorption in obese hyperinsulinaemic individuals.

The molecular mechanisms responsible for decreased insulin effectiveness are currently under debate. A decreased translocation of GLUT4 in response to insulin may be involved, and this may be the consequence of alterations in the insulin receptor or signalling cascade. There is evidence that insulin resistance in skeletal muscle, which accounts for the major portion of the decreased insulin-mediated glucose disposal in obese diabetic patients, may be secondary to alterations of adipose tissue metabolism. This concept is supported by the observation that elevated free fatty acid concentrations acutely decrease insulin sensitivity in humans by decreasing muscle glucose transport and oxidation. In addition, activation of peroxisome proliferator-activated receptor gamma (PPARγ), which is essentially expressed in adipose cell, increases insulin sensitivity *in vivo*. Our present understanding is that it is tightly linked to altered lipid metabolism. As a consequence of increased body fat mass, the total flux of non-esterified fatty acids (NEFA) is frequently increased in obese subjects. This is especially marked in subjects with visceral obesity because omental adipocytes, which constitute visceral fat depots, are particularly lipolytic. Furthermore, lipolysis in visceral adipocytes releases NEFA directly in the portal vein, thus exposing the liver to an excess of NEFA. NEFA reesterification in the liver can in turn produce both an accumulation of intrahepatic lipids and an enhanced secretion of very low-density lipoprotein triglycerides (VLDL-TGs). While the bulk of VLDL-TGs are subsequently delivered and stored in the adipose tissue, some may be taken up by muscle and accumulate as intramyocellular lipids. An excess accumulation of triglycerides in liver cells (now recognised as NAFLD, a highly prevalent disease in obese subjects) and in muscle can then occur. This excess fat load may exert so-called 'lipotoxic effects' in tissue, which impair insulin signalling. Intracellular metabolites, such as di-acyl-glycerol and ceramides, may be involved.

6.6 The role of affluence in diabetes, dyslipidaemia, and essential hypertension

We will only briefly review here the role of nutritional changes associated with affluence and insulin resistance in the pathogenesis of these disorders.

Type 2 diabetes mellitus

Until now, this disorder has been highly prevalent in Europe and North America but uncommon in

> **Box 6.3 Pathogenesis of hyperglycaemia in type 2 diabetes**
>
> - impaired glucose-induced insulin secretion;
> - insulin resistance (skeletal muscle, adipose tissue);
> - increased endogenous glucose production (hepatic insulin resistance).

emergent countries. However, recent data indicate a sharp increase of this disorder in South America, North Africa, and South-East Asia. Type 2 diabetes is a complex disease, in which genetic factors, nutritional factors, and environment are involved. It is frequently, but not invariably, associated with overweight or obesity. The development of hyperglycaemia in type 2 diabetes results in an increase in fasting glucose production and a decreased postprandial glucose utilisation. The latter is the consequence of impaired glucose-induced insulin secretion and of insulin resistance (Box 6.3). Nutritional factors may impact both processes.

Insulin secretion is impaired in type 2 diabetes. Plasma insulin and C peptide concentrations may be decreased, normal, or even increased. The first phase of insulin secretion in response to intravenous glucose is impaired, while insulin secretion after oral glucose is delayed. When insulin secretion is related to plasma glucose concentration, a decreased glucose-induced insulin secretion is observed. The mechanism at the origin of a decreased insulin secretion in type 2 diabetes remains unknown. Based on the observation that a low glucose-induced insulin secretion is a familial trait, genetic factors can be suspected. Several monogenic forms of diabetes are due to a reduced insulin secretion secondary to mutations of beta cell transcriptional factors (HNF1α, HNF4α, HNF4β, PDX-1). It is therefore possible that alterations of other transcription factors are also involved in type 2 diabetes but have not yet been identified.

Nutritional factors may also be involved, and there is considerable evidence that fatty acids are involved in the control of insulin secretion. Long-chain fatty acids increase insulin secretion of islet cells *in vivo* and *in vitro* in the short term. This effect is due to a stimulation of insulin release by long-chain fatty acid CoA. In contrast, incubation of islet cells in the presence of elevated levels of fatty acid over several days impairs insulin release. This effect is concomitant with accumulation of triglyceride in the islet cells. It is therefore possible that energy and fat overfeeding decrease insulin secretion through a lipotoxicity on islet beta cells.

Insulin resistance is observed at various degrees in type 2 diabetes. It is severe in obese patients and moderate to low in lean patients. Although the inhibition of insulin actions may in part be genetically determined, evidence suggests that much of it is acquired. Weight loss significantly improves insulin resistance in obese type 2 diabetic patients. Energy restriction rapidly enhances insulin sensitivity before any significant changes in body composition take place. This indicates that energy intake may be as important as, or more important than, body fat in determining insulin actions.

Part of the insulin resistance observed in obese type 2 diabetes may be related to the increased free fatty acid concentrations. As a consequence of increased body fat mass, the rate of whole-body lipolysis is increased in obese patients, resulting in elevated free fatty acid concentrations. Elevated free fatty acid concentrations in turn inhibit insulin-mediated glucose disposal by decreasing insulin-mediated glucose transport and oxidation. The exact mechanism by which fatty acid exerts these effects is not known. Nonetheless, a role of fatty acid in the insulin resistance of obese type 2 diabetic patients is substantiated by the observation that antilipolytic agents improve insulin sensitivity.

Infusion of lipid emulsion, which increases free fatty acid concentrations, acutely inhibits insulin-mediated glucose disposal and hence produces insulin resistance in humans. No such effect is observed after addition of fat to a carbohydrate meal. This can be explained by the fact that dietary lipids reach the circulation as chylomicrons, which are hydrolysed locally in adipose tissue capillaries. The free fatty acids liberated are essentially used for triglyceride resynthesis in the adipocyte, and the plasma free fatty acid concentrations do not increase. High-fat feeding is nonetheless associated with the development of insulin resistance in animal models and in humans, but the mechanisms remain unclear. A high intake of saturated fat may increase intracellular lipid stores, particularly in skeletal muscle. Alternatively, it has been proposed that changes in plasma-membrane lipid composition may be involved.

Apart from its actions on intracellular metabolism, insulin also results in vasodilation of skeletal muscle and adipose tissue. This facilitates the stimulation of glucose metabolism by increasing the delivery of glucose and of insulin itself to insulin-sensitive tissues. This effect is mediated by an endothelial release of nitric oxide (NO). NO is produced by endothelial cells from arginine through the action of endothelial NO synthase in response to various local stimuli, including shear stress. The released NO diffuses within the vascular wall and is a major factor in relaxing vascular smooth-muscle cells. The vasodilatory effects of insulin are decreased in obese and type 2 diabetic patients, which may contribute to insulin resistance. Again, a role of free fatty acids has been postulated in this impairment of NO synthesis by endothelial cells of obese patients.

Insulin resistance and dyslipidaemia

Overweight and obesity are frequently associated with elevated plasma triglyceride concentrations and decreased high-density lipoprotein (HDL) concentrations. High carbohydrate feeding can induce such changes in plasma lipid profile. It appears that insulin resistance may play a role in the pathogenesis of these alterations. In insulin-resistant obese subjects, free fatty acids are released from the adipose tissue as a result of both insulin resistance in adipose tissue and enhanced body fat mass. Activation by insulin of lipoprotein lipase is reduced, resulting in decreased clearance of triglyceride-rich lipoprotein particles. Insulin resistance also results in increased insulin secretion and hyperinsulinaemia. In the liver cells, high insulin concentrations in the presence of an increased free fatty acid supply lead to increased triglyceride synthesis and secretion of very low-density lipoproteins (VLDLs). In addition, insulin may stimulate liver conversion of carbohydrate to fat or hepatic *de novo* lipogenesis.

Dietary management of the metabolic syndrome

Given the key role played by insulin resistance in the pathogenesis of this syndrome, its dietary management and that of directly related metabolic disorders are essentially aimed at improving insulin sensitivity (Box 6.4).

The keystone of this dietary management is to avoid overfeeding and hence to provide a daily amount of energy corresponding to the energy need of an individual with a normal BMI between 20 and 25. It is important to note that an obese individual expends substantially more energy than a nonobese individual of similar height, and hence will progressively lose weight if fed the corresponding amount of energy.

Diet composition also affects insulin sensitivity. A diet high in simple carbohydrates is associated with high postprandial plasma glucose, high insulin concentrations, and low insulin sensitivity. Excessive amounts of simple sugars such as sucrose and fructose are associated with the development of insulin resistance, dyslipidaemia, and hypertension. On the other hand, diets high in saturated fat also induce the development of insulin resistance and dyslipidaemia. The current concepts favour two alternative approaches: high-carbohydrate, fibre-rich diets and high-monounsaturated fat diets, the relative benefits of which remain debated. A low saturated fat and sugar intake is the common denominator of these two diets and appears to be of importance in preventing insulin resistance, together with a low salt intake to prevent high blood pressure.

Encouragement of regular physical activity should be an integral part of the dietary management of the metabolic syndrome. The improved physical fitness associated with physical activity leads to enhanced insulin sensitivity, increased levels of protective HDL cholesterol, and prevention of excess weight gain.

Insulin resistance and hypertension

Hypertension is frequently encountered in insulin-resistant patients. Moreover, essential hypertension (but not secondary hypertension) is associated with decreased insulin sensitivity even in lean individuals. Several mechanisms may be involved in increasing blood pressure in insulin-resistant patients. Hyperinsulinaemia stimulates muscle sympathetic nerve activity and this may increase arterial vasoconstrictive tone. Hyperinsulinaemia also stimulates Na^+ reabsorption in the kidney, which may contribute to the pathogenesis of hypertension. Finally, as mentioned in the previous section, insulin resistance is often associated with increased plasma fatty acid concentrations. Such increased fatty acid concentrations have been shown to produce endothelial dysfunction, and may be responsible for the absence of insulin-induced vasodilation. This mechanism may contribute to insulin resistance. In addition, endothelial dysfunction may be responsible for enhanced responses to sympathetic stimulations, such as mental stress, and therefore contribute to the pathogenesis of hypertension (Figure 6.3).

6.7 Alcohol

As a consequence of affluence, the consumption of drugs, tobacco, and alcohol has increased. This is likely to have a significant impact on public health. Alcohol consumption shows large interindividual variability, ranging from 0 to more than 100 g/day. On average, however, it represents up to 10% of total calorie intake in many European countries. Alcohol is essentially metabolised in the liver, where it can be converted into acetaldehyde through the actions of three distinct enzymatic systems: alcohol dehydrogenase, the microsomial

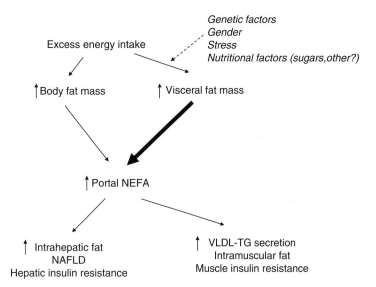

Figure 6.3 Possible mechanisms linking insulin resistance with the metabolic syndrome.

ethanol-oxidising system, and catalase. In most nonhabitual drinkers, alcohol dehydrogenase represents the major pathway for alcohol metabolism. In habitual drinkers, the contribution of the microsomial ethanol oxidation system increases due to its induction by ethanol. A small amount of ethanol is metabolised by catalase. After ethanol administration, plasma ethanol concentration first increases rapidly and then decreases more or less linearly, indicating a constant rate of conversion into acetaldehyde and acetate. The average rate of alcohol metabolism is about 100 mg/kg/hour, but shows considerable interindividual variability.

Excess ethanol intake has well-known deleterious effects on the liver, resulting in hepatic steatosis, steatohepatitis, and alcoholic liver cirrhosis. Alcohol consumption is also associated with gastritis and peptic ulcer disease and can lead to acquired cardiomyopathy, myopathy, and neuropsychiatric disorders. This chapter will deal briefly with the effect of alcoholic consumption on body-weight control and cardiovascular risk factors.

Alcohol and body weight

The net effect of alcohol consumption on body weight remains poorly understood. Both retrospective dietary surveys and experimental prospective studies indicate that addition of alcoholic calories to the diet does not inhibit consumption of nonalcoholic calories. As a consequence, alcohol consumption is estimated to increase total calorie intake. On the other hand, epidemiological studies show no clear association between alcohol intake and excess body weight. Some studies even show a negative correlation between alcohol intake and body weight in women. This discrepancy may suggest that alcohol calories are not efficiently utilised and may be wasted as heat loss. If this were the case, however, one would expect that energy expenditure would increase unduly after alcohol consumption. Experimental studies do not support this concept. The increase in energy expenditure observed after ingestion of alcohol corresponds to about 20% of its energy content. This can largely be attributed to the expected energy cost of alcohol metabolism. There is indeed an obligatory consumption of ATP for conversion of alcohol into acetaldehyde. Based on this ATP consumption, it can be calculated that the thermic effect of alcohol metabolism through the alcohol dehydrogenase pathway is about 15%, and that through the microsomial ethanol-oxidising system about 30%. The measured thermic effect of alcohol falls between these two values, suggesting that there are no significant additional heat losses. This indicates that alcoholic calories are used efficiently to provide energy to the organism.

Further studies indicate that alcoholic calories essentially replace fat as a fuel source when available. The reasons for the absence of a relationship between alcohol intake and body weight therefore remain unknown. It is possible that alcohol consumption stimulates the energy expended in physical activity, or exerts other unrecognised effects on energy intake or expenditure.

Alcohol and blood lipids

Moderate alcohol consumption increases plasma HDL cholesterol concentrations through unknown mechanisms. This effect improves the atherogenic risk profile, and may be involved in the reduction of cardiovascular and overall mortality observed in moderate drinkers.

Alcohol consumption has also been associated with increased plasma triglyceride levels. This effect is particularly observed in overweight individuals. The rise in triglycerides is mainly associated with the VLDL fraction. The exact mechanism remains unknown, but is thought to involve increased free fatty acid reesterification and VLDL secretion in hepatocytes. Decreased VLDL clearance may also be involved. Like simple sugars, alcohol consumption stimulates *de novo* fatty acid synthesis in the liver, but this represents only a minor pathway of alcohol metabolism.

Alcohol and glucose metabolism

Acute alcohol administration has been shown to impair glucose tolerance in healthy individuals. Acute ethanol intoxication has even been associated with overt diabetic decompensation in predisposed individuals (presumably with latent diabetes or a low insulin secretory response). This appears to be due to an alcohol-induced inhibition of insulin sensitivity, the mechanism of which remains unknown. Alcohol has also been associated with hypoglycaemia. This may be due to potentiation by alcohol of the hypoglycaemic effect of drugs (insulin or sulphonylureas), or it may occur in fasting individuals, particularly after carbohydrate deprivation. Acute inhibition of hepatic gluconeogenesis is the main mechanism responsible for this effect.

Alcohol and blood pressure

Administration of a single dose of ethanol produces vasorelaxation and induces a modest drop in blood pressure. In contrast, heavy habitual alcohol consumption produces a dose-dependent increase in blood pressure. The mechanisms remain disputed, but may involve a stimulation of the sympathetic nervous system.

6.8 Concluding remarks

There is strong evidence that the lifestyle in the West is associated with an increased risk of major non-communicable diseases. Dietary factors are clearly involved, and future research will allow a better understanding of the role of specific nutrients, such as sugar and saturated fat, in the interactions between various nutrients, and will lead to practical dietary recommendations. It is also likely that the genetic background of individuals plays an important role. Genetic factors may explain why some individuals increase their cardiovascular risk factors or develop diseases as a consequence of their way of life, while other individuals do not. In the future, it is likely that identification of the genes involved will lead to novel, possibly individualised, therapeutic and preventive strategies. In the meantime, it appears reasonable to provide guidelines aimed at increasing physical activity and preventing excess calorie and saturated fat intake.

References and further reading

Canto C, Auwerx J. Caloric restriction, SIRT1 and longevity. Trends Endocrinol Metab 2009; 20: 325–331.

Duffey KJ, Popkin BM. Energy density, portion size, and eating occasions: contributions to increased energy intake in the United States, 1977–2006. PLoS Med 2011; 8(6): e1001050.

Flegal KM, Carroll MD, Ogden CL, Curtin LR. Prevalence and trends in obesity among US adults, 1999–2008. JAMA 2010; 303: 235–241.

Fontaine KR, Redden DT, Wang C, Westfall AO, Allison DB. Years of life lost due to obesity. JAMA 2003; 289(2): 187–193.

Harris JA, Benedict FG. A Biometric Study of Basal Metabolism in Man. Washington, DC: Carnegie Institution of Washington, 1919.

Jéquier E, Tappy L. Regulation of body weight in humans. Physiol Rev 1999; 79: 451–480.

Nield L, Summerbell CD, Hooper L, Whittaker V, Moore H. Dietary advice for the prevention of type 2 diabetes mellitus in adults. Cochrane Database Syst Rev 2008. CD005102.

Preston SH, Stokes A. Contribution of obesity to international differences in life expectancy. Am J Public Health 2011; 101(11): 2137–2143.

Reaven GM, Lithell H, Landsberg L. Hypertension and associated metabolic abnormalities – the role of insulin resistance and the sympathoadrenal system. N Engl J Med 1996; 334: 374–381.

Swinburn B, Sacks G, Ravussin E. Increased food energy supply is more than sufficient to explain the US epidemic of obesity. Am J Clin Nutr 2009; 90: 1453–1456.

Szendroedi J, Roden M. Ectopic lipids and organ function. Curr Opin Lipidol 2009; 20: 50–56.

Tappy L, Le KA. Metabolic effects of fructose and the worldwide increase in obesity. Physiol Rev 2010; 90: 23–46.

Westerterp KR, Prentice AM, Jéquier E. Alcohol and body weight . In: Health Issues Related to Alcohol Consumption (Macdonald I, ed.). Brussels: ILSI Europe, 1999, pp. 104–123.

Westerterp KR, Speakman JR. Physical activity energy expenditure has not declined since the 1980s and matches energy expenditures of wild mammals. Int J Obes (Lond) 2008; 32: 1256–1263.

Wright J, Marks V. Alcohol. In: The Metabolic and Molecular Basis of Acquired Disease (Cohen RD, Lewis B, Alberti KGMM, Denman AM, eds). London: Baillière Tindall, 1990, pp. 602–633.

7
Eating Disorders

Kate Williams

South London and Maudsley NHS Foundation Trust, London, UK

Key messages

- Individuals with eating disorders often feel ambivalent about recovery, so need a collaborative and motivational approach to treatment.
- Eating disorders can result in severe nutritional problems, which must be addressed as part of a multidisciplinary approach to treatment and recovery.
- The aims of nutritional interventions in eating disorders are to promote a safe and effective recovery of healthy weight and nutritional status, to abolish disordered eating behaviours, and to support the development of the knowledge,

skill, and confidence required for long-term normal, healthy eating.
- Major nutritional problems arise in anorexia nervosa as a result of restriction of the amount and variety of food consumed. This can lead to life-threatening starvation.
- The early stages of nutritional rehabilitation in anorexia nervosa carry risks, which must be managed safely.
- Nutritional assessment and management in eating disorders must place the management of body weight in the context of overall nutrition management, which includes all aspects of nutrition.

7.1 Introduction

Eating disorders are conditions in which abnormalities of eating behaviour, driven largely by psychological factors, are severe and persistent enough to impair nutrition, physical health, and social functioning, as well as cause psychological distress for the sufferer and their carers.

Broadly, the disordered eating may be a restriction of the amount, variety, and frequency of food and fluid consumed, or excessive overeating, or alternating episodes of restriction and overeating. In some individuals, there may additionally be efforts to prevent or compensate for the effects of eating, most usually by self-induced vomiting, excessive use of laxatives, or over-exercising. All of these symptoms give rise to significant physical and nutritional problems, which need to be addressed as part of the management of the condition.

7.2 Classification and features

Both the World Health Organization (WHO) and the American Psychiatric Association (APA) have published diagnostic criteria for eating disorders, which are broadly similar (see Tables 7.1, 7.2 and 7.3). The WHO and APA diagnostic criteria both recognise two major eating disorders: anorexia nervosa and bulimia nervosa. In the APA criteria – the *Diagnostic and Statistical Manual of Mental Disorders* (DSM IV-TR) – anorexia nervosa is divided into two subtypes: restricting and binge–purge. There are additional diagnoses, classified in the DSM as Eating Disorders Not Otherwise Specified (EDNOS), which include partial syndromes and binge-eating disorder.

These criteria demonstrate the difficulties inherent in separating disordered eating from the range and variety of normal eating, and in separating eating disorders from one another. These separations are

---

Clinical Nutrition, Second Edition. Edited by Marinos Elia, Olle Ljungqvist, Rebecca J Stratton and Susan A Lanham-New.
© 2013 The Nutrition Society. Published 2013 by Blackwell Publishing Ltd.

necessary for precision in communication and research. In practice, it may sometimes be more realistic to regard eating disorders as a spectrum along which individuals can move during the course of their illness. Nevertheless, there are clear differences between the major syndromes, not only in the presenting features but also in the predisposing and maintaining factors, and so it is useful to distinguish between them in examining aetiology, epidemiology and management.

Anorexia nervosa

The central feature of anorexia nervosa is restriction of food intake, which is severe and persistent enough to maintain body weight well below normal. Diagnostic criteria set 15% below normal weight, or body mass index (BMI) $17.5\,kg/m^2$, as the cut-off in adults (Table 7.1). Ideally, the normal weight would be the pre-morbid healthy weight for the individual, if this were known, but practitioners often find they must rely on standard body-weight tables for whole populations, or normal BMI ranges. In such cases,

care is needed to use standards for the appropriate ethnic group. In children and young people below the age of eighteen, some skill is needed to interpret the comparison of an individual with anorexia with norms shown on standard growth charts, as height as well as weight may be affected by under-nutrition.

Usually, the foods most stringently avoided are those perceived to be most likely to cause weight gain – typically high-fat and high-sugar foods – and there may be an escalating reduction in the variety of foods eaten as the illness progresses. This may typically begin with exclusion of the high-fat and -sugar foods, then other foods containing fat such as red meat, cheese, and eggs, and at its most severe it can leave little more than fruit and vegetables. Vegetarianism is common.

The restriction is almost always driven by overvaluation of shape and weight as a basis for self-worth, driving a persistent and overwhelming wish to lose weight, in spite of having a body weight below – sometimes severely below – normal. Restriction of food intake may also be driven by a wish for control, often in the context of a life with many stressful and

Table 7.1 Diagnostic criteria for anorexia nervosa. Reprinted with permission from the Diagnostic and Statistical Manual of Mental Disorders, Fourth Edition, Text Revision, (Copyright 2000). American Psychiatric Association.

DSM IV-TR	ICD-10 (F50)
Refusal to maintain body weight at or above a minimally normal weight for age and height; weight loss leading to maintenance of body weight below 85% of that expected or failure to make expected weight gain during a period of growth, leading to body weight below 85% of that expected	Significant weight loss (BMI at or below $17.5\,kg/m^2$) or failure of weight gain or growth
Intense fear of gaining weight or becoming fat, even though underweight	Weight loss self-induced by avoiding fattening foods and one or more of the following: (a) vomiting (b) purging (c) excessive exercise (d) appetite suppressants (e) diuretics
Disturbance in the way in which one's body weight, size, or shape is experienced; undue influence of body weight and shape on self-evaluation; or denial of seriousness of the current low body weight	A dread of fatness as an intrusive overvalued idea and the self-imposition of a low weight threshold
Amenorrhea (at least three consecutive cycles) in post-menarchal girls and women	Widespread endocrine disorder: (a) amenorrhea (b) raised growth hormone (c) raised cortisol

uncontrollable events; by anxiety reduction and seeking of illusory safety; and by perfectionistic pursuit of compliance with rigid rules. There is commonly a distortion of body image, characterised by a conviction of being fat in spite of low body weight; and resistance to accepting that the behaviour is harmful. Occasionally, however, the wish to lose weight is not the primary driver, which may instead be overzealous striving for religious or spiritual purity, an attempt to manage physical symptoms perceived to be food-related – for example, the conviction of having multiple food allergies or sensitivities – or extreme and distorted pursuit of healthy eating.

Female athletes may exhibit the so-called 'athlete's triad' of disordered eating, amenorrhoea, and low bone mineral density, especially in sports where low weight is necessary, such as distance running and gymnastics. Ballet dancers may be similarly affected.

Other diagnostic features result from the starvation itself. The endocrine disorder is mediated by the hypothalamus and the pituitary, affecting the gonads, thyroid, and adrenal glands. The reduction in oestrogen in females results in the cessation of menstruation, which is a diagnostic feature. The reduction in thyroid function contributes to a range of physical abnormalities, including bradycardia, hypotension, and hypothermia. There is failure of growth and pubertal development in children and adolescents.

Some individuals with anorexia nervosa may make additional efforts to reduce body weight by vomiting, especially if an eating is, or is perceived to be, a binge, unplanned, uncontrolled, inappropriate food, or otherwise unacceptable. Laxatives, diuretics, and excessive exercise may also be employed.

In some individuals, there may be persistent cycles of restriction, binge eating, and purging. The DSM distinguishes two subtypes: restricting and binge–purge, though purging behaviour may occur without any bingeing.

Bulimia nervosa

The defining feature of bulimia nervosa is a cycle of restriction of eating, which may be very severe, followed by food craving and uncontrolled excessive eating. This raises anxiety about the possible weight increase the binge might cause, provoking attempts to compensate, most commonly by self-induced vomiting, excessive use of laxatives, or excessive exercise, and further restriction of eating (Table 7.2). This binge–starve cycle is driven by over-valuation of thinness and by attempts to lose weight as a means to improve low self-esteem. BMI must be above 17.5 kg/m^2, or the diagnosis would be anorexia nervosa. It is most usually in the normal range, but may be above or below normal, and is often erratic.

Table 7.2 Diagnostic criteria for bulimia nervosa. Reprinted with permission from the Diagnostic and Statistical Manual of Mental Disorders, Fourth Edition, Text Revision, (Copyright 2000). American Psychiatric Association.

DSM IV-TR	ICD-10 (F50.2)

Recurrent episodes of binge eating characterised by both:
  eating, in a discrete period of time, an amount of food that is definitely larger than most people would eat in a similar period of time and under similar circumstances
  a sense of lack of control over eating during the episode, defined by a feeling that one cannot stop eating or control what or how much one is eating
	A preoccupation with food, and an irresistible craving for food; the person succumbs to episodes of overeating in which large amounts of food are consumed in a short period of time

Recurrent inappropriate compensatory behaviour to prevent weight gain, such as self-induced vomiting; misuse of laxatives, diuretics, enemas, or other medications; fasting; or excessive exercise	Attempts to 'counterbalance' the 'fattening' effects of food by one or more of the following: self-induced vomiting; purgative abuse; alternating periods of starvation; use of drugs such as appetite suppressants, thyroid preparations, or diuretics
The binge eating and inappropriate compensatory behaviour both occur, on average, at least twice a week for 3 months	The psychopathology consists of a morbid dread of fatness and the person holds themselves at a sharply defined weight threshold, well below the pre-morbid weight that constitutes the optimum or healthy weight in the opinion of the physician
Self-evaluation is unduly influenced by body shape and weight The disturbance does not occur exclusively during episodes of anorexia nervosa	

Table 7.3 Diagnostic criteria for partial syndromes and binge-eating disorder. Reprinted with permission from the Diagnostic and Statistical Manual of Mental Disorders, Fourth Edition, Text Revision, (Copyright 2000). American Psychiatric Association.

DSM IV-TR

All diagnostic criteria for anorexia nervosa are met, except the menstrual cycle is normal

All diagnostic criteria for anorexia nervosa are met, except weight is normal for height and age, even after considerable weight loss

All diagnostic criteria for bulimia nervosa are met, but the frequency of binges is less than twice weekly and they have a duration of less than 3 months

Recurring efforts to compensate (such as self-induced vomiting) for eating only small amounts of food, but body weight is normal for height and age

Regular chewing and spitting out of large quantities of food without swallowing

Binge-eating disorder: regular episodes of binge eating, but with no recurring efforts to compensate, such as purging or excessive exercise

---

EDNOS and binge-eating disorder

As shown in Table 7.3, the DSM IV-TR diagnostic criteria include a number of partial syndromes.

Diagnostic criteria for binge-eating disorder were first proposed and tested by Spitzer *et al.* (1992). Binge-eating disorder is characterised by repeated episodes of binge eating, without significant compensatory behaviours, though there may be a history of repeated attempts at dieting. There is no objective measure of a binge, though some individuals report eating several thousand calories in a short period of time. Episodes of eating large amounts are a normal response to a period of restricted eating, and are also normal in most cultures as part of social celebration. In binge-eating disorder, the binges do not have these normalising contexts, and are associated with severe distress. Levels of concern about weight and shape are similar to those in the other eating disorders, and higher than in obese people without binge-eating disorder. Binge-eating disorder is usually associated with weight cycling and obesity, which may be severe.

7.3 History

Disordered eating has been described for centuries, though the details of presentation and contemporary interpretations have varied.

From antiquity onwards, there are descriptions of extreme, apparently deliberate, restriction of food intake resulting in severe weight loss. In mediaeval and Renaissance European cultures, this seems to have presented most commonly as overzealous religious fasting. In early modern times, belief in magic and witchcraft was widespread, and regarded as part of the natural order of the world. The appearance of living without eating was viewed as a 'natural wonder' in a culture where many such apparent miracles were described, including for example young women giving birth to rabbits and boys vomiting pins. A view of self-starvation as a natural illness emerged at this time, exemplified in Morton's famous description of a condition recognised as 'nervous atrophy'. In 1694 he described a young woman unable to eat and losing flesh, which he ascribed to 'violent passions of the Mind'. This view moved in to mainstream medicine in the late nineteenth century, with descriptions in the medical literature by Lasègue in France and Gull in England. In 1888 Gull coined the term 'anorexia nervosa', and by then he clearly considered it a primarily psychological or 'nervous' condition. In the twentieth century, pursuit of slimness emerged in Europe and North America as a widespread cultural phenomenon, and as the predominant driver of restriction of eating in anorexia nervosa, to the extent that it has been included as a diagnostic criterion since the 1960s.

Likewise, binge eating associated with loss of control has been described from antiquity. This is arguably a natural and appropriate response to food deprivation, and also social celebration. Self-induced (or doctor-induced) vomiting has also been described for thousands of years, often in attempts to prevent or treat illness.

In 1979, Gerald Russell described a new eating disorder, linking binge eating and purging in the context of a drive for thinness, and coined the term 'bulimia nervosa' for it. He described this disorder as characterised by a cycle of restriction of eating, followed by an episode of uncontrolled and extreme overeating, then attempts to prevent the weight-gaining effect of the binge by self-induced vomiting, use of laxatives, over-exercise, or other means. He related it to anorexia nervosa, as he recognised that the disorders share the underlying fear of fatness and over-valuation of thinness. Although Russell viewed it as a variant of anorexia nervosa, it rapidly became clear that bulimia nervosa can occur at any weight, and most usually at or close to normal weight. In later diagnostic criteria, bulimic features in people with a BMI below 17.5 kg/m^2 are allocated the diagnosis of anorexia nervosa, binge–purge subtype.

7.4 Aetiology

Biological, psychological, and environmental factors interact to increase vulnerability to eating disorders.

There is clear evidence of heritability in all eating disorders, most strongly in anorexia nervosa. It may be that some of the genetic vulnerability is shared with other psychiatric disorders, such as depression, anxiety, obsessive–compulsive disorder, and substance misuse, and many individuals with eating disorders also have these conditions.

The genetic predisposition may be mediated by personality traits. Personality traits are discernible from childhood, and persist after recovery from the illness. Perfectionism, rigid and rule-bound thinking, and compulsivity are associated with eating restraint. Novelty-seeking and impulsivity are associated with binge eating. These traits may arise from genetic influences on brain neurotransmitters, with serotonin of particular interest because of its role both in eating behaviour and in mood. These distinct thinking styles influence the individual's response to environmental factors such as parenting style, stressful events such as childhood sexual abuse, bereavement and loss, or bullying, and also cultural influences such as the over-valuation of thinness.

Puberty seems to be a particularly vulnerable time for these factors to come together to bring about the development of an eating disorder, as body changes, in particular increase in weight and, for girls, adiposity, interact with increasing social awareness and sensitivity.

Dieting to attempt to reduce body weight is very widespread behaviour among girls in Western cultures, and is a common precursor of eating disorders, often, though not always, in the absence of clinical overweight or obesity. It has been suggested that cultural over-valuation of thinness, especially as promoted by advertising and other media, has a role in promoting eating disorders. It is not clear exactly what this contribution is, but one way it may operate is by increasing the number of young people, especially girls, who diet.

This view of eating disorders arising typically during or shortly after puberty, from a multiplicity of factors, is supported by some elements in the epidemiology, in particular the age of incidence, and the very much higher prevalence in females than in males.

7.5 Incidence and prevalence

Authors considering the epidemiology of eating disorders often urge caution, and suggest that published figures may be underestimates, for a number of reasons, including secrecy about symptoms and reluctance to seek treatment. For example, in one community sample, half of the cases of anorexia nervosa had not been detected by healthcare services. A study of young people in America found that 34% of boys and 43% of girls has some signs of disordered eating. Individuals may move over time from one diagnostic classification to another.

Anorexia nervosa

The highest incidence of anorexia nervosa is at age 15–19. In Europe and the USA, prevalence of anorexia in that age group is around 0.3%, and lifetime prevalence is about 0.6–0.9%. Overall incidence in these populations is at least 8 per 100 000 per year for anorexia nervosa. The female-to-male ratio is generally found to be about 10 : 1, though this difference is less marked in children and adolescents than in adults. Outside Western societies, prevalence is lower, and the exact presentation differs, but there is some evidence that it is increasing with the spread of Western cultural norms.

Bulimia nervosa

Incidence of bulimia nervosa is much higher than that of anorexia nervosa, at about 1–1.5% among young women in Europe and North America. For young men, as in anorexia nervosa, the prevalence is about 10% of that for females. Over whole populations, incidence rates of about 12 per 100 000 per year have been found.

EDNOS and binge-eating disorder

It is likely that partial syndromes are more commonly seen in clinical practice than presentations of disorders meeting the full diagnostic criteria for anorexia or bulimia nervosa. The prevalence of binge-eating disorder is probably about 3% of whole populations in Western societies, with a more even distribution between males and females. It may be as much as 25% among people seeking treatment for severe obesity.

7.6 Medical complications of eating disorders

Starvation and low weight

The malnutrition arising from anorexia nervosa can be severe and life-threatening.

Anorexia has long been recognised as having the highest mortality of any mental disorder. A meta-analysis in 1995 included 42 published studies, and found a crude mortality rate from anorexia nervosa of 5.9%. In 2007, a review of 10 reports found a similar rate of 5.25%. Significant causes of death include suicide and cardiac complications. There are concerns about the risk of death resulting from inappropriate refeeding practice.

There is no organ or tissue that is not affected by the deficient nutrition. Some of these changes cause significant functional impairment. Many reverse quickly with refeeding, though some may have life-long impact.

Musculoskeletal system

Muscle strength and stamina are reduced. In severe cases, this can be demonstrated by an inability to stand from a squatting position without using the hands for support. Some individuals are strikingly able to over-exercise in spite of this.

Osteoporosis is the commonest cause of pain and disability in anorexia nervosa, and in adults is not entirely reversible with nutritional rehabilitation. Because anorexia develops most commonly during puberty, when bone mineral density would normally be increasing, osteopaenia can develop rapidly in young people, within the first 12 months of illness. Osteoporosis in anorexia nervosa probably has multiple causes, including suppression of oestrogen and androgens, deficiency of insulin-like growth factor 1, raised cortisol production, and nutritional deficiencies of calcium and vitamin D. Low body weight reduces the stimulus of impact on bones during physical activity, which would result in increasing bone density at normal weight.

Central nervous system

There is reduced tissue mass in the brain, which may not be fully restored by recovery of normal nutrition and body weight.

There is related functional cognitive impairment, with deficits in memory tasks, flexibility, and inhibitory tasks, which may persist despite weight recovery.

Cardiovascular system

In prolonged restriction of food intake with severe weight loss, there is loss of muscle tissue from the heart and blood vessels. This, combined with general, thyroid-mediated, slowing of physiological processes, results in reduced pulse rate and blood pressure, and impaired peripheral circulation. Symptoms related to this are sensitivity to cold, peripheral oedema, and fainting, and death may result from cardiac complications.

Endocrine system

The activity of the hypothalamic–pituitary–gonadal axis is suppressed, causing regression of the gonads, with loss of sexual interest and function. Long-term fertility in recovered anorexic women is lower than average, possibly because of a tendency to maintain a lower proportion of adipose tissue in their bodies by residual restriction of food intake.

The activity of the hypothalamic–pituitary–thyroid axis is also suppressed, so that metabolic activity is generally reduced, with hypothermia, bradycardia, and hypotension.

The hypothalamic–pituitary–adrenal axis is overactive, and circulating cortisol is increased. This may contribute to perpetuation of the disorder by raising anxiety.

Gastrointestinal tract

There is a general reduction of motility of the gastrointestinal tract, probably associated with loss of muscle function in the gut wall. This results in delayed gastric emptying and constipation, so that eating provokes early satiety and bloating. This discomfort adds to the individual's reluctance to eat, so may impede recovery.

There may be damage to the teeth and soft tissues of the mouth from malnutrition and vitamin deficiency, or excessive use of low-sugar fizzy drinks.

Bone marrow and immune function

White cell count is reduced in relation to loss of adipose tissue, and the immune system is compromised, with impaired response to infection.

Compensatory behaviours

Frequent, persistent self-induced vomiting and excessive use of laxatives or diuretics can result in loss of fluid and electrolytes, leading to dehydration and low blood levels of electrolytes, in particular low potassium, which may lead to life-threatening cardiac or renal complications.

Vomiting can cause direct damage to the gastrointestinal tract. There may be acid erosion of the teeth from frequent contact with regurgitated stomach contents, and this damage may extend to the soft tissues of the mouth and lead to swelling of the parotid glands. Frequent vomiting can cause gastric reflux or Mallory–Weiss tear.

Binge eating

In the absence of significant compensatory behaviours, the most prevalent complication of binge eating is obesity, which often develops as a pattern of weight cycling, with gains greater than losses. The impact of obesity on health in binge-eating disorder seems to be similar to that of obesity in the absence of disordered eating (see Chapter 4).

There are occasional reports of gastric dilatation following massive binges, and rarely this has resulted in death. This may be more likely to occur in people with a gut wall weakened by starvation.

7.7 Nutritional problems in eating disorders

The most serious problems with nutrition arise in anorexia nervosa, in association with restricted amount and variety of food intake. Overeating in the context of binge eating may lead to weight gain and obesity, with its related problems. Compensatory behaviours such as vomiting and laxative abuse cause disturbances in fluid and electrolyte balance.

Disruption of appetite regulation further drives abnormal eating behaviour and impaired nutrition.

Appetite regulation in eating disorders

People with eating disorders find it very difficult to judge confidently when and how much to eat. All aspects of appetite regulation are disrupted. It is central to eating disorders that emotional states are primary drivers of eating behaviour. In both anorexia nervosa and bulimia nervosa, restriction of eating may be used to try to avoid intolerable emotional states of anxiety, guilt, or loss of control. Binge eating may be a response to an emotional trigger such as anger or loneliness. This dominance of emotional eating may overwhelm other regulatory signals.

Physiological appetite control depends on a number of factors, including neural signals from the gut and the cascade of polypeptides and hormones produced by the gut and the central nervous system in response to nutrients. There are long-term signals from energy stores, in particular leptin from adipose tissue and glucose released from glycogen stores in the liver. In anorexia, a paradoxical rise in polypeptide Y (PYY) has been observed, suggesting a possible aetiological role of a pre-existing abnormality of PYY production creating abnormal appetite signals. This raises the intriguing possibility of other analogous abnormalities. Slow peristalsis and delayed gastric emptying may result in early satiety and discomfort after eating. Even the normal sensation of food in the stomach may elicit guilt, shame, and anxiety, because it signals that food has been consumed, and so provokes self-induced vomiting or other compensatory behaviour to deflect the emotional distress.

Persistent vomiting of ingested food creates paradoxical appetite-control signals. Vomiting abolishes the neural signals of gastric fullness. Insulin production in response to a binge which included a large amount of carbohydrate may result in a rapid drop in blood glucose if the food is then vomited, stopping the flow of glucose into the blood and the normal satiety associated with rising blood glucose.

The normal response to eating as a pleasurable experience may also be distorted. In anorexia, food and eating may become associated with shame, disgust, anxiety, and guilt, or with powerful aversive experiences, and these may overwhelm pleasure as a driver of eating. If there is a cycle of restriction and binge eating, eating persistently follows a period of eating restriction, producing a heightened reward sensation from food, which then increases the drive to binge again, escalating and entrenching the restriction–binge–purge cycle.

Learned aspects of eating control are abolished as eating behaviour is increasingly deranged, and social benchmarking is lost if social eating is avoided.

In these ways, many of the normal regulators of eating behaviour are impaired. This leaves emotional drivers, which are often distorted, dominating the drivers of eating behaviour, and perpetuating the disorder.

Nutritional impact of starvation and low weight

The malnutrition of anorexia nervosa is distinct from malnutrition in other contexts. In clinical practice, malnutrition is often seen in the context of physical disease, surgery, or injury, when it interacts with the disease processes, each worsening the other. In these situations, the body may be severely catabolic, leading to rapid worsening of nutritional status and to high risks associated with refeeding. Severe malnutrition also occurs in famine. This situation is also distinct from anorexia nervosa, because in such situations there is often an additional burden of infection and parasite infestation due to associated poor living conditions, including poor quality and limited quantity of food. Anorexia nervosa arises in young people who are generally otherwise physically well. The amount of food eaten is far below requirement, but the quality is often good in some aspects; for example, fruit and vegetables are often eaten in normal or above-normal quantities. The nutritional complications are therefore in some ways different from these other contexts of malnutrition and weight loss.

Electrolytes and refeeding syndrome

Refeeding syndrome is the constellation of symptoms that occurs in a person who is severely malnourished when nutritional intake, particularly of carbohydrate, is increased. It arises primarily because of shifts of fluid and electrolytes, but other

problems may occur, including heart failure and acute thiamine deficiency.

In severe starvation, carbohydrate stores are depleted, and intake of carbohydrate may be very low. Carbohydrate metabolism is therefore minimal, and the body makes a metabolic change to using ketone bodies (mostly acetone, aceto-acetic acid, and hydroxybutyric acid), derived from fatty acids and amino acids, as a major energy substrate. Body stores of the micronutrients necessary to metabolise carbohydrate are also depleted, and insulin production is low. Increasing carbohydrate intake provokes rapid changes. Insulin release from the pancreatic beta-cells increases, driving anabolism. Under its influence, uptake of phosphate to synthesise adenosine triphosphate (ATP) is increased, and potassium, phosphate, and magnesium are taken up into cells. Blood levels of these electrolytes can fall rapidly as a result of these shifts, and this may precipitate acute on chronic electrolyte depletion if there has been long-term low intake prior to the refeeding.

Increasing carbohydrate metabolism increases demand for thiamine, which catalyses reactions in the chain of carbohydrate metabolism, and so can precipitate acute thiamine deficiency, as Wernicke–Korsakoff syndrome.

Fluid retention arises for a number of reasons. Activity of the sodium potassium pump is suppressed in starvation. With increasing availability of energy, active transport of sodium and potassium ions across cell membranes increases, creating shifts in fluid, leading to fluid retention. This may be increased in individuals who have vomited or used laxatives, as these behaviours result in losses of water from the body. There is renal compensation for this, by increased production of antidiuretic hormone (ADH), and so renal conservation of water. When the purging behaviour stops, it takes some time for ADH production to return to normal, so until then water is retained.

Blood volume may increase rapidly because of these shifts in fluid balance. This may lead to peripheral oedema, because of poor peripheral circulation, and overload cardiac capacity, which may already be diminished by wasting of the cardiac muscle.

Refeeding syndrome can cause distressing and uncomfortable fluid retention, which may cause severe clinical problems if it extends to vital organs such as the lungs or heart. Fluid overload and electrolyte depletion may lead to muscle weakness and cardiac failure, which at worst can be fatal.

Energy and macronutrients

Major changes in body composition occur with inadequate energy intake, with loss of adipose tissue and muscle mass and tone, leading to the characteristic wasted appearance and associated loss of muscle function. The depletion of adipose tissue contributes to hypothermia and cold sensitivity, loss of physical protection for bony prominences, and consequent discomfort sitting and lying down. Reduction in leptin production and some other endocrine abnormalities are proportional to loss of adipose tissue.

Low carbohydrate intake depletes glycogen stores, with the loss of the associated water. Thus any increase in carbohydrate intake large enough to replete this loss, for example a binge, results in rapid weight gain, reinforcing the belief that food intake must be strictly limited to prevent rapid and uncontrolled weight gain, and further entrenching the psychopathology. The reduced carbohydrate metabolism and low blood glucose forces the shift to ketone bodies as an energy substrate, particularly for the brain, which is unable to utilise fatty acids directly for energy. As a result of this shift, people with anorexia nervosa may be unusually tolerant of low blood glucose and not experience the usual symptoms of acute hypoglycaemia.

Protein intake is often adequate in the earlier stages of anorexic restriction of eating, as low-fat milk products, fish, white meat, and pulses may continue to be eaten when many other foods are excluded. Protein deficiency may develop in very chronic anorexia nervosa, reflected in low blood urea, and this may contribute to poor wound healing and impaired immune response.

Vitamins

Frank, symptomatic vitamin deficiency is unusual in anorexia nervosa, in spite of severe and chronic malnutrition. This relates to a number of protective factors.

Restriction of intake may develop slowly, allowing time for adaptation and conservation of vitamins, though extreme fat avoidance may impair absorption of fat-soluble vitamins. This can result in normal blood levels of vitamins in spite of depleted body stores.

Although the quantity and variety of food may be restricted, fruit and vegetables are often perceived as safe foods because they are low in energy density, so intakes of vitamin C, folate, and carotene may be high. In some individuals, excessive intake of fruit and vegetables may lead to visible yellowing of the skin, especially the palms of the hands, associated with hypercarotenaemia and accumulated deposits of carotene in subcutaneous tissue.

As carbohydrate metabolism is reduced by low carbohydrate intake, the requirement for B vitamins associated with energy release from carbohydrate is reduced, so symptoms of deficiency do not occur.

Many individuals with anorexia take vitamin supplements, and so compensate for low intake.

Vitamin D intake may be low because of vegetarianism, which excludes foods rich in vitamin D such as oily fish and offal. Avoidance of dairy products, or limitation of intake to very low-fat dairy products, further reduces vitamin D intake. This may contribute to the development of osteoporosis.

Subclinical deficiency and depleted body stores of vitamins are widespread in anorexia nervosa. Blood levels may remain in the normal range because of metabolic conservation and dehydration. Individuals with a history of restriction over periods of years, or of idiosyncratic food avoidance, may have specific vitamin deficiencies and related symptoms.

Minerals

The minerals of most clinical significance in anorexia nervosa are calcium, iron, and zinc.

Calcium intake is commonly inadequate because of overall low food intake and specific avoidance of dairy products, especially those that contain fat. The low-calcium status is generally not seen in low blood calcium levels because of calcium leaching from bones into the blood. Calcium deficiency contributes to the complex aetiology of osteoporosis in anorexia nervosa.

Because iron is not widespread in foods, even normal diets may not provide adequate iron intakes, and iron deficiency is not unusual in normal-weight women. Iron intake in anorexia nervosa is therefore typically low, especially in individuals who avoid red meat. There may also be impaired absorption because of high consumption of tea or coffee (in an attempt to suppress hunger) or of high-fibre cereal foods. This can generally be seen as low blood ferritin, reflecting depleted iron stores. Haemoglobin may remain in the normal range, as losses are reduced by cessation of menstruation, and the body becomes highly adapted to the conservation of iron. Some individuals do become anaemic, adding to the symptoms of tiredness and weakness typical of underweight and loss of muscle tissue generally.

Low zinc intake is common in anorexia, especially associated with avoidance of red meat and cheese. As zinc is released from muscle cells as they break down in the starvation process, blood zinc may remain normal. A symptom of zinc deficiency is altered taste perception, but this may also be caused by smoking or by prescribed medication such as antidepressants. The common overuse of condiments and spices may suggest loss of taste sensation, though it may be a result of a drive to increase the sensory stimulation derived from a very limited amount of food. Whatever the cause, the loss of normal flavour appreciation may further reduce the motivation to eat. As zinc is necessary for protein synthesis, zinc deficiency may inhibit nutrition rehabilitation, but it is not clear that supplementation with high doses is helpful.

It is likely that intake of other essential minerals is low.

Antioxidants and essential fatty acids
Blood levels of antioxidants may be low in anorexia nervosa. This may be due to low intake, and to additive factors such as increased demand for antioxidants associated with heavy exercise. There is some evidence that blood levels of essential fatty acids remain normal in anorexia, at least when the duration of food restriction is relatively brief.

Fluid and electrolytes
Some individuals may restrict fluid intake in order to reduce body weight or try to manage abdominal bloating. Others may drink excessively to suppress hunger or falsify weight, and this may lead to low electrolyte levels in the blood. Fluid may be taken in the form of drinks with caffeine, sometimes leading to very high caffeine intake, and excessive quantities of artificial sweeteners may also be used. Attempts to reduce caffeine intake may inadvertently reduce potassium intake from coffee.

Blood levels of sodium and potassium may be low because of vomiting and excessive use of laxatives, and this may lead to dangerous complications requiring urgent medical intervention. This risk may be increased by chronic low intake. Low sodium is most commonly caused by water loading. Magnesium intake is often adequate, as magnesium is present in foods that are often eaten in normal or even excessive amounts, such as green leafy vegetables and high-fibre cereals. As many people with anorexia are vegetarian, they may get adequate magnesium form eating wholegrain cereals, nuts, and seeds. However, magnesium may be depleted because of vomiting or laxative use. Shifts of fluid and electrolytes are a major feature of refeeding syndrome (see earlier in this section).

Compensatory behaviours
Both vomiting and excessive use of laxatives and diuretics cause losses of fluid, potassium, and sodium from the body. Excessive exercise increases the breakdown of muscle cells, and in the absence of adequate energy and protein, these cannot be restored, so iron and zinc are lost from the body.

Binge eating
Persistent binge eating, even without alternating periods of restriction, may result in a nutritionally poor-quality diet. Foods used in binges are generally those that the individual believes should be avoided and those that are highly pleasurable, usually high-fat, high-sugar foods with a relatively low content of essential nutrients. If a high proportion of energy intake comes from binges of foods and drinks of low nutritional quality, the whole diet may be deficient in fibre, vitamins, minerals, essential fatty acids, and antioxidants. There may be excessive intake of energy, fat, saturated fat, sugar, and sodium.

Overall energy intake may be high if there is no compensatory vomiting or exercise and there are no periods of restriction, as in binge-eating disorder. Obesity may arise, or pre-existing obesity may be worsened by this.

7.8 Nutritional management of eating disorders

Eating disorders have physical, psychological, and social components, which all need to be addressed by a multidisciplinary approach. Psychotherapy is central to recovery, and this may be supported with medication and help to restore normal social functioning and to recover normal healthy eating. Nutrition management must be delivered alongside appropriate medical, psychological, and social monitoring and management. It aims not only to reduce or abolish eating-disordered symptoms, but also to help develop the knowledge, skills, and confidence to recover healthy, normal eating and good nutritional status in the long term.

Ambivalence, or even hostility, to recovery is characteristic of eating disorders. This challenges every member of the professional multidisciplinary team involved in treatment and care, and family and other carers. A collaborative, motivational approach is therefore essential to engaging and maintaining a person with an eating disorder in the work towards recovery.

Restoring appetite regulation

An eating disorder may be very destructive of a person's ability to recognise and respond to hunger and satiety. Although normal eating may be a response to emotional factors as part of a complex and fluctuating mix of internal and external influences, in eating disorders emotions become a very dominant driver of eating, restriction of eating, or purging.

Restriction of eating involves persistent over-riding of the drive to eat. Responding to hunger by eating may be psychologically reframed as unacceptable weakness or loss of control. Individuals may use strategies to suppress hunger – such as exercise, work, or other frantic activity; excessive consumption of calorie-free fluid, in particular drinks with caffeine; or smoking or chewing gum – and so confuse hunger signals. They may find social eating very difficult, and avoid it, so losing contact with social benchmarks of eating behaviour. As the eating disorder persists, normal learned eating behaviour is lost. A normal feeling of fullness may be interpreted as a disastrous loss of control and potential cause of unacceptable weight gain, severely raising anxiety, and triggering efforts to compensate, such as vomiting, taking large doses of laxatives, or exercise. Persistent vomiting means the normal sensations of satiation are rarely experienced and come to feel abnormal. Those who binge without purging constantly over-ride the normal sensation of fullness and lose the ability to recognise it, and may be able to stop eating only when feeling bloated and nauseous. An individual with an eating disorder may be aware of appetite and the constant struggle to suppress it, or feel quite unable to recognise hunger or fullness, and unable to trust their own body.

It may be that it is not always possible to restore entirely normal appetite regulation in an individual with an eating disorder. Abnormalities in the physiological systems may exist before development of the disorder, and contribute to its development, and may thus be expected to persist after recovery. However, there is benefit in seeking to optimise physiological appetite control and restore the individual's ability to understand it and to respond appropriately to internal and external cues. This can help to reduce eating-disorders symptoms, improve confidence, and reduce anxiety and distress associated with eating.

Signals from normal body energy reserves (adipose tissue and glycogen) contribute to satiety, so restoration of healthy weight is fundamental to appetite control. Maintenance of body weight below normal will therefore tend to perpetuate a persistent drive to eat. Vomiting interferes with normal appetite regulation, so needs to be abolished in order to restore it.

Once healthy body weight is achieved, and vomiting is abolished, a normal rhythm of hunger, satiation, and satiety can be established. This is helped by regular meals of normal size and energy density, which provide a healthy cycle of fullness and emptying of the stomach. Adequate amounts of low-energy-density foods – such as vegetables and fruit – and fluid should be included to trigger the sensation of gastric fullness, but excessive use should be reduced.

Stabilisation of insulin production and blood glucose level can be achieved with regular carbohydrate intake, and with a choice of foods with a low glycaemic index. Meals should include protein and fat to help keep the glycaemic load low.

A mixture of protein, fat, and carbohydrate will stimulate the production of the range of gut hormones that regulate satiation and satiety.

Eating with others in normal social situations can help the recovering individual to learn and practise normal eating.

Many aspects of this process may be very challenging, and it needs to be planned in small steps, with achievable goals and sensitive support.

Weight recovery

In anorexia nervosa, recovering from a very low weight to a healthy weight occurs in three stages: initial stabilisation and management of refeeding risk; restoration of healthy body composition, body weight, and general nutritional status; and maintenance of good nutrition in the long term.

Stabilisation and management of refeeding risk

There is some controversy about how best to manage refeeding risk in anorexia nervosa. There may be an urgent need to reverse life-threatening malnutrition, but reintroducing food too quickly may precipitate life-threatening electrolyte disturbances. In practice, if the process can be closely medically monitored, and electrolyte replacement delivered promptly, safely, and effectively, more aggressive refeeding can be safely undertaken. Where this level of monitoring and replacement therapy cannot be provided, a more cautious approach is needed.

At this stage, feeding may be by ordinary food or oral liquid nutritional supplements, by tube, or by a mixture of these. The decision to use tube feeding as a supplement to, or in place of, oral nutrition presents practical, ethical, and legal challenges, especially if it is to be implemented without the consent of the individual. It must be made after careful consideration by the multidisciplinary team, bearing in mind local policies and protocol, staff skills, and the wishes of the individual. In the UK, it is generally a last resort, to be used only after every effort has been made to restore nutrition orally. There is a risk of long-term dependence on tube feeding, and to help prevent this, oral feeding should be maintained, even if minimally, or reintroduced as soon as possible. Tube feeding may be used very successfully for individuals who find eating adequately to be an insurmountable psychological challenge, or who are too physically frail or compromised to be able to eat adequately. It can be used alongside efforts to help the individual to restore normal eating.

The mainstays of restoring nutrition safely at this stage are:

- Delivery of thiamine and other B vitamins before beginning any feeding, and continuing to give them for the first 10 days, to ensure that vitamins necessary for carbohydrate metabolism are available, and in particular to prevent Wernicke–Korsakoff syndrome.

- Vitamin and mineral supplement to correct subclinical and minor deficiencies and restore depleted body stores. This may need to be provided for several weeks. Unless there are deficiency symptoms, there is no justification for high doses of any specific vitamin or mineral, which may cause side-effects or problems of competitive absorption.

- Gradual reintroduction of calories, especially carbohydrate, delivered either continuously as a tube feed at a slow rate or as very small and regular snacks of food. Minimising glycaemic load by including fat and protein, and low-glycaemic-index carbohydrate foods where possible, moderates the rate of carbohydrate absorption and reduces metabolic stress. With good monitoring and medical support, it should be possible to reach intake equivalent to resting energy expenditure within 24–48 hours, and so prevent further nutritional loss.

- High potassium and phosphate intake, with additional supplements if necessary, according to blood levels. Because of the relatively high sodium levels in food, low sodium is usually best managed by controlling fluid intake rather than supplementing sodium, except in very severe cases, usually associated with severe vomiting and laxative use. Caution is needed when interpreting blood levels of electrolytes, as low levels due to low intake and purging may be counterbalanced by dehydration, resulting in normal blood levels. Rehydration can therefore result in very rapid falls in blood electrolytes.

- Controlled fluid intake to prevent cardiac overload, providing enough fluid to prevent worsening dehydration, with gradual increases according to cardiac function.

- Limited volume of food and fluid, to minimise gastric bloating.

For individuals who are able to eat ordinary food, it should be in a form that is not physically demanding to eat, and foods that cause the most severe psychological distress – usually very fatty and sweet foods – should be avoided.

The rate of increase of nutritional intake should be judged according to medical condition. In practice, it is usually possible to achieve positive energy balance within 3–5 days, unless complications arise.

Restoration of weight and nutritional status

UK National Institute of Clinical Excellence (NICE) guidance advises aiming for a weight gain of about

0.5 kg per week for out-patients, and 0.5–1.0 kg per week for those being treated in hospital. This can be achieved with energy intake of maintenance-energy requirement plus 500–1000 calories per day. Achieving and maintaining this is likely to need a high level of very skilled support from those caring for the individual.

At this stage, the aims are recovery of healthy weight, normal nutritional status, and normal healthy eating behaviour. For those using tube feeding or nutritional supplements, normal food can be reintroduced, working towards a normal and healthy diet.

Vitamin and mineral supplements should be continued to recover body stores of micronutrients. At this stage, calcium and vitamin D supplements do not seem to promote restoration of bone mass, but it may be appropriate to ensure that adequate amounts of bone mineral nutrients are available as soon as endocrine recovery allows them to be utilised to improve bone mineral density.

The nutritional quality of the diet should be good, to ensure recovery of protein, micronutrient, and antioxidant status, and to support learning about healthy eating.

Maintenance of recovered nutritional status

Relapse is common in anorexia nervosa, and so attention needs to be given to maintaining health gains in the long term.

Education about healthy eating and nutrition may be needed to correct distorted beliefs about food, eating, and nutrition, and to enable long-term maintenance of good nutritional health. Improved understanding of normal appetite regulation can reduce anxiety and improve confidence.

Most aspects of nutritional health recover with weight restoration and good-quality diet. However, after even a brief episode of anorexia nervosa, there is a risk to long-term bone health. Those with a history of low weight for more than 6 months should have a bone scan to assess bone mineral density and appropriate management, which may include medication and appropriate exercise. High calcium and vitamin D intake in the long term, possibly including supplements, may help optimise bone recovery, though appropriate levels of intake are not known.

For individuals whose nutritional recovery is not complete, supplements of vitamins, minerals, and essential fatty acids may be useful in the long term.

Compensatory behaviours

Those individuals who use self-induced vomiting or laxatives to try to compensate for the weight-gaining effects of food need education alongside psychotherapy to abolish these behaviours and prevent relapse.

Many people with bulimia nervosa may be unable to tolerate normal meals without purging. The impulse to purge may be reduced by establishing a regular intake of small meals and snacks, which do not result in excessive feelings of fullness. The use of foods which feel safe for the individual, usually low-fat and low-sugar foods, as well as temporary avoidance of foods which trigger purging, may be helpful.

Rapid weight increase may occur when the use of vomiting, laxatives, or diuretics is reduced or stopped, and may provoke a relapse of purging. This weight gain is largely fluid. It may result from repletion of low glycogen stores and associated fluid. There may also be temporary renal retention of fluid because of a delay in adjusting production of ADH, and rebound over-hydration may occur. This may result in rapid weight increase and a feeling of bloating, and this may provoke relapse of purging. Careful explanation of this self-limiting effect can help prevent this.

An understanding of the effects on blood electrolyte levels, physical damage to the mouth and gastrointestinal tract, and impairment to natural appetite regulation will help the individual to manage the effects of purging. Until these practices are stopped, it is necessary to protect the teeth and replace loss of potassium and fluid. Potassium and fluid can be replaced by using products such as milk or fruit juice, or prescribed supplements, though excessive or frequent use of fruit juice may damage the teeth. After vomiting, rinsing the mouth with plain water increases pH and so reduces the risk of erosion to enamel.

Excessive exercise causes loss of muscle cells, so it may be useful to supplement zinc and iron alongside the increase in energy and protein in order to promote replacement.

Binge eating

The abolition of binge eating relies on the reduction of hunger and hyper-reward of food as drivers of overeating, alongside psychotherapeutic work.

Reduction in hunger as a driver requires the abolition of loss of calories through self-induced vomiting and excessive exercise, and the restoration of normal appetite regulation. This can be achieved by establishing a regular eating pattern, with frequent, relatively small meals that provide enough energy to prevent the excessive hunger that may trigger binge eating. For those who are underweight, energy intake should be sufficient to promote gradual return to healthy weight. Even obese individuals may need to eat enough to maintain a stable weight while they work to reduce bingeing. This may require energy intake well above average. Some overweight or obese binge eaters may feel an overwhelming need to reduce their weight, and may be better able to abolish bingeing if their body weight is falling, as this improves confidence and self-efficacy, but energy restriction of more than 200–500 calories per day below maintenance requirement may provoke hunger and overeating, so this needs careful management.

Stable blood glucose level helps to reduce insulin-induced hunger, so regular intake of low-glycaemic-index carbohydrate and avoidance of high-gylcaemic-index foods is helpful.

Drugs which affect appetite control, such as alcohol, cannabis, and amphetamines, will impede progress, so their use should be stopped or carefully controlled. For individuals who do not sleep well, especially if they binge during the night, small, planned snacks to have during the night may be helpful until a more healthy sleep pattern is restored.

To reduce the overstimulating effect of high-reward foods, it may be helpful for binge eaters to limit the use of high-fat and high-sugar foods, and of other foods that have become binge triggers. These foods can be reintroduced to the diet in modest amounts, in a controlled way. For example, a person who has habitually binged on chocolate may plan to have a small amount of it as a dessert, in order to ensure that they are not excessively hungry, in a café with a friend, so that the situation is one in which bingeing would be difficult. In this way, they can build confidence in using this foods safely and without anxiety, which is an essential element of recovery.

In restoring a stable eating pattern, attention must be given to establishing healthy food choices in order to ensure good nutrition and stable, healthy body weight in the long term.

7.9 Concluding remarks

Recent years have brought increased understanding of the genetics of eating disorders and the physiological control of appetite and its disturbance, and advances in psychological approaches to achieving recovery from eating disorders. These all show promise in improving the identification of disordered eating, and the speed and effectiveness of treatment. This has great potential for reducing the toll of nutritional damage that eating disorders can incur.

Acknowledgements

This chapter was revised and updated by Kate Williams, based on the original chapter by Janet Treasure and Tara Murphy.

References and further reading

American Dietetic Association. Position of the American Dietetic Association: nutrition intervention in the treatment of eating disorders. Journal of the American Dietetic Association 2011; 111: 1236–1241.

APA. Diagnostic and Statistical Manual of Mental Disorders, 4th edn. Washington, DC: American Psychiatric Association, 2000.

Barada K, Azar C, Al-Kutoubi A, Harb S, Hazimeh Y, Abbas J, Kahnir M, Al-Amin H. Massive gastric dilatation after a single binge in an anorectic woman. International Journal of Eating Disorders 2006; 39(2): 166–169.

Bell R. Holy Anorexia. Chicago, IL: University of Chicago Press, 1985.

Birmingham C, Treasure J. Medical Management of Eating Disorders. Cambridge, UK: Cambridge University Press, 2010.

Birmingham CL, Alothman A, Goldner E. Anorexia nervosa: refeeding and hypophosphatemia. International Journal of Eating Disorders 1995; 20(2): 211–213.

Brumberg JJ. Fasting girls: the emergence of anorexia nervosa as a modern disease. Cambridge, MA: Harvard University Press, 1988.

Caregaro L, Di-Pascoli L, Favaro A, Nardi M, Santonastaso P. Sodium depletion and hemoconcentration – overlooked complications in patients with anorexia nervosa? Nutrition 2005; 21(4): 438–445.

Chaudhri O, Field B, Bloom S. Editorial: From gut to mind – hormonal satiety signals and anorexia nervosa. Journal of Endocrinology and Metabolism 2006; 91(3): 797–798.

Collier DA, Treasure JL. The aetiology of eating disorders. British Journal of Psychiatry 2004; 185(5): 363–365.

Davis C, Patte C, Levitan R, Reid C, Tweed S, Curtis C. From motivation to behaviour: a model of reward sensitivity, overeating and food preferences in the risk profile for obesity. Appetite 2007; 48(1): 12–19.

Fairburn C. Overcoming Binge Eating. New York: Guilford Press, 1995.

Fairburn CG, Harrison PJ. Eating disorders. Lancet 2003; 361: 407–416.

Fisher M, Simpser E, Schneider M. Hypophosphataemia second-ary to oral refeeding in anorexia nervosa. International Journal of Eating Disorders 2000; 28(2): 181–187.

Hart S, Abraham S, Luscombe G, Russell J. Fluid intake in patients with eating disorders. International Journal of Eating Disorders 2005; 38(1): 55–59.

Hearing S. Refeeding syndrome. BMJ 2004; 328: 908–909.

Herrin M. Nutrition Counselling in the Management of Eating Disorders. New York: Brunner-Routledge, 2003.

Hoek HW. Incidence, prevalence and mortality of anorexia ner-vosa and other eating disorders. Current Opinion in Psychiatry 2006; 19(4): 389–394.

Hoek HW, van Hoeken D. Review of the prevalence and incidence of eating disorders. International Journal of Eating Disorders 2003; 34: 383–396.

Keys A, Brozek J, Henschel A, Mickelsen O, Taylor H. The Biology of Human Starvation. Minneapolis, MN: University of Minnesota Press, 1950.

Kingston K, Szmukler G, Andrewes D, Tress B, Desmond P. Neuropsychological and structural brain changes in anorexia ner-vosa before and after refeeding. Psychol Med 1996; 26(1): 15–28.

Lawson E, Klibanski A. Endocrine abnormalities in anorexia ner-vosa. Nature Clinical Practice: Endocrinology and Metabolism 2008; 4(7): 407–414.

Mehanna H, Moledina J, Travis J. Refeeding syndrome: what it is, and how to prevent and treat it. BMJ 2008; 336: 1495–1498.

Melchior JC. From malnutrition to refeeding during anorexia ner-vosa. Current Opinion in Clinical Nutrition and Metabolic Care 1998; 1: 481–485.

Mitchell J, Crow S. Medical complications of anorexia nervosa and bulimia nervosa. Current Opinion in Psychiatry 2006; 19(4): 438–443.

Morton R. Phthisologia, or a Treatise of Consumptions wherein the Difference, Nature, Causes, Signs and Cure of all Sorts of Consumptions are Explained. London: Samuel Smith and Benjamin Walford, 1694.

Moyano D, Sierra C, Brandi N, Artuch R, Mira A, Garcia-Tornel S, Vilaseca M. Antioxidant status in anorexia nervosa. International Journal of Eating Disorders 1999; 25(1): 99–103.

National Collaborating Centre for Acute Care (2006) National Clinical Practice Guideline 32, Nutrition Support in Adults.

National Collaborating Centre for Mental Health (2004) National Clinical Practice Guideline 9, Eating Disorders.

Peters T, Parvin M, Petersen C, Faircloth V, Levine R. A case report of Wernicke's encephalopathy in a pediatric patient with ano-rexia nervosa – restricting type. Journal of Adolescent Health 2007; 40(4): 376–383.

Prince A, Brooks S, Stahl D, Treasure J. Systematic review and meta-analysis of the baseline concentrations and physiologic responses to gut hormones to food in eating disorders. American Journal of Clinical Nutrition 2009; 89: 755–765.

Robinson P, Clarke M, Barrett J. Determinants of delayed gastric emptying in anorexia nervosa and bulimia nervosa. Gut 1988; 29: 458–464.

Royal College of Psychiatrists. CR162: Management of Really Sick Patients with Anorexia Nervosa (MARSIPAN). 2010.

Russell GFM. Bulimia nervosa: an ominous variant of anorexia nervosa. Psychological Medicine 1979; 9: 429–448.

Schmidt U. Aetiology of eating disorders in the 21st century: new answers to old questions. European Child & Adolescent Psychiatry 2003; 12(Suppl. 1): 30–37.

Setnick J. Micronutrient deficiencies and supplementation in anorexia and bulimia nervosa: a review of the literature. Nutrition in Clinical Practice 2010; 25(2): 137–142.

Solomon SM, Kirby DF. The refeeding syndrome: a review. Journal of Parenteral and Enteral Nutrition 1990; 14: 90–97.

Spitzer RL, Devlin MJ, Walsh BT, Hasin D, Wing R, Marcus M, Stunkard A, Wadden T, Yanovski S, Agras S, Mitchell J, Nonas C. Binge eating disorder: a multisite field trial of the diagnostic criteria. International Journal of Eating Disorders 1992; 11: 191–203.

Swenne I, Rosling A, Tengblad S, Vessby B. Essential fatty acid sta-tus in teenage girls with eating disorders and weight loss. Acta Paediatrica 2011; 100(5): 762–767.

Teng K. Premenopausal osteoporosis, an overlooked consequence of anorexia nervosa. Cleveland Clinic Journal of Medicine 2011; 78(1): 50–58.

Treasure J. Eating disorders. Medicine 2008; 36(8): 430–435.

Treasure J, Cardi V, Kan C. Eating in eating disorders. Eur Eat Dis Rev 2011. DOI: 10.1002/erv/1090.

Treasure J, Claudino A, Zucker N. Eating disorders. Lancet Online 2009. Available from: http://www.thelancet.com/journals/lancet/article/PIIS0140-6736(09)61748-7/abstract.

Treasure J, Schmidt U, van Furth E, editors. The Essential Handbook of Eating Disorders. Chichester: Wiley, 2005.

Treasure J, Smith G, Crane A. Skills-based Learning for Caring for a Loved One with an Eating Disorder: The New Maudsley Method. Hove: Routledge, 2007.

Whyte E, Jefferson P, Ball D. Anorexia nervosa and the refeeding syndrome. Anaesthesia 2003; 58(10): 1025–1026.

Wilfley D, Schwartz MB, Spurrell EB, Fairburn CG. Using the Eating Disorder Examination to identify the specific psychopa-thology of binge eating disorder. International Journal of Eating Disorders 2003; 27(3): 259–269.

Yanovski S, Agras S, Mitchell J, Nonas C. Binge eating disorder: to be or not to be in DSM-IV. International Journal of Eating Disorders 1991; 10: 627–629.

8
Adverse Reactions to Foods

Simon H Murch

Warwick Medical School, University of Warwick, Coventry, UK

Key messages

- Increasing dietary allergies have been most apparent in children, with an estimated 5% demonstrating allergy to cow's-milk protein.
- As dietary exposures in early life have broadened in the developed world, previously rare adverse reactions have become increasingly common.
- It is important to differentiate between the different forms of adverse reactions to foods, in particular between food intolerance and food allergy.

- There are two major classes of food allergic reaction: IgE-mediated and non-IgE-mediated. Within these classes, reactions may be divided clinically as localised or generalised.
- There is now increasing understanding of the mechanisms of oral tolerance to food antigens and of the importance of infectious exposures, particularly gut bacteria, in imprinting these in early life.

8.1 Introduction

In recent decades, dietary allergies have become increasingly common in privileged countries. This increase has been most apparent within the childhood population, with an estimated up to 5% of children demonstrating allergy to cow's milk protein. In addition to this remarkable increase in frequency, there has been a change in patterns of presentation. As dietary exposures in early life have broadened for the children of the developed world, previously rare adverse reactions to antigens such as peanut and sesame seeds have become increasingly common.

There are significant geographical differences, dependent on patterns of dietary intake, including reports of anaphylaxis in response to birds' nest soup in Singaporean infants. Early life exposures, which have changed substantially for developed-world children in the last 50 years, appear particularly important. Children born in disadvantaged conditions within the developing world have a much lower incidence of dietary allergies. Early life exposures appear to be a major determinant of allergic sensitisation, with genetic predisposition appearing to have an influence only after a certain threshold of improved material conditions is passed. Later in this chapter, the basic mechanisms of oral tolerance to dietary antigens underpinning such demographic change will be discussed. Because such tolerance is mediated by immunological mechanisms, there will be some overlap with concepts discussed in Chapter 17, on 'Nutrition and Immune and Inflammatory Systems'.

First, it is important to differentiate between the different forms of adverse reactions to foods, particularly between food intolerance and food allergy. Only the latter is mediated by an immune response, whereas the former may be a consequence of a variety of non-immune mechanisms. There is often overlap in the symptoms displayed, and an accurate history is thus a vital component of the assessment of a patient suspected of adverse food reactions.

Clinical Nutrition, Second Edition. Edited by Marinos Elia, Olle Ljungqvist, Rebecca J Stratton and Susan A Lanham-New.
© 2013 The Nutrition Society. Published 2013 by Blackwell Publishing Ltd.

8.2 Food intolerance

This is by definition a reproducible adverse reaction to ingested food that is not mediated by immune hypersensitivity. This intolerance may be a response to the whole food, for example an aversion to its appearance, taste, or smell. It may be a consequence of an inability to process specific components of individual foods – the most common worldwide is lactose intolerance. Lactose is a disaccharide composed of glucose and galactose monosaccharides, which requires breakdown of the bond between the two component sugars by the intestinal enzyme lactase in order to allow their absorption. If lactase is deficient, the unabsorbed lactose passes down the gut and is fermented by gut bacteria, producing gas and acid by-products. This often causes uncomfortable abdominal distension and diarrhoea.

Humans are in fact the only mammal in which lactase persists into adult life, and such persistence has arisen by mutation since farming began. Many population groups, including those with ancestral origins in southern Europe and Africa, do not show lactase persistence and are thus lactose intolerant as adults. By contrast, in infancy low lactase expression is always abnormal, usually due to immune reactions in the intestine. Thus lactose intolerance in adults may be physiological, whereas in infants it is always pathological, and their food intolerance is caused by an underlying immune-mediated (allergic) mechanism.

Potentially more serious, and thankfully much rarer examples occur in infants with inborn errors of metabolism. In these disorders, lack of individual metabolic enzymes leads to damaging build-up of toxic metabolites of initially dietary origin. The best-known disorder is phenylketonuria, in which brain damage occurs if dietary phenylalanine is not excluded.

A third mechanism of food intolerance may occur when foodstuffs contain components with definite pharmacological effects, such as tyramine in cheeses and red wines. While most people are usually able to tolerate these, use of certain medications, such as monoamine oxidase inhibitors, may interfere with innate detoxication mechanisms and lead to potentially dangerous toxicity if these foods are consumed. Some people are sensitive to the histamines naturally occurring in strawberries, and rapidly develop rash or wheezing after eating them.

Although these symptoms appear similar to immediate allergic reaction, they are mediated by non-immunological mechanisms and are thus due to food intolerance and not allergy.

Direct effects of foods are common, particularly those due to bacterial contamination. In most cases, this is sporadic, and clustering only occurs if large numbers of people eat the same contaminated food (e.g. wedding guests, airline passengers). However, the advent of modern food-handling practices increases the potential for very widespread transmission of such infections. This has occurred with recent outbreaks of life-threatening *E. coli* infections in Europe and North America. While considerable epidemiological detective work is necessary to trace the source of such epidemic food poisoning, there is usually little doubt of the involvement of food ingestion. This may not be so obvious if the foodstuff is contaminated by nonbacterial toxins or chemicals. In recent decades there have been epidemics of irreversible neural damage due to contamination of cooking oils in Spain and mercury poisoning in Japanese fishermen, and in neither case was it initially obvious that food contamination was to blame.

Detection of inborn errors of metabolism in early life is particularly important, as appropriate removal of dietary components in infancy can completely prevent serious brain damage. Recognition of the importance of early diagnosis led to the introduction of routine heel-prick testing of all newborn infants for phenylketonuria. Other rare disorders are not routinely tested for, and it is important to consider these diagnoses in any infants with early abnormal symptoms, including vomiting, poor feeding, enlarged liver and spleen, prolonged jaundice, failure to thrive, hypoglycaemia, floppiness, or impaired consciousness. The onset of such symptoms after weaning of a breast-fed infant to sucrose-containing foods may occur in hereditary fructose intolerance. Rapid diagnosis is the key, and delays usually occur because a metabolic cause is not included in the differential diagnosis of an unwell infant.

8.3 Food allergy

Allergies occur as a consequence of a breakdown in immunological tolerance. The immune system has continually to differentiate between myriad foreign molecules, recognising and responding to those which pose a threat to the organism – such as pathogens or their toxins – while remaining largely unresponsive (tolerant) to those necessary for survival and health – such as foods and the commensal bacterial flora in the intestine. Recent evidence suggests that the role of the bacterial flora in establishing immune tolerance is considerable, as discussed in Section 8.10.

Allergies are a varied group of conditions induced by inappropriate immune reactivity to foreign antigens; these are called allergens if they reproducibly cause symptoms on exposure. Food allergic responses by definition require an abnormal immunologically mediated reaction to ingested dietary antigens. However, there may well be overlap in the clinical manifestations of allergies and nonallergic food intolerance, and there is much potential for confusion if true allergy is mistaken for intolerance or vice versa. The nature of an allergic response is that initial sensitisation is required, and that the first exposure will not lead to obvious response, but that hypersensitivity reactions will occur on later challenge. Recent changes in the presentation of infant allergies suggest that such initial sensitisation may occur without such an obvious history. Indeed, even exclusively breastfed infants may sensitise to minute amounts of dietary antigen passing into their mother's breast milk.

8.4 Types of food allergy

There are two major classes of food allergic reactions: *IgE-mediated* and *non-IgE-mediated*. The former are generally obvious, present soon after ingestion, and are thus relatively easy to investigate and diagnose (Box 8.1). They can be more violent than non-IgE-mediated reactions, and can cause death through anaphylaxis in severe cases. Non-IgE-mediated food allergies tend to present rather later and can be more subtle, but may be an important (and often unrecognised) cause of ill-health (see Table 8.1). The immunological basis of such reactions is discussed in more depth in Section 8.10.

Food-allergic reactions may also be divided clinically into those of *quick onset* (within minutes to an hour of food ingestion) and those of *slow onset* (taking hours or days). In general, quick-onset symptoms

tend to be IgE-mediated and slow-onset symptoms non-IgE-mediated. However, this is by no means invariable, and many children with clear quick-onset responses to foods have a low or undetectable serum total IgE and absent food-specific IgE (radio allergosorbent test, RAST). This may be because there is local IgE response within the intestine that is not matched by systemic response. IgE responses may be compartmentalised, often being limited to the intestine and not occurring elsewhere. This may explain discordance between positive clinical responses and negative 'allergy test' results.

In a study of 120 children with multiple food allergies, we identified a significant increase of

---

Box 8.1 The classical forms of hypersensitivity. After Gell & Coombs (1968)

Type I: anaphylactic or immediate hypersensitivity
This occurs within minutes of exposure, and is characteristic of quick-onset food allergy. The reaction occurs when an allergen reacts with IgE (or in certain circumstances, IgG1) on the surface of activated mast cells. This leads to mast-cell degranulation and release of vasoactive agents such as histamine, proteases, and cytokines such as TNFα. Peanut hypersensitivity is a classic type I response.

Type II: cytotoxic hypersensitivity
This reaction occurs when antibody binds to a cell or tissue component and fixes complement, which leads to complement-mediated cell death. It is thus not usually thought to play a role in food allergic responses, although complement activation itself is seen in some forms of food-induced enteropathy, such as coeliac disease.

Type III: immune-complex hypersensitivity
In this type of reaction, also known as the Arthus reaction, antigens and antibodies (IgG or IgM) form complexes in the presence of antigen excess to induce complement fixation and consequent local inflammatory response, several hours after exposure to antigen. Recent evidence suggests that the Fc receptors for immunoglobulin, rather than the complement itself, are important for such tissue damage.

Type IV: delayed hypersensitivity or cell-mediated immunity
This reaction is mediated by T-lymphocytes and macrophages. Much evidence has accrued since the publication by Gell & Coombs to suggest that T-cell responses (e.g. T_H1 or T_H2 secretion patterns) may determine overall immunopathology. The classic type IV reaction is a T_H1 response, as in coeliac disease; less is known about T_H2 immunopathology in food allergy.

Table 8.1 Clinical manifestations in food-allergic responses.

1. Quick onset	2. Late onset	3. Less-clear responses	4. Secondary general effects
• wheezing • urticaria • angio-oedema • rashes • vomiting • gastro-oesophageal reflux • anaphylaxis	• diarrhoea • abdominal pain • allergic rhinitis • atopic eczema • food-sensitive enteropathy or colitis • rectal bleeding • constipation • protein-losing enteropathy	• irritable bowel syndrome • chronic fatigue • attention-deficit hyperactivity disorder(ADHD)	• eosinophilia • iron-deficiency anaemia • other micronutrient deficiencies

Notes:
(1) Those who make a clear quick-onset response may go on to show secondary worsening after a period of some hours, and it is important to institute appropriate medical therapy and/or supervision.
(2) The conditions in group 3 are ones in which there are a number of reports of favourable clinical responses to exclusion of dietary antigens, sometimes impressive. However, these have yet to be established in the lists of true food allergies, and probably only a proportion of such patients will benefit. An open-minded approach, and joint management with a skilled dietitian, would nevertheless appear reasonable at present. As with every dietary exclusion, the clinical response should be sufficiently good to make it worthwhile continuing with the exclusion.

serum IgE in children who had early-onset symptoms compared to those with late-onset symptoms. What was notable was that the great majority (>90%) of those with early-onset symptoms additionally demonstrated late-onset symptoms. Both groups shared a pattern of immune deviation (including low IgG subclasses and IgA) consistent with reduced responses of the innate immune system to infectious exposures. This concords with data from several other countries, which link delayed immune maturation with early-life food allergies. These data suggest that there may be a consistent pattern of minor immunodeficiency associated with the process of sensitisation in early life, and that the manifestation of that sensitisation (quick- or slow-onset) may depend on whether a child has inherited a tendency to high IgE production. In other words, high IgE does not cause food allergy *per se*, but may determine how that allergy is expressed. Most of the early literature on food allergy focuses on IgE and quick-onset responses, which is understandable as it is so much more obvious to detect.

8.5 Patterns of food-allergic responses

Quick-onset symptoms

These often follow the ingestion of a single food, such as egg, peanut, or sesame. Within minutes, the sufferer may notice tingling of the tongue, and there may be a rapid development of skin rash, urticaria, or wheezing. Angioneurotic oedema, with swelling of the mucous membranes, can develop extremely fast, and the airway may become compromised. Anaphylactic shock may also occur, with dramatic systemic hypotension accompanying the airway obstruction.

Specific therapy for mild cases of immediate hypersensitivity would include antihistamines such as chlorpheniramine, together with inhaled bronchodilators as appropriate. It is notable that some patients can make a biphasic response, with a relatively modest initial reaction followed several hours later by a more profound and potentially life-threatening response, and thus care should be taken in the assessment to ensure that adequate instructions and therapy are administered before allowing the patient to go home. The presence of wheezing on examination should suggest caution, and a bronchodilator should certainly be prescribed, in many cases alongside a few days' course of oral corticosteroids.

More severe reactions should be assessed very rapidly. Any evidence of airway obstruction or systemic hypotension warrants the immediate use of intramuscular adrenaline. If the patient has a preloaded adrenaline syringe pen, such as an EpiPen, this should be administered prior to urgent transfer to an appropriate medical setting, such as an Accident and Emergency department. There, it is likely that other measures, including oxygen, intravenous hydrocortisone, and intravenous or

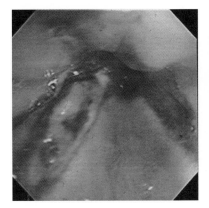
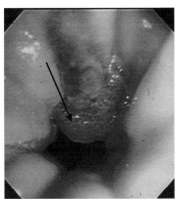

Figure 8.1 Endoscopic appearances in food-allergic gastro-oesophageal reflux in infants. Both cases show endoscopic evidence of oesophagitis, with linear reddening of the mucosa and contact bleeding. The case on the right demonstrates an oesophageal 'pearl' (arrowed), which is found on histological assessment to contain multiple eosinophils. Both cases failed to resolve with conventional medical therapy, but normalised on exclusion diet.

intramuscular chlorpheniramine, should be administered, and the requirement for inhaled bronchodilator therapy assessed. Supportive treatment for hypotension or cardiac dysrrhythmia may be required, and in the most severe cases the patient may need to be transferred to an intensive therapy unit.

In the follow-up of a patient who has had an immediate hypersensitive response to food antigens, a decision needs to be taken about the level of prophylaxis required, and whether or not to prescribe an adrenaline pen. Clearly the severity of the first response will inform this decision, and it is probably better to err on the side of caution if foods such as peanuts are implicated, because of their propensity for triggering particularly severe episodes. If there is doubt about the specific food involved, both skin-prick tests and specific IgE tests (RASTs) may be very helpful: these should be postponed for several weeks after an episode of anaphylaxis as they may be artefactually negative in the immediate aftermath of a severe reaction.

Late-onset symptoms

Symptoms may appear slowly and insidiously, and their true allergic nature may not be recognised (Table 8.1). These may include failure to thrive or chronic diarrhoea due to enteropathy or colitis, eczema, rhinitis, or rectal bleeding. As these are likely to be mediated by T cells in a delayed hypersensitive reaction, they may not be so clearly linked to food ingestion. More recently, the concept of food-allergic intestinal dysmotility has been sug-

gested in paediatric patients, with dietary antigen (most commonly cow's milk, soya, or wheat) inducing gastro-oesophageal reflux (Figures 8.1 and 8.2) or constipation (Figure 8.3). On gastrointestinal investigation of children with delayed responses, antigen-induced dysmotility or mucosal pathology such as small-intestinal enteropathy or colitis may often be found. However, it can be the case that both skin-prick tests and RASTs are negative but food elimination relieves all the symptoms and challenge with the food causes return of symptoms. If a child with severe eczema, failure to thrive, or intractable reflux has been transformed by an exclusion diet, it may be appropriate to defer such challenge until after a period of stability. Much more common is the problem of a patient with a genuine food-induced reaction who is refused appropriate treatment because the 'investigations are negative' – that is, specific IgE or skin-prick tests – and thus it 'can't be allergy'. Thankfully, recognition of non-IgE-mediated allergy is improving, although this does rely on clinical awareness of the diagnostic possibility.

Both types of reaction may occur individually or together: as mentioned above, a careful history will often uncover delayed in addition to immediate food reactions. The slow response is likely to be T cell-mediated, and the frequency of patients with low circulating immunoglobulins in the food-allergic population means that patients may have clinically important dietary responses without detectable antibodies.

*Failure to detect specific antibodies does **not** rule out food allergy.*

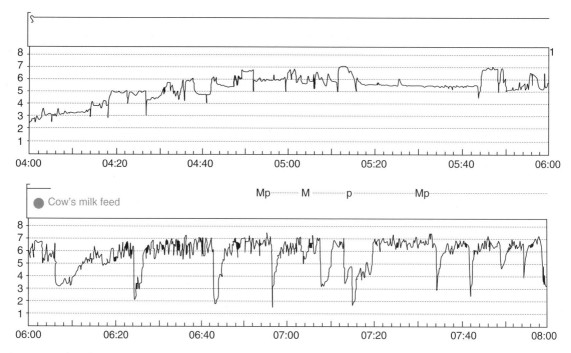

Figure 8.2 Evidence from a 24-hour pH study of the triggering of gastro-oesophageal reflux by cow's milk in a 3-year-old child. Episodes of reflux are seen when the pH dips below 4. During the course of 24 hours, the reflux episodes only occurred after milk, and not after taking equal volumes of an amino acid formula.

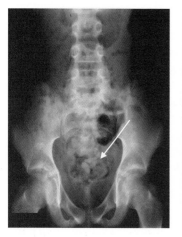
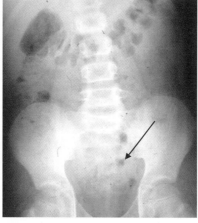

Figure 8.3 Allergic dysmotility with chronic constipation. Abdominal X-ray is often helpful, as the constipation may not be clinically obvious if the characteristic impaction within the rectum (acquired megarectum, arrowed) is the only feature. These cases were chronically unresponsive to conventional therapy, but remitted after cow's milk and wheat were excluded from the diet for a period of several months.

8.6 Diagnostic criteria for food allergy

Whatever the results of tests, an essential criterion for secure diagnosis of food allergy is a response to an elimination diet. Ideally there should be relief of all symptoms, with restoration of normal growth if the patient is a child. A positive response to challenge is strongly supportive but is not always essential in routine practice, particularly when other diagnostic tests were positive at diagnosis.

In childhood allergy, there is often reacquisition of tolerance with age, and a challenge may then reasonably be performed when the child is older (usually over 2 years, often rather later, especially in multiply allergic children). Various bodies, including EAACI (European Academy of Allergy and Clinical

Immunology) and ESPGHAN (European Society for Paediatric Gastroenterology, Hepatology and Nutrition), have made recommendations for diagnostic criteria.

In children with multiple food allergies, the response to elimination of a single antigen may be incomplete, and inpatient assessment with a very restricted diet may be required. Such situations can become very challenging, and it may be difficult to persuade some parents to broaden their child's diet. If the patient is manifesting non-IgE-mediated allergy, it may be difficult for anyone concerned (including the allergist) to achieve diagnostic certainty. As such affected children typically relapse symptomatically when suffering intercurrent viral infections, and have a propensity for prolonged viral infections related to minor immunodeficiency, it is imprudent to make any definitive statements about the extent of allergies, or even to perform food challenges, while the child is unwell.

In cases where there remains uncertainty or controversy about potential reactions, blinded food challenges may be needed. Close teamwork with an experienced dietitian is absolutely required. The 'gold-standard' double-blind placebo-controlled food challenge (DBPCFC) is a cumbersome and time-consuming intervention that nevertheless may have a very useful and important role in sorting out such cases. If there is real uncertainty about a single food, and the child makes immediate responses, it may be possible to repeat the challenge and withdrawal, and to truly establish tolerance or persistent reactivity in a way that no other test can. Its value decreases markedly when there are large numbers of foods to be tested and the child makes delayed responses only. Normal day-to-day variation may then be over-interpreted, stress will increase due to prolonged hospital admission, and the child may acquire a viral infection, rendering interpretation difficult. As non-IgE-mediated responses may take up to a week to manifest, this testing scenario can become very complex in cases of likely multiple-food allergy. Lack of a reliable biomarker for non-IgE-mediated food allergy makes such management particularly difficult.

In adult practice, similar principles may apply, and indeed similar problems may occur. Food allergy can be invoked as a cause of an almost unlimited spectrum of symptoms, and such beliefs will be given apparent credence by any number of internet Web sites. Conversely, there are many people with genuine delayed hypersensitive reactions – food-allergic dysmotility is a good example – in whom the opportunity for clinical improvement is missed because of a lack of immediate hypersensitive responses and negative skin-prick and specific IgE tests. The time-consuming nature of extensive DBPCFC testing is difficult to reconcile with most full-time occupations.

8.7 Food-sensitive enteropathy

In food-sensitive enteropathy, there is an immune-mediated abnormality of the small-intestinal mucosa, which may include excess lymphocyte infiltration, epithelial abnormality, or architectural disturbance with crypt lengthening or villous shortening. This can often impair absorption or even cause a frank malabsorption syndrome. This continues while the food remains in the diet and remits on an exclusion diet. In cases of diagnostic uncertainty, it may be necessary to confirm the return of mucosal abnormality by food challenge. The two most common causes of such enteropathy in childhood are cow's milk (cow's milk-sensitive enteropathy, CMSE) and wheat (coeliac disease). Unlike in coeliac disease, the mucosa in CMSE may show relatively subtle changes, such as villous blunting or mild increase in mucosal eosinophils (Figure 8.4).

8.8 Specific food allergies

Allergic responses to many food proteins have been described. The most common in childhood are cow's milk, soya, eggs, and fish, with peanut allergy rapidly becoming more common. Intolerance to fruits, vegetable, meats, chocolate, nuts, shellfish, and cereals have also been described. In adult life there is a different spectrum, with allergy to nuts, fruits, and fish relatively more common than in childhood. However, as the dietary exposures of UK children broaden, the range of reported allergens also increases: thus sesame, kiwi fruit, mango, avocado, and other allergies have increased in frequency. As mentioned in the introduction, such sensitisation appears to depend more on genetics, infectious challenges, and patterns of exposure than on the innate antigenicity of

(a)   (b)

(c)

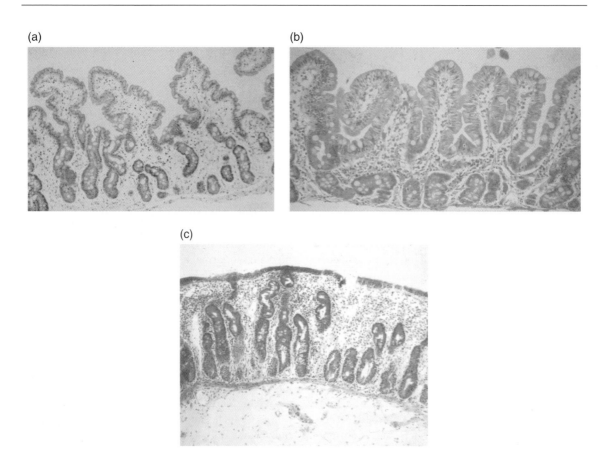

Figure 8.4 Histological changes occur within the small intestine in food-sensitive enteropathy. In specimen (a), which is from a nonallergic child with poor growth who did not eventually have a gastroenterological diagnosis (thus likely to represent normal findings at this age), there are long villi with no lengthening of the crypts, and no evidence of excess inflammatory infiltrate within the epithelium or lamina propria. Specimen (b) was obtained from a child with cow's milk-sensitive enteropathy (CMSE). There are subtle abnormalities, including some shortening and blunting of the villi and a modest increase in lymphocyte density within the lamina propria. However, it is easy to see why specimens are sometimes labelled 'within normal limits', particularly in centres where there are no paediatric pathologists. Specimen (c), by contrast, is grossly abnormal and shows the characteristic features in coeliac disease, with complete loss of villous architecture and lengthening of the crypts (crypt hyperplastic villous atrophy). There is a dense infiltrate of lymphocytes and plasma cells.

individual foodstuffs, with the possible exception of some highly allergenic foods such as peanuts.

There is no consistent association between any particular food and specific syndromes, although some foods are more likely to induce enteropathy, particularly cow's milk and soya. This may simply be a reflection of the dose ingested. The incidence of gastrointestinal food allergy is greatest in early life and appears to decrease with age. In early life, the enteropathy associated with dietary allergy may sometimes be relatively subtle (Figure 8.5), but it can cause profound failure to thrive (Figure 8.6). However, complex dietary allergy can occur with quite normal growth (Figure 8.7). Some recent reports

suggest that CMSE may indeed occur in adult life, but the whole area remains under-studied.

Cow's milk

Cow's milk hypersensitivity may manifest as described above, either as an immediate response, sometimes including anaphylaxis, or with delayed responses within the gut or skin. These sensitisations can follow an episode of gastroenteritis and may manifest as 'lactose intolerance'. As mentioned above, lactose intolerance in infants and young children is most commonly a secondary consequence of a food-sensitive enteropathy. Use of reduced-lactose

(a)   (b)

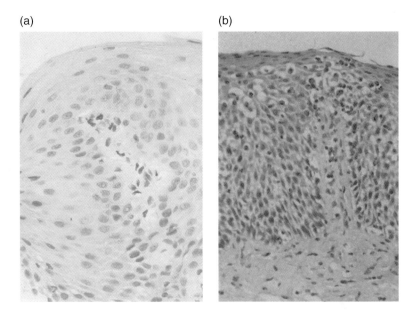

Figure 8.5 Histological findings in the oesophagus in food-allergic dysmotility. (a) Infiltration of lymphocytes within the papillae, from the lamina propria underlying the epithelium. (b) Large numbers of eosinophils, showing their characteristic red cytoplasm, within the epithelium.

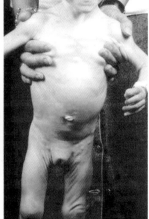

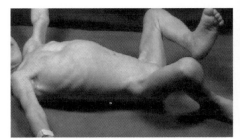

Figure 8.6 Potential severe nutritional consequences of dietary allergies. The child on the left, who suffered from cow's milk-sensitive enteropathy (CMSE), shows severe wasting without abdominal distension. The child on the right, who has coeliac disease, shows gross wasting with the classical abdominal protuberance. The majority of cases of coeliac disease show much less obvious abnormality, hence the phrase 'the coeliac iceberg' – most cases are hidden out of sight.

cow's milk simply masks this problem, without addressing the basic lesion. Few would advocate treating lactose intolerance in coeliac disease by a lactose-free gluten-containing diet.

CMSE may induce protein-losing enteropathy or iron-deficiency anaemia. Cow's milk colitis may also occur, and can induce occult or overt gastrointestinal bleeding. Usually CMSE and cows' milk-induced colitis do not coexist in the same patient. Cow's milk allergy is now recognised to induce oesophageal reflux in many infants, which in severe cases can also induce haematemesis or anaemia.

Soya

Soy-based formulas have for some years been used in infants with cow's milk allergy, although not usually by paediatric gastroenterologists or allergists. They are not currently recommended by EAACI or ESPGHAN as first-line treatment for infants with cow's milk allergy, both instead recommending hydrolysates (with amino acid formulas for the subgroup of infants who are sensitised to hydrolysates). Soy formulas appear to be at least as antigenic as cow's milk-based formulas, and there are numerous reports of intolerance to soy protein. Such reactions

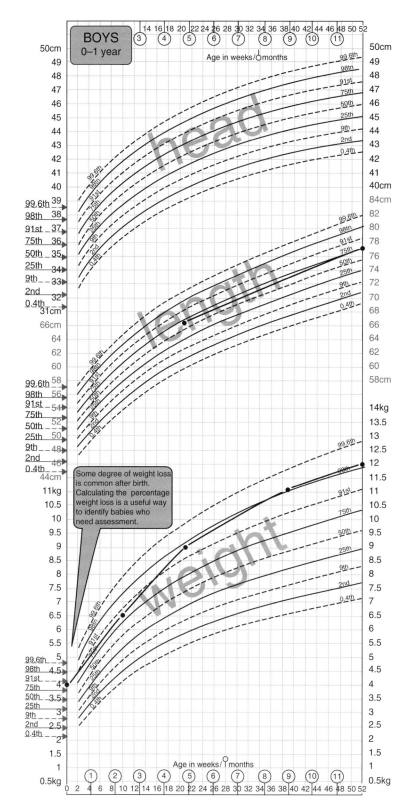

Figure 8.7 Dietary allergy does not always cause failure to thrive. This child, who had both IgE-mediated and non-IgE-mediated allergies to multiple dietary antigens, nevertheless showed good growth despite chronic eczema, colic, gastro-oesophageal reflux, and constipation. In well-grown children without an IgE-mediated component, who have negative skin-prick tests and RASTs, the diagnosis of allergy is often missed and the parents are labelled 'neurotic' or 'demanding'. Chart developed by RCPCH/WHO/Department of Health, Copyright © 2009 Department of Health.

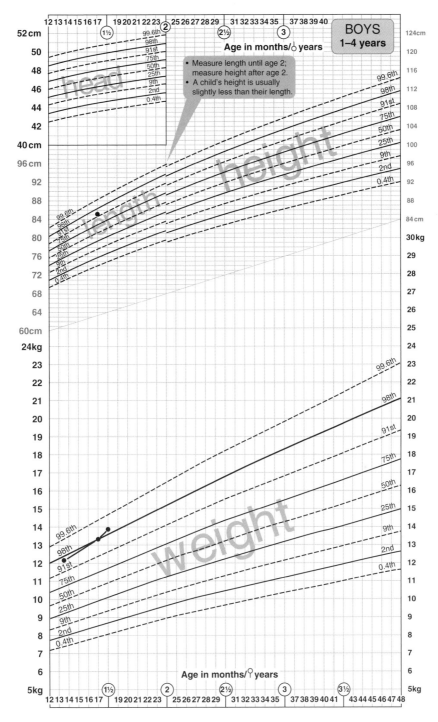

Figure 8.7 (*Continued*)

have varied from anaphylaxis to chronic enteropathy, as well as eczema, asthma, and colitis. They may be useful in older infants and children with milk allergy, as they are more palatable than hydrolysates or amino acid formulas.

Egg

In contrast to cow's milk, egg allergy usually presents as an acute response or with exacerbation of infant eczema, and there is no real evidence of egg enteropathy. Vomiting within a few minutes to an hour after ingestion is characteristic, but diarrhoea, abdominal pain, and nausea may also occur. Delayed responses are most likely to occur in the lungs (asthma) and skin (eczema). RAST and skin-prick responses to egg are more likely to be positive than for many other allergens.

Wheat

While acute allergic reactions to wheat are much more rare, acute wheat anaphylaxis has been described. Delayed hypersensitive reactions are both common and clinically important. Of particular importance is the role of wheat gluten in causing coeliac disease (Figure 8.4), which is not only common (now recognised to occur in >1% of European populations) but very variable in manifestation – from the classic child with profound failure to thrive and malabsorption to a thriving child with unexplained neurological problems or anaemia. While in-depth discussion of coeliac disease is beyond the scope of this review, it is important to recognise that its incidence is increased in children with other dietary allergies, partly because IgA deficiency is a shared risk factor, and it is advisable that serological testing for coeliac disease (currently based on IgA antibodies to tissue transglutaminase) be performed in all food-allergic patients if blood is being taken for other tests.

Subtle forms of wheat intolerance

Less well understood is the role of wheat in precipitating intestinal dysmotility, which can manifest as gastro-oesophageal reflux and particularly constipation. Allergic dysmotility represents part of the spectrum of non-IgE-mediated food allergy and is receiving increasing recognition. There is now increasing evidence that both gastro-oesophageal reflux and constipation may be features of the food-allergic dysmotility syndrome (Figures 8.1, 8.2, 8.3, and 8.4), which may present as infant colic and then continue well beyond infancy to cause chronic symptoms that require prolonged dietary exclusions. There are so far few studies of food-allergic dysmotility in adults, but this area may become directly relevant to irritable bowel syndrome in atopic patients.

The histological characteristic of food-allergic dysmotility is local infiltration of eosinophils within tissue (Figure 8.5). In addition, both wheat and cow's milk may sometimes be implicated in childhood behavioural disturbances, although the literature is still inadequate to provide clinical certainty. The effects of wheat exclusion in such children may sometimes be very striking, but it is mandatory to screen for coeliac disease before commencing such a diet.

Peanuts

Peanut allergy is concerning because of its rising incidence and its propensity to induce severe anaphylaxis. Even trace amounts of peanut can cause death in those severely sensitised. The reasons for the surge in peanut-hypersensitive cases may relate to different patterns of exposure, with sensitisation via low-dose exposure in breast milk, or even by the percutaneous route in children with eczema, if skin creams containing peanut-derived oils are used.

It is now recommended that UK children, particularly from an atopic background, are not given peanut products until after the age of 6 years. However, as most children now appear to be sensitised very early in life by nonclassical routes, this may not be as effective as hoped. The LEAP study is currently underway, aiming to determine whether early high-dose administration of peanut antigens to infants at risk of allergy may be better at preventing peanut allergies, through induction of immune tolerance, than the current policy of exclusion.

One encouraging point is that at least some early-sensitised infants may reacquire tolerance to peanuts with age. The skin-prick test is extremely useful in peanut allergy, particularly the size of response. Children with a >7 mm wheal have a >95% chance of remaining sensitised, and thus rechallenge is inadvisable. By contrast, those with a <4 mm response have a similar chance of being tolerant. However, peanut challenge should always be undertaken with extreme caution, by experienced personnel with full resuscitation equipment and appropriate drugs to hand.

8.9 Multiple-food allergy

Increasing numbers of infants and children develop gastrointestinal and other symptoms related to a wide variety of foods. These may be immediate or delayed, and do not differ significantly from those described above for individual foods. Patients often have an individual and family history of atopy, and may have increased eosiniphils in peripheral blood, with elevated serum IgE and positive RAST and skin tests to specific foods. In this circumstance, there is overlap with eosinophilic gastroenteritis, where eosinophils are found within gastric and intestinal biopsies but where a clear history of dietary triggering may not be obtained. Many such cases sensitise by the evolutionarily novel route of maternal breast milk, with the trace amounts of dietary proteins apparently sufficient to sensitise or insufficient to tolerise: a specific defect in oral tolerance for low-dose antigen has been postulated as a cause of this phenomenon. Diets involving the elimination of single foods are usually ineffective.

It was first shown that infants can be sensitised to cows' milk via trace amounts in maternal breast milk of a cow's milk-drinking mother, and more recently it has become clear that sensitisation to many other antigens can occur in this way. One important clinical point is that many infants show continued responses to trace amounts of cow's milk protein in conventional hydrolysate formulas, and may require an amino acid-based formula. Such propensity to sensitise during breastfeeding would clearly have been maladaptive in evolutionary terms. This novel response is thought likely to be a consequence of recent changes in nondietary exposures (e.g. altered gut bacteria in the first week of life, related to changed perinatal management of infants and antibiotic use), which may be preventing the normal induction of immune tolerance to low-dose antigens. We identified evidence that infants who sensitise in this way show low numbers of immune cells in the small intestine producing transforming growth factor (TGF)-β, the cytokine involved in low-dose oral tolerance. Gut bacteria play a critical role in inducing such regulatory cells within the mucosa, as described in Section 8.10.

8.10 Scientific background: the basic mechanisms of immune response to dietary antigen

Innate immunity and the importance of evolutionary heritage

Much progress has been made in the last 3 decades in understanding the basic mechanisms of immune responses to dietary components. There is one important difference in the overall set-up of the mucosal immune system of the intestine when compared to the systemic immune system, essentially due to evolutionary longevity. This relates to a relative dominance of innate immune mechanisms, preserved within the intestines of multiple species for hundreds of millions of years. Long before the earliest development of adaptive immune systems, which can recognise antigen in a specific way and respond more vigorously on reacquaintance, the basic mechanisms of host defence through innate immunity were in place within the gut. The explorations of comparative immunology in primitive organisms by Ilya Metchnikoff in the late nineteenth century established a clear cellular basis for host defence within the gut, which has considerably more resonance today than it appeared to have for his peers at the time. Much current work focuses on the molecules and receptors, such as Toll-protein receptors, that integrate initial innate immune responses with a subsequent specific lymphocyte reaction.

The pattern of evolutionary change in the intestine appears to be one of adding on new levels of control, rather than of abandoning the older, established mechanisms. The intestine contains disproportionately large numbers of primitive lymphocytes that arose substantially earlier than classic T cells and B cells. These include B1 cells, B cells which produce antibody of broad affinity for bacterial products but generally of low specificity for individual antigens. Amongst the T cell population, similarly archaic γδ cells (which express γ and δ chains instead of the α and β chains of classic T cells), are also highly over-represented within the intestinal epithelium.

Although animal data suggest that they play an important role in intestinal immune responses, little is yet known about the role of these numerous cell types in the maintenance of enteric tolerance in humans.

Lymphocytes may differentiate within the intestine and not the thymus

The great majority of circulating T cells mature within the thymus, where cells do not survive if they either fail to react adequately to self-major histocompatibility complex molecules (MHCs) or if they overreact to self-antigen. In this way, the tendency towards autoimmunity is minimised, although this is clearly unlikely to affect potential reactivity towards dietary antigen. However, it is apparent that a very substantial portion of the body's T cells do not undergo this process, but mature instead within the epithelium of the intestine (so-called extrathymic differentiation). Thus T cells may be detected at several stages of immaturity in the epithelium. It is fair to say that very little indeed is known about the interaction of these cells with dietary antigens, yet given their huge numbers and their situation – right at the very interface with luminal antigens of all types – it is extremely likely that these reactions are very important. It is notable that infants with immunodeficiencies of all kinds have an extraordinarily high incidence of dietary sensitisations, chronic enteropathy, and failure to thrive. Much is yet to be learned, which may give insight into the basic mechanisms of acquiring or regaining tolerance to dietary antigens.

Antigen presentation by the epithelium

In recent years, some light has been shed on the role of gut epithelial cells (enterocytes) within the mucosal immune system. Enterocytes line the lumen of the gut and represent the first cellular component of the mucosal barrier to antigens, separating the immune system of the gut from both dietary antigens of all kinds and massive numbers of bacteria. Apart from their function in the absorption of nutrients, enterocytes are now recognised for their ability to process antigens and present them to the immune system. They also secrete immunoregulatory cytokines, affecting the way the immune system reacts. Therefore, a role for intestinal epithelial cells in the induction of tolerance has been suggested, and it is suspected that

enterocytes are of major importance in downregulating immunologically-mediated intestinal inflammation, either by induction of tolerogenic lymphocyte subsets (regulatory T cells) or through direct effects on lymphocyte activity.

In support of this contention, it is now recognised that disturbed epithelial function leads to immunopathology. Animal models with increased gut permeability demonstrate marked secondary inflammation around leaky epithelium. In the context of allergy, it is notable that sensitisation to cow's milk formulas often occurs in the aftermath of gastroenteritis, where epithelial integrity has been damaged by pathogens.

Distribution of T cells within the intestine

It is likely that T-cell responses are critical in determining tolerance or sensitisation to dietary antigens, and there are intriguing differences in genetically determined patterns of sensitisation to individual antigens. This is seen particularly well in East Asia and Australasia, although little is known still about the mechanisms underlying this in humans.

There are clear differences between the T cells of the lamina propria (the tissue beneath the epithelium) and the epithelium itself in the small intestine. CD8 cells may have both suppressor and cytotoxic functions, whereas CD4 cells control functions of other cell types by secretion of individual cytokines. CD8 cells predominate within the epithelial compartment, where they are known as intraepithelial lymphocytes (IELs), whereas CD4 cells are uncommonly seen within this compartment. By contrast, CD4 cells predominate within the lamina propria. Great advance has been made in dissecting the patterns of secretion of inflammatory messenger molecules (cytokines), and two broad patterns of cytokine production are now recognised. This is of major importance in controlling allergic responses.

The $T_H1/T_H2/T_H17$ paradigm of T-cell responses and infectious exposures

T helper cells coordinate the immune response by both direct cell–cell contact and secretion of cytokines. Three major groups of T helper cells are now recognised, directing immune reactions towards either cell-mediated (T_H1/T_H17) or humorally mediated

(T_H2) responses. T_H1 cells produce cytokines such as IL-2, interferon-γ, and TNFα and β, which induce chronic cell-mediated responses and suppress IgE production. Such reactions occur in Crohn's disease, sarcoidosis, and probably coeliac disease. T_H2 cells produce a contrasting combination of cytokines (IL-4, IL-5, IL-6, IL-10, and IL-13) that promote humoral responses, including IgE production, and suppress cell-mediated responses. T_H17 cells produce IL-17 and IL-22 and are predominantly concerned with defence against extracellular pathogens. In contrast to systemic allergic responses, which are often T_H2-dominated, intestinal allergic reactions may also involve the other types of immune reaction. At its core, allergic responses in the gut are determined by a reduction in the generation of regulatory T cells, which damp down potential reactions of T_H1, T_H2, or T_H17 type, rather than by excess production of one pro-inflammatory cell type.

Control of B-cell responses, and the importance of mucosal IgA production

Antibodies are produced by plasma cells, which are terminally differentiated B cells, and this may occur either independently of T cells or following specific interactions between T cells and B cells. Only after such specific interaction can high-affinity antibodies be produced. However, within the intestine there is also large-scale production of T cell-independent antibodies, directed against bacterial components, by the primitive B1 cell population. It remains unclear whether this response is involved in dietary tolerance.

T cells play an important role in shaping the type of antibody response, and T cell-derived cytokines and surface molecules directly affect the shift in antibody isotype (from the default IgM response) towards either the protective IgA response or the pro-allergic IgE response. TGF-β is highly important in this regard, as a molecule that induces IgA production. Recent evidence suggests that pathways leading to mucosal IgA production are shared with those inducing a T regulatory response and are influenced critically by gut bacteria.

The pattern of antibody production within the gut immune system is significantly different from systemic responses, in that IgA predominates, and this is important in protecting the mucosal surface and limiting allergic sensitisation. Within the lamina propria, IgA plasma cells dominate, and even in allergic children the number of IgE plasma cells is relatively low. IgA is secreted actively into the lumen in a dimeric form called secretory IgA, following its complexing with secretory component, a glycoprotein synthesised by the enterocytes. As IgA antibodies complex with luminal antigen, they are important regulators of dietary antigen entry.

Detection of serum IgG antibodies to food antigens implies either that ingested immunogenic molecules have entered the systemic circulation and induced a response there or that local intestinal skewing towards the IgA isotype has been disrupted. Small amounts of food IgG antibodies, particularly to cow's milk or wheat gliadin, are often found in the serum of normal children. These may not indicate clinically relevant intolerance, although high titres suggest a problem with mucosal permeability, as seen in small-intestinal enteropathy.

Skewing of B cells towards IgE

While it is now increasingly accepted that non-IgE-mediated responses to dietary antigen may be an important cause of chronic symptomatology, IgE-mediated mechanisms account for the majority of immediate hypersensitive reactions to foods. Transient IgE responses to foods are seen in normal children, but their clinical relevance is uncertain. By contrast, high-level IgE responses are usually pathological and may be important in severe food allergies and anaphylaxis.

Production of IgE is favoured by a dominance of T_H2 responses, particularly due to IL-4 and IL-13 secretion. By contrast with T_H2 cytokines, products of T_H1 cells (particularly IFN-γ and IL-2) directly inhibit IgE production, as do other T_H1-associated cytokines such as IL-12 and Il-18. As T_H1 responses are upregulated by infectious exposures, this may partly explain the protection against allergy that childhood within the developing world gives.

Mucosally produced IgE may also be transported into the gut lumen (or airway), like IgA, but by a mechanism that does not utilise secretory component. Such compartmentalisation of response may explain why skin-prick testing or serum-specific IgE tests (RASTs) may be negative in some cases where there is a clear history of rapid-onset responses to dietary antigens.

Mast cells and eosinophils in food allergies

As mentioned above, there is a clear link between food-allergic responses within the intestine and the infiltration of eosinophils: white blood cells which produce a number of vasoactive and proinflammatory mediators. Both eosinophils and mast cells, which also produce such mediators, have been particularly implicated in dysmotility responses, and it is likely that these products directly affect the function of enteric nerves. Elevated levels of eosinophil cytokines have been detected in the stools of infants with food allergies associated with eczema. Although mast cells and eosinophils produce a similar spectrum of mediators, with similar effects upon gut motility, they may mediate two quite different responses: rapid responses are induced by immediate degranulation of mast cells (which store 'pre-packed' mediators in intracellular granules), whereas delayed responses may occur after recruitment of eosinophils from the peripheral circulation. As eosinophil accumulation within the mucosa is a hallmark of chronic food-allergic responses, there has been great interest in their recruitment mechanisms. Two molecules are very clearly implicated: the chemokine (chemotactic cytokine) eotaxin and the cytokine IL-5. There is increasing evidence for a final common pathway in the mucosal allergic response to dietary antigen, which is dependent on upregulation of IL-5 production and expression of the chemokine eotaxin. These may be amenable to specific therapy in the future.

Oral tolerance to dietary antigens

Oral tolerance is an actively maintained phenomenon which extends beyond the confines of the mucosal immune system, so that systemic immunological tolerance to an antigen is induced by taking it orally. The molecular mechanisms of oral tolerance to dietary antigens have been the subject of intense study. The nature of the antigen is to a certain extent important, and some foods are undeniably more sensitising than others. However, as in so much of immunology, the most critical components appear to be antigen dosage, timing of first administration, and input from innate immunity.

The dose of ingested antigen appears to be particularly important in determining how tolerance is established. Clearly the bulk of dietary antigen needs to be absorbed by enterocytes for nutritional purposes, and this is presented by the epithelium to the immune system in such a way that lymphocyte reactivity is suppressed and the lymphocytes are rendered anergic. Potential mechanisms include the known absent expression of co-stimulatory molecules by enterocytes and more direct inhibition of the lymphocytes by suppressor-cell populations or cytokines. Epithelial barrier function is critical, and this form of tolerance may be abrogated by epithelial damage and consequent presentation of dietary antigen by activated antigen-presenting cells. This explains the post-gastroenteritis sensitisation to cow's milk that is well-recognised in bottle-fed infants.

Tolerance to low-dose antigen is thought to be mediated separately, and requires uptake by the antigen-sampling M cells in the epithelium overlying the organised lymphoid tissue of Peyer's patches. This process depends on the active generation of regulatory lymphocytes within the lymphoid tissues of the intestine. Two cytokines are particularly important in the generation of regulatory T cells (of which several types have been recognised), namely TGF-β and IL-10. Although probably produced within Peyer's patches and mesenteric lymph nodes, regulatory T cells home back to the intestinal lamina propria via the circulation. Once there, they act to suppress intestinal immune reactivity by a process termed 'bystander tolerance', in which they release TGF-β or IL-10 upon encountering antigen, thereby inhibiting the potential reactivity of all surrounding lymphocytes. If these cells are not generated, spontaneous gut inflammation may occur in response to the enteric flora, and tolerance cannot be established.

The major clue to the role of infectious challenge in preventing food allergies comes from recognition that both gut colonisation and local inflammation appear to be required to establish oral tolerance. Mice maintained germ-free – that is, without gut colonisation – do not establish normal enteric tolerance for antigen and require about 30% additional calories to gain weight compared to colonised mice. The sheer extent of gene induction now known to occur within enterocytes via the commensal flora is an important recent finding and is probably quite central in concepts of mucosal tolerance. Probiotics may represent a promising approach to establishing oral tolerance mechanisms. However, although most probiotic studies have focused on bifidobacteria and lactobacilli, recent data in mice point towards clostridia and bacteroides as the critical species that induce mucosal tolerance. So far, the human equivalents are unknown, but their identification will be extremely important in offering new directions for specific therapy of food allergies.

8.11 Concluding remarks

These substantial recent findings from the basic science arena promise a shift in emphasis in food allergy from the downstream effector mechanisms of IgE response towards a broader consideration of mucosal tolerance. Does a genetic tendency to high IgE response simply mean that adverse immune reactions are more noticeable? Certainly doctors are happier to have specific tests to use, and non-IgE-mediated allergy is thus an uncomfortable area for many. The absence of specific tests can also lead to overdiagnosis, as a few minutes on the Internet will testify.

However, a time in which paradigms are shifting is also an exciting time, with major opportunities for real advance. The whole area of basic research, now seen to involve both intestinal inflammation and allergy due to shared tolerance mechanisms, begin to explain many of the important demographic shifts in allergy. We can say with some justification that a lack of appropriate early immune infectious priming may specifically hinder the development of normal gut tolerance. Such events may occur right at the start of life, and infant handling at the time of initial colonisation may have impact on allergic sensitisation. Further studies focusing more specifically on the role of specific infectious exposures within the gut on the development of food allergies are likely. It is therefore possible that future therapeutic approaches to food allergy will be as strongly based on stimulation of innate immune responses in early life in order to optimise tolerance as in antigen exclusion.

References and further reading

Agostoni C, Decsi T, Fewtrell M, Goulet O, Kolacek S, Koletzko B, Michaelsen KF, Moreno L, Puntis J, Rigo J, Shamir R, Szajewska H, Turck D, van Goudoever J. Complementary feeding: a commentary by the ESPGHAN Committee on Nutrition. J Pediatr Gastroenterol Nutr 2008; 46: 99–110.

American Academy of Pediatricsl, Committee on Nutrition. Hypoallergenic infant formulas. Pediatrics 2000; 106: 346–349.

Barth B, Furuta GT. These FADS are here to stay – clinicopathological patterns of food allergic diseases. Gastroenterology 2004; 126: 1481–1482.

Carroccio A, Montalto G, Custro N, Notarbartolo A, Cavataio F, D'Amico D, Alabrese D, Iacono G. Evidence of very delayed clinical reactions to cow's milk in cow's milk-intolerant patients. Allergy 2000; 55: 574–579.

ESPGHAN. Diagnostic criteria for food allergy with predominantly intestinal symptoms. J Pediatr Gastroenterol Nutr 1992; 14: 108–112.

Fox AT, Lloyd K, Arkwright PD, bhattacharya D, Brown T, Chetcuti P, East M, Gaventa J, King R, Martinez A, Meyer R, Parikh A, Perkin M, Shah N, Tuthill D, Walsh J, Waddell L, Warner J. The RCPCH care pathway for food allergy in children: an evidence based national approach. Arch Dis Child 2011; 96(Suppl. 2): i25–i29.

Gell PGH, Coombs RRA. Classification of allergic reactions responsible for hypersensitivity and disease. In: Clinical Aspects of Immunology (PGH Gell, RRA Coombs, eds). Oxford: Blackwell, 1968. p. 575.

Hepatology and Nutrition (ESPGHAN) Committee on Nutrition. Dietary products used in infants for treatment and prevention of food allergy. Arch Dis Child 1999; 81: 80–84.

Høst A, Halken S, Muraro A, Dreborg S, Niggemann B, Aalberse R, Ashad SH, von Berg A, Carlsen KH, Duschén K, Eigenmann PA, Hill D, Jones C, Mellon M, Oldeus G, Oranje A, Pascual C, Prescott S, Sampson H, Svartengren M, Wahn U, Warner JA, Warner JO, Vandenplas Y, Wickman M, Zeiger RS. Dietary prevention of allergic diseases in infants and small children. Pediatr Allergy Immunol 2008; 19: 1–4.

Iacono G, Cavataio F, Montalto G, Florena A, Tumminello M, Soresi M, Notarbartolo A, Carroccio A. Intolerance of cow's milk and chronic constipation in children. New Engl J Med 1998; 339: 1100–1104.

Kalliomaki M, Salminen S, Arvilommi H, Kero P, Koskinen P, Isolauri E. Probiotics in primary prevention of atopic disease: a randomised placebo-controlled trial. Lancet 2001; 357: 1076–1079.

Latcham F, Merino F, Lang A, Garvey J, Thomson MA, Walker-Smith JA, Davies SE, Phillips AD, Murch SH. A consistent pattern of minor immunodeficiency and subtle enteropathy in children with multiple food allergy. J Pediatr 2003; 143: 39–47.

Matricardi PM, Rosmini F, Riondino S, Fortini M, Ferrigno L, Rapicetta M, Bonini S. Exposure to foodborne and orofecal microbes versus airborne viruses in relation to atopy and allergic asthma. BMJ 2000; 320: 412–417.

Murch S. Allergy and intestinal dysmotility – evidence of genuine causal linkage? Curr Opin Gastroenterol 2006; 22: 664–668.

Murch SH. Clinical manifestations of food allergy: the old and the new. Eur J Gastroenterol Hepatol 2005; 17: 1287–1291.

Murch SH. Gastrointestinal mucosal immunology and mechanisms of inflammation. In: Pediatric Gastrointestinal and Liver Disease, 4thedn (Wyllie R, Hyams JS eds). Philadelphia, PA: Elsevier, 2011, pp. 50–63.

Rook GA. Hygiene and other early childhood influences on the subsequent function of the immune system. Dig Dis 2011; 29(2): 144–153.

Sampson HA, Sichere SH, Bimbaum AH. AGA technical review on the evaluation of food allergy in gastrointestinal disorders. American Gastroenterological Association. Gastroenterology 2001; 120: 1026–1040.

Simon D, Wardlaw A, Rothenberg ME. Organ-specific eosinophilic disorders of the skin, lung, and gastrointestinal tract. J Allergy Clin Immunol 2010; 126: 3–13.

von Mutius E, Vercelli D. Farm living: effects on childhood asthma and allergy. Nat Rev Immunol 2010; 10: 861–868.

9
Nutritional Support

Esther van den Hogen,[1] Marian AE van Bokhorst-de van der Schueren,[2]
and Cora F Jonkers-Schuitema[3]

[1] Maastricht UMC, Maastricht, The Netherlands
[2] VU University Medical Centre, Amsterdam, The Netherlands
[3] Academic Medical Centre, Amsterdam, The Netherlands

Key messages

- Disease-related malnutrition is a frequent clinical finding in hospital populations.
- Improvement in nutritional intake can be achieved with food fortification and dietary counselling, oral nutritional supplements, enteral feeding, parenteral nutrition, or a combination of these approaches.

- Nutritional support can effectively contribute to improved functional and clinical outcomes, not only in hospitals, but also in the community setting.

9.1 Introduction

'Nutritional support' refers to the provision of adequate nutrients to meet the requirements of patients at risk of developing malnutrition. This can be in the form of oral diet, diet and nutritional supplements, or artificial nutritional support, such as enteral or parenteral feeding. Identifying people at risk of undernutrition is the first step in management. Many studies have shown that a substantial proportion of hospitalised patients are at risk of developing malnutrition. This proportion may increase in certain population groups. Assessing nutritional status and assessing nutritional requirements is necessary before optimal nutritional support can be instigated.

Causes and consequences of malnutrition and the process of assessing nutritional status are discussed in Chapter 2. Specific guidelines for disease groups are discussed in the chapters specific to those conditions. Ethical issues should always be considered before considering nutritional support, and these are covered very comprehensively in Chapter 10. This chapter aims to outline general considerations in providing nutritional support and the methods and products available to do so.

9.2 Meeting nutritional needs

Energy, macronutrients, minerals, vitamins, trace elements, fluid, and electrolytes are all necessary for optimal body function. Without sufficient energy, fat and protein stores will be mobilised and these fuels will be oxidised in order to meet energy needs. Since the loss of protein stores directly affects body

---

Clinical Nutrition, Second Edition. Edited by Marinos Elia, Olle Ljungqvist, Rebecca J Stratton and Susan A Lanham-New.
© 2013 The Nutrition Society. Published 2013 by Blackwell Publishing Ltd.

function, it is important to administer sufficient amounts of energy and protein. Protein synthesis and protein degradation occur simultaneously in all body tissues; the difference between these two processes determines whether the body is anabolic or catabolic. Whereas in the diseased patient protein synthesis can be stimulated by feeding, protein intake cannot influence whole-body protein breakdown that occurs during inflammation. In severely ill patients, an increased protein intake of 1.5 g/kg body weight per day (normally 0.8 g/kg body weight/day) optimally stimulates protein synthesis, resulting in the least-negative nitrogen balance.

Carbohydrates are not essential nutrients as they can be produced from amino acids and glycerol. However, carbohydrates yield energy, and delivering carbohydrates in food prevents unnecessary stimulation of gluconeogenesis and thus slows down the rate of protein breakdown.

Fat is an excellent energy source that yields, on a weight basis, more than twice the energy of carbohydrates (9 vs. 4 kcal/gram). Dietary fat is also a source of essential fatty acids that cannot be synthesised by the body. Essential fatty acids maintain biomembrane structure, influence coagulation characteristics, and are precursors for leukotrienes and prostaglandins. The minimal fat allowance to ensure an adequate intake of fat-soluble vitamins and essential fatty acids is 10–15% of energy intake.

During disease, fluid and electrolyte balances can become disturbed. Fluid retention will affect body weight, and if not accounted for, can lead to inaccuracies in assessing nutritional requirements. Therefore, fluid/electrolyte balance should be carefully monitored and intake should be adapted accordingly (see Chapter 3).

In the past, hyperalimentation (the delivery of energy in excess of requirements) was thought to be efficient in improving nutritional status. However, hyperalimentation has been shown to induce severe metabolic abnormalities such as hyperglycaemia, hyperlipidaemia, and increased carbon dioxide production. Patients receiving nutritional support should be fed to meet their requirements. In clinical practice, basal energy expenditure is often calculated using empirical formulas, which are often regression equations, computed on the basis of energy expenditure and some anthropometric variables. Selected methods for estimating energy requirements are

---

Box 9.1 Selected methods for estimating energy requirements

There are several equations to predict energy requirements. The most frequently used are:

1. *Harris–Benedict equation* (1919)

Men: $66.4730 + (13.7516 \times W) + (5.0033 \times H) - (6.7550 \times A)$
Women: $655.0955 + (9.5634 \times W) + (1.8496 \times H) - (4.6756 \times A)$
W, weight in kg; H, height in cm; A, age in years.
To predict total energy expenditure (TEE), add an illness/activity factor of 1.2–1.8, depending on the severity and nature of illness.

2. *FAO/WHO/UNU equation*

Age (years)	kcal/day	Age (years)	kcal/day
men		*women*	
0–3	$60.9W - 54$	0–3	$61.0W - 51$
3–10	$22.7W + 495$	3–10	$22.5W + 499$
10–18	$17.5W + 651$	10–18	$12.2W + 745$
18–30	$15.3W + 679$	18–30	$14.7W + 496$
30–60	$11.6W + 879$	30–60	$8.7W + 829$
>60	$13.5W + 487$	>60	$10.5W + 596$

W, weight in kg.

3. *Owen's equation*

Men: $879 + (10.2 \times W)$
Women: $795 + (7.18 \times W)$

4. *Mifflin (equation for obese subjects)*

For adults aged from 19 to 77 years.
Men: $10W + 6.25H - 5A + 5$
Women: $10W + 6.25H - 5A - 161$
W, weight in kg; H, height in cm; A, age in years.

---

shown in Box 9.1. The Schofield equation is another frequently used formula; it is used in Chapter 25 (Table 25.1). An often-used simple guideline for estimating the daily energy needs of a patient is 25–35 kcal/kg body weight. One should realise that all of the equations, including the fixed factor of 25–35 kcal/kg, provide only rough estimates of the resting energy requirements, providing accurate predictions in only ~50% of patients and prediction errors as large as 20–30% (200 kcal/day or more). In addition, the extra factor for activity and disease needed to obtain an idea of total energy expenditure also carries large uncertainties. Therefore, the equations can be used as a starting point for nutritional therapy, but monitoring the effects of the therapy is of greater importance.

Energy requirements are strongly dependent on body composition. The body can be divided into fat mass and fat-free mass. Of the fat-free mass, the body cell mass is metabolically the most active; it consumes, on a weight basis, more energy than the fat mass. Patients with a higher body cell mass have higher energy needs than patients with a lower body cell mass. For example, young adult men who are tall and heavy need more energy compared with women or elderly, small, or slim people. This can be explained by the fact that men have a higher body cell mass than women and need more energy even if they are of the same age, height, and weight. Women have 10% more fat mass than men. During ageing, both men and women lose body cell mass, which is replaced by fat mass, leading to a decrease in overall energy expenditure. Obese people have considerable amounts of fat mass but their body cell mass is also increased, resulting in a higher energy requirement than they would have if they had a normal body weight. When applying equations in obese persons, a correction for optimal body weight does not seem to be necessary; the current body weight is the best predictor of energy expenditure.

Basal energy expenditure, together with additional factors such as physical activity levels, has to be assessed to calculate total energy expenditure. In the clinical situation, additional disease-associated factors should be taken into account during the calculation of the required energy needs. These include disease stress factor, activity factor, and temperature factor. During fever, basal energy expenditure is raised approximately 10% per degree of body temperature. Energy and nutrient losses from malabsorption should be taken into account when present.

In view of differences in nutritional needs between patients, it is always important to assess needs on an individual basis.

9.3 Oral feeding and oral nutritional supplements

Nutritional screening is an effective way of identifying patients at nutritional risk. Once these patients are identified, a decision can be made with regard to oral feeding and nutritional supplements.

Regular hospital food should contain sufficient energy and nutrients for the vast majority of people, and this should be the first option for feeding wherever possible. The macronutrient ratio of standard hospital food (the general menu), for hospital patients not at risk of malnutrition, corresponds to the requirements of optimal nutrition and should consist of 45–55% carbohydrate (of which 20–30 g is fibre), 30–35% fat, and 15–20% protein. Energy should be distributed as follows: 20% at breakfast, 30% at lunch, and 25% in the evening. The remaining 25% should be distributed over the course of the day in the form of snacks.

If a patient can be fed orally and is malnourished or at risk of developing malnutrition, oral intake must be optimised. The purpose of this diet is to increase energy and protein intake in order to meet the recommended nutritional needs. Consumption of food rich in protein and fat should be encouraged due to the high energy density of fat, and the fact that illness is often accompanied by an increased energy and protein need. The energy and protein intake can be improved by the supply of additional appetising and nourishing normal foods and snacks, supply of modular products, and alteration of food consistency or sip feeding. Other solutions to improve intake include tailoring food provision to meet the demands of patients (i.e. guaranteeing that the hospital meals meet the requirements of patients) and having patients make their food choice at the point of consumption, for example by changing food catering from a plated system (ordering choices and portion size in advance) to a bulk system (ordering at the moment of consumption).

One novel way of ensuring at least 30 minutes of undisturbed meal time is the 'protected meal times' policy, which has been promoted by the UK Hospital Caterers Association (HCA). Protected meal times require a minimisation of interruptions, such as medical or drug rounds and cleaning, and the rescheduling of procedures to avoid the three appointed times. Nursing staff are thus able to provide assistance and encouragement with eating where necessary, and will have immediate knowledge of patients' eating habits or difficulties.

In Figure 9.1, the different options for feeding are shown. All patients should be screened at admittance, and nutritional intake should be assessed by

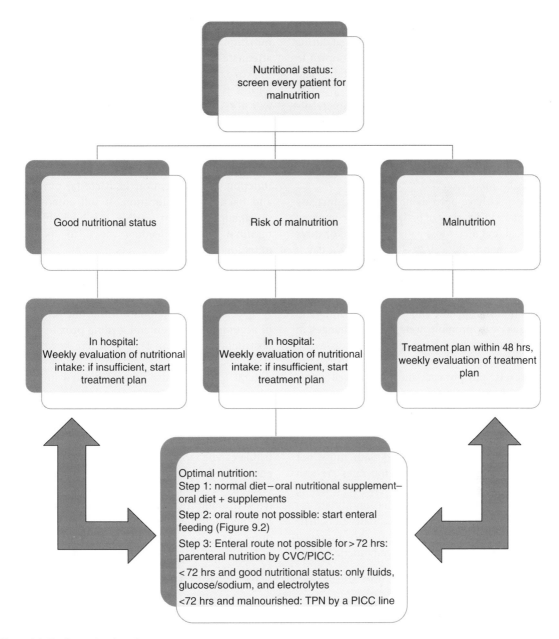

Figure 9.1 Feeding options in patients.

a dietitian/clinical nutritionist at regular intervals so that nutritional support can be adjusted if necessary.

If the addition of normal foods does not improve nutritional intake, commercially available modular products can be used. Modular products are single macronutrients and are used to augment oral feeding. They exist as glucose polymers, protein powders, and fat emulsions. Typically modular products do not provide a source of micronutrients.

If sufficient energy intake cannot be achieved with fortified foods, many nutritional supplements are available which can be taken in addition to the diet to provide extra macro- and micronutrients. Most of these oral nutritional supplements (ONS) are supplied in the form of a drink and are nutritionally complete, providing protein, carbohydrate, fat, vitamins, and minerals. These drinks can be used during the day in between meals and have been shown to have beneficial effects on nutritional status and outcome.

The majority of ONS formulas are commercially available either over the counter in supermarkets and pharmacies or on prescription. Homemade liquidised supplements have the advantage of being more palatable but the disadvantage of being of unknown nutritional composition.

ONS drinks have been demonstrated to increase energy intake in a variety of patient groups compared to a normal oral diet. Most patients use two or three portions (around 500 kcal/20–40 g protein) a day if they use normal meals as well. In most studies they have had little suppressive effect on food intake, and in some patients groups they have been shown to actually stimulate appetite and food intake. Although ONS drinks can promote weight gain, changes in body composition have been infrequently assessed. Functional changes, for example in muscle strength, activity levels, and physical and mental well-being, have been shown to improve with supplementation. Although the impact of supplements may be limited in patients with severe end-stage disease, mortality rates are significantly lower in other malnourished patients receiving ONS compared with those not receiving supplements. Complication rates are also lower and length of hospital stay is reduced, resulting in considerable cost savings with the appropriate use of ONS. They have also been shown to have a beneficial role in the community setting, with improved intake and weight as well as improved functional and clinical outcomes.

9.4 Enteral tube feeding

If oral intake is insufficient to meet nutritional requirements, or if it is contraindicated due to dysphagia, obstruction, facial injuries, artificial respiration, GI operation, malabsorption, or lack of consciousness, enteral tube feeding (ETF) should be considered (Figure 9.2). In both hospitals and the community, tube feeding is used in a variety of clinical conditions and ages and over varying periods of time, from weeks to years. It can be used as the sole source or as a supplementary source of nutrition. ETF has been shown to increase nutritional intake compared to a normal oral diet, attenuate loss of body weight and lean tissue, and improve functional and clinical outcomes. Patients with a functional gastrointestinal (GI) tract who will not, cannot, or should not eat, and are candidates for nutritional support, should be fed enterally. If possible, enteral feeding is always preferred over parenteral nutrition because of the benefits of feeding the gut, such as stimulation of the immune function and prevention of bacterial overgrowth and bacterial translocation. If full enteral nutritional support is not feasible, it is advisable to use minimal enteral feeding next to parenteral nutrition.

ETF is contraindicated in patients with intestinal obstruction distal to the tube, high-output fistulas (>1000 ml/day), GI bleeding, or bowel ischaemia. A mechanical obstruction distal to the tube results in accumulation of enteral feeding proximal to the obstruction. This can lead to severe bowel extension, abdominal pain and even bowel rupture. Enteral feeding is also contraindicated in patients with paralytic ileus due to the lack of peristalsis. Enteral feeding in patients with a high-output fistula or enterostomy stimulates the production of GI juices. Losses of water and electrolytes through the fistula can be replaced, but stimulation of the gut by enteral feeding can lead to a high fistula output, resulting in considerable losses of fluids and electrolytes through the fistula or enterostomy. These patients should be limited in their enteral intake in order to reduce electrolyte and fluid losses, in spite of feelings of thirst, to a maximum of 10–15 ml/kg. Fluids can be given by infusion. During bowel ischaemia there should be no enteral provocation, as the feed cannot be absorbed and may increase ischaemia. Enteral nutrition should be avoided in patients with active GI bleeding and nutritional support should only commence once a patient is haemodynamically stable.

Enteral nutrition should be given as early as possible. In critically ill patients, starting enteral nutrition within 24 hours after admission to the intensive care unit (ICU) seems to have positive effect on several outcome parameters. Although there is currently insufficient evidence, early enteral nutrition in an appropriate amount and with the aim of avoiding gut failure is recommended.

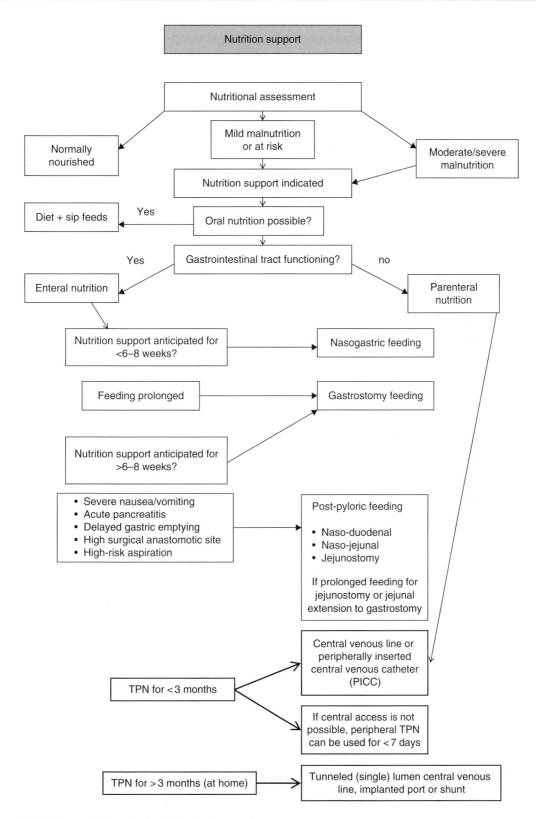

Figure 9.2 Decision tree for the optimal route for nutrition support.

Feeding routes

Access routes for enteral feeding vary according to the individual patient. In deciding which route to use, the anticipated length of feeding and the presence of delayed gastric emptying are two major considerations. Access to the GI tract via the nasal route, by for example nasogastric (into the stomach), nasoduodenal (into the duodenum), or nasojejunal (into the jejunum) tubes, is usually short-term (less than 8 weeks). During tube placement, patients are asked to swallow the tube after advancing it through the nose. Nasogastric tubes are usually placed at the bedside. Naso small-bowel tubes can be placed in the endoscopy unit or under fluoroscopic guidance in the X-ray department, but some units have success in placing small-bowel feeding tubes at the bedside with the aid of a motility agent such as erythromycin or metoclopramide hydrochloride. The latest technique is the use of an electromagnetic guidance system to guide the tube through the pylorus.

Feeding tubes can increase the incidence of gastroesophageal aspiration, as the cardiac sphincter at the top of the stomach cannot fully close. Placing the patient's bed at an angle of 30° can reduce the incidence of aspiration. With ongoing problems, a motility agent can be given or the tube can be placed post-pylorically.

Box 9.2 Contraindications for gastrostomy tube placement

- disturbed coagulation;
- neoplasms in the stomach;
- morbid obesity;
- gastric varices;
- progressive ascitis or peritonitis.

When enteral feeding is anticipated for a longer period of time, a percutaneous endoscopic gastrostomy or jejunostomy (PEG/PEJ – see Table 9.1) should be considered. This is a more-invasive category of enteral feeding, in which the tube accesses the GI tract through the abdominal wall. This procedure can be carried out in the endoscopy unit or the radiology department. Access can be to the stomach or small bowel. Complications associated with these procedures are infrequent, but include reaction to anaesthesia, perforation of adjacent organs, bleeding, and infection. Special precautions should be taken when feeding into the small bowel, due to the lack of gastric volume or acidity. Contraindications for enterostomy access are summarised in Box 9.2.

Table 9.1 Choice of artificial enteral access.

Type of access	Position	Material	In situ	Placement by
Nasogastric tube	Nose–stomach	Polyvinyl chloride	Maximum 7 days	Nurse at ward Patient self
Nasogastric tube	Nose–stomach	Polyurethane silicone	Maximum 6 weeks; if longer, consider PEG	Nurse at ward Patient self
Nasoduodenal tube	Nose–duodenum	Polyurethane silicone	Maximum 6 weeks; if longer, consider PEJ	Gastroenterologist, by scope Trained nurse Magnetic guidance Self-migrating tube X-ray department
Nasojejunal tube	Nose–jejunum			Gastroenterologist, by scope Trained nurse Magnetic guidance Self-migrating tube X-ray department
Needle jejunostomiy	Abdomen–jejunum	Polyurethane	Maximum 6 weeks	Surgeon, during operation
Percutaneous endoscopic gastrostomy (PEG)	Abdomen–stomach	Silicone	Long-term	Gastroeneterologist X-ray department
Percutaneous endoscopic jejunostomy (PEJ)	Abdomen–jejunum (sometimes PEG, with tube passing pylorus)	Silicone	Long-term	Gastroeneterologist X-ray department

Post-pyloric feeding

A specific problem with post-pyloric feeding is the so-called dumping syndrome, which results from the administration of a high-osmolar solution directly into the small bowel. This leads to an increased fluid secretion from the bowel in order to dilute the solution. Dumping syndrome may cause diarrhoea, dizziness, and an exaggerated insulin response and ensuing hypoglycaemia. This situation is worsened when the administration rate is increased too quickly. It is generally recommended that the infusion rate of small-bowel feeding in adults does not exceed 125 ml/hour.

Complications of enteral feeding

Aspiration pneumonia

Many patients experience problems with swallowing, which can cause aspiration pneumonia. It is very important to identify these as soon as possible to minimise the risk. Patient groups at risk include those with head and neck cancer and those with a tracheostomy, stroke, or a neurological disease such as motor neurone disease or multiple sclerosis. A swallowing assessment should be carried out by qualified personnel (ideally a speech and language therapist) and the consistency of the diet should be altered as necessary. It was former practice to check for possible aspiration by adding blue food dye to feeds. This has been shown to be ineffective as a clinical tool and potentially life threatening, and should not be used. Although postpyloric feeding reduces the chance of aspiration, it can not fully exclude aspiration, so all patients with artificial enteral feeding should be monitored in order to prevent this complication.

Diarrhoea and constipation

Following the introduction of ready-to-use feeding systems, bacterial contamination of feeds is rarely seen. Some feeds may need to be decanted or reconstituted prior to feeding, which increases the incidence of bacterial contamination. The manufacturer's guidelines on feed hanging times should be referred to in all cases. Usually, giving sets should be changed every 24 hours, but they may need to be changed more frequently in critically ill or immunocompromised patients.

Diarrhoea in the enterally fed patient can be drug-related, infection-related (due to *Clostridium difficile*), disease-related, or caused by hyperosmolar feeds being administered too fast. The offending cause should be removed, if possible. The key medications which cause diarrhoea include antibiotics, sorbitol-containing medications often present in syrups, and magnesium-containing medications. First-line treatment of diarrhoea should be fluid and electrolyte replacement. If *C. difficile* infection is suspected, a stool sample should be sent for analysis and the patient should be started on treatment as required.

Constipation may be caused by many drugs. A typical and common example is opioids. If possible, the offending agent should be discontinued. Factors that can be used to reduce constipation include:

- increased water intake;
- the use of a high-fibre feed to increase faecal bulk;
- laxatives and stool softeners.

Nausea and vomiting

This should be assessed medically. Patients who have an impaired gastric function are at risk of aspiration if they vomit. It is important to confirm placement of the feeding tube. The patient may just need a couple of hours with the feed disconnected, but long periods of discontinuation of the feed should be avoided to prevent malnutrition. Antiemetic drug can be used, and in extreme cases post-pyloric feeding or parenteral nutrition may be required. Long-term diabetes mellitus patients and neurological patients are at risk for gastric-emptying disturbances.

Physical characteristics of enteral feeding tubes

Clinical nutritionists and dietitians will need a working knowledge of the physical characteristics of enteral access devices, including tubes, connectors, giving sets, and feeding pumps, in order to be able to identify the devices best suited to the needs of a patient. Nasoenteric tubes for adults are available in lengths from 94 cm (36 in) (enteral) to 156 cm (60 in) (the longest for feeding postpylorically). Gastrostomy tubes are shorter and are available in different options, including very-short gastrostomy skin-level devices called 'buttons', which are very useful for GI

Table 9.2 Advantages and disadvantages of different enteral feeding routes.

Feeding route	Advantages	Disadvantages
Nasogastric tube or nasoenteral tube	Less invasive Quick Cheap Feeding can be initiated immediately after tube placement and confirmtion of tube location	Oropharyngeal and esophageal irritation Increased risk of sinusitis, esophagitis, nasopharyngitis Swallowing may be painful and difficult Increased risk of reflux Coughing, vomiting, or sneezing may result in migration of the tube into the oesophagus or pharynx, with an increased risk of aspiration Abnormalities in the nose, neck, or oesophagus area may prevent tube placement Tube can be placed in the trachea The tube can easily be removed by disoriented patients Stigmatising Tubes should be replaced on a regular basis (PVC 7 days, PUR 6 weeks) Location of the nasoenteral tubes often requires an endoscopic approach and/or X-ray confirmation

Through abdominal wall:
  Percutaneous endoscopic gastrostomy
  Gastrostomies
  Enterostomies
  Jejunostomy catheters
	Less stigmatising
	Better psychosocial acceptance
	Less migration of tube
	Less tube removal
	Less reflux or aspiration
	No oropharyngeal and oesophageal irritation
	Surgical options can be performed when disorders in the nose, neck, or oesophagus are present
	No difficulties with swallowing
	Rare replacement of tubes
		Invasive access method with increased risks of postoperative complications
		Sedation and antibiotics may be necessary
		Placement may be time-consuming
		Skin around the tube can be irritated
		Leakage of nutrients or intestinal juices into the abdomen
		Translocation of the bowel around the jejunostomy catheter
		Occlusion of the bowel, caused by haematomas
		Jejunostomy catheter can dislocate and clog
		Jejunostomy catheter requires X-ray confirmation
		Abnormalities in the oropharyngeal-oesophageal area may prevent percutaneous endoscopic gastrostomy placement

access in patients who are young or aware of the cosmetic appearance of the tube, or in agitated, confused patients who are at risk of pulling out the tube.

Feeding tubes have variable diameters, measured in French size (the higher the French size, the wider the tube). Wider-bore tubes should be used in post-operative or critical-care situations where the feed is aspirated to monitor gastric emptying when enteral feeding is being established. Feeding solutions with a high viscosity may require a larger-diameter tube to prevent blockages. For the comfort of the patient, tubes with a maximum of Fr 12 should be used. When enteral feeding is administered with a pump, tube occlusions occur less frequently and a smaller diameter can be used. Finer-bore tubes are more comfortable for the patient, but measuring residual volume can be more complicated.

Enteral feeding tubes are made from a variety of materials, including silicone, polyvinyl chloride (PVC), latex, and polyurethane (PUR). PVC and latex tubes should only be used for a maximum of 7 days as they become stiff during use and can lead to perforations of the stomach. PUR and silicone tubes are more comfortable and can be used for a period of 6 weeks. In case of difficult placement of the tube, this period can be prolonged until the material of the tube is worn down. The advantages and disadvantages of different feeding routes are shown in Table 9.2.

Enteral feeding solutions

The selection of enteral nutrition should depend on the nutritional needs of the individual patient, taking into account fluid and energy requirements and renal function, as well as the absorptive capacity of the

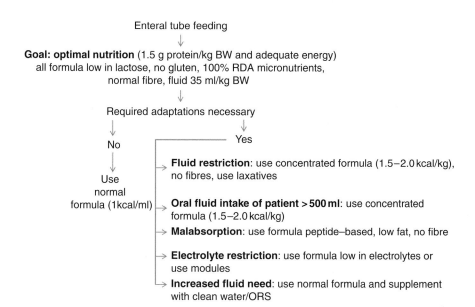

Figure 9.3 Enteral tube feeding (ETF) options.

gastric tract. Nowadays, ETF containing fibre is regarded as the standard feed, and all commercially available enteral formulas are appropriate for use in patients with lactose intolerance. Figure 9.3 shows the decision tree for using specialised enteral formulas. Attention should also be paid to the osmolarity of the solution. Administration of a high-osmolar solution directly into the bowel lumen leads to an increased fluid secretion of the bowel in order to dilute the solution. This can lead to diarrhoea and dizziness, and other symptoms of dumping syndrome.

The micronutrient profile of feeds is usually in line with recommended levels. These levels may be adjusted in some disease-specific formulas in line with recommendations for specific disease states. Meeting energy as well as protein requirements should be the goal in enteral feeding. In many cases, enteral feeding with an energy/protein rate of about 20 can be necessary.

Disease-specific supplements

The majority of patients can be given 'standard' enteral feeds, but some will benefit from a disease-specific product. The market for disease-specific supplements is growing fast and changing quickly.

Box 9.3 gives an overview of disease-specific products (either ONS or enteral tube feeds).

Box 9.3 Overview of disease-specific supplements

- Products based on short-chain peptides or amino acids: for patients with malabsorption (sometimes also enriched with glutamine or arginine).
- Diabetes-specific products for optimal glucose regulation (no mono- or disaccharides, rich in monosaturated fatty acids).
- Products for patients with pressure sores: containing extra vitamins and minerals, antioxidants, and zinc.
- Products for cancer patients: usually containing omega-3 fatty acids and antioxidants.
- Low-fat products, containing medium-chain triglycerides: for patients with malabsorption.
- Carbohydrate-rich supplements: to be used shortly before an operation.
- Immune-enhancing products: often containing omega-3 fatty acids, arginine, RNA nucleotides.
- Products for patients with pulmonary disease: low in fat, high in carbohydrates and protein.
- Protein-restricted, electrolyte-restricted, energy-enriched products: for patients suffering from renal diseases.
- Products to slow down the progression of Alzheimer's disease: containing omega-3 fatty acids, antioxidants, B vitamins, choline, and uridine monophosphate.
- Products to support elderly/geriatric patients: enriched in vitamin D, protein, folic acid, etc.

Feeding rate

The duration of enteral feeding depends on the patient's needs and tolerance, as well as local practices. Time should also be allocated in the day for washing, physiotherapy, and X-ray when a patient is not connected to the feed. If the patient is given antacids, the feeding can continue over a period of 24 hours if required, as the gastric acidity is already altered. Particular care should be taken with patients requiring insulin treatment where glucose levels need to be closely monitored.

If a patient is tolerating enteral feeding well, the length of time for which they are fed can be reduced. The key factor to remember in this situation is that as the time of feeding is reduced, the infusion rate must increase to make sure all requirements are met. In situations where adult patients are well established on feeding, feeds can be administered at a rate of up to 200 ml/hour by pump or bolus. This can facilitate a mobile patient to be disconnected from the feed for several hours at a time. Patients requiring supplementary nutrition can receive feeds overnight that maximise their oral intake during the day.

Monitoring and complications of enteral nutrition

Monitoring of patients on ETF should be carried out by professionals with knowledge of nutritional requirements, feeding routes, feeding devices and enteral solutions, as well as the associated risks and complications of enteral feeding. Clinical, anthropometric and biochemical parameters should be monitored before the start and throughout the period of feeding (see Chapter 2).

Complications associated with ETF may be of a mechanical, GI or metabolic nature. The most common complications of enteral feeding and advice about how to minimise them are shown in Table 9.3. Severe complications, such as bowel necrosis and GI perforation, rarely occur.

9.5 Administration of drugs and enteral feeding

If a patient cannot take medication orally, they will need to be administered through the feeding tube. This section outlines considerations for the administration of drugs through a feeding tube. Liasion with a pharmacist is advised, in order to decide on the most appropriate method of drug administration.

Drugs that are liable to cause gastric irritation, or those that are better absorbed with food, should ideally be given while the patient is being fed. Drugs which should be given on an empty stomach are ideally given during a feeding break of at least 30 minutes.

If patients can swallow tablets and capsules, they should be encouraged to take them orally. If a patient cannot swallow, a liquid formulation of the drug should be tried. Viscous liquids should be diluted with water for injection, to aid passage through the tube. The enteral feed should be stopped and the tube cleared by flushing with 10–30 ml of water before and after drug administration. Consideration of the sorbitol or lactose content of liquid medication is important, as it can cause diarrhoea. Elixirs and suspensions can be extreme hypertonic.

Dispersible tablets and effervescent granules do not need to be crushed and are the least likely option to cause obstruction. They are more cost-effective than liquid formulations.

Many drugs are only available as tablets or capsules. For optimum drug absorption, and to minimise tube occlusion, a mortar and pestle is recommended for crushing. A tablet crusher or serrated syringe may also be used. Most tablets, if left in water for 10–15 minutes, will soften sufficiently to allow them to be mixed to a slurry using a mortar and pestle. Alternatively, a compressed tablet may be crushed to a fine powder and mixed to a suspension with water. The coating of sugar-coated or film-coated tablets will dissolve if crushed finely. Small, compressed tablets may be difficult to crush in a serrated crushing syringe but a mortar and pestle may be used.

Drugs formulated as hard gelatin capsules containing a fine powder may be twisted open and have their contents mixed in 10–15 ml of water for injection. There is no need to crush the contents. One exception to this is phenytoin. Mixing the contents of phenytoin capsules with water may cause clumping and obstruction of the tube, so the suspension form of the drug should be used.

Drugs formulated as soft gelatin capsules may be delivered by piercing a hole at one end of the capsule,

Table 9.3 Possible complications of enteral tube feeding (ETF).

Complication	Probable causes	Actions/advice
Mechanical complications		
Tube clogging	Displacement or kink in tube	Check tube for displacements or kinks, change tube if necessary
	Administration of medications	Flush the tube with water when medication is administered
	Diameter too small	Employ a larger diameter when highly viscous formulas are used
	Nutritional residue adhering to tube	Flush the tube frequently – every 4 hours – with water
Tube displacement	Coughing, sneezing, vomiting	Reposition the tube
	Migration of tube	Replace the tube and consider placement of a tube with a larger diameter
	Dislodgement by patient	Replace the tube, if necessary restraining the patient
	Inadequate taping of tube	Consider another feeding route; replace the tube and fasten it properly
Irritations of nose, throat, and oesophagus	Tube diameter is too large	Use a tube with a smaller diameter
	Tube is stiff	Use a flexible tube
	Improper positioning of tube	Reposition the tube properly; replace the tube through the other nostril
	Tube is placed too long	Consider other feeding routes
	Inadequate taping of tube	Tape the tube properly; it should be able to move during swallowing
Gastrointestinal complications		
Problems in the oral cavity	Decreased or no stimulation of salivary glands	Advise patient to rinse their mouth regularly or sip fluids if possible; advise chewing on sugar-free gum or peppermints if allowed
	Dry mouth	Advise proper mouth care and regular rinsing of the mouth
	Tube placed for too long	Replace tube or consider other feeding route
Nausea or vomiting	Formula too cold	Only administer enteral formulas at room temperature
	Rate of infusion too high	Decrease rate of infusion
	Volume too high	Decrease volume; consider a more concentrated formula
	Formula too concentrated	Decrease concentration of formula
	Disturbed gastric emptying	Check gastric residuals; monitor for diseases or drugs that might influence gastric motility; advise prokinetics if possible; consider nasoenteral feeding
	No bowel movements	Exclude an ileus; if indicated, stimulate bowel movements with a clysma
	Ileus	Immediately stop enteral feeding; if indicated, advise parenteral nutrition
	Dislocation of tube	Replace the tube and confirm its position
	Possible lactose intolerance	Switch to lactose-free formula
	Infectious origin	Check performance of infection-control protocol
Aspiration	Delayed gastric emptying	Check gastric residuals; monitor for diseases or drugs that might influence motility; advise prokinetics if possible
	Patient only in lying position	Elevate head of bed through 30°
	Administration of bolus feeding	Alter bolus to continue feeding or decrease bolus volume
	High infusion rate	Decrease infusion rate; consider concentrated solutions
	Displaced feeding tube	Replace tube; consider nasoenteral feeding
Constipation	Inadequate fluid intake	Monitor fluid balance; if necessary, increase fluid administration
	Medication	Check medication use which might cause a decrease in bowel motility
	Inactivity	Advise more physical activity, if possible
	Inadequate fibre intake	Consider a formula rich in dietary fibre
Diarrhoea	Formula too cold	Only administer formula at room temperature
	Infusion rate too fast	Decrease infusion rate
	Hyperosmolar formula	Change to isotonic formula
	Bolus feeding	Decrease bolus volume or change to continuous feeding
	Infectious origin	Evaluate tube-feeding handling and infection-control strategies

(Continued)

Table 9.3 (cont'd)

Complication	Probable causes	Actions/advice
	Malabsorption	Monitor malabsorption; change to elemental formula, if indicated
	Lactose or gluten intolerance	Switch to lactose-free or gluten-free formula
	Increased bowel motility	Review possible effects of medication or diseases on bowel motility; if possible, advise starting medications that slow bowel motility
	Extremely low albumin levels	Since adequate enteral feeding is difficult to achieve, advise parenteral nutrition; if possible, a small amount of enteral tube feeding can be administered; check fluid and electrolyte balance
	Medications	Monitor medications which might induce diarrhoea, such as antibiotics
Metabolic complications (see also refeeding and overfeeding)		
Dehydration	Inadequate water supply	Monitor fluid balance, with special interest in kidney function, serum values of electrolytes, urea, and creatinine; check changes in body weight; if indicated, increase volume or add sterile water or a sodium hydroxide solution next to the enteral formula through the tube (portions of 50–100 ml by syringe 4–6 × per day)
Hyper-/hypoglycaemia	Feeding and insulin therapy incompatible	Adjust feeding or insulin therapy; considerations about bolus or continuous feeding depend on insulin therapy; monitor blood sugar frequently; if necessary, stop nutrition
Serum electrolyte and mineral disturbances	Disease-related	Adjust enteral formula to abnormalities; add sodium to enteral formula
Deficiencies of essential nutrients	Insufficient supply of nutrients	Administer the recommended daily allowances of all essential nutrients; if indicated, advise supplying
	Losses of nutrients	Monitor nutrient losses; check serum values and advise supplementation, if necessary
	Disease-related deficiencies	Check deficiencies when they can be expected and advise supplying them, if indicated

squeezing out the contents, and mixing them with water for injection. If this is not possible, it is advisable to dissolve the capsule in a glass of warm water, taking care to avoid administration of the not-dissolved gelatin, which may clog the tube.

The purpose of an enteric coating is to bypass dissolution of the drug in the stomach, so that the active compound is released into the small intestine. If the enteric-coated tablet is crushed, it loses this property and may cause undesirable side effects (e.g. gastric irritation with aspirin), or it may lose effectiveness if it is degraded by stomach acid. However, if the drug is only available as an enteric-coated formulation, crushing it may be unavoidable.

Controlled-release products

Controlled-release products are described by a variety of names, including long-acting (LA), retard, modified-release (MR), and sustained-release (SR).

These formulations are designed to release the active ingredient over an extended period of time. Tablets, hard gelatin capsules containing granules, and sachets may contain drugs in a controlled-release formulation. Crushing SR products to facilitate passage through the enteral tube will alter the drug absorption profile and pharmacokinetics. The pharmacist should be contacted for advice in these situations.

Cytotoxic drugs

Crushing cytotoxic drugs is hazardous, due to the risk of powder inhalation and skin contact. These should be administered parenterally. Some cytotoxic drugs should not be opened for enteral administration.

Hormonal drugs

Hormonal drugs should be crushed using a closed system. To avoid powder inhalation, a tablet crusher or a serrated crushing syringe is recommended. They may also be wet-crushed.

Alternative routes of delivery

In some instances, alternative routes of drug delivery for the enterally fed patient may be worth considering. These include the topical, rectal, transdermal, buccal, sublingual, nebulised, and parenteral routes.

To minimise drug–nutrient interactions, special precautions should be taken when administering phenytoin, carbamazepine, warfarin, fluoroquinolones, and proton-pump inhibitors via feeding tubes. Care should be taken to prevent tube occlusions, and immediate intervention is required when blockages occur.

Adding drugs to the formula

Drugs should not be added directly to the enteral formula. There is a potential risk of microbiological contamination of the feed, and there are difficulties in predicting the effect medication may have on the physical characteristics of the enteral feed. This may lead to complications like tube obstruction.

9.6 Parenteral nutrition

Parenteral nutrition is used to provide nutrition support when the oral or enteral route cannot be used. Indications for parenteral feeding are listed in Box 9.4. Total parenteral nutrition (TPN) consists of a hypertonic solution (>1200 Mosmol/l) with glucose, amino acids, fat, electrolytes, vitamins, trace elements, and minerals. It should be administered to patients where oral or enteral intake is impossible or insufficient to meet the nutritional needs.

One of the indications for TPN is short-bowel syndrome. The most important feature of this syndrome is insufficient absorption of nutrients, indicating the need for parenteral nutritional support. Adaptation of the bowel is possible in the 1–3 years after the resection. If the remaining bowel is smaller than 50 cm and the ileocaecal valve has been resected, lifetime TPN will be nescesary.

In case of malabsorption caused by severe inflammation of the bowel, we speak of 'functional short

Box 9.4 Indications for parenteral nutrition

- Inflammatory bowel disease where enteral nutrition has failed to prevent or reverse malnutrition (i.e. severe malabsorption).
- Patients with multiorgan failure where nutritional requirements cannot be met by the enteral route alone.
- Intestinal atresia.
- Radiation enteritis.
- Severe mucositis following chemotherapy.
- Motility disorders such as sclerodermia or chronic idiopathic intestinal pseudoobstruction syndromes.
- Extreme short-bowel syndrome (e.g. trombogenic), trauma, resection due to tumour.
- High-output stoma (>1000 ml).
- *Enterocutaneous fistulas.*
- Inborn error of the bowel surface, such as microvillis inclusion disease.
- Motility disorders.
- Adynamic ileus.
- Malnourshed dialysis patients (interdialytic parenteral nutrition, IDPN).

bowel', since there is only loss of function. After successful treatment of the inflammation, the function of the bowel is expected to return.

Another indication for TPN is multiple organ failure, often caused by sepsis, a condition in which several organs malfunction or do not function at all. The bowel is often involved and does not tolerate full enteral nutrition. In this situation, complete or supplementary parenteral nutrition is again indicated.

Since delivery of parenteral nutrition requires a catheter in a central vein, parenteral nutrition is contraindicated in patients with an increased risk of pneumothorax (as discussed later in this section). Percutaneous puncture of a central line is also contraindicated in patients with clotting abnormalities, since they have an increased risk of bleeding.

It is especially important with parenteral nutrition not to exceed the body's metabolic handling capacity of glucose (5 mg/kg per minute), fat (1 g/kg body weight), or energy (>40 kcal/kg body weight). Hypermetabolic feeding is the main cause of parenteral nutrition-associated liver failure. In insulin-resistant patients, the amount of glucose administered by parenteral nutrition (250 g and more) can cause hyperglycaemia. Treatment with insulin (if possible, inserted in the TPN bag) is recommended in this case.

Catheter access

Parenteral delivery of nutrients can be executed via central venous access. Parenteral nutrition via a central vein with a large blood flow ending in the right atrium results in a quick dilution of the solution and is the most frequently employed option. This can be maintained for longer periods of time, even at home. The central vein that is used most often is the subclavian vein. Other suitable veins are the internal and external jugular veins. Peripheral inserted central venous catheters (PICC) are a good option for administering TPN.

In rare instances when upper veins are not available, the femoral vein is used, which has a great impact on the mobility of the patient. An indwelling catheter or implanted port is another option. This device is placed under the skin, in the upper part of the chest. It has a small reservoir that is connected to a major vein inside the chest. This device facilitates the administration of parenteral nutrition into the venous system.

Peripheral access is also possible, but is not the first option, and should only be used for short periods, as hypertonic parenteral solutions irritate small veins with a low blood flow, causing phlebitis or thrombosis of the vein.

The basilic vein is mostly used for peripheral access.

In long-term TPN, arterio venous shunts are employed with success. Sterile techniques must be used in the cleaning and maintenance of sites in order for feeding to be successful.

Parenteral nutrition solutions

Parenteral nutrition solutions are complex ready-to-use formulas which include macronutrients (glucose, protein, and fat) and micronutrients (electrolytes, vitamins, and trace elements). Single nutrients such as sodium and glucose solutions can be given intravenously as well, but will not be referred to as 'parenteral nutrition'. When using such intravenous fluids next to parenteral nutrition, their content should be considered alongside the content of the parenteral nutrition solution. For instance, calories from the use of intravenous lipids (Propofol) and glucose (5–10%) could have an impact on the total energy intake of the patient.

There are commercially available two-in-one bags with glucose and amino acids and three-in-one bags containing glucose, amino acids and fat emulsion. These all vary in macronutrient content and come with or without electrolytes.

(Hospital) pharmacies can mix parenteral nutrition from single nutrient solutions (glucose, amino acids, and/or fat), normally if the commercially available products don't cover the needs of a patient, such as the neonatal and paediatric patient. There are strict regulations about the possibilities of mixing these solutions. In particular, the use of lipids, calcium, phosphate, and magnesium should be carefully monitored for stability and compatibility. Compounding machines and software are available and can prevent instable solutions.

During the preparation of a parenteral solution, several aspects should be taken into account. To control bacterial and fungal contamination, trained personnel should produce intravenous nutrition in an aseptic work area, using aseptic techniques under laminar flow conditions. Routine microbiological testing of the prepared solution should also be performed. Nowadays, (hospital) pharmacies have to work under strict hygiene rules concerning rooms and the storage of preparations, and require certification in order to be able to compound parenteral nutrition.

The vitamin and trace-elements given to patients using parenteral nutrition are different from those provided by the enteral route as there is no enteral compensation for these products. As the route of access of the micronutrients is different, frequent monitoring is necessary, even if sufficient micronutrients are provided (see Tables 9.4 and 9.5 for recommendations).

Vitamins and trace elements are usually provided in the TPN bags in commercially available mixtures. These mixtures do not always provide the required amount of these micronutrients.

Not all essential nutrients (e.g. iron, calcium) can be mixed in optimal amounts in a parenteral solution and supplementation of micronutrients next to the TPN should be considered if necessary.

Monitoring and complications of parenteral nutrition

Given the risks and complications associated with parenteral nutrition and the fact that they are often critically ill and immunosuppressed, patients

Table 9.4 Recommendations for supplementation of parenteral vitamins.

Ingredient	Amount
Fat-soluble vitamins	
A (retinol)	1 mg (3300 IU)
D3 (ergocalciferol or cholecalciferol)	200 IU
E (α-tocopherol)	10 mg (10 IU)
K (phylloquinone)	150 μg
Water-soluble vitamins	
C (ascorbic acid)	200 mg
Folic acid	600 μg
Niacin	40 mg
B_2 (riboflavin)	3.6 mg
B_1 (thiamine)	6.0 mg
B_6 (pyridoxine)	6.0 mg
B_{12} (cyanocobalamin)	5 μg
Pantothenic acid	15 mg
Biotin	60 μg

Table 9.5 Recommendations for parenteral supplementation of trace elements.

Element	Recommendation
Zinc	2.5–4 mg
Selenium	60 μg
Copper	0.3–1.2 mg
Manganese	0.2–0.8 μg
Iron	1–1.5 mg
Iodine	1–1.5 mg
Molybdenum	100–200 μg
Chromium	10–20 μg

receiving parenteral feeding should be carefully monitored. Fluid balance, electrolytes, glucose, vitamins, biochemical parameters (liver, kidney), and anthropometric measurements should be performed frequently.

Complications associated with parenteral nutrition can be mechanical, metabolic, or infectious. The most frequent infectious complication of parenteral nutrition is catheter-related sepsis, with incidence rates up to 25% in the ICU. The catheter hub is the most common site of origin of organisms that cause catheter-tip infection and bacteraemia. Catheter care is one of the most important factors influencing the incidence of catheter sepsis. Performed strictly according to protocol, catheter care achieves a significant decrease in infectious complications.

Possible differences in infectious risk between single and multilumen catheters remain controversial. Other factors that can contribute to catheter sepsis are catheter insertion and the thrombogenic properties of the catheter, related to the texture of the catheter and the tendency of platelets to adhere to it.

Patients should not be intravenously fed in excess of their requirements as this can lead to a variety of metabolic problems, such as:

- Disorders in fat metabolism (hypertriglyceridaemia – evaluation of tryglycerides should be carried out if TPN is disconnected for at least 6 hours, in order to have the body clear the lipids from the infusion).
- Glucose metabolism (hyperglycaemia).
- Electrolyte (sodium, potassium) imbalance.
- Mineral (magnesium, phosphate) imbalance.
- Hepatic disorders.

Monitoring of patients on TPN in hospital settings should be carried out according to Table 9.6. If the patient is stable but still depending on TPN, this therapy can be continued at home. Monitoring of a stable patient is less intensive; for such patients, the parameters of Table 9.6 should be considered on a weekly basis and every 1–4 months.

9.7 Special considerations with nutritional support

There is now good evidence to demonstrate that perioperative nutritional support is of benefit, particularly for patients with severe malnutrition. Enteral feeding is usually considered to be the preferred route of feeding as it is more physiological, as well as cheaper and safer. However, it is increasingly recognised that enteral nutrition often fails to achieve targeted caloric requirements, especially in critically ill patients, as a consequence of a poor tolerance of feeding manifested by large gastric aspirates.

Maintaining gut-barrier function is often quoted as a reason for enteral feeding. The gut barrier is not a single entity, but instead a number of factors, including mechanical defences, intestinal microflora, immunological defences, bile salts and gastric acids. These all work to prevent the movement of bacteria and endotoxins from the lumen of the gut through the intestinal lumen to extra-intestinal sites. The evidence

Table 9.6 Parameters that should be evaluated during parenteral nutrition.

Parameter	Daily	1–2 per week	Once every 2 weeks
Fluid balance	×		
Anthropometry		×	
Biochemical parameters			
Haemoglobin		×	
Leukocytes		×	
Thrombocytes		×	
Sodium		×	
Potassium		×	
HCO$_3$		×	
Chloride		×	
Calcium		×	
Magnesium		×	
Phosphate		×	
Urea		×	
Creatinine		×	
Alkaline phosphatase		×	
Gammaglutamyl transpeptidase		×	
Bilirubin total		×	
Triglycerides			×
Albumin		×	
Glucose	×		
Zinc			×
Copper			×
Folate			×
Iron			×

25 OH vitamin D2 + D3 (on start once, repeat if supplementation is requested)
PTH (on start once, repeat if calcium and vitamin D status is out of range)
Hydroxycobalamin (on start once, repeat every 6 months)

in support of the theory of bacterial translocation has been extensively discussed, and it now seems that bacterial translocation can occur in humans and is associated with an increase in septic morbidity.

There is little or no evidence supporting the theory that short-term parenteral nutrition results in mucosal atrophy or that intestinal permeability is a valid measurement of barrier function. Although ETF is always preferred when the GI route is functional, one should consider that disease alters GI function. During critical illness such as sepsis, patients are often haemodynamically unstable and blood supply to the GI intestinal tract can be insufficient. Enterocyte integrity and function may be compromised by the response to sepsis induced by cytokines and other modulators. Decreased pancreatic function, fat malabsorption, glucose and lactose malabsorption, delayed gastric emptying, decreased hydrogen ion production and prolonged colonic transit time have all been described during sepsis.

Also, bacterial overgrowth can cause extreme complications and the use of enteral feeding does not have positive influence on this. Administration of enteral nutrition to patients with disturbed GI function may cause bowel distension, delayed gastric emptying, paralytic ileus and diarrhoea.

The mode of nutritional support should be chosen based on intestinal tolerance. In many instances, a combination of enteral and parenteral feeding may be necessary to meet nutritional requirements. If oral nutrition fails completely and long-term artificial nutrition is necessary at home, it is wise to use either the enteral or the parenteral route, as the impact on quality of life with two types of artificial nutritional access is extreme.

Clinical nutrition at home

With a trend towards reduction of length of stay for in-hospital care in order to reduce costs, improve quality of life and reduce complications (hospital infections), the use of clinical nutrition at home (both enteral and parenteral) has increased over the years. Enteral nutrition at home is a well-accepted therapy in which the patient, their caretaker, or a specially trained home-care nurse manages the feeding. Specialised home-care services take care of pumps, formula, and other equipment to make the therapy safe and easy to deliver at home. Mobility of the patient is often extremely important, and to support this, overnight feeding and special carry-on pumps are used. Every hospital can discharge patients with enteral nutrition at home and even home physicians use this therapy with success. Evaluation of the therapy should be taken care of by a specialised team that is able to detect and cure complications.

Parenteral nutrition is rarely used at home and should only be provided by specialised centres. These home TPN teams take care of training the patient, caretakers, and specialised home-care nursing staff. If commercially available solutions are not used, preparation of the TPN can be done by a specialised pharmacy or by giving instructions to the patient at home. For hygiene reasons, TPN prepared at home can only be used for 24 hours, as complications are far more severe than in enteral nutrition (sepsis, liver failure, osteoporosis, dehydration, hypoglycaemia, electrolyte disturbances, anaemia). These need to be monitored by an experienced team (physician, nurse, dietitian). Quality of life and mobility are of extreme importance. Overnight TPN and small infusion pumps make the lives of these patients bearable. In the long term, home-TPN patients can consider transplantation if the complications of TPN (infections, liver failure, severe loss of quality of life) increase. For patients who are in need of temporary TPN at home (e.g. enterocutanous fistulas, bowel rest), 3–6 months can improve outcome on further surgery.

Complications of clinical nutrition

Feeding of an undernourished patient warrants particular caution (see Chapter 5). Refeeding syndrome is defined as severe fluid and electrolyte shifts in malnourished patients, precipitated by the introduction of nutrition. Refeeding syndrome can occur after the start of both enteral and parenteral nutrition. In starvation, the secretion of insulin is decreased in response to a reduced intake of carbohydrates. Instead, fat and protein stores are catabolised to produce energy. This results in an intracellular loss of electrolytes, particularly phosphate. When these patients start to feed, a sudden shift from fat to carbohydrate metabolism occurs, and secretion of insulin increases. This stimulates the cellular uptake of phosphate, potassium, and magnesium, and concentrations in plasma can fall dramatically and must be supplemented.

Phosphate is directly related to intermediates in energy metabolism, such as ATP. Potassium, one of the most important intracellular minerals, is a significant component of cellular metabolism. Magnesium, also a relevant intracellular mineral, is a co-factor in many enzyme systems. Decreased plasma levels of such important minerals may lead to serious disorders, such as altered myocardial function, cardiac arrhythmia, haemolytic anaemia, liver dysfunction, neuromuscular abnormalities, acute ventilatory failure, GI disturbances, renal disorders, and even death.

Identifying patients at risk of refeeding syndrome helps to prevent the syndrome. Patients at greatest risk are those with chronic alcoholism, oncology patients on chemotherapy, chronic diuretic users, chronic antacid users, those with chronic malnutrition (patients with a low BMI, elderly patients and anorexia nervosa patients), and patients totally unfed for 7–10 days. Postoperative patients have an incidence of severe hypophosphataemia at least twice that of other groups of patients.

Guidelines for preventing refeeding syndrome are summarised in Box 9.5.

Nutrition support team

Since clinical nutrition, especially TPN, is an invasive method of feeding, associated with possible

---

Box 9.5 Practical guidelines to help prevent refeeding syndrome

- Patients identified as requiring nutritional support should start feeding as soon as possible; however, electrolyte disturbances should be corrected before nutritional support is commenced.
- Electrolyte levels should be monitored before starting nutritional support and daily during the first week of refeeding until levels stay normal, and twice weekly thereafter.
- Food and fluid intake and output should be monitored.
- Feeding should be introduced slowly: 10 kcal/kg for the first 24 hours, stepwise increased with 5 kcal/kg per day until the required amount of calories is reached.

severe complications, a specialised team is necessary to support these patients. A nutrition support team should be a consulting service with knowledge in the field of nutritional and metabolic support of patients. To achieve such expertise, an interdisciplinary approach (including a medical doctor, nurse, dietitian and pharmacist) is essential. The primary goals of a nutrition support team should be the identification of patients who have nutrition-related problems, the performance of nutritional assessment, the provision of effective nutritional support under continuous guidance, and the creation of guideliness to increase impact. It has been shown that a nutrition support team encourages nutritional support in depleted patients, prevents not-indicated or short-term parenteral nutrition, reduces metabolic and mechanical complications and decreases the incidence of catheter sepsis.

9.8 Concluding remarks

In this section, some aspects of nutritional support which may be of importance in the future will be discussed. All clinicans working in the field of nutrition support should keep updated as to current evidence-based practice in the area.

Immunonutrition

In the last decade, the use of so-called immune-modulating nutrition formulas in different patient groups, in the form of ONS, enteral nutrition and parenteral nutrition, has been extensively researched and discussed. Immunonutrients can come in the form of vitamins, minerals, fatty acids, nucleotides, or specific amino acids and have been suggested to accelerate recovery or to positively alter metabolic responses to illness. Most often, formulas are mixtures of several of these. The most important nutrients and their related immune-modulating functions are discussed briefly here; further reading of the extensive literature is recommended for those who are interested.

Glutamine
Glutamine is a non-essential amino acid. It is also the most abundant free amino acid in the body. Glutamine is a precursor of nucleotides, proteins, and glutathione (involved in the antioxidant defence

system), serves as fuel for enterocytes and lymphocytes, and plays a role in the regulation of the acid–base balance. It is hypothesised that under certain circumstances, such as severe nutritional depletion or stress, glutamine is insufficiently produced, making it a conditionally essential amino acid. Organ systems that require glutamine, such as the immune system and the gut, may lack it, resulting in more complications in these severely depleted patients. Clinical studies have shown beneficial clinical outcome with better survival rates and less complications when glutamine-enriched nutritional support is administered in trauma and ICU patients and in patients undergoing large (GI) operations.

Arginine
Arginine, also a non-essential amino acid, is produced by the kidneys and stimulates the secretion of several hormones, such as growth hormone, glucagon, and insulin. Arginine supplementation is associated with positive effects on nitrogen balance and immune response. However, the clinical relevance of arginine supplementation has not been fully elucidated. The use of arginine supplementation in critically ill patients should be avoided.

n-3 fatty acids
It is hypothesised that *n*-3 fatty acids (present in fish oil) positively influence the inflammatory response, resulting in a less-severe inflammation and the production of anti-inflammatory cytokines. It has been shown that oral or enteral supplementation of *n*-3 fatty acids contributes to maintaining body weight and quality of life, but does not prolong survival in cancer patients. Postoperative parenteral supplementation in surgical oncology may reduce the length of hospital stay. In critical care, enteral supplementation of *n*-3 fatty acids has beneficial effects on clinical outcome. Supplementation in these specific patient populations can be considered, taking the route of administration into account.

Acknowledgements

This chapter has been revised and updated by Esther van den Hogen, Marian A.E. van Bokhorst-de van der Schueren and Cora F. Jonkers–Schuitema, based on the original chapter by Karin Barendregt and Peter Soeters.

References and further reading

Background clinical nutrition

Boateng AA, Sriram K, Meguid MM, Crook M. Refeeding syndrome: treatment considerations based on collective analysis of literature case reports. Nutrition 2010; 26: 156–167.

Cahill NE, Dhaliwal R, Day AG, Jiang X, Heyland DK. Nutrition therapy in the critical care setting: what is 'best achievable' practice? An international multicenter observational study. Critical Care Medicine 2010; 38(2): 395–401.

Strack van Scheijndel RPJ, Weijs PJ, Koopmans RH, Sauerwein HP, Beishuizen A, Girbes AR. Optimal nutrition during the period of mechanical ventilation decreases mortality in critically ill, long-term acute female patients: a prospective observational cohort study. Crit Care 2009; 13(4): R132.

Access

Al Raiy B, Fakih MG, Bryan-Nomides N, Hopfner D, Riegel E Nenninger T, Rey J, Szpunar S, Kale P, Khatib R. Peripherally inserted central venous catheters in the acute care setting: a safe alternative to high-risk short-term central venous catheters. Am J Infect Control 2010; 38(2): 149–153.

Mathus-Vliegen EM, Duflou A, Spanier MB, Fockens P. Nasoenteral feeding tube placement by nurses using an electro-magnetic guidance system (with video). Gastrointest Endosc 2010; 71(4): 728–736.

Phillips MS, Ponsky LJ. Overview of enteral and parenteral feeding acces techniques: principles and practice. Surg Clin North Am 2011; 91(4): 897–911.

Versleijen MW, Huisman-de Waal GJ, Kock MC, Elferink AJ, van Rossum LG, Feuth T, Willems MC, Jansen JB, Wanten GJ. Arteriovenous fistulae as an alternative to central venous catheters for delivery of long-term home parenteral nutrition. Gastroenterology 2009; 136(5): 1577–1584.

Disease specific nutrition

Marik PE, Zaloga GP. Immunonutrition in critically ill patients: a systematic review and analysis of the literature. Intensive Care Med 2008; 34(11): 1980–1990.

Meij van der BS, van Bokhorst-de van der Schueren MAE, Langius JAE, Brouwer IA, van Leeuwen PAM. n-3 polyunsaturated fatty acids: systematic review on clinical effects of oral, enteral and parenteral supplementation in cancer, surgery and critical care Am J Clin Nutr 2011; 94(5): 1248–1265.

Requirements

Milne AC, Potter J, Vivanti A, Avenell A. Protein and energy supplementation in elderly people at risk from malnutrition. Cochrane Database 2009. DOI: CD003288.

Sriram K, Lonchyna VA. Micronutrient supplementation in adult nutrition therapy: practical considerations. JPEN J Parenter Enteral Nutr 2009; 33(5): 548–562.

Weijs PJ, Kruizenga HM, van Dijk AE, van der Meij BS, Langius JA, Knol DL, Strack van Schijndel RJ, van Bokhorst-de van der Schueren MA. Validation of predictive equations for resting energy expenditure in adult outpatients and inpatients. Clin Nutr 2008; 27(1): 150–157.

Weijs PJ. Validity of predictive equations for resting energy expenditure in US and Dutch overweight and obese class I and II adults aged 18-65 y. Am J Clin Nutr 2008; 88(4): 959–970.

Enteral nutrition

ASPEN Board of Directors; Bankhead R, Boullata J, Brantley S, Corkins M, Guenter P, Krenitsky J, Lyman B, Metheny NA, Mueller C, Robbins S, Wessel J. Enteral nutrition practice recommendations. JPEN J Parenter Enteral Nutr 2009; 33(2): 122–167. Comment in: JPEN J Parenter Enteral Nutr 2010; 34(1): 103; author reply 104.

Chen Y, Peterson SJ. Enteral nutrition formulas: which formula is right for your adult patient? Nutr Clin Pract 2009; 24(3): 344–355.

Kreymann KG, Berger MM, Deutz NEP, Hiesmayr M, Jolliet P, Kazandjiev G, Nitenberg G, van den Berghe G, Wernerman J, Ebner C, Hartl W, Heymann C, Spies C. ESPEN guidelines on enteral nutrition: intensive care. Clinical Nutrition 2006; 25: 210–223.

Lochs H, Allison SP, Meier R, Pirlich M, Kondrup J, Schneider S, van den Berghe G, Pichard C. Introductory to the ESPEN guidelines on enteral nutrition: terminology, definitions and general topics. Clinical Nutrition 2006; 25: 180–186.

van den Bemt PM, Cusell MB, Overbeeke PW, Trommelen M, van Dooren D, Ophorst WR, Egberts AC. Quality improvement of oral medication administration in patients with enteral feeding tubes. Qual Saf Health Care 2006; 15(1): 44–47.

Williams NT. Medication administration through enteral feeding tubes. Am J Health Syst Pharm 2008; 65(24): 2347–2357.

Parenteral nutrition

Cano NJ, Aparicio M, Brunori G, Carrero JJ, Cianciaruso B, Fiaccadori E, Lindholm B, Teplan V, Fouque D, Guarnieri G; ESPEN. ESPEN guidelines on parenteral nutrition. Clin Nutr 2009; 28(4).

Korez RL, Lipman TO, Klein S. AGA technical review on parenteral nutrition. Gastroenterology 2001; 121: 970–1001.

Pironi L, Joly F, Forbes A, Colomb V, Lyszkowska M, Baxter J, Gabe S, Hébuterne X, Gambarara M, Gottrand F, Cuerda C, Thul P, Messing B, Goulet O, Staun M, Van Gossum A; Home Artificial Nutrition & Chronic Intestinal Failure Working Group of the European Society for Clinical Nutrition and Metabolism (ESPEN). Long-term follow-up of patients on home parenteral nutrition in Europe: implications for intestinal transplantation. Gut 2011; 60(1): 17–25.

Singer P, Berger MM, Van den Berghe G, Biolo G, Calder P, Forbes A, Griffiths R, Kreyman G, Leverve X, Pichard C; ESPEN. ESPEN guidelines on parenteral nutrition: intensive care. Clin Nutr 2009 Aug; 28(4): 387–400.

Wanten G, Calder PC, Forbes A. Managing adult patients who need home parenteral nutrition. BMJ 2011; 342: d1447. DOI: 10.1136/bmj.d1447.

Useful web sites

American Journal of Clinical Nutrition, www.ajcn.org.

American Society for Parenteral and Enteral Nutrition, www.nutritioncare.org.

Arbor Nutrition Guide, www.arborcom.com.

British Association for Parenteral and Enteral Nutrition, www.bapen.org.uk.

British Nutrition Foundation, www.nutrition.org.uk.

European Society for Clinical Nutrition and Metabolism, www.espen.org.

Federation of American Societies for Experimental Biology, www.faseb.org/ascn.

Fight Malnutrition, www.fightmalnutrition.eu.

Nutritional Assessment, www.nutritionalassessment.english.azm.nl.

10
Ethics and Nutrition

Clare McNaught and John MacFie

Scarborough Hospital, Scarborough, UK

Life is short; and the art long; and the right time an instant; and treatment precarious; and the crisis grievous. It is necessary for the physician not only to provide the needed treatment but to provide for the patient himself, and for those beside him, and to provide for his outside affairs.

Attributed to Hippocrates, circa 400 BC
(translation by Dickinson Richards)

Man is an animal with primary instincts of survival. Consequently, his ingenuity has developed first and his soul afterwards. Thus, the progress of science is far ahead of man's ethical behaviour.

Sir Charles Spencer Chaplin (1899–1977)

Let the doctors work out the ethical implications; let them face the problems in the context of ethics. I think the courts have given the medical profession the opportunity to get their ethical house in order. If they do, the common law will follow the guidance of the ethical solutions reached.

Lord Scarman, 1984

Key messages

- The four principals of medical ethics are autonomy, nonmaleficence, beneficence, and justice.
- Artificial nutrition and hydration is a medical treatment which can be withheld or withdrawn if it is in the best interests of the patient.
- The concept of capacity and best interests has been defined in law through the Mental Capacity Act 2005.
- The application of ethical principles to artificial nutritional support can guide clinical decision-making.

10.1 Introduction

Medicine is inherently a moral enterprise; the very practice of medicine involves making decisions between good and bad, right and wrong. This has been part of the practice of medicine for centuries. Nonetheless, it is only in relatively recent years that the principles of ethics applied to medicine have come to dominate contemporary practice. Traditionally, doctors are seen as experts in addressing the 'can we?' questions, which are technical questions, but the ethics questions, the 'should we?' questions, are comparatively new to clinical practice.

The term 'bioethics' was coined in the early 1970s to denote a new, rapidly expanding discipline in medicine. There were many stimuli for this growth, the most important of which can be summarised as follows:

- *The explosion of medical technology and pharmacology.* As patients, researchers, and technicians discover newer and improved methods of treatment, each development is matched by an extension of the ethical dilemmas that surround each new innovation.
- *The changing doctor–patient relationship.* Traditionally, the paternalistic physician unilaterally made decisions about what was appropriate for a particular patient. Paternalism, however, has been seen to be flawed and current case law in most countries recognises the essential principle of autonomy and the fact that the competent patient is empowered to participate in medical decisions.

Clinical Nutrition, Second Edition. Edited by Marinos Elia, Olle Ljungqvist, Rebecca J Stratton and Susan A Lanham-New.
© 2013 The Nutrition Society. Published 2013 by Blackwell Publishing Ltd.

- *Concerns about cost containment.* Medical decisions used to be made by one physician, who would provide the professional service almost irrespective of cost. This inevitably resulted in dramatic increases in utilisation of new medical technologies. As third-party payers (insurance companies, governments, health authorities) became alarmed about increasing costs, they demanded not only accountability but also some voice in decisions about the use of expensive technology. In addressing this dilemma about costs, there are two different perspectives. The medical-practice perspective attempts to maximise the good of the individual patient. This perspective looks at personal concerns on a case-by-case basis, and is particularly concerned about the ethical principles of beneficence (doing good for the patient) and autonomy (the patient's right to self-determination). In contrast, the health-policy perspective seeks to maximise the good of society rather than of the individual. This perspective reflects the importance of the ethical principles of utilitarianism and justice.

The issue of nutritional support in clinical practice exemplifies these changing attitudes to ethical dilemmas. The administration of artificial nutrition and hydration (ANH) was originally intended as a temporary bridge to the restoration of a patient's normal digestive functioning. It is now, however, often given to patients who have irretrievably lost all higher brain function. It is a strange paradox that society and many members of the medical profession frequently recommend nutritional support in those with severe neurological disease or terminal illness but at the same time fail to recognise or treat malnutrition in hospitalised patients. An analysis of the ethical issues surrounding malnutrition and nutritional support serves to emphasise not only the changing face of bioethics but also how the ethical issues themselves have influenced the clinical application of nutritional support techniques.

10.2 Brief history of medical ethics

Hippocrates is considered the father of medical ethics. He is thought to have been born around 460 BC, but little is known of his life, and there may, in fact, have been several men of this name. Whether Hippocrates was one man or several, the works attributed to him mark the stage in Western medicine at which disease was coming to be regarded as a natural rather than a supernatural phenomenon and doctors were encouraged to look for physical causes of illness. Hippocrates laid much stress on diet in the treatment of disease and the use of few drugs. He emphasised the importance of the natural history of disease, recognising the futility of treatment in many instances. Perhaps his greatest legacy was the charter of medical conduct embodied in the so-called Hippocratic oath, which has been adopted as a pattern for physicians throughout the ages. It was not strictly an oath, but rather an ethical code or ideal, an appeal for right conduct. In one or other of its many versions, it has guided the practice of medicine for more than 2000 years.

The fundamental tenets of the Hippocratic tradition were to do away with suffering, to lessen the violence of disease, and to refuse to treat those who were overwhelmed by their disease, in the realisation that in such cases medicine or treatment was powerless. Nontreatment was not considered to violate the concept of doing no harm because the physicians accepted a limit to their abilities. Provision of food and water was not deemed 'necessary' in the face of overwhelming disease. The Hippocratic concepts of beneficence – the providing of benefit – and nonmaleficence – the avoidance of harm – remain fundamental to contemporary medical ethics.

This Hippocratic tradition remained largely unchallenged for the best part of the next 2 millennia. Comparatively little was written on the subject of ethics until the fifteenth and sixteenth centuries, when contemporary theologians recorded their thoughts for posterity. The sixteenth-century theologian Bonez, for example, was the first to expound the theory of ordinary versus extraordinary treatment in prolonging life. It is important to emphasise here that 'extraordinary' does not refer to the techniques employed but rather to the condition of the patient. Historically, even the most simple remedy was deemed extraordinary if it offered no hope to the patient. Such remedies were, therefore, morally optional. Even food and water were considered to be extraordinary therapies and therefore, as in the Hippocratic tradition, morally optional.

The British physician Thomas Percival was arguably the first to formulate a doctrine of medical ethics. In 1803 he published a treatise entitled *Code of Institutes and Precepts Adapted to the Professional Conduct of*

Physicians and Surgeons. This treatise was to be the most influential document on ethics on both sides of the Atlantic for over 100 years. It work served as a prototype for the American Medical Association's first code of ethics in 1847. Percival believed that the welfare of the patient was governed by the good and virtuous behaviour of doctors. He believed in the assets of a strong interprofessional relationship achieved through the propriety and dignity of the conduct of doctors. His was the philosophy of the doctor–doctor relationship: the doctor knows best. This philosophical approach to medical care is termed 'paternalism'.

While there are many different aspects to paternalism, the fundamental principle of this philosophy is the presumption that the doctor is in the best position to make decisions on behalf of the patient. Percival argued that nonmaleficence and beneficence fix the physician's primary obligations and triumph over the patient's preferences and rights in any circumstance of serious conflict. It was accepted that doctors determined by themselves, or in conjunction with colleagues, the most appropriate care for their patients. This rendered unnecessary the inconvenience of discussing with either the patient or their surrogates the relative merits or demerits of any given therapy. Percival failed to foresee the power of the principles of autonomy and distributive justice, which in the twentieth century became ubiquitous in discussions of biomedical ethics.

One catalyst to the dramatic shift away from paternalism towards acceptance of the critical importance of autonomy was the publication of the Nuremberg Code, which followed the unpleasant discovery of human experiments performed during World War II. The doctor–doctor relationship was seen to be flawed and the Nuremberg Code established the importance of the doctor–patient relationship. Implicit in this is the recognition of a patient's right to self-determination: the right to know, the right to choose, and the right to be informed.

Another important principle in contemporary ethical debate relates to justice. Common to all theories of justice is a minimal requirement that equals are treated equally, a concept originally attributed to Aristotle. These days the principle of distributive justice refers to fair, equitable, and appropriate distribution in society, determined by justified norms that structure the terms of social cooperation. Most

governments today and certainly all democracies would claim to support the principles inherent in distributive justice.

10.3 Medical ethics: the four-principle approach

From the foregoing discussion, it can be seen that four principles underpin present approaches to medical ethics (Box 10.1):

- Autonomy is the principle of self-determination and is a recognition of patient rights. This is now the preeminent theme in law in most democratic states.
- Nonmaleficence is the deliberate avoidance of harm.
- Beneficence is the concept that the patient is provided with some kind of benefit.
- Justice is the fair and equitable provision of available medical resources to all.

Application of these four principles offers a systematic and relatively objective way to approach ethical dilemmas. The advocates of this 'four-principle' approach to biomedical ethics stress that these principles should be seen not as specific precise action guides that will inform doctors of the appropriate action for any circumstance, but rather as a framework of virtues or values that are relevant to ethical debate. It is important to note that there are alternative ethical approaches, including virtue-based theories, the ethics of caring, casuistry, narrative ethics, and others. These are outwith the scope of this chapter and the interested reader is referred to standard texts on ethical theory and moral philosophy.

Analysis of ethical dilemmas employing principalism as outlined above results in three common themes that distinguish different individuals' perspectives on ethical debate:

- The duty-based moralist is concerned predominantly with the intrinsic merits or otherwise of a medical decision, rather than its consequences.

Box 10.1 The four principles of medical ethics

- Beneficence
- Nonmaleficence
- Justice
- Autonomy

A wholly committed duty-based moralist would support the sanctity of life at all costs.

- The utilitarian or goal-based moralist requires the doctor to judge the general aggregate of good according to the consequences of an action rather than the act itself. Thus, this doctor would stand by the principles of a controlled clinical trial, thereby justifying the morbidity and even mortality of a few patients by the potential benefit to be gained by a majority of patients.
- The rights-based moralist is, as already pointed out, the dominant contemporary theme and is now the fundamental principle of medical law. This doctor would condemn an action if it wronged someone or if it violated the right of a patient to determine their own destiny.

Application of these themes to the issue of nutritional support gives very different recommendations for treatment. The duty-based moralist would always feed the patient, whatever the anticipated outcome, on the basis that this was the right and responsibility of the doctor. The goal-based or utilitarian doctor would feed when appropriate in their healthcare setting and if the results of such intervention were justified on the basis of scientific evidence. The rights-based moralist would argue that the patient should always be offered nutritional support and that, if requested by the patient on the basis of information given, the moral responsibility must be to provide nutritional support. Equally, if the patient or their surrogate refuses nutritional support, the patient's wishes must be respected.

Obviously there is some conflict between these three themes, as well as with the four principles of autonomy, beneficence, nonmaleficence, and justice. These conflicts serve to emphasise that ethics is a process of reasoning whereby a morally respectable and defensible position can be reached which protects the best interests of the patient. There are no absolutely satisfactory resolutions of ethical dilemmas and the most that one can hope to achieve is a balance between the conflicting interests and goals of different individuals involved in patient care. While this is a very simplistic approach to a complex area, it is hoped that the foregoing discussion will have provided the reader with an insight into how these ethical principles have evolved and given some feeling for their relative importance.

10.4 Definitions and ethical terms

The definitions and terms described here are adopted from the British Medical Association (BMA)'s publication *Withholding and Withdrawing Life-prolonging Medical Treatment* (BMA, 2007). This text is highly recommended.

Oral nutrition and hydration: 'basic care'

The provision of food or water by mouth, whether simply by moistening a patient's mouth for comfort, or by the use of cup, spoon, or other assistance, is deemed part of basic care. 'Basic care' means those procedures deemed essential to keeping a patient comfortable. It is a health professional's duty to ensure the provision of basic care to all patients unless actively resisted by the patient. Food and water should therefore always be offered, unless the process of feeding produces an unacceptable burden to the patient. Many patients, such as babies, young children, and people with disability, may require assistance with feeding but retain the ability to swallow if the food is placed in their mouths; this forms part of basic care. Evidence suggests that when patients are close to death, however, they seldom want nutrition or hydration, and its provision may exacerbate discomfort and suffering. Good practice should include moistening the mouth as necessary to keep the patient comfortable.

Artificial nutrition and hydration

The term 'artificial nutrition' should be used specifically for those techniques for providing nutrition that are used to bypass a pathology in the swallowing mechanism. All parenteral and the majority of enteral feeding techniques (except perhaps sip-feeding oral supplements) are forms of provision of artificial nutrition. In North America and in most European countries, ANH is considered a medical treatment, as opposed to simply an aspect of basic care, and therefore subject to same ethical constraints in its instigation or withdrawal, just like any other life-prolonging therapy. Some people continue to argue that tube feeding should be regarded as part of basic care, while others have made a distinction between the insertion of a feeding tube, which is classed as treatment, and the administration of fluid or nutrients through a tube, which they consider basic care. If this view were generally accepted then decisions not to insert a feeding tube or not to reinsert it if it became dislodged would be legitimate medical decisions, whereas a decision to stop providing nutrition through an existing tube would not. This distinction is not generally accepted.

Consent and competence

All individuals have the right to agree to or decline medical treatment, including nutritional support. For consent to be valid in law, three principles must be fulfilled: the consent must be informed, the patient must be competent to make the decision, and the decision must be voluntary. The amount of information given to the patient and how this is delivered will vary depending on the clinical situation and requires careful judgement on the part of the doctor. The patient must understand the nature of the nutritional support and the benefits and risks of the intervention. There is no definite legal guidance on the level of risk that needs to be disclosed to patients, but serious complications, such as pneumothorax or haemorrhage in the placement of feeding lines, must be discussed. It is customary to take written consent for invasive procedures, such as central-line or percutaneous endoscopic gastrostomy (PEG) placement, as evidence that consent has been given. More often, consent for nutritional support is given verbally, and the concept of 'implied consent' is well established in law. It is important to remember that patients have the right to withdraw consent at any time.

Many decisions relating to ANH occur in patients who have a temporary or permanent impairment of cognitive function, for example after a stroke. For many years, health professionals have made treatment judgements based on the notion of patients' 'best interests', influenced by the UK General Medical Council's guidelines. This involves balancing the treatment options, taking into consideration any preferences stated by the patient in the past – either through an advanced directive or from evidence given by a third party who knows the patient well – and choosing the intervention which least restricts the patient's future choices. The concept of what constitutes capacity and 'best interest' has now been defined in law through the Mental Capacity Act 2005 (MCA). The five main principles of the act are listed in Box 10.2. The MCA states unequivocally that a doctor must assume that the patient has the capacity to make decisions unless a lack of capacity has been clearly demonstrated (Box 10.3). The act acknowledges that patients with impaired mental capacity may still have the ability to make some decisions

---

Box 10.2 The principles of the Mental Capacity Act 2005. © Crown Copyright 2007, Mental Capacity Act 2005, Code of Practice

1. A person must be assumed to have capacity unless it is established that they lack capacity.
2. A person is not to be treated as unable to make a decision unless all practicable steps to help them to do so have been taken without success.
3. A person is not to be treated as unable to make a decision merely because they make an unwise decision.
4. An act done, or decision made under this Act for or on behalf of a person who lacks capacity must be done, or made, in their best interests.
5. Before the act is done, or the decision is made, regard must be had to whether the purpose for which it is needed can be as effectively achieved in a way that is less restrictive of the person's rights and freedom of action.

Box 10.3 The Mental Capacity Act 2005: lack of mental capacity. © Crown Copyright 2007, Mental Capacity Act 2005, Code of Practice

1. A person is unable to make a decision for himself if they are unable—
   (a) to understand the information relevant to the decision,
   (b) to retain that information,
   (c) to use or weigh that information as part of the process of making the decision, or
   (d) to communicate their decision (whether by talking, using sign language, or any other means).
2. A person is not to be regarded as unable to understand the information relevant to a decision if they are able to understand an explanation of it given to them in a way that is appropriate to their circumstances (using simple language, visual aids, or any other means).
3. The fact that a person is able to retain the information relevant to a decision for a short period only does not prevent them from being regarded as able to make the decision.
4. The information relevant to a decision includes information about the reasonably foreseeable consequences of—
   (a) deciding one way or another, or
   (b) failing to make the decision.

about their care and states that efforts should be made to facilitate this where possible. This idea of 'enhancing capacity' may involve the treatment of intercurrent illness to resolve an acute confusional state or the use of simple visual aids to assist patient comprehension.

Advanced decisions/directives/proxies

If the patient does lack capacity then the doctor must establish whether the patient has made an advanced decision indicating their preference for treatment or nontreatment. Except in the case of life-sustaining treatments, this does not have to be a formal, written, witnessed document but must specify the treatment that is to be refused and under which circumstance (this can be made in lay terms as long as it is understood clearly). If the patient has fully comprehended the implication of their advanced decision then the decision will be binding. In the case of ANH, a number of criteria must be met to make an advanced decision compulsory. It must be in writing and the maker and a witness must sign it at the same time. It must also include a statement that ANH should not be given 'even if life is at risk'. This statement must also be signed by the patient and a witness. The advanced decision can be invalidated if the patient withdraws it while they have capacity or if there is a change of circumstances that could not have been predicted by the patient which casts doubt on the decision. Clinicians must use their judgement carefully in these circumstances and seek legal advice if there is any uncertainty.

The MCA has also introduced two situations in which a designated person can make decisions on behalf of incapacitated individuals. Some patients may have appointed a Lasting Power of Attorney (LPA), who is usually a relative or close friend. They can make proxy decisions relating to personal health, financial, and property matters when the patient becomes incapacitated. They can also make choices pertaining to medical interventions, but are only permitted to make judgements on life-sustaining treatments if this power was specifically granted to them. The Court of Protection, which acts as the final arbiter for capacity matters, can also appoint a Deputy to make decisions on behalf of the patient, but not in the scenario of life-saving treatments.

Time-limited trials of treatment

Considerable anxiety is produced by reports of mistaken diagnosis or a belief that, had a treatment been provided, a patient might have recovered to a level that would have been acceptable to that individual. One of the difficulties for health professionals is that it is often not possible to predict with certainty how any individual will respond to a particular treatment or, in the final stages of an illness, how long the dying process will take. Doctors have an ethical obligation to keep their skills up to date and to keep abreast of new developments in their speciality so that they can make decisions based on a reasonable assessment of the facts available. There will, however, always remain some areas of doubt, and empirical judgments may be made founded on probability rather than certainty.

In the acute medical setting, clinicians often have to make rapid decisions and commence treatment based on the evidence available to them. As the clinical scenario unfolds and more information becomes obtainable, it may become clear that the treatment is unjustified and that it is futile to continue it. When there is genuine doubt about possible benefit, treatment should be given, but it may be withdrawn if on subsequent review it is found to be inappropriate or not beneficial. The uncertainty about patient outcome from a disease may lead to a reticence to commence therapy, in order that dilemmas upon stopping the treatment are avoided. In these cases it is worth considering a time-limited trial of therapy. This involves setting specific goals and carefully monitoring progress over a previously specified period of time. End points may vary, but can include, for example, objective signs of recovery or deterioration in multi-organ failure for patients in intensive care, or neurological status in patients following stroke. It would be reasonable to assess these on a weekly basis. Ideally, clinicians should determine the goals of therapy or response to illness after discussion with colleagues, as well as with relatives, in order to minimise ethical conflicts. In the case of nutritional support, it would seem sensible to involve a nutrition team. Time-limited trials of therapy facilitate decision-making as they permits wider consultation over complex problems and acknowledge that clinical situations evolve with time, diminishing uncertainty in medical treatment.

Futility and the concept of net patient benefit

There are many aspects to medical futility and many definitions of it. In considering the principle of futility, it is important to differentiate between effect and benefit. In patients with persistent vegetative states (PVSs), nutritional therapy will maintain organ function and keep the patient alive. However, nutritional therapy is unlikely to restore the patient to a conscious and sapient life. It is arguable, therefore, that nutritional therapy, in these instances, is futile. This is certainly the view accepted by British Courts of Justice. The BMA has defined benefit for patients as treatment conferring a net gain or advantage. Benefit does not necessarily equate with simply achieving certain physiological goals. This principle might apply for example to the perioperative patient with multi-organ failure who is being sustained on long-term haemodialysis and artificial ventilation. It is worthy of emphasis, with regard to assessment of futility in clinical practice, that the courts in the UK have made clear on a number of occasions that doctors are not obliged to provide treatment contrary to their clinical judgment.

10.5 Application of ethical principles to artificial nutritional support: clinical scenarios

Stroke

The World Health Organization (WHO) definition of stroke is a neurological deficit of cerebrovascular cause that persists beyond 24 hours or is interrupted by death within 24 hours. Stroke is the third leading cause of death in the UK, affecting 150 000 people every year. One-third of the patients will die after the event and the majority of survivors will be left with permanent disabilities. At presentation, over 40% of stroke victims will suffer from dysphagia, leaving them at risk of malnutrition and aspiration pneumonia. Malnutrition is associated with poorer medical outcome after stroke and also impaired long-term functional recovery. There is, therefore, a strong rationale for artificial feeding in stroke patients, but considerable debate surrounds the optimal time for initiating therapy and the route that this should be delivered.

In 2005, the FOOD Trial Collaboration published the results of two multicentre randomised controlled trials in dysphagic patients. In one, patients were randomised to early enteral nutrition or no enteral nutrition for 7 days. In the other, patients were allocated to nasogastric feeding and compared to those with PEG feeding. They reported a nonsignificant trend towards survival in the early-feeding group versus the delayed-feeding group, but this small survival benefit was offset by a 4.7% excess of survivors in the severely disabled state who might have otherwise died. Early enteral nutrition was not associated with reduced length of stay and did not influence the rates of long-term institutional care. In the PEG versus tube study, 10% of the deaths in PEG patients were directly attributable to the technique versus 3% in the nasogastric-feeding group, although the rate of gastrointestinal haemorrhage was higher in the tube-fed group. For this reason, the authors suggested that nasogastric feeding should be the preferred route of nutrition, at least for the first 2–3 weeks.

When faced with the dilemma of ANH in a stroke patient, a powerful case can be made for delaying the instigation of feeding for 5–7 days. This will allow time to carefully assess the prognosis of the patient, which can be predicted by the early signs of recovery, and also provides opportunities for frank discussions with the relatives and the members of the multidisciplinary team. More importantly, delay for a week may permit recovery from aphasia or dysarthria such that the patient's views can be carefully considered. Dysphagia rates can fall to 16% a week after the event, and many patients may be able to tolerate oral feeding, using strategies such as food and fluid texturing and patient positioning. Where reasonable doubt exists over outcomes, time-limited trials of therapy should be considered. A recent report, published jointly by the Royal College of Physicians and British Society of Gastroenterology (2010), has established guidelines for the care of patients with oral feeding difficulties. This report suggests that nutritional support should be delivered via a fine-bore nasogastric tube. If this is well tolerated and is required for less than 6 weeks, a PEG is not necessary. If the tube is required for longer than 6 weeks, a PEG should be fitted prior to discharge to the community.

The application of the four ethical principles can guide decision-making by clinicians when considering ANH in stroke patients. First, the principles of beneficence and nonmaleficence. There is no doubt that harm will result from inadequate dietary intakes and that some patients will benefit from some form of nutritional support. The duty of the doctor is to employ those feeding techniques which are most effective and impose least burden on the patient. The concept of justice necessitates the attending physician to make a judgment of outcome. Allocation of resources is justified if recovery is anticipated, particularly if a good quality of life is expected. The problem for the ethicist arises when recovery is uncertain. This raises the question of medical futility. In practice, it is often impossible to know what progress the patient may or may not make. In these circumstances, there is much to recommend the instigation of time-limited trials of therapy. This facilitates decision-making and acknowledges that clinical situations evolve with time. Nutritional support may be justified early in the course of the disease, but after weeks without tangible progress or with actual deterioration, the clinician is ethically justified to discontinue therapy on the basis of medical futility. Finally, recognising the principle of autonomy, the clinician must ensure that all efforts have been made to assess what the patient would have wanted had they been in a position to express a view. If an advanced decision has been made, the doctor must accept the patient's right to self-determination.

Dementia

'Dementia' is the term used to describe a range of clinical conditions, including Alzheimer's disease and vascular dementia, which cause progressive neurodegeneration and result in reduced mental, social, and physical functioning. It is estimated that 750 000 people in the UK suffer from this condition and that this number will double over the next 3 decades. The UK government currently spends £17 billion per year on dementia care and has recently launched a National Dementia Strategy to promote early diagnosis and improve the quality of life of dementia sufferers. Over 60 000 deaths per year in the UK are directly attributable to dementia, with a median survival of 10 years if diagnosed in the seventh decade of life, but only 3 years if over 90. In patients with advanced dementia, where patients are doubly incontinent and rely on others for all activities of daily living, the prognosis is poor and survival rates are comparable to other terminal illnesses, such as metastatic breast cancer. Inadequate nutrition can occur early in the clinical course of dementia, as patients lose the normal physiological drives of appetite and satiety and cognitive impairment leads to an indifference to food. In advanced dementia, physical disabilities predominate, with patients becoming bedbound and muscular incoordination leading to the development of dysphagia, apraxia, and aspiration. Many relatives and carers will react intuitively to the inevitable weight loss and request nutritional support, often by the placement of an enteral feeding tube or PEG, in the belief that it will reduce their loved one's suffering.

The commonly held conviction amongst carers that enteral feeding may benefit dementia patients is also shared by many in the medical professions. It is often stated that enteral feeding may prevent aspiration and, through the correction of nutritional deficiencies, prevent mortality, infection, and the development of pressure sores. There is very little evidence in the literature to support this opinion. To date, no prospective randomised trial has been performed comparing ANH with best supportive care in advanced dementia. This topic has recently been the subject of a Cochrane review, which analysed seven observational cohort studies, the majority of them from the USA. There was no conclusive evidence that enteral nutrition had any beneficial effect on survival, nutritional status, pressure sores, or any other outcome measure. It has long been recognised that enteral nutrition can have adverse effects: it may be associated with aspiration pneumonia and occasionally with diarrhoea, which may worsen decubitus ulcers in the immobile patient. The short-term mortality rate for PEG placement is no higher in dementia patients than in those with other neurological conditions, but it remains a significant risk given that there is little evidence of benefit. Finally, patients with dementia do not have the cognitive capacity to understand the purpose of feeding tubes, whether nasogastric or transabdominal, with the result that they may need restraining to prevent them from pulling them out.

The decision to initiate enteral feeding in dementia patients remains a contentious, highly emotive issue. Clinicians must assess each case individually and take into consideration any advanced directive, and, if one does not exist, explore the opinions of the relatives and carers. There may be situations where doctors feel pressured to initiate ANH in order to appease relatives or to aid discharge from acute hospital wards to institutional care establishments. These situations can often be resolved by educating carers and offering advice on alternative feeding techniques which might improve oral intake. These include the use of hand feeding with finger foods, personal assistance with meals, giving frequent reminders to swallow and cough, and using thickened spoon feeds as required. Where conflict or uncertainty prevails, time-limited trials of enteral nutrition using therapies with minimal morbidity may be justified.

Wasting disorders: cancer and terminal illness

Many patients with advanced cancer experience weight loss and reduced appetite, which may lead to weakness, fatigue, and reduced quality of life. In recent years, many studies have been performed to understand the pathophysiology behind this anorexia/cachexia syndrome (ACS). It is clear that there are many reasons why patients become cachexic, including the presence of gastrointestinal obstruction, the effects of nausea and pain associated with the primary tumour, and the side effects of chemotherapy and radiotherapy. There is increasing evidence that intermediary metabolism is also altered in these patients, driven by cytokine and hormonal release, which leads to pronounced loss of skeletal muscle and fat. Weight loss has major prognostic significance in cancer patients, with shorter survival in those who have had the greatest weight reduction. This association between wasting and death has led to the assumption that prevention or reversal of wasting with artificial nutritional support might delay or prevent death and be associated with improved quality of life. Regrettably, there is little evidence to support this view.

An excellent summary of the evidence on ANH in the treatment of adult patients during anticancer treatment and haemopoietic cell transplantation was published by the American Society of Parenteral and Enteral Nutrition. They made a number of recommendations, which are summarised in Box 10.4. In general, it has been repeatedly demonstrated that

> **Box 10.4 Nutritional support guideline recommendations during adult anticancer treatment and in haemopoietic cell transplantation. August & Huhmann (2009), JPEN (Vol. 33, No. 5) pp. 472–500. © 2009 by SAGE Publications. Reprinted by Permission of SAGE Publications**
>
> 1. Nutrition support therapy should not be used *routinely* in patients undergoing major cancer operations.
> 2. Perioperative nutrition support therapy may be beneficial in moderately or severely malnourished patients if administered for 7–14 days preoperatively, but the potential benefits of nutrition support must be weighed against the potential risks of the nutrition-support therapy itself and of delaying the operation.
> 3. Nutrition support therapy should not be used *routinely* as an adjunct to chemotherapy.
> 4. Nutrition support therapy should not be used *routinely* in patients undergoing head and neck, abdominal, or pelvic irradiation.
> 5. Nutrition support therapy is appropriate in patients receiving active anticancer treatment who are malnourished and who are anticipated to be unable to ingest and/or absorb adequate nutrients for a prolonged period of time.
> 6. The palliative use of nutrition support therapy in terminally ill cancer patients is rarely indicated.
>
> **In patients undergoing haematopoietic cell transplantation**
>
> 7. Nutrition support therapy is appropriate in patients undergoing haematopoietic cell transplantation who are malnourished and who are anticipated to be unable to ingest and/or absorb adequate nutrients for a prolonged period of time.

the use of supplemental feeding, by either the parenteral or the enteral route, does not reduce the morbidity or mortality rates from cancer. Any weight gain seen in patients is likely to be secondary to peripheral oedema and an increase in total body water. There are, however, a few exceptions to this. In patients with head and neck cancers who are malnourished and unable to eat, or in some patients with gastrointestinal obstruction who are not in the terminal phase, adjuvant nutritional therapy may prolong survival, improve tolerance to anticancer treatment, and enhance quality of life. This is also true for patients undergoing haematological stem-cell transplantation.

In the terminal phase of cancer, the increasing cachexia is often distressing to the patient and to those who care for them. The view that the correction of obvious malnutrition or dehydration must bring about improved quality of life is difficult to substantiate, but is fundamental to the ethical debate that surrounds the withholding or withdrawing of artificial nutrition from terminally ill patients. In essence, the critical question is whether or not the absence of feeding leads to or causes a cruel and painful demise. There is little in the literature that addresses this question, but existing documentation suggests that death accompanied by starvation and dehydration is in fact painless and humane. Many studies from palliative care hospices have shown that terminally ill patients do not experience more than transient hunger and that any thirst can be easily offset by careful mouth care. This is one of the main priorities set out in the Liverpool Care Pathway for the Dying Patient. The paucity of evidence for a benefit of nutritional support in these patients and the fact that any nutritional intervention can itself be associated with harm does not mean that nutritional support is never indicated, however. Basic care in the form of offered oral nutrients should never be withdrawn and there will often be cases in which the clinician feels that the patient has not entered the terminal phase of their illness where nutritional support might be indicated to achieve specific short-term goals. This merely serves to emphasise that patients need to be assessed on an individual basis. Decisions over nutritional therapy must be discussed with the patient and their relatives in the context of available evidence. The responsibility of clinicians is to avoid interventions that they know to be futile. Clinical judgment must decide whether the patient's inability to eat is irreversible and a consequence of overwhelming disease. If so, nutritional support can at best delay the dying process and at worst will result in discomfort or morbidity with no benefits in terms of quality or quantity of life. Inappropriate feeding has resource implications, but more importantly is unfair on the individual patient, who is given unrealistic expectations of therapy.

Persistent vegetative states: withdrawing and withholding nutritional support

A PVS is state of profound unresponsiveness caused by severe brain injury. Patients may be in a 'wakeful state' but are unable to speak, move, or signal when confronted with environmental stimuli. The mortality rate in the first year is considerable, but patients may survive for many decades with the administration of ANH. There have been a few well-publicised instances of patients emerging from a PVS after many years, but this is extremely rare. Landmark 'right to die' cases of patients diagnosed as being in a PVS, both in this country and elsewhere, have generated much ethical debate and established important legal precedent. In the UK, the Bland case was the first of these judgments. Tony Bland was a 21-year-old man who suffered anoxic brain damage when a football stadium collapsed. He was subsequently confirmed as being in a PVS. Nutrition and hydration were maintained by tube feeding. After some months in this condition, his attending physicians approached the courts to enquire as to the legality of withdrawing nutritional support. They were informed that this would constitute judicial murder. The case was ultimately heard in the House of Lords, which constitutes the highest court in the UK, and the Lords authorised the removal of the feeding tube. Tony Bland died 11 days later. This case clarified the law relating to withholding and withdrawing life-prolonging treatments and highlighted several important legal points:

- Medical decisions for a mentally incapable patient should be made in the best interests of the patient.
- If a decision to withdraw or withhold treatment is in the best interests of the patient then it is lawful.
- There is no legal difference between withdrawing and withholding treatment.
- Artificial nutrition and hydration constitute medical treatments and can be withdrawn if it is in the best interests of the patient to do so.

The situation in the USA and the UK is now similar to that which already exists in many European countries, in that there is no legal or ethical restraint on the discontinuation of feeding in a patient with an established PVS if this can be shown to accord with the patient's wishes and if no doubt exists as to the diagnosis of PVS. These patients are unable to express a view and, therefore, the weight of evidence in all such court cases has revolved around a discussion with relatives, proxies, or surrogates. On each occasion, the courts have taken the view that the weight of evidence must show clearly that a decision to discontinue feeding would accord with the patient's wishes were they able to express them. In other words, the principle of patient autonomy and right to self-determination is preeminent in any ethical debate. This also applies to the withholding or withdrawing of any medical therapy. The BMA's report on *Withholding and Withdrawing Life-prolonging Medical Treatment* (BMA, 2007) provides a comprehensive overview of all the issues involved and the current legal position.

Two recent events have reopened the debate of the withdrawal of ANH from patients with PVS. The first was the statement by Pope Benedict XVI in the Congregation for the Doctrine of the Faith. When asked if ANH could be removed from a patient with PVS, he stated that a 'patient in a permanent vegetative state is a person with fundamental human dignity and must, therefore, receive ordinary and proportionate care, which includes, in principle, the administration of water and food even by artificial means'. The second was the recent discovery of wilfully stimulated cortical motor responses, detected by MRI scanning, in patients in a minimally conscious state. As technology advances and new medications or treatments become available, the futility of ANH in this situation may be further challenged. Indeed, Italy's parliament has just passed a law that explicitly excludes the option for people to refuse ANH.

In clinical practice, at least in the UK, there is now the paradox that there is clear legal precedent for withdrawal of artificial nutrition in patients confirmed as being in a PVS but not for the many patients with severe neurological illness who are not designated as being in a vegetative state. For those in a PVS, a declaration to the courts must be sought to authorise discontinuation of feeding, but for other patients whose death is not imminent and for whom it is deemed that their best interests are served by cessation of nutritional therapy, there is currently no requirement for court review. It is clearly important for these patients that additional safeguards should be implemented, including the use of a routine second opinion and the establishment of systems to record and monitor decisions and progress.

Malnutrition in the hospitalised patient

Many patients in hospital suffer malnutrition. These include the preoperative patient, the postoperative patient, the cancer patient, and the chronically ill. In all of these groups, starvation and subsequent malnutrition may occur as a complicating factor during the course of the patient's illness. Nutritional therapy, like ventilatory or renal support, is not a disease-specific treatment, and assessment of benefit should be based primarily on the correction of nutritional abnormality. In other words, it is important to weigh up the risk of nutritional support in order to allay the effects of starvation separately from the treatment of the underlying disease. There is no doubt that starvation is harmful; death from protein-energy malnutrition occurs within 60–70 days of total starvation in normal adults. Functional metabolic deficits occur after some 10–15 days of semi-starvation in previously healthy adults, and in shorter periods in those already compromised by disease. The consequences of starvation are well known and include impairment of the immune response, alterations in organ function, malaise, lethargy, and changes in cognitive function. Against this background of information on the causes and consequences of malnutrition, it is a relatively simple matter to make recommendations for treatment. For example, the UK National Institute for Health and Clinical Excellence published guidelines in 2006 (due to be reviewed 2011) for the use of parenteral and enteral nutritional support in adults. It recommended routine screening of hospital inpatients for malnutrition, and nutritional intervention in those who have not eaten/are not expected to eat for more than 5 days. Any patient with a recalled weight loss of 10% in the recent past should also be considered as having an indication for nutritional support.

What then is the ethical situation in those patients who have already been or who are anticipated to be subjected to inadequate intakes of 7 days or more? Considering the principles of beneficence and non-maleficence, one is immediately confronted with the dilemma that no consensus exists as to the advantage of nutritional support therapy in many patient groups. This probably reflects the use of inappropriate outcome measures in many studies. There is no doubt that nutritional deprivation causes harm and that nutritional repletion by whatever means will prevent this. It is reasonable, therefore, to assume that the nutritional support therapy provides benefit. On the other hand, certain techniques of nutritional support, such as total parenteral nutrition (TPN) in inappropriate patients, can be harmful. The small percentage of complications arising from tube or PEG feeding, some of which can be serious or fatal, must be considered within the clinical background of each patient. This emphasises the importance of the clinician tailoring the method of nutritional support, which for a given patient will provide maximal benefit for minimal morbidity. The expected clinical benefit of feeding must always outweigh the significant risks and suffering caused to the patient.

Consideration must also be given to the principle of justice. If it is accepted that some form of nutritional support should be considered in all patients with significant weight loss or in those who have sustained 7 or more days of inadequate oral intake then the resource implications are clearly enormous. Recent evidence suggests that up to one-fifth of all hospital admissions may be malnourished and up to one-half of all hospital patients have one or more abnormal parameter of nutritional status. Application of the ethical principle of justice requires that health professionals assess the cost–benefits of their treatments and that these are based on sound evidence. It is well established that malnourished patients have longer hospital stays and a greater incidence of morbidity and death than well-nourished individuals. The hospital cost associated with the treatment of a malnourished patient is significantly greater than that of a well-nourished patient without complications. Clinical trials have demonstrated that nutritional intervention improves clinical outcome, enhances wound healing, facilitates return of normal physiological function, and reduces hospital stay. It is worth reiterating that there is no precedent, legal or ethical, that justifies the absence of resources as a reason not to treat. The inability of clinicians to provide nutritional support because of either personal beliefs or institutional policy will necessitate the clinician making reasonable efforts to arrange for the prompt transfer of the patient's care to a practitioner or facility willing to implement appropriate treatment. This does not, however, permit the clinician to abrogate his or her responsibility to ensure that every effort is made to provide cost-effective nutritional support.

The principle of autonomy must always take precedence. Given the deleterious consequences of short-term starvation, it would seem reasonable to conclude that, if patients are informed of these, they will request active measures to prevent harm. Unlike sophisticated medical therapies, patients understand the principles of nutritional support. The provision of food and water to the sick has a symbolic and an emotional role that transcends cultural, ethnic, and socioeconomic barriers. Patients already ask about antimicrobial therapy and other well-publicised treatments and will surely do the same with regards to nutrition therapy when there is a greater public awareness of the dangers of malnutrition, as well as an appreciation of the options for nutritional support. There may be patients who specifically object to artificial means of nutritional support and in these cases the wishes of the patient will have to be respected.

10.6 Ethical conflict

The case of Ms Terri Schiavo clearly demonstrates the destructive effects of ethical conflicts between relatives, medical professionals, and the law in relation to artificial nutrition and hydration. Ms Schiavo collapsed and suffered a cardiac arrest in 1990, related to severe hypokalaemia secondary to an eating disorder. She suffered extensive hypoxic brain damage, was diagnosed to be in a PVS, and was kept alive by tube feeding for 15 years. After 3 years, Ms Schiavo's husband asked for her feeding tube to be removed and for Terri to be allowed to die. This was contested by her parents and siblings and led to many well-publicised legal cases and court rulings, which were subsequently appealed and denied. The media attention this case received was heightened by the involvement of religious and other interest groups. Ms Schiavo's PEG tube was removed and replaced three times before she died in 2005.

When a patient lacks the capacity to make a decision, doctors have a legal responsibility to speak to the relatives, carers, and any LPA. It is important to gain as much information as possible in relation to the patient's views and beliefs, what their quality of life was like before the illness, and what the future is likely to hold for them, as well as to clarify what the relatives' opinion is in regard to treatment. The main issue, however, is not what the relatives want for themselves or for the patient, but to try and understand what the patient would want if they had the capacity to express it. The ethical principle of autonomy remains the preeminent theme in law. The opinions of the relatives are very important and often assist in determining what is best for a patient, but they carry no legal weight. It should also be noted that clinicians are not obliged to offer useless interventions and these do not need to be discussed with patients. In a situation in which a relative demands artificial nutrition against medical advice, the clinician is not legally obliged to accede. Such cases have already come to the courts in North America. Clearly, the clinician must act in what he or she considers the best interests of the patient, and where possible decisions should be evidence-based. Many authors have referred to this potential conflict between relatives and carers. Most now agree that doctors have little to fear in the legal arena when withholding therapy if the clinical judgment is made in the best interests of the patient. There is a consensus that doctors remain the final arbiters of treatment decisions in patients who lack capacity. It must be recognised, however, that the massive increase in medical litigation worldwide may reflect a growing public opinion that challenges the appropriateness of doctors taking decisions in isolation. There is undoubted pressure on the medical establishment to involve patients, their carers, and patient interest groups in difficult or controversial treatment decisions.

Conflicts might also arise because of strongly held cultural or religious beliefs. When religious principle conflicts with medical opinion, legal judgments have ruled that personal conviction cannot override public policy. Thus a doctor cannot be forced to treat against the dictates of his or her professional conscience, especially when acting according to a widely held professional view.

10.7 Clinical guidelines in ethical care

The decision-making process surrounding the provision or withdrawal of artificial nutrition can be difficult. A clear understanding of the clinical goals of therapy, together with an appreciation of the ethical issues involved, facilitates resolution of dilemmas. Application of the four principles of autonomy, beneficence, nonmaleficence, and justice is one approach and is recommended. Figure 10.1 illustrates how these principles may be used to assist the clinician in the decision as to whether to feed or not to feed. Contemporary thinking, both ethical and legal,

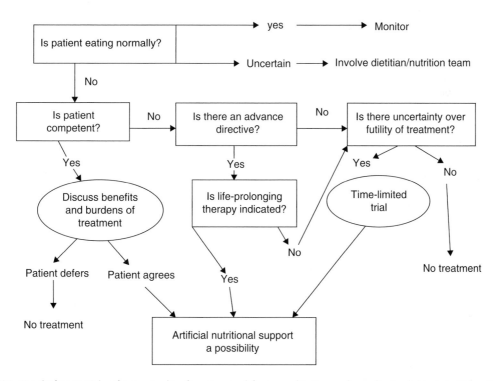

Figure 10.1 How the four principles of autonomy, beneficence, nonmaleficence, and justice may be used in the clinician's decision as to whether to feed a patient.

places most emphasis on the patient's right to self-determination – autonomy – which is reflected here.

The first question that must be asked is whether or not the patient is eating normally. Clearly, if they are, they must be encouraged to maintain adequate intakes, and ideally these should be monitored by the healthcare team. If uncertainty exists, formal assessment of intakes is appropriate. In these situations, no ethical dilemmas occur. If the patient is not eating adequately, the next decision must be to involve the patient. Is the patient competent? If so, the pros and cons of feeding must be discussed, with clear expositions as to possible outcomes and potential morbidity. The patient has the right to refuse therapy. If they do so then respect for the patient's wishes is paramount. If appropriate, all palliative care must be offered together with unforced offers of oral hydration. The patient should have the opportunity to change their mind at any point. Doctors have a responsibility to outline the futility of treatment if this is relevant to the given situation. If the patient is deemed incompetent, the next enquiry should be to establish whether they have an advanced decision or directive. If this exists and applies specifically to life-prolonging therapy, the wishes of the patient must be observed. Not to do so renders the attending physician liable to the charge of assault. In the absence of an advanced decision, the doctor must make a judgement as to whether or not the treatment is futile. This necessitates a clear decision as to the objectives of therapy. Doctors are not obliged to instigate therapies which they perceive will do no good for the patient.

Genuine uncertainty over the futility of treatment necessitates discussions with other members of the healthcare team, possible second opinions, and involvement of the relatives. All endeavours must be made to attempt to establish what a patient might have wanted were they in a position to express a view. The overriding factor must be to do what is in the best interests of the patient. Continuing uncertainty is a good reason for a time-limited trial of therapy. The goals and time span of such trials must be clearly recorded, and frank, open discussions with relatives and other carers are essential. When a decision is made to consider artificial nutritional support, whether indefinitely or as a time-limited trial, the following questions must be asked: Is swallowing normal? Is the gut functioning? Are there specific nutrient requirements? Have outcomes been decided?

Has it been recorded in the notes? Are the relatives and other members of the team involved? Is the intention to have hospital or community care? In this way, optimal nutritional support appropriate to an individual patient that ensures minimal morbidity is more certain.

Throughout this process, patients should be encouraged to state their preferences. If this is not possible, the views of the patient's surrogates, relatives, friends, or medical or legal representative should be sought. The most important factor is the best interests of the patient. In some circumstances there will be disagreement between members of the healthcare team and patient surrogates as to what is in the best interests of the patient. This might reflect conflicts in religious, ethnic, or other value systems. These must be discussed openly before the instigation or withdrawal of therapy. Clinicians must be seen to be transparently honest in their discussions with all concerned. They must avoid the temptation to arbitrarily impose their value systems or preferred biases in feeding modality in the absence of evidence. It is not for the individual clinician to make recommendations for treatment or its withdrawal on the basis of resource considerations. When doubt persists as to the validity of treatments, it is the patient's preferences, when fully informed, or their presumed preferences, based on discussions with others, that take precedence over healthcare systems or an individual doctor's opinions, providing this serves the patient's best interests.

10.8 Concluding remarks

The implications of recognising nutritional support as a medical therapy and of assessing its provision on the basis of accepted ethical principles are far-reaching. First, there would seem to be a sound philosophical argument that dictates that all patients who have inadequate intakes for 7 days or more should at least be offered advice on nutritional care. A documented dietetic referral may suffice. Second, failure to appraise and document nutritional status may, in the future, have medico-legal consequences. Third, there is an urgent need to raise awareness about nutritional problems and their treatment in both medical and nursing professions. Finally, the financial implications of these recommendations are enormous. While dietetic advice, sip feeding, and certain techniques of enteral nutrition are not in themselves expensive, the inevitable consequence of an increased awareness of nutritional problems will be an increase in the use of expensive nutritional support techniques.

The giving of artificial nutrition, where indicated, is not sufficient in itself. It must also be done well and conducted according to nationally accepted standards and guidelines. Failure to do this or to provide resources and expert staff to carry this out may be construed as unethical and may leave doctors and hospitals, in the future, open to legal action in the courts. Clinical decision-making, including the provision of nutritional support, is increasingly informed by ethical and legal as well as clinical considerations. The ethical principles of beneficence, nonmaleficence, autonomy, and justice must be applied to all patients in need of nutritional support. Doctors must practice on the basis of evidence concerning the efficacy of nutritional support and the means of providing it, moderated by compassion and consideration for the patient and their family. In conclusion, the application of simple ethical principles to the use of nutritional support is likely to have a significant impact on clinical practice, particularly in Western society, where the morality of different treatment strategies is increasingly being subjected to public scrutiny.

References and further reading

Arras JD, Steinbock B, editors. Ethical Issues in Modern Medicine, 4th edn. California: Mayfield Publishing, 1995.

August D, Huhmann M. ASPEN Clinical Guidelines: nutritional support therapy during adult anticancer treatment and in hematopoietic cell transplantation. JPEN 2009; 33(5): 472–500.

Beauchamp TL, Childress JF, editors. Principles of Biomedical Ethics, 4th edn. Oxford, New York: Oxford University Press, 1994.

BMA. Withholding and Withdrawing Life-prolonging Medical Treatment. Guidance for Decision Making. London: BMA Books, 2007.

Clarke J, Cranswick G, Dennis MS, *et al.* for the FOOD Trial Collaboration. Effect of timing and method of enteral tube feeding for dysphagic stroke patients (FOOD): a multicenter randomised trial. Lancet 2005; 365: 764–772.

Gillon R, Lloyd A. Principles of Health Care Ethics. London: John Wiley & Sons, 1993.

Hope T, Savulescu J, Hendrick J, editors. Medical Ethics and the Law. Edinburgh: Churchill Livingstone, 2008.

Leaning J. War crimes and medical science. BMJ 1996; 313: 1413–1415.

Monti MM, Vanhaudenhuyse A, Coleman MR, Boly M, Pickard JD, Tshibanda L, Owen AM, Laureys S. Willful modulation of brain activity in disorders of consciousness. New Engl J Med 2010; 362: 579–589.

National Collaborating Centre for Acute Care. Nutrition Support for Adults: Oral Nutrition Support, Enteral Tube Feeding and Parenteral Nutrition. London: National Collaborating Centre for Acute Care, 2006. Available from www.rcseng.ac.uk.

Percival T. Medical Ethics; or a Code of Institutes and Precepts Adapted to the Professional Conduct of Physicians and Surgeons. 1803. In Percival's Medical Ethics (Leake CD, ed.). Philadelphia, PA: The Williams & Wilkins Company, 1927.

Royal College of Physicians and British Society of Gastroenterology. Oral Feeding Difficulties and Dilemmas. A Guide to Practical Care towards the End of Life. London: Royal College of Physicians, 2010.

Sampson EL, Candy B, Jones L. Enteral tube feeding for older people with advanced dementia. Cochrane Database of Systematic Reviews 2009, Issue 2. Art. No.: CD007209. DOI: 10.1002/14651858. CD007209.pub2.

11
The Gastrointestinal Tract

Miquel A Gassull and Eduard Cabré

Hospital Universitari Germans Trias i Pujol, Spain

Key messages

- Coeliac disease is an intestinal mucosal disorder caused by hypersensitivity to gluten present in several cereal grains, such as wheat, barley, rye, and possibly oats. Symptoms may range from severe malabsorption to oligosymptomatic cases, often with extradigestive symptoms (anaemia, osteopaenia), which are particularly frequent in adults.
- The only effective treatment for coeliac disease is the absolute withdrawal of gluten from the diet for life. This is particularly important to minimise the risk of late complications, such as intestinal lymphoma and other gastrointestinal malignancies.
- Tropical enteropathy and tropical sprue are a group of disorders mainly affecting the small intestine of individuals living in, or visiting, the tropics. Correction of water and electrolyte imbalances and nutritional replacement are the basis for the management of tropical sprue.

- Protein–energy malnutrition and other micronutrient deficiencies are frequent in patients with inflammatory bowel disease (IBD) and result from a combination of poor nutrient intake, increased metabolic demands, increased intestinal protein losses, and nutrient malabsorption.
- If patients with IBD are severely malnourished or suffering from severe inflammatory bouts of the disease, they will need to be treated with artificial nutrition.
- Many patients with irritable bowel syndrome (IBS) believe that their symptoms are triggered by specific foods, but this is difficult to prove scientifically. However, specific sugar malabsorptions should be investigated, by means of the hydrogen breath test, in those patients in whom diarrhoea and/or bloating continue to occur.

11.1 Introduction

The majority of the diseases of the gastrointestinal tract are not fatal but are significant causes of poor health, responsible for large proportions of patients attending hospital and local medical services. The major conditions associated with the gastrointestinal tract are summarised in Box 11.1.

Infectious diseases of the gastrointestinal tract are covered in Chapter 21, pancreatitis in Chapter 13, and liver disease in Chapter 12. Management of food allergy is covered in Chapter 8.

Dysphagia

Dysphagia (difficulty in swallowing) is a common consequence of many different types of illness or injury, resulting in mechanical or neurological impairment of the swallowing process. Swallowing occurs in two phases – oropharyngeal and oesophageal. In the oropharyngeal phase, food in transferred from the mouth via the pharynx to the upper oesophagus. The oesophageal phase carries food from the pharynx to the stomach. Some of the most common causes of dysphagia are listed in Table 11.1.

Attempting to swallow foods or liquids without the ability to do so carries a high risk of aspiration pneumonia and is potentially fatal. If dysphagia is suspected, it is very important that the patient's swallow is assessed by a health professional qualified to do so. Dysphagia is almost always accompanied by a reduced food intake, leading to significant weight loss, compromised immune function, and a high risk

Clinical Nutrition, Second Edition. Edited by Marinos Elia, Olle Ljungqvist, Rebecca J Stratton and Susan A Lanham-New.
© 2013 The Nutrition Society. Published 2013 by Blackwell Publishing Ltd.

Box 11.1 The major conditions associated with the gastrointestinal tract

- diarrhoea and vomiting;
- dyspepsia;
- peptic and duodenal ulcers;
- constipation, abdominal pain, and irritable bowel;
- haemorrhoids and anal fissure;
- dysphagia;
- hernia;
- gallstones;
- appendicitis;
- malabsorption syndromes;
- ulcerative colitis and Crohn's disease;
- diverticular disease of the colon;
- pancreatitis;
- liver disease;
- food intolerance.

Box 11.2 The primary aims of management of dysphagia

- Assess the nature of the swallowing problem.
- Determine a safe and adequate feeding route.
- Determine the appropriate texture and consistency of foods and fluids.
- Meet nutritional needs.
- Ensure adequate hydration status.
- Educate patient and/or carers.
- Monitor progress and ensure continuity of care.

Box 11.3 Causes of GORD

- oesophageal sphincter weakness;
- increased pressure within the stomach;
- high pressure from the abdominal area (obesity or pregnancy);
- hiatus hernia.

Table 11.1 The most common causes of dysphagia.

Oropharyngeal	
Neuromuscular	Stroke
	Head injury
	Muscular disorders
	Motor neuron disease
	Parkinson's disease
Physical obstruction	Pharyngeal pouch
	Goitre
Psychological	Globus hystericus
Infections	Tonsillitis
Oesophageal	
Neural	Achalasia
	Multiple sclerosis
	Diffuse oesophageal spasm
Muscular	Scleroderma
	Dystrophia myotonica
Physical obstruction	Stricture:
	cancer
	chronic oesophagitis
	Diverticulum
	External compression (aortic aneurysm)
	Postoperative
Infections	Candida

Box 11.4 Some dietary methods of managing GORD

- Eat smaller meals more frequently.
- Avoid eating late at night.
- Avoid bending, lifting, or lying down after meals.
- Reduce weight if overweight.
- Avoid excessive consumption of caffeine-containing drinks and alcohol.
- Avoid highly spiced foods or those foods known to exacerbate symptoms.

of dehydration. The primary aims of management of dysphagia are listed in Box 11.2.

Gastro-oesophageal reflux disease

Gastro-oesophageal reflux disease (GORD) occurs as a normal event, and clinical features only occur when antireflux mechanisms fail enough to allow gastric contents to make prolonged contact with the lower oesophageal mucosa. The presence of acid and enzymes irritates the mucosa and causes pain, and repeated injury may cause mucosal damage and inflammation (oesophagitis). This in turn increases the risk of oesophageal adenocarcinoma. The causes of GORD are listed in Box 11.3.

About 50% of patients can be treated successfully with simple antacids. Other need proton-pump inhibitor drugs. Antireflux surgery may be indicated in patients where medical treatment is insufficient. Loss of weight and raising of the head of the bed at night are caadjuvant measures in some patients. Some dietary methods of managing GORD are summarised in Box 11.4.

Cancer of the oesophagus and stomach

Surgical treatment of cancer of the oesophagus may be partial or total oesophagectomy, oesophagogastrectomy, or partial or total gastrectomy, depending on the site and extent of the cancer. Since many oesophageal cancer patients may be severely nutritionally compromised, preoperative and early postoperative nutritional support is often necessary (see Chapter 9). Weight loss, iron-deficiency anaemia, B_{12} deficiency, and osteomalasia may all occur after gastric surgery and must be identified and managed.

Short-bowel syndrome

Short-bowel syndrome occurs after small-bowel resection where less than 1 m of the bowel remains. The management of short-bowel syndrome patients depends on the extent of bowel resection, the site of the resection, and the presence or absence of the ileocaecal valve. Intestinal adaptation can occur postoperatively, leading to hypertrophy of the mucosal surface and lengthening of the villi, leading in turn to a substantial increase and recovery of the absorptive surface.

The fact that gastrointestinal disease is a major cause of malnutrition for patients both in hospital and in the community is not surprising given its pivotal role in digestion and absorption. In some conditions, such as coeliac disease and some food allergies, the illness is caused by the intolerance of some nutrient, and treatment is based on the withdrawal of the offending foodstuff. In others, such as gastrointestinal infections and tropical enteropathy, the causative agent is not dietary, but the consequences of the illness are nonetheless nutritional and metabolic in nature and need to be managed.

In other conditions, such as inflammatory bowel disease (IBD) (ulcerative colitis and Crohn's disease), where the aetiology is unknown, not only may nutritional support provide macro- and micronutrients, but certain elements may play a pharmacological role in the management of the disease itself. Finally, in functional intestinal diseases, dietary management may play a role in alleviating or reducing symptoms.

This chapter will focus on the nutritional consequences and management of some non-neoplastic diseases of the small bowel and the colon. These include:

(1) coeliac disease;
(2) tropical enteropathy and tropical sprue;
(3) inflammatory bowel disease;
(4) irritable bowel syndrome and diverticular disease.

11.2 Coeliac disease

Coeliac disease – also termed coeliac sprue or gluten-sensitive enteropathy – is a disease of the small bowel characterised by:

(1) malabsorption of nutrients by the damaged portion of the small intestine;
(2) a characteristic, although unspecific, lesion of the intestinal mucosa;
(3) prompt clinical and histological improvement after withdrawal of gluten from the diet.

Epidemiology

The true prevalence of coeliac disease is probably unknown, since many patients have mild or no symptoms, and in these cases the disease often remains undiagnosed. In most European countries, the prevalence of the disease ranges from 0.05 to 0.2%. Some studies report an increased incidence of coeliac disease in recent decades. This must be due, at least in part, to an increasing awareness of the disease and the recognition of oligosymptomatic patients. Classically, coeliac disease used to seem to be less frequent in the USA. However, recent studies of serological screening in blood donors suggest that the frequency is the same as that in Europe.

Although some areas – including Scandinavia, the British Isles, and the Mediterranean basin – are particularly at risk, coeliac disease is considered a worldwide phenomenon. However, it is rare in Africa, East Asia, and the Caribbean.

Pathogenesis

Coeliac disease is a hereditary illness. Its development is strongly associated (90–95% of cases) with the human leukocyte antigen (HLA) haplotype DQw2 on chromosome 6. However, environmental factors also play a role in the development of the disease.

The most important environmental factor for developing coeliac disease in susceptible individuals is gluten, a protein component of several cereal grains. Some alcohol-soluble fractions of gluten, termed prolamines, are particularly harmful. These are α, β, γ, and Ω gliadins (from wheat), hordeins (from barley), secalins (from rye), and possibly avidins (from oats). In contrast, rice and corn are not harmful to the intestinal mucosa.

Some factors may play a role in precipitating symptoms. These include gastrointestinal surgery, pregnancy, high-dose or early gluten challenge, and viral infection. Breast-feeding seems to delay the age of onset of coeliac disease, but there is no clear evidence that it reduces the lifetime risk for developing the disease.

There is now evidence that coeliac disease is an intestinal immunological disease. In brief, selected prolamin peptides are presented by distinctive surface-HLA heterodimers to specific T cells. T-cell activation then results in a cascade of proinflammatory cytokines. At the same time, B cells and plasma cells produce antibodies that stimulate the release of other noxious mediators, possibly causing cell-mediated cytotoxicity. As a result of this process, the intestinal mucosa is damaged.

Coeliac disease may occur in association with other immune-based diseases (Box 11.5). Individuals suffering from these conditions should be screened for coeliac disease. Amongst these associated diseases, dermatitis herpetiformis deserves special mention. This is an itchy bullous skin rash that involves the extensor surfaces of the limbs, trunk, and scalp, characterised histologically by the deposition of IgA granules in the dermal–epidermal junction. The disease is accompanied by intestinal damage, sometimes asymptomatic, but indistinguishable from that seen in coeliac disease. In fact, both the intestinal and cutaneous lesions regress with dietary gluten withdrawal. Thus, dermatitis herpetiformis is at present considered part of the spectrum of gluten sensitivity rather than a mere associated condition to coeliac disease.

Magnitude of the problem: the spectrum of gluten sensitivity

Coeliac disease involves the mucosa of the small bowel, while the submucosa, muscularis, and serosa are usually unaffected. Proximal segments of the bowel (duodenum and jejunum) are damaged more

---

Box 11.5 Diseases associated with coeliac disease

Well-established association

- dermatitis herpetiformis;
- type I diabetes mellitus;
- autoimmune thyroid disease;
- selective IgA deficiency.

Suggested but not fully proven association

- autoimmune connective-tissue disease;
- Sjögren syndrome;
- IgA nephropathy;
- IBD;
- sclerosing cholangitis;
- primary biliary cirrhosis;
- Down's syndrome.

---

frequently, while ileal involvement is less frequent. The mucosal damage in coeliac disease varies from almost normal morphology (latent coeliac disease) to the classical picture of villous atrophy and 'flattened mucosa'.

Traditionally, coeliac disease has been considered a paediatric disease, but it is also frequently diagnosed in adult life. Classical symptoms in children include diarrhoea, vomiting, anorexia, irritability or apathy, and failure to thrive. In adults, the 'complete' coeliac syndrome consists of chronic diarrhoea, weight loss, malabsorption and iron-deficiency anaemia. In most severe cases, the so-called 'coeliac crisis' would ensue if left untreated – with tetany, haemorrhagic diathesis, and oedema – constituting a true gastrointestinal emergency.

In recent decades it has become evident that coeliac disease may present with only scarce and/or mild symptoms. This is particularly true in the adult. Diagnosis of the disease may thus be delayed. Digestive symptoms can include recurrent abdominal pain in children and complaints of indigestion and bloating in adults. A number of patients have only extradigestive symptoms. Some of the most frequent manifestations, which may occur (alone or in combination) in the absence of the classic malabsorptive syndrome in coeliac disease, are listed in Box 11.6. Coeliac disease may remain clinically silent for years despite the existence of histological lesions. This situation has been reported to occur in first-degree relatives of coeliac patients and other risk groups.

Box 11.6 Symptoms and signs of coeliac disease other than the classical malabsorptive syndrome

- unespecific dyspepsia (recurrent abdominal pain, bloating, etc.);
- iron-deficient anaemia, refractory to oral iron therapy;
- low bone-mineral density, osteoporosis, and its consequences (particularly if excessive for the age);
- peripheral neuropathy;
- intellectual deterioration, epilepsy with posterior cerebral calcifications;
- dental-enamel hypoplasia;
- recurrent oral aphtous ulcerations;
- amenorrhoea, delayed menarche, female infertility;
- repeated miscarriages;
- male impotence and/or infertility;
- arthritis and other joint symptoms;
- 'unexplained' mild–moderate increase in serum liver enzymes.

Diagnosis and screening

The diagnosis of coeliac disease is based on a demonstration of the characteristic histological findings in a well-orientated jejunal biopsy specimen, followed by clinical remission when the patient is put on a gluten-free diet. In 1990, the European Society of Paediatric Gastroenterology and Nutrition (ESPGAN) revised its diagnostic criteria, stating that a single jejunal biopsy could be enough for the diagnosis of coeliac disease. The old ESPGAN criteria required a second biopsy after withdrawing gluten from the diet (which must be normal), followed by a third one after gluten challenge (where histological lesion must reappear). At present a demonstration of normalised histology following a gluten-free diet is no longer required for a definitive diagnosis of coeliac disease.

Based on very high sensitivities and specificities, the best available tests are the IgA antihuman tissue transglutaminase (TTG) and IgA endomysial antibody immunofluorescence (EMA) tests, which appear to have equivalent diagnostic accuracy (TTG is the specific protein that is identified by the IgA-EMA). Antigliadin antibody (AGA) tests are no longer routinely recommended because of their lower sensitivity and specificity.

Serological screening should be made in patients with clinical suspicion of coeliac disease, in first-degree relatives of coeliac patients, or in individuals suffering from any of the associated conditions to the disease (Box 11.5). However, it must be stressed that serological tests do not replace intestinal biopsy in the diagnosis of coeliac disease. Moreover, patients with malabsorptive symptoms or signs must undergo jejunal biopsy irrespective of the results of the serological tests, in order to rule out an enteropathy other than coeliac disease. Negativisation of antibodies can be used as a monitoring test for compliance to the gluten-free diet.

Treatment

Coeliac disease is perhaps the one disease above all other gastrointestinal disorders in which diet is the key to management. Patients with coeliac disease and/or dermatitis herpetiformis must adhere to a strictly gluten-free diet for life. Cutaneous manifestations of dermatitis herpetiformis usually respond to treatment with sulphones (dapsone), but such a therapy fails to reverse the intestinal disease. A major reason for recommending absolute removal of gluten from the diet is prevention of late development of malignancies. Coeliac patients have been found to have an increased risk for malignancy – particularly T-cell lymphoma of the small bowel, oesophageal cancer, and cancer of the oropharynx – as compared to the general population. A strict gluten-free diet for life decreases such a risk, although unfortunately this is not fully eliminated in the case of lymphoma.

Avoiding gluten is easier to say than to do. Follow-up studies indicate that only 50–70% of coeliac patients maintain a strict gluten-free diet later in life. Noncompliance is more frequent in children and, particularly, in teenagers. Removal of obvious sources of the offending grains (wheat, rye, barley, and oats), such as bread, breakfast cereals, pasta, cakes, and pastry, is relative easy. However, hidden sources of gluten are frequent, as wheat flour is added in many manufactured food products. Adequate food labelling is very important in this setting. Lists of foods which obviously contain gluten (and are thus forbidden), are positively gluten-free (and thus permitted), and may be surreptitious sources of gluten (to be considered with caution) are provided in Table 11.2.

The institution of an effective gluten-free diet requires extensive education of the patient by their physician, as well as the advice of an experienced professional dietitian. Recipe books are also available in some countries. In addition, patients should be encouraged to contact and join the coeliac societies

Table 11.2 Food chart for coeliac patients.

Forbidden (obviously contain gluten)	Permitted (obviously gluten-free)	Surreptitiously contain gluten (not to be eaten unless explicitly labelled as gluten-free by the manufacturer)
Bread and flour from wheat, rye, barley, and oats[a]	Milk and other dairy products	Manufactured foodstuffs which might contain cereal flours as additive, thickening, or flavouring agents
Cakes, pastry, biscuits, pies, and other baked goods made with these flours	Any kind of fresh meat, fish, or other seafood	Sausages, pâtés, luncheon meats, canned meats, and poultry
Italian pasta (spaghetti, macaroni, etc.), wheat semolina	Eggs	Meat sauces (soy, Worcestershire, etc.)
	Rice, corn, millet, buckwheat, sorghum, and any foodstuff made with flour from these cereals	Cheese spreads
Manufactured products with the above flours (flans, custard, ice-cream, jelly, etc.)	Tapioca, soybean	Salad dressings, mustard, ketchup, tomato sauce, etc.
	Fruits, vegetables, potatoes	Instant and canned soups, bouillon cubes
	Butter, margarine, oils, and other fats	Instant coffee and tea
	Salt, pepper, vinegar	Candy bars, chocolate mixes
	Sugar, honey	As a rule, **_any canned food_**
Malted foods (e.g. malted milk)	Coffee made with ground coffee beans, tea, and other herbal infusions	Any food possibly contaminated with flour during harvesting, packaging, storage, or in the kitchen
Drinks containing cereals (beer, ale)	Homemade cakes and pastry without the offending flours	Residual gluten in 'gluten-free' wheat starch used in baked products
		Nonfood items with trace amounts of gluten
		Excipients of some medications (either prescriptions or over-the-counter)
		Communion wafers
		Grain-derived alcoholic drinks (whisky, vodka, etc.)
		Anything with misleading labelling

[a]Some patients can probably tolerate certain amounts of oats without risk (see text).

or other support groups existing in many countries, which produce up-to-date lists of brands of gluten-free foods.

Commercially available brands of gluten-free foods (e.g. pasta, biscuits, bread) help to diversify the diet of coeliac patients. These brands are internationally identified with a special logo (Figure 11.1). The Codex Alimentarius defines a food as gluten-free when '…the total nitrogen content of the gluten containing cereal grains used in the product does not exceed 0.05 g/100 g of these grain on a dry matter basis'. It is important to note that this norm does not refer to the minimal amount of gluten tolerated by a coeliac patient. In some particularly susceptible patients, even this small amount could induce insidious symptoms. In addition, gluten-free brands are expensive. Therefore, they should be used merely as a complement of the coeliac diet, which must be essentially based on naturally occurring gluten-free foods.

In recent years, there has been increasing evidence to suggest that some coeliac patients can tolerate moderate amounts of oats. The source of oats must be free of gluten contamination (in harvesting, storing, or packaging) in order to be safe, and it is uncertain whether larger and long-term oats challenges would be harmless in these patients. Thus, if a coeliac patient is

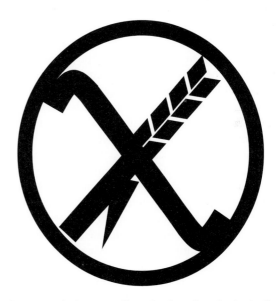

Figure 11.1 The international logo identifying gluten-free foodstuffs.

going to consume oats, a pure source should be used, and monitoring for relapse should be maintained.

Besides avoiding gluten, coeliac patients must eat an otherwise balanced diet, with normal amounts of nitrogen, fat, and carbohydrates. In most symptomatic cases, the administration of iron, folate, fat-soluble vitamins (parenterally), and oral medium-chain triglycerides (MCTs) (as a caloric supplement) at the beginning of therapy is useful. Epithelial damage leads to the loss of brush-border enzymes and then to hypolactasia. In this setting, transient withdrawal of milk and its derivatives from the diet may be advisable. Patients with 'coeliac crisis' will need intravenous fluid and electrolyte replacement, as well as calcium and magnesium administration to prevent tetany. Severely malnourished cases will benefit from enteral nutrition. These formulas may accelerate recovery, since most of them are absolutely free of both gluten and lactose.

Therapeutic failure

The great majority of coeliac patients will recover both clinically and histologically on a strict gluten-free diet. Clinical improvement is usually apparent after only 1 or 2 weeks on the diet, although complete recovery may take several months.

A minority of patients (about 15%) do not improve with the diet, or their symptoms relapse after a variable period of time. The most important cause of therapeutic failure is incomplete removal of gluten from the diet. On many occasions, the patient themselves will be unaware of this circumstance and an in-depth dietary interview is required to reveal it. As mentioned before, TTG and EMA usually become negative with total gluten withdrawal and are a useful tool for monitoring dietary compliance.

Recent studies indicate that a number of patients with coeliac disease and persistent diarrhoea suffer from another coexisting disease, such as exocrine pancreatic insufficiency, microscopic colitis, lactose or fructose malabsorption, intestinal bacterial overgrowth, or irritable bowel syndrome (IBS). This fact should be taken into account in assessing unresponsive coeliac patients.

Another cause of therapeutic unresponsiveness in coeliac disease is the development of an associated intestinal malignancy (mostly T-cell lymphoma), particularly if the patient has low-grade fever. The risk for this neoplasm is increased in coeliac patients despite a complete adherence to a gluten-free diet.

In a minority of coeliac patients with therapeutic failure (either *de novo* or after initial response), none of the above circumstances can be demonstrated. This situation is arbitrarily termed 'refractory sprue'.

Some, but not all, of these patients will respond to steroids or other immunosuppressors.

11.3 Tropical enteropathy and tropical sprue

Concept and epidemiology

Aside from infectious intestinal diseases with known aetiology, there is a group of gastrointestinal disorders mainly affecting the small intestine of individuals predominantly living in – and less often visiting or returning from – the developing world, usually the tropics. These disorders range from asymptomatic or oligosymptomatic structural and/or functional abnormalities of the intestinal mucosa (tropical enteropathy) to a fully symptomatic condition with malabsorption of nutrients, nutritional deficiencies, and a 'coeliac-like' appearance of the intestinal mucosa (tropical sprue). It has been suggested that tropical enteropathy and tropical sprue may be the two ends of the same clinical and pathological spectrum, but this is far from being proven.

Epidemiological distribution of both conditions is one of the arguments against this view. Tropical enteropathy has been detected in most tropical regions of Asia, Africa, the Middle East, the Caribbean, and Central and South America. Tropical sprue, however, has a much more restricted geographical distribution, occurring in southern and South East Asia, the Caribbean and, to a much lesser extent, Central and South America. It almost never occurs in Africa.

Pathology and clinical relevance

Tropical enteropathy is characterised by some reduction in intestinal villi height, often associated with hyperplasia of the intestinal crypts. This results in a reduction of the absorptive surface, cellular infiltration of the lamina propria, and cytological changes in the enterocytes. The clinical repercussion of tropical enteropathy is usually mild, so that it has been argued it would be the 'normal state' for individuals living in these tropical developing areas.

In contrast to tropical enteropathy, tropical sprue is a much better defined clinical entity. Tropical sprue is a syndrome of chronic diarrhoea often associated with steatorrhoea, anorexia, abdominal cramps and bloating, weight loss, megaloblastic anaemia, and oedema. It may occur in epidemics, in which the illness begins as an acute attack of watery diarrhoea with fever and malaise preceding the chronic phase. When the situation has been maintained for months or even years, the clinical picture is dominated by nutritional deficiencies, sometimes in the absence of diarrhoea.

Histopathological changes in tropical sprue vary in intensity depending on the duration and severity of the illness. In well-established cases, the small-intestinal histology mostly resembles that of coeliac disease. In fact, coeliac disease was formerly known as nontropical sprue. Severe cases may also cause chronic atrophic gastritis (leading to vitamin B_{12} malabsorption due to the lack of intrinsic factor) and changes in the colonic mucosa similar to those of the small bowel, which lead to impaired absorption of water and sodium.

Pathogenesis

Tropical enteropathy is an acquired condition, since newborns in the developing world have intestinal villi as high as those of newborns in Western countries. The intestinal abnormalities begin to appear at between 4 and 6 months of age, and may be due to a relatively hostile post-weaning environment for the small intestine. The most plausible environmental factors are either an intestinal infection and/or bacterial overgrowth, or a nutritional deficiency. However, studies in British Indians and Afro-Caribbeans living for more than 30 years in the UK revealed the persistence of intestinal abnormalities, suggesting that a genetic predisposition to development of this disease may play a role.

As in tropical enteropathy, the cause of tropical sprue has not been clearly defined, but nutritional and infectious mechanisms seem to be involved. An important role has been proposed for bacterial colonisation of the small bowel by both aerobic and anaerobic bacteria, but protozoal infection by agents such as *Cryptosporidium parvum*, *Isospora belli*, *Blastocystis hominis*, and *Cyclospora cayetanensis* may also be involved. Initial infectious damage would induce hormonal and functional abnormalities in the gut that would lead to active secretion of water and electrolytes and impaired intestinal motility, thus perpetuating the disease.

Treatment

Correction of water and electrolyte imbalance and nutritional replacement are the mainstays of the early management of cases of tropical sprue. In fact, nutritional intervention alone is responsible for the dramatic decrease in mortality of epidemic bouts of tropical sprue in southern India. Oral supplements of folic acid, iron, and parenteral vitamin B_{12} should be promptly administered, leading to a rapid recovery of anaemia and a marked appetite gain.

There is no specific pharmacological treatment for tropical sprue, but the long-term use of a broad-spectrum antibiotic (such as tetracycline 250 mg four times daily for from 4 weeks to several months) is recommended. However, subclinical malabsorption remains in a significant proportion of patients for many years after being apparently cured with tetracyclines.

11.4 Inflammatory bowel disease

Definition

IBD includes ulcerative colitis and Crohn's disease. In both entities there is inflammation of the bowel mucosa, with different patterns and degrees of severity. In ulcerative colitis, the inflammatory phenomena only occur in the mucosa and submucosa of the colon, whereas the whole thickness of the bowel wall, from mucosa to serosa, is involved in Crohn's disease. In contrast to ulcerative colitis, which involves only the colon, Crohn's disease may affect any portion of the gastrointestinal tract, from the mouth to the anus, often in a segmentary pattern, although involvement of the terminal ileum and the right colon is most frequent. In some cases of IBD involving only the colon, features of both ulcerative colitis and Crohn's disease are observed, so that a clear-cut diagnosis cannot be established. For these cases, the term 'unclassified colitis' is used.

Epidemiology

Incidence rates range between 2 and 12 per 100 000 population for ulcerative colitis, and 0.1 and 7 per 100 000 population for Crohn's disease. Both diseases are more frequent in northern countries (e.g. the UK, Scandinavia, the USA) that in southern countries (e.g. Mediterranean countries, South Africa, Australia), but in recent years these differences have been decreasing. The incidence of ulcerative colitis remains stable, while the occurrence of Crohn's disease appears to be increasing.

Whites are more often affected than non-whites, and in some ethnic groups (e.g. Askenazi Jews) the frequency of the disease is particularly high. In most studies, the incidence of IBD peaks in subjects between 15 and 30 years of age. A second smaller peak in incidence has been observed between 60 and 80 years, particularly for Crohn's disease.

Pathogenesis

The aetiology of IBD is unknown. In both diseases there is a pattern of family aggregation, suggesting a genetic basis which is not fully elucidated. Genetic linkage and, more recently, genome-wide studies have identified a number of susceptibility genes for both ulcerative colitis and Crohn's disease. It is thought that IBD occurs in genetically susceptible individuals as the result of a combination of:

(1) An exaggerated intestinal immune response to gastrointestinal antigens or normal bacterial flora.
(2) A normal immunological response to noxious and as-yet unknown stimuli.
(3) Autoimmune involvement.

All of these will trigger the release of inflammatory mediators (cytokines, eicosanoids, etc.) that will be responsible for the clinical and histological manifestations of the disease.

Clinical features and diagnosis

A detailed description of the clinical features of IBD is beyond the scope of this chapter. Both involved diseases typically have a chronic relapsing course. Bloody diarrhoea is the main symptom of ulcerative colitis, whereas patients with Crohn's disease may present with different combinations of diarrhoea, weight loss, abdominal pain, fever, and other digestive complaints. Fistulae between the intestinal loops, or between the gut and the skin or any hollow viscus in its vicinity, as well as perianal disease (abscess, fistulae), often occur in Crohn's disease. Moreover, both diseases may be associated with extraintestinal complaints, including rheumatological, ophthalmological, cutaneous, and hepatobiliary diseases.

IBD is diagnosed by a set of clinical, endoscopic, and histological characteristics. In ulcerative colitis, only the colon is involved, and colectomy, either with permanent ileostomy or with an ileo-anal pouch anastomosis, is considered to be curative. In contrast, Crohn's disease may involve any part of the gastrointestinal tract, often two or more segments at the same time. Moreover, after the surgical removal of the involved segment, the disease may recur at any level of the gastrointestinal tract. Thus, although necessary in some cases, surgery cannot be envisaged as a curative therapeutic approach for Crohn's disease.

The chronic relapsing character of IBD, its predominance in young people, and the fact that the disease has no cure (except for colectomy in ulcerative colitis) contribute to a very negative socioeconomic impact of the disease, as well to a poor quality of life for patients.

Treatment

As there is not a curative medical therapy for IBD, the standard therapy, both in ulcerative colitis and Crohn's disease, relies on corticosteroids or aminosalicylates, depending of the severity and extent of the attack. A number of patients become resistant to these therapies or require long-term steroid therapy to remain asymptomatic. For these patients, a number of therapeutic strategies have been developed in the last two decades, including immunosuppressors (azathioprine, 6-mercaptopurine, cyclosporine, methotrexate), antibiotics (metronidazole, ciprofloxacin), and, more recently, the so-called biological therapies, such as monoclonal anti-tumour necrosis factor alpha (TNFα) antibodies. In recent years, there has been a trend toward using immunesuppressors and biological agents earlier in the disease course (the so-called top-down strategy), mainly in Crohn's disease.

Malnutrition in IBD

Nutritional deficits are frequently observed in IBD, especially in Crohn's-disease patients with extensive involvement of the small bowel. Malnutrition may manifest as weight loss, growth retardation and delayed sexual maturation, anaemia, asthenia, osteopaenia, diarrhoea, oedema, muscle cramps, impaired cellular immunity, or poor wound-healing.

The prevalence of protein–energy malnutrition in IBD ranges from 20 to 85%. This wide range is due to the fact that most studies put ulcerative colitis and Crohn's disease together, as well as hospitalised and ambulatory patients. This results in a marked heterogeneity of disease extension, inflammatory activity, and organ involvement (small and/or large bowel). It is believed that irrespective of steroid use, around 20–30% of children will become adults with abnormally short stature.

Two factors, seldom mentioned, may be relevant regarding the severity and type of malnutrition in IBD:

(1) The time elapsed since the onset of the disease, which is usually longer in Crohn's disease.
(2) The acuteness of the attack, which is usually greater in ulcerative colitis.

These factors are related to the type of protein–energy malnutrition developed, which is predominantly marasmatic or mixed in Crohn's disease and hypoalbuminaemic (kwashiorkor-like) in ulcerative colitis.

Pathogenesis of malnutrition in IBD

Several factors are involved in the development of malnutrition in IBD (Box 11.7). The most important are (i) poor nutrient intake, (ii) increased metabolism, (ii) increased intestinal protein losses, and (iv) nutrient malabsorption.

Poor nutrient intake

Inadequate intake of nutrients is common in IBD. Anorexia, nausea and vomiting, abdominal pain or discomfort, and/or medical restrictions on some foods are frequent in acute attacks of ulcerative colitis and Crohn's disease. In addition, in almost one-third of patients with Crohn's disease the upper gastrointestinal tract (oesophagus, stomach, and duodenum) may be involved, and approximately the same proportion will suffer from one or more episodes of intestinal obstruction during the course of their disease. In addition, drugs used in the treatment of active disease may induce gastric upset (sulphasalazine, metronidazole, 5-ASA). All these factors negatively impact on food intake.

The possibility that alimentary antigens might act as triggering factors for the inflammatory response

> **Box 11.7 Pathogenic mechanisms for malnutrition in inflammatory bowel disease (IBD)**
>
> - poor nutrient intake;
> - anorexia;
> - upper-GI tract involvement;[a]
> - drug-induced dyspepsia;
> - intestinal obstruction;[a]
> - inadequate or restrictive diet;
> - 'therapeutic' fasting;
> - increased metabolism;
> - increased energy expenditure;
> - increased protein turnover (mainly breakdown);
> - increased intestinal protein losses;
> - mucosal inflammation and ulceration;
> - enteric fistulae;[a]
> - impaired intestinal lymph drainage (mesenteric involvement);[a]
> - malabsorption;
> - extensive small-bowel involvement;[a]
> - multiple intestinal resections (short bowel);[a]
> - intestinal bacterial overgrowth;[a]
> - bile salt malabsorption (ileal dysfunction or resection);[a]
> - impaired intestinal lymph drainage (mesenteric involvement).[a]
>
> [a]Only in Crohn's disease

in IBD, and the fact that diarrhoea is the most prominent symptom of these patients, led to the use of fasting as part of the treatment of acute attacks of both ulcerative colitis and Crohn's disease, in order to achieve 'bowel rest'. The consequence of this therapeutic approach was the deterioration of nutritional status, and this treatment should no longer be advocated. Decreased food intake is still sometimes erroneously reinforced by attendants' and physicians' advice: in almost one-third of patients, a reduction in food intake could be related to an inadequate, restricted diet, which prescribes a reduction of fat- and fibre-rich foods. Adequate dietary assessment may be crucial in preventing malnutrition in these patients. This can be achieved by offering palatable energy- and protein-rich foods that do not exacerbate the disease or symptoms of obstruction.

Increased metabolism

Reports on energy metabolism in patients with IBD have been contradictory. Energy expenditure has been reported to be either increased or reduced in these patients as compared to healthy subjects. This may be partly due to the fact that patients with different disease extensions, inflammatory activities, and nutritional statuses were put together in the studies. However, when adjusted for body composition, an increase in resting energy expenditure is generally disclosed.

Protein turnover is also enhanced in IBD. Increase in both synthesis and breakdown of protein accounts for accelerated turnover. However, protein breakdown usually exceeds synthesis, the result being protein depletion.

Increased intestinal protein losses

An increased blood and protein loss through the inflamed intestinal mucosa is another contributing factor in the development of malnutrition in IBD. Protein losses parallel the degree of inflammation of the intestinal mucosa, and the quantification of this phenomenon has been used as an index of disease activity. Moreover, the possible existence of intestinal bacterial overgrowth, abnormalities in the intercellular tight junctions of the mucosal epithelium, and difficulties in the lymphatic drainage of the intestine may contribute to the protein-losing enteropathy associated with IBD.

Nutrient malabsorption

When Crohn's disease involves the small intestine, malabsorption of various nutrients can occur. This may be an important contributing factor to the development of protein–energy malnutrition in these patients. However, the inflamed mucosa itself is seldom the primary cause of gross nutrient malabsorption in Crohn's disease, except when the disease involves a very extensive area of the small intestine, or successive surgical resections have led to a short-bowel syndrome. Nutrient malabsorption is more often secondary to bile-acid malabsorption or intestinal bacterial overgrowth. Bile-salt malabsorption often occurs when the terminal ileum is extensively diseased or has been resected. In such a situation, spillover of bile salts through the colon produces diarrhoea and decreases the bile-salt pool, leading to abnormal micellar solubilisation and fat malabsorption. Intestinal bacterial overgrowth occurs in 30% of Crohn's-disease patients, as a result of strictures in the small bowel or the resection of the ileo-caecal valve. In addition to an increased consumption of vitamin B_{12}, small-intestine bacterial overgrowth deranges carbohydrate and protein absorption and bile-salt metabolism.

Micronutrient deficiencies in IBD

Deficiencies of micronutrients in IBD, as well as their possible role in its pathogenesis, have been little documented in the literature. The main problems in interpreting the reported results are:

(1) The absence of reference values in healthy individuals from the same geographical area.
(2) The lack of agreement about the type of sample to be analysed for a particular micronutrient (whole blood, plasma, urine, or other tissue).
(3) The concept of subclinical deficiency or inadequacy for a given element.

This concept may be of importance in IBD, since clinically apparent vitamin or trace-element deficiencies do sometimes appear (except for iron and folate). However, micronutrient inadequacies may play an important role in the metabolic pathways relevant to the pathogenesis of the disease.

Vitamins

It is well known that patients on sulphasalazine can develop folate deficiency. Also, vitamin B_{12} malabsorption may occur in Crohn's-disease patients with ileal involvement or resection, or intestinal bacterial overgrowth. Deficiencies of individual vitamins have been reported in IBD patients. In many cases, clinical signs of vitamin deficiency do not accompany low plasma vitamin levels. The pathophysiological and clinical implications of suboptimal vitamin status found in active IBD are unknown. However, some vitamin-dependent enzyme systems are presumably altered in these patients. Low folate levels were associated with epithelial dysplasia in ulcerative colitis. Inappropriate levels of antioxidant vitamins (β-carotene, vitamins A, E, and C), as well as biotin and vitamin B_2 – involved in the scavenging of reactive oxygen metabolites and in the polyunsaturated fatty acid biosynthesis – may prove to be of pathobiological importance in the future.

Minerals and trace elements

Iron-deficient anaemia because of acute or chronic blood loss is frequent in patients with IBD. Deficiencies of many other minerals and trace elements, including magnesium, zinc, selenium, copper, chromium, manganese, and molybdenum have been also described in these patients. Of these, zinc and selenium deserve special mention.

The clinical interest in evaluating zinc status in IBD relates to its role in growth retardation and to the fact that overt zinc deficiency associated with total parenteral nutrition (TPN) can occur. Low serum zinc levels have been found in active and inactive Crohn's disease and in active ulcerative colitis.

Serum selenium is low in patients with severe attacks of IBD, associated malnutrition, and/or long-standing disease. Glutathione peroxidase is a selenium-dependent enzyme with antioxidant functions whose activity has been found to be decreased in the plasma of patients with both ulcerative colitis and Crohn's disease. However, overt symptoms of deficiency, which include myopathy and cardiomyopathy, are rare.

Consequences of impaired nutrition in IBD

The general consequences of malnutrition in IBD (Box 11.8) do not differ from those in other disease states. Malnutrition in the second most common cause of secondary immunodeficiency (the first is AIDS). Thus malnutrition renders patients with ulcerative colitis and Crohn's disease immunodepressed and hence more susceptible to infectious complications. A well-demonstrated effect of malnutrition in children with IBD is growth retardation and delayed sexual maturation. Both in children and in adults, malnutrition contributes to the osteopaenia associated with Crohn's disease. Additional consequences of malnutrition include delayed fistula healing, increased surgical risk and impaired healing of wounds, deficient transport of drugs by plasma proteins, and hypoplasia of the intestinal epithelium, which contributes to autoperpetuating the nutritional derangement. Recent years have seen growing evidence that some specific nutritional derangements may even play a role in the pathogenesis of the abnormal immune response of IBD patients.

Nutritional support in IBD

In previous sections, a rationale for nutritionally supporting patients with active IBD has been provided. Patients with mild to moderate attacks can be managed with an oral conventional diet. No major dietary restrictions should be prescribed in active disease, except for avoidance of coarse fibre (particularly in

> **Box 11.8 Consequences of impaired nutrition in inflammatory bowel disease (IBD)**
>
> - immunosuppression (increased susceptibility to infection);
> - growth retardation and delayed sexual maturation (children);
> - osteopaenia;
> - delayed healing of fistulae;
> - increased surgical risk;
> - impaired healing of wounds;
> - deficient transport of drugs by plasma proteins;
> - impaired trophism of the intestinal mucosa (autoperpetuation of malnutrition itself);
> - a possible role for some nutritional deficiencies in the pathogenesis of the disease.

patients with ulcerative colitis, and in the presence of bowel strictures in Crohn's disease). Milk and its derivatives should not be restricted unless overt intolerance (e.g. increase in diarrhoea) is observed.

Patients with inactive disease must eat a normal, well-balanced diet. Coarse fibre has to be restricted in those patients with persistent intestinal strictures. The use of exclusion diets to maintain remission in Crohn's disease has been advocated by some authors but, with few exceptions, does not seem to be effective.

A significant number of patients with either ulcerative colitis or Crohn's disease may need to be nutritionally supported with artificial nutrition at any time during the course of their illness. This is a major issue that will be discussed in more detail in the following sections.

Artificial nutrition as adjuvant therapy in IBD

As in other disease states, TPN was the first modality of artificial nutrition to be used in patients with acute attacks of IBD. The rationale for this was the concept that 'bowel rest' was a cornerstone of the treatment of these patients. However, current available data indicate that 'bowel rest' is by no means necessary to induce remission in either Crohn's disease or ulcerative colitis. Randomised controlled trials in patients with both Crohn's disease and ulcerative colitis treated with steroids indicated that the remission rate was the same when patients received either TPN or total enteral nutrition (TEN). Moreover, the frequency of side effects related to artificial nutrition is usually lower with TEN than with TPN. Interestingly enough, in ulcerative colitis patients who were unresponsive to steroids and required to be colectomised, the rate of postoperative complications was also lower among those who had received TEN.

In the light of these data, TEN should be preferred to TPN in patients with IBD in whom artificial nutrition is indicated. In fact, enteral feeding has physiological advantages, as it contributes to the maintenance of intestinal trophism and it is cheaper and safer than TPN. However, TPN must be used in patients who do not tolerate enteral feeding or in those situations where enteral feeding is contraindicated. These are:

(1) toxic megacolon;
(2) intestinal perforation;
(3) complete intestinal occlusion;
(4) massive gastrointestinal bleeding;
(5) fistulae arising in the mid-jejunum, where the enteral diet cannot be infused far enough (either proximally or distally) from the origin of the fistula.

Short-term enteral nutrition should be used in patients with active IBD (both ulcerative colitis and Crohn's disease) who are malnourished or at risk of become rapidly malnourished (e.g. those with severe attacks). In these cases, diet infusion through a fine nasoenteric tube, with the aid of a peristaltic pump, improves tolerance. Long-term enteral feeding (either nocturnal or cyclic) is a well-established treatment for the prevention or reversal of growth retardation in children and adolescents with Crohn's disease. Patients with complicated Crohn's disease may need long-term home enteral nutrition to maintain their nutritional status. In these circumstances, the insertion of a percutaneous endoscopic gastrostomy has to be considered. Prior to performing this procedure, a careful endoscopic and histological study must always be performed in order to rule out the possibility of gastric involvement in the disease, since a permanent fistulous tract may be favoured if percutaneous gastrostomy is carried out on a previously diseased gastric wall.

Repeated or extensive intestinal resections may lead some patients with Crohn's disease to a status of intestinal insufficiency, termed 'short-bowel syndrome'. In the early phases of short-bowel syndrome, protein and energy requirements should be provided with TPN, but small amounts of enteral feeding should also be administered in order to favour intestinal adaptation. In most patients, progressive weaning from TPN will be possible. A minority, however, will become dependent on home TPN for life. Factors influencing the adaptation of short-bowel syndrome to enterally administered foods include the extent and site of the resected segment and the presence of residual disease in the remnant bowel.

Enteral nutrition as primary treatment in Crohn's disease

Since the early 1980s, the possibility of enteral feeding being used as the primary treatment (i.e. able to induce remission *per se*) in this disease has been a matter of debate.

Meta-analyses of the published randomised controlled trials comparing TEN with steroids in the treatment of active Crohn's disease have concluded that steroids are better than any type of enteral feeding. In spite of that, the overall remission rate with TEN is about 60%, a figure that is substantially higher than the 20–30% placebo response obtained in placebo-controlled therapeutic trials in Crohn's disease. This suggests that enteral nutrition would indeed have a role as primary treatment in active Crohn's disease. In addition, enteral feeding has been shown to be useful in preventing relapse in inactive Crohn's disease, particularly in children.

On the other hand, meta-analysis of the randomised trials comparing elemental (e.g. amino acid-based) and non-elemental (e.g. peptide- or whole protein-based) diets as primary therapy in Crohn's disease showed that both types of diet were equally effective. In other words, the primary therapeutic effect of TEN does not appear to depend on the type of nitrogen source.

The remission rates of 26 studies (both controlled and uncontrolled), including 673 compliant adult patients with active Crohn's disease treated with enteral diets for at least 2 weeks, ranged from 36 to 100%, with a mean value of 75%. This wide range of remission indicates that not every enteral diet is equally effective. It has been hypothesised that differences in the amount or type of fat may partly account for this, but it is far from proven. Hence, identifying the nutrient (or nutrients) responsible for the therapeutic effect of enteral diets in Crohn's disease will be a hard task for the future. On the other hand, it could well be that some patients are more susceptible than others to the effect of enteral diet. Reliable assessment of disease-related predictive factors in response to enteral feeding will require the performance of large-scale trials. While such studies are not available, TEN should be attempted as primary therapy for active Crohn's disease in those patients in whom steroids are especially harmful (i.e. children and adolescents, osteopenic elder patients, and post-menopausal women). In any case, TEN should be kept in mind as a possible therapeutic alternative for steroid-resistant and, particularly, steroid-dependent Crohn's-disease patients.

11.5 Irritable bowel syndrome and diverticular disease

Definition

IBS – also referred to as irritable or spastic colon – is one or the most common disorders seen at gastro-enterology clinics (20–50% of all referrals). IBS is a combination of chronic and recurrent gastrointestinal symptoms not explained by structural or biochemical abnormalities. A variety of criteria have been developed to identify a combination of symptoms in order to diagnose IBS, the most widely used being the Rome criteria, which have undergone three versions over 15 years (Table 11.3). Recently, the American College of Gastroenterology Task Force has promoted a simple, pragmatic, and clinically useful definition incorporating the key features of previous diagnostic criteria. They have defined IBS as 'abdominal pain or discomfort that occurs in association with altered bowel habits over a period of at least 3 months'. In general, three subtypes of IBS are recognised: (i) IBS with (predominant) constipation; (ii) IBS with (predominant) diarrhoea; and (iii) IBS with mixed (alternate) constipation and diarrhoea.

Other symptoms include bloating, excess of flatus, passage of mucus in the stools, a sensation of incomplete rectal emptying, and proctalgia fugax (fleeting rectal pain).

In addition to symptom assessment by means of the Rome criteria, a limited screening for organic disease seems mandatory. This includes complete physical examination, haematology counts and routine biochemistry analysis (including erythrocyte sedimentation rate and, probably, serum thyroid hormones), a search for ova and parasites in the stool, and a flexible sigmoidoscopy plus barium enema

Table 11.3 Evolution of the Rome criteria for irritable bowel syndrome (IBS).

Rome I	Abdominal pain or discomfort relieved with defecation, or associated with a change in stool frequency or consistency, *PLUS two or more of the following* on at least *25% of occasions or days for 3 months*: (1) altered stool frequency (2) altered stool form (3) altered stool passage (4) passage of mucus (5) bloating or distension
Rome II	Abdominal discomfort or pain that has had *two of three features for 12 weeks (need not be consecutive) in the last 1 year*: (1) relieved with defecation (2) onset associated with change in stool frequency (3) onset associated with change in stool form
Rome III	Recurrent abdominal pain or discomfort *3 days per month in the last 3 months associated with two or more of*: (1) improvement with defecation (2) onset associated with change in stool frequency (3) onset associated with change in stool form

(or total colonoscopy in patients older than 50). Additional tests may be necessary according to the syndromic subtype or the particular characteristics of the patient.

Epidemiology

As mentioned, IBS is one of the most frequent causes of referral to the gastroenterologist. However, many patients do not seek medical care. Thus, the true prevalence of IBS must be estimated using symptom questionnaires in population surveys. A recent review of the published studies indicates that, in the UK and the USA, IBS affects 14–24% of women and 5–19% of men. In general, IBS is more common in females. In studies that stratified groups by age, there is a decrease in frequency among older subjects. The prevalence seems to be equal in white and black people, but may be lower in Hispanics. However, data on the racial prevalence of IBS are confounded by cultural influences. There are few epidemiological studies in non-Western countries. The available data suggest that IBS is rare in sub-Saharan Africa but common in Japan, China, the Indian subcontinent, and South America.

Pathogenesis

A detailed description of the pathogenic mechanisms thought to be involved in the development of IBS exceeds the purpose and scope of a textbook devoted to clinical nutrition. A neurobiological pathophysiological model for IBS, which includes alterations in autonomic, neuroendocrine, and pain-modulatory mechanisms, is currently being developed. Altered viscerosomatic sensitivity (the so-called 'visceral hyperalgesia') seems to play a key role in this model, leading to the development of symptoms of irritable bowel. Psychological stress and/or specific psychological disturbances (anxiety/depression) contribute to the exacerbation of symptoms. Intestinal infections have also been incriminated as a triggering factor. The role of dietary components in this pathogenic network will be discussed next.

Food intolerance and IBS

Many patients with IBS believe that their symptoms are triggered by specific foods but this causative relationship is difficult to prove. Many studies have investigated the role of a variety of foodstuffs in the development of symptoms of irritable bowel, with controversial results. Positive response to an elimination diet ranges from 15 to 71%, and double-blind placebo-controlled challenges identify problem foods in 6–58% of cases. Milk, wheat, and eggs, as well as foods high in salicylates (coffee, nuts, corn, wine, tomato, etc.) or amines (chocolate, bananas, wine, tomato, etc.) are most often identified as causing symptom exacerbation. However, studies had major limitations in their design, so that it is unclear whether adverse reactions to foods are a key factor in exacerbating symptoms, or whether dietary manipulation is a valid therapeutic option.

The role of individual sugar (i.e. lactose, fructose, sorbitol) malabsorption in the development of symptoms of irritable bowel deserves particular comment. Lactose malabsorption has been reported to occur in about 25% of patients with IBS in the USA and Northern Europe, whereas the prevalence may be as high as 52–68% in Mediterranean countries. In addition to geographical influences, patient selection may account for these differences. Lactose malabsorption can cause osmotic diarrhoea and bloating, and hence may be more frequent in the subset of patients in whom these symptoms predominate. In a series of

unselected Finnish patients, there was a poor relationship between lactose malabsorption, lactose intolerance, and symptoms of irritable bowel. In the light of these data, routine investigation of lactose malabsorption in every patient with IBS does not seem advisable. However, lactose malabsorption should be investigated, by means of a hydrogen breath test after an oral load of lactose, in those patients in whom diarrhoea and/or bloating predominate, particularly in countries where lactase deficiency is highly prevalent.

Fructose and sorbitol malabsorption also occur among patients with IBS. The prevalence of malabsorption is particularly high when both sugars are administered together (31–92%). Although these figures do not differ from those found in healthy controls, the intensity of symptoms after the ingestion of these sugars is significantly higher in IBS patients. Such a difference does not appear to be due to intestinal dysmotility or hypersensitivity to distension, but to an increased fermentative capacity in patients with IBS. As in the case of lactose, hydrogen breath tests using fructose, sorbitol, and fructose + sorbitol mixtures as substrate should be performed in IBS patients with predominant diarrhoea and/or bloating symptoms.

Nutritional consequences

Fortunately, malnutrition is not particularly prevalent among IBS patients. In fact, the diagnosis of IBS must be questioned in the presence of marked nutritional deficiencies or weight loss. In this setting, the diagnostic work-up for organic disease must be expanded with specific imaging and laboratory tests to rule out IBD, coeliac disease, gastrointestinal neoplasm, chronic pancreatitis, pancreatic cancer, and so on.

Despite the rarity of malnutrition in IBS, some patients attribute all their symptoms to the 'last meal they ate'. Thus, they begin to eat a more and more restrictive and imbalanced diet, which can lead them to protein–energy malnutrition or micronutrient deficiencies.

Dietary management of IBS

The treatment of IBS should be based on the nature and severity of the symptoms, the degree of physiological disturbance and functional impairment, and the presence of psychosocial disturbance affecting the course of the illness. Patients with mild symptoms respond to education and reassurance, whereas antispasmodic (anticholinergics) drugs or low-dose antidepressant agents (either tricyclic or serotonin-reuptake inhibitors) are recommended in more symptomatic patients. However, it should be kept in mind that 40–70% respond to placebo alone.

In this setting, it is important to avoid restrictive and monotonous diets, since, as mentioned, many patients tend to exclude from their diet a great number of foodstuffs without a firm reason to do so. After an accurate dietary interview, most patients will realise that a given foodstuff which apparently caused symptoms on one occasion was well tolerated in many other instances. In general, most patients with IBS can (and should) eat a balanced diet without restrictions. However, in some patients, in whom symptoms are repeatedly triggered by eating, an exclusion diet may be of benefit. Also, a substantial percentage of patients with associated sugar malabsorption will improve after excluding the offending sugar from their diet.

For years, high-fibre diets and/or the addition of bulking agents (e.g. bran) have been accepted as effective therapeutic measures for IBS patients. In fact, such a recommendation still appears in the more recent editions of authoritative gastroenterology textbooks. However, several randomised crossover trials have shown that the administration of 12–15 g of bran or 20 g of corn fibre per day was not better that placebo in improving symptoms of irritable bowel. In fact, more than half of patients from a large uncontrolled series felt that they get worse after bran supplementation. High-fibre diets might, at least in part, aggravate symptoms through an increase in gas production, because, as mentioned before, patients with IBS appear to have an increased fermentative capacity.

In spite of these considerations, high-fibre diets or fibre supplements should not be totally withdrawn from the therapeutic armament for IBS. Fibre supplements will be particularly useful in patients with constipation. Hydrophilic colloids such as psyllium derivatives and methylcellulose tend to produce less gas (or to produce it at a slower rate). In addition, due to their hydrophilic properties, these agents bind water and prevent both excessive stool dehydration and excess liquidity. They may thus be equally effective for patients in whom either constipation or diarrhoea predominates.

Diverticular disease

Definition and epidemiology

Although diverticula (pouches protruding out from the wall of the bowel) may occur anywhere in the gut, the term 'diverticular disease' usually denotes the presence of diverticula in the large intestine, particularly in the sigmoid colon. In fact, 95% of cases of colonic diverticular involve this segment, and it is exclusively affected in 65% of patients.

Diverticular disease is very common, particularly in industrialised countries. The prevalence of this condition increases with age, being rare in individuals younger than 40 but occurring in more than a third of subjects over 65. Diverticular disease is rare in people who live in developing countries. However, the risk rapidly increases when they migrate to Western societies.

About 80% of patients with diverticular disease never have any symptoms. When symptomatic, patients complain about pain in the left lower quadrant of the abdomen, usually colic, and changes in bowel habit. These symptoms mostly resemble those of IBS. Complications occur in about 5% of cases, and mainly consist of infection of a diverticulum (diverticulitis), which may lead to bowel perforation or abscess formation. Gastrointestinal bleeding can also occur, particularly from diverticula arising in the right colon.

Dietary fibre and diverticular disease

Colonic hypersegmentation resulting in intraluminal hypertension has been incriminated as the primary cause of diverticular disease. Increased intraluminal pressure (myochosis) will result in mucosal herniation and diverticula production, but these motility disturbances are not present in all patients with diverticula.

While there is no direct evidence to prove it, a number of data sets suggest that diverticular disease is caused by a fibre-deficient diet. In fact, it occurs more often in omnivores than in vegetarians, and individuals consuming a high-meat, low-fibre diet are particularly at risk. The essential pathology in diverticular disease is colonic muscular hypertrophy. This is thought to be due to the need to propel hard faecal contents. Once muscular thickening occurs, the bowel lumen becomes narrowed, forming a small chamber with high pressure, leading to diverticula formation.

Treatment of uncomplicated diverticular disease relies on the use of a high-fibre diet. Bran supplements have proven to be effective in both uncontrolled and controlled trials. Bran appears to be more effective than other sources of non-starch polysaccharides or bulk-forming agents. As in IBS, however, fibre supplements may increase flatus production and bloating. A high-fibre diet alone should therefore always be tried first.

11.6 Concluding remarks

Future research on the role of nutrition and nutrients in the gastrointestinal tract is likely to focus on the effects of individual nutrients on gene expression. Over recent years, the hypothesis has emerged that digestive end products and/or their metabolic derivatives regulate pancreatic gene expression directly, independently of hormone stimulation. The role of fatty acids in the control of gene expression is now at an early stage of understanding. Whether or not this mechanism is related to pancreatic adaptation to dietary fat is unknown and will have to be discovered by additional research.

Current information on developmental gene expression in the intestine and on the dietary regulation of genes expressed in the developing intestinal epithelium is limited to only a handful of genes – primarily highly expressed genes involved in differentiated cellular functions (see Chapter 10 of *Nutrition and Metabolism* in this series). The carbohydrate structure and amount in many foods and ingredients can be manipulated to achieve specific physiochemical properties of benefit to food structure, and to produce a diverse range of physiological effects. It can be expected that many functional foods of the future will contain such specially selected or modified carbohydrates, but the metabolic and health consequences of these carbohydrates should be examined in more detail before health claims can be justified (see Chapter 4 of *Nutrition and Metabolism* in this series).

Probiotics is another area of ongoing research, and manipulation of colonic microflora has real potential for therapeutic management of gastrointestinal disease.

Increased knowledge in all of these areas will lead to a better understanding of the mechanisms through which nutrients affect gastrointestinal health.

References and further reading

American Gastroenterological Association. American Gastroenterological Association medical position statement: short bowel syndrome and intestinal transplantation. Gastroenterology 2003; 124: 1105–1110.

Brandt LJ, Chey WD, Foxx-Orenstein AE, Quigley EMM, Schiller LR, Schoenfeld PS, *et al.* An evidence-based systematic review on the management of irritable bowel syndrome. Am J Gastroenterol 2009; 104(Suppl. 1): S8–S35.

Buchman AL, Scolapio JS, Fryer J. AGA technical review on short bowel syndrome and intestinal transplantation. Gastroenterology 2003; 124: 1111–1134.

Cabré E. Irritable bowel syndrome: can nutrient manipulation help? Curr Opin Clin Nutr Metab Care 2010; 13: 581–587.

DiBaise JK, Young RJ, Vanderhoof JA. Intestinal rehabilitation and the short bowel syndrome: part 1. Am J Gastroenterol 2004; 99: 1386–1395.

DiBaise JK, Young RJ, Vanderhoof JA. Intestinal rehabilitation and the short bowel syndrome: part 2. Am J Gastroenterol 2004; 99: 1823–1832.

Dziechciarz P, Horvath A, Shamir R, Szajewska H. Meta-analysis: enteral nutrition in active Crohn's disease in children. Aliment Pharmacol Ther 2007; 26: 795–806.

Farthing MJG. Tropical malabsorption and tropical diarrhoea. In: Sleisenger & Fordtran's Gastrointestinal and Liver Disease, 8th edn (Feldman M, Friedman LS, Brandt LJ, eds). Philadelphia: Saunders-Elsevier, 2006, pp. 2307–2318.

Fox JM, Stollman NH. Diverticular disease of the colon. In: Sleisenger & Fordtran's Gastrointestinal and Liver Disease, 8th edn (Feldman M, Friedman LS, Brandt LJ, eds). Philadelphia: Saunders-Elsevier, 2006, pp. 2613–2632.

Gassull MA, Cabré E. The role of nutrition in the pathogenesis of inflammatory bowel disease. In: Falk Symposium 106: Advances in Inflammatory Bowel Disease (Rutgeerts P, Colombel J-F, Hanauer S, Schölmerich J, Tytgat GN, Van Gossum A, eds). London: Kluwer Academic Pub., 1999, pp. 80–88.

Gassull MA. Review article: the role of nutrition in the treatment of inflammatory bowel disease. Aliment Pharmacol Ther 2004; 20(Suppl. 4): 79–83.

Lochs H, Dejong CHC, Hammarqvist F, Hébuterne X, León-Sanz M, Schütz T, *et al.* ESPEN guidelines on enteral nutrition: gastroenterology. Clin Nutr 2006; 25: 260–274.

Sands BE. Crohn's disease. In: Sleisenger & Fordtran's Gastrointestinal and Liver Disease, 8th edn (Feldman M, Friedman LS, Brandt LJ, eds). Philadelphia: Saunders-Elsevier, 2006, pp. 2459–2498.

Su C, Lichtenstein GR. Ulcerative colitis. In: Sleisenger & Fordtran's Gastrointestinal and Liver Disease, 8th edn (Feldman M, Friedman LS, Brandt LJ, eds). Philadelphia: Saunders-Elsevier, 2006, pp. 2499–2548.

Van Gossum A, Cabré E, Hebuterne X, Jeppesen P, Krznaric Z, Messing B, *et al.* ESPEN guidelines on parenteral nutrition: gastroenterology. Clin Nutr 2009; 28: 415–427.

Various Authors. Proceedings of the NIH Consensus Conference on Celiac Disease. Gastroenterology 2005; 128(Suppl. 1): S1–S141.

Zachos M, Tondeur M, Griffiths AM. Enteral nutritional therapy for inducing remission in Crohn's disease. Cochrane Database Syst Rev 2007; DOI: CD000542.

12
Nutrition in Liver Disease

Mathias Plauth[1] and Tatjana Schütz[2]

[1]*Staedtisches Klinikum (Municipal Hospital Dessau), Germany*
[2]*Leipzig University Medical Centre, Germany*

Key messages

- In chronic liver disease (CLD), patient malnutrition is frequent and an independent negative prognostic factor. Protein depletion in particular is associated with loss of vital physiological functions and impaired liver function. Malnutrition can be detected by simple clinical methods.
- In CLD, patients' glycogen stores are depleted and therefore even short periods of fasting are noxious and must be avoided. In general, spontaneous food intake is overestimated and in fact is very often totally insufficient.
- In CLD, trace element and vitamin deficiencies are frequent. Measures to prevent refeeding syndrome or Wernicke's encephalopathy must be adopted.
- In CLD, the goal of nutrition therapy is to ensure the adequate provision of energy, protein, and micronutrients, making use of oral nutritional supplements, tube feeding, or parenteral nutrition.
- Nutrition therapy improves the liver function, body composition, morbidity, and mortality of CLD patients.
- CLD patients require a protein provision higher than that recommended for healthy, well-nourished individuals. In encephalopathy,

especially after gastrointestinal haemorrhage, the use of branched-chain amino acid-enriched solutions is beneficial.
- Obese patients with nonalcoholic steatohepatitis (NASH) benefit from sustained weight reduction, irrespective of the medical strategy (dietary counselling, orlistat, bariatric surgery, etc.) by which this is achieved.
- In acute liver failure (ALF), the treatment goals are to ensure: (i) the adequate provision of energy, and especially ensuring euglycaemia by giving glucose, lipid, vitamins, and trace elements; and (ii) optimal rates of protein synthesis, by providing an adequate intake of protein or amino acids. In the majority of patients, these goals can be achieved by enteral nutrition.
- In many respects (energy requirement, utilisation of exogenous glucose and lipids, use of early enteral nutrition), ALF patients are not different from critically ill patients suffering from other entities. Hypoglycaemia is a frequent problem in ALF, meriting particular attention.
- Irrespective of the modality of nutrition (enteral, parenteral), tight metabolic monitoring is warranted in order to avoid cerebral oedema of ALF.

12.1 Introduction

Nutrition has long been recognised as a prognostic and therapeutic determinant in patients with chronic liver disease (CLD), and was therefore included as one of the variables in the original prognostic score proposed by Child and Turcotte. Nutritional status, however, was not included in the widely used modified Child–Pugh score, and not all hepatologists consider nutrition issues relevant in the management of their patients. In this chapter, the scientific and

evidence base of nutrition management of patients with liver disease is reviewed, in order to give recommendations for nutrition therapy.

12.2 Nutritional risk in liver-disease patients

Adequate nutrition is a complex process, which in healthy organisms is regulated in an adaptive response according to the prevailing condition. Therefore,

Clinical Nutrition, Second Edition. Edited by Marinos Elia, Olle Ljungqvist, Rebecca J Stratton and Susan A Lanham-New.
© 2013 The Nutrition Society. Published 2013 by Blackwell Publishing Ltd.

the assessment of nutritional risk of patients must include variables indicative of the physiologic capabilities – the nutritional status – and the burden inflicted by the ongoing or impending disease and/or medical interventions. A meaningful assessment of nutritional status should encompass not only body weight and height, but also information on energy and nutrient balance, as well as body composition and tissue function, reflecting the metabolic and physical fitness of the patient facing a vital contest. Such information can best be interpreted when viewed dynamically (e.g. weight loss over time).

Numerous descriptive studies have shown higher rates of mortality and complications, such as refractory ascites, variceal bleeding, infection, and hepatic encephalopathy (HE), in cirrhotic patients with protein malnutrition, as well as reduced survival when such patients undergo liver transplantation. In malnourished cirrhotic patients, the risk of postoperative morbidity and mortality is increased after abdominal surgery.

In cirrhosis or alcoholic steatohepatitis (ASH), poor oral food intake is a predictor of increased mortality. In nutrition-intervention trials, patients with the lowest spontaneous protein intake showed the highest mortality. Dietary intake should be assessed by a skilled dietitian, and a three-day dietary recall can be used in outpatients. Appropriate tables for food composition should be used for the calculation of proportions of various nutrients. As a gold standard, the energy content of food servings and leftovers can be measured by bomb calorimetry.

Simple bedside methods such as the 'Subjective Global Assessment' (SGA) or anthropometry have been shown to identify malnutrition adequately. Composite scoring systems have been developed based on variables such as actual/ideal weight, anthropometry, creatinine index, visceral proteins, absolute lymphocyte count, delayed-type skin reaction, absolute CD8+ count, and hand grip strength. Such systems, however, include unreliable variables such as plasma concentrations of visceral proteins and 24-hour urine creatinine excretion, and do not confer an advantage over SGA.

The accurate measurement of nutritional status is difficult in the presence of fluid overload or impaired hepatic protein synthesis (e.g. reduced synthetic rate of albumin in cirrhosis). Sophisticated methods are required to assess body cell mass (BCM) by total body potassium counting, lean body mass by dual-energy X-ray absorptiometry (DXA), total body protein by *in vivo* neutron activation analysis (IVNAA), or total body water by isotope-dilution techniques. Among bedside methods, the measurement of phase angle α or determination of BCM using bioimpedance analysis is considered superior to methods such as anthropometry and 24-hour creatinine excretion, despite some limitations in patients with ascites.

Muscle function is reduced in malnourished CLD patients and, as monitored by hand grip strength, is an independent predictor of outcome. Plasma levels of visceral proteins (albumin, prealbumin, retinol-binding protein) are heavily influenced by hepatic synthetic capacity, alcohol intake, or acute inflammatory conditions. Immune status, which is often considered a functional test of malnutrition, may be affected by hypersplenism, abnormal immunological reactivity, and alcohol abuse.

12.3 Effect of nutritional state on liver disease

Under-nutrition

Severe under-nutrition in children can cause fatty liver, which in general is fully reversible upon refeeding. In children with kwashiorkor, there seems to be a maladaptation associated with less-efficient breakdown of fat and oxidation of fatty acids compared to children with marasmus. An impairment of fatty acid removal from the liver could not be observed. Under-nutrition impairs specific hepatic functions, such as phase-I xenobiotic metabolism, galactose elimination capacity, and plasma levels of c-reactive protein in infected children. In nutrition-intervention trials in cirrhotic patients, quantitative liver-function tests improved more, or more rapidly, in the treatment groups. This included antipyrine, aminopyrine, and ICG clearance, as well as galactose elimination capacity. It is unknown whether fatty liver of malnutrition can progress to CLD.

Quantitative liver-function tests can be used to monitor the effects of nutritional intervention on liver function. They are not useful, however, for the identification of patients who will benefit from nutritional intervention, since none of the tests can differentiate whether loss of liver function is due to reduced hepatocellular mass or lack of nutrients. A simple test is needed that can distinguish between these two alternatives, in analogy to the intravenous (IV) vitamin K test, in order to estimate the potential benefit of nutritional support in individual patients.

Over-nutrition

In obese humans subjected to total starvation, weight-reducing diets, or small-bowel bypass, the development of transient degenerative changes with focal necrosis was described in the 1970s. Nonalcoholic steatohepatitis (NASH) was initially described in weight losing-individuals; currently insulin resistance and obesity are its most common causes. It is estimated that in Europe, 20% of the population with moderate or no alcohol consumption has nonalcoholic fatty liver (NAFL), of which 20% progress to NASH. Analyses of dietary habits in NASH patients do not show a uniform pattern. Increased consumption of fat and *n*-6 fatty acids and increased consumption of carbohydrate and energy have been observed. The occurrence of insulin resistance has been attributed to a high fructose consumption from corn syrup, as used in soft drinks. Body mass index (BMI) and total body fat are predictors for the presence of NASH in the obese, and in patients undergoing bariatric surgery NASH is diagnosed on average in 40%, with a range of 24–98%. The key role of obesity is illustrated by the observation that weight reduction, regardless of whether it is achieved by dietary counselling, bariatric surgery, or drug treatment, has the potential to ameliorate or even cure NASH.

12.4 Effect of liver disease on nutritional state

Acute liver disease

Minor or moderate acute liver disease induces the same metabolic effects as any disease associated with an acute-phase response. In more severe acute liver disease, such as acute liver failure (ALF), there are profound changes in carbohydrate and protein metabolism. The effect on nutritional status depends on the duration of the disease and the presence of an underlying CLD which might have already compromised the patient's nutritional status. In ALF, in

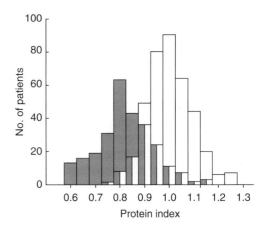

Figure 12.1 Protein depletion in patients with liver cirrhosis, as measured by *in vivo* neutron activation analysis. The graph shows the distribution of the protein index (ratio of measured to estimated pre-illness total body protein) in 268 patients with liver cirrhosis (■) and in 386 healthy volunteers (□). Am J Clin Nutr 2007; 85: 1257–1266. Copyright © American Society for Nutrition.

particular hyperacute liver failure, a so-far healthy individual is struck by a fulminant disease which leads to spontaneous recovery, liver transplantation, or death within days. On the other hand, patients with subacute liver failure are at considerable risk of becoming malnourished and suffer from severe changes in body composition during the protracted course of their illness.

Cirrhosis

Mixed-type protein-energy malnutrition with coexisting features of kwashiorkor-like malnutrition and marasmus is commonly observed in patients with cirrhosis. The prevalence and severity of malnutrition are related to the clinical stage of CLD, increasing from 20% of patients with well-compensated disease up to more than 60% of patients with severe liver insufficiency. Patients with cirrhosis frequently suffer from substantial protein depletion (Figure 12.1), and the resulting sarcopenia is associated with impaired muscle function and survival. Recovery from this loss in BCM can be achieved by the control of complications such as portal hypertension and by adequate nutrition. The aetiology of liver disease *per se* does not seem to influence the prevalence and degree of malnutrition and protein depletion, and the higher prevalence and more

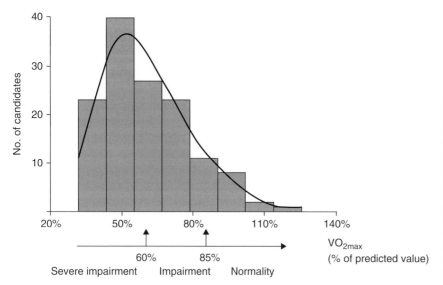

Figure 12.2 Loss of tissue function, exemplified by severe limitation of cardiopulmonary exercise capacity in cirrhotics. The graph shows the distribution of peak VO_2 within the study population ($n = 135$). Peak VO_2, expressed as percentage of predicted value, was normal ($\geq 85\%$) in only 11.9% of cases and impaired in 88.1% of cases. Impairment was severe ($<60\%$) in 54% of cases. With kind permission from Dharancy *et al.* (2008).

profound degree of malnutrition in alcoholics obviously results from unhealthy lifestyle and low socioeconomic conditions.

In hospitalised cirrhotics, fatigue, somnolence, and psychomotor dysfunction often lead to insufficient oral nutrition, even in the absence of overt HE.

Surgery and transplantation

After successful liver transplantation, in many patients there is an enormous weight gain in the first year following surgery and, unfortunately, a considerable number put their regained health in jeopardy by the development of full-blown metabolic syndrome. In the first year after transplantation, patients expand their body fat mass with no gain in lean body mass, and there is persisting impairment of nonoxidative glucose disposal in skeletal muscle. Even long-term survivors after liver transplantation exhibit an abnormal body composition with the phenotype of sarcopenic obesity. Preoperatively, cardiorespiratory exercise capacity is severely compromised in many cirrhotics (Figure 12.2), and this loss of physical function is associated with reduced survival after transplantation. The metabolic trauma of liver transplantation is associated with a loss in total body protein, irrespective of the nutritional management prior to the operation. This loss is associated with loss of tissue function, such as respiratory muscle function. There is growing evidence that in solid

organ-transplanted patients, skeletal muscle deconditioning persists from the time of decreased physical performance prior to transplantation, which should be addressed by appropriate comprehensive rehabilitation programmes, including physiotherapy.

Taken together, these observations indicate that upon restoration of hepatic function and cessation of portal hypertension, full nutritional rehabilitation is possible and should be aimed at.

12.5 Pathophysiology and nutrient requirement in liver disease

Energy

Acute liver failure

In healthy individuals, hepatic energy expenditure contributes 25% to whole-body energy expenditure, and in ALF one would expect a reduction in oxygen-consuming processes like hepatic ketone body production and lactate elimination due to the loss of functioning hepatocyte mass. Indirect calorimetry in patients with ALF, however, showed an increase in resting energy expenditure (REE) of 18–30% when compared to healthy controls. Most likely, the accompanying systemic inflammatory-response syndrome has caused an increase in energy expenditure that more than outweighs the reduced oxygen consumption of hepatocytes. Thus, in terms of energy expenditure, patients with ALF are not different from critically ill patients with other aetiologies.

Table 12.1 Energy requirements in various types of liver disease, as calculated from measured or predicted resting energy expenditure (REE), on the basis of body weight, or as total energy requirement, including the energy content of amino acids or protein as given in recommended amounts.

Liver disease	Energy requirement (non-protein kcal/day)	Energy requirement (non-protein kcal/kg BW/day)	Energy requirement (kcal/kg BW/day)
Acute liver failure	1.2–1.3 × REE	30	35
Alcoholic steatohepatitis	1.2–1.3 × REE	30	35
Liver cirrhosis	1.2–1.3 × REE	30	35
Liver transplantation	1.2–1.3 × REE	30	35

Cirrhosis

On average, measured REE is of the same magnitude as energy expenditure predicted by the use of formulas (Harris–Benedict, Schofield, etc.). Likewise, in ASH patients, one study showed the same relationship between measured REE and predicted REE as in healthy individuals. Whenever available, indirect calorimetry should be used to measure REE, since in an individual patient measured REE may differ considerably from predicted values.

The question of hypermetabolism has been addressed in cirrhosis and ASH patients. ASH patients may be considered hypermetabolic when measured REE is related to their reduced muscle mass. Measured REE is increased by more than 20% above predicted REE in up to 35% of cirrhotic patients (hypermetabolism), and decreased by more than 20% below the predicted value in 18% of patients. In cirrhosis, hypermetabolism has been shown to be associated with reduced event-free survival and unfavourable outcome after transplantation, and seems to regress with improvement of body composition and after liver transplantation. For the diagnosis of hypermetabolism, however, indirect calorimetry is required, so that in daily practice most clinicians cannot use this approach.

Measurements of total energy expenditure indicate that the 24-hour energy requirement of cirrhotic patients amounts to about 130% of the basal metabolic rate (BMR) (Table 12.1). Diet-induced thermogenesis and the energy cost of defined physical activity in stable cirrhosis patients are not different from values obtained in healthy individuals. The spontaneous physical activity level, however, is considerably lower in cirrhotic patients. Obviously, the increased REE in advanced illness is balanced by diminished physical activity, reflecting the poor physical condition, and thus total energy expenditure is typically normal.

In cirrhotics without ascites, the actual body weight should be used for the calculation of the BMR when using formulas such as that proposed by Harris and Benedict. In patients with ascites, the ideal weight according to body height should be used, despite the suggestion from a series of 10 patients with liver cirrhosis, of whom only four were completely evaluated, in which it was suggested that ascites mass should not be omitted when calculating energy expenditure on the basis of body weight.

Surgery and transplantation

Liver-transplant patients on average have the same energy requirements as the majority of patients undergoing major abdominal surgery. In general, the provision of non-protein energy at 1.3 × REE is sufficient. In a longitudinal study, postoperative hypermetabolism peaked on day 10 after the transplantation at 124% of the predicted REE. By 6–12 months posttransplant, there was no longer a difference between the measured and predicted REE.

Carbohydrate metabolism

Acute liver failure

Hypoglycaemia is a clinically relevant and common problem in ALF, resulting entirely from loss of hepatic gluconeogenetic capacity, lack of glycogen, and hyperinsulinism. As a standard procedure, hypoglycaemia is treated by infusing glucose at a rate of 1.5–2 g/kg BW/day. Infection and cerebral oedema resulting from astrocyte swelling are the two key factors in the prognosis of ALF. Therefore, the rigorous control of blood glucose and tight metabolic monitoring may prove beneficial in this condition, where the central organ of metabolism is failing. Considering the facts that (i) glucose infusion is aimed at providing the critically ill with oxidative fuel essential for vital tissues such as CNS and erythrocytes, (ii) exogenous insulin at rates above 4 IU/hour cannot increase glucose oxidation, and (iii) in ALF there is insulin hypersecretion, hyperinsulinaemia, and insulin resistance, there seems to be little reason for insulin administration above 4 IU/hour in order to control glycaemia.

Cirrhosis

The utilisation of oxidative fuels is characterised by an increased rate of lipid oxidation in the fasting state and the frequent occurrence of insulin resistance (even in Child–Pugh class A patients). In the fasting state, glucose oxidation rate is reduced and hepatic glucose production rate is low despite increased gluconeogenesis due to a depletion of hepatic glycogen. Insulin resistance affects skeletal muscle metabolism: glucose uptake and non-oxidative glucose disposal such as glycogen synthesis are reduced, while glucose oxidation and lactate production are normal after glucose provision. It is not known to what extent glucose deposition as glycogen is impaired in skeletal muscle alone versus in both muscle and liver. Some 15–37% of patients develop overt diabetes, indicating an unfavourable prognosis.

Surgery and transplantation

In the early postoperative phase, there is often a disturbance of glucose metabolism, associated with insulin resistance. In this situation, hyperglycaemia should be managed by reducing glucose intake, because higher insulin doses are unable to increase glucose oxidation.

Fat metabolism

Acute liver failure

The oxidation of fatty acids and ketogenesis are the main energy-yielding processes for hepatocytes. Thus, adequate provision of lipid will be a plausible therapeutic objective provided there is sufficient oxygen supply to the hepatic tissue. It must be kept in mind, however, that some cases of ALF, in particular those with microvesicular steatosis and mitochondrial dysfunction, are caused by an impairment of hepatic beta-oxidation. In such a case, exogenous

lipid, even from administering propofol as a sedative, cannot be metabolised and may be harmful. Unlike the situation in septic patients, the splanchnic organs of ALF patients do not take up but rather release free fatty acids. This may result from either mobilisation of mesenteric fat or, more likely, the compromised hepatic utilisation of fatty acids as a consequence of loss of parenchymal mass. Apart from these physiological data, there are no systematic studies available regarding the role of fat as a nutrient in ALF. Anecdotal data and data from a European survey demonstrate that exogenous fat seems to be well tolerated by many patients. It should be kept in mind, however, that the use of fat may be harmful in cases of ALF due to the group of microvesicular steatosis conditions, where mitochondrial dysfunction may be predominant, leading to severely impaired oxidation of fatty acids. In the absence of data from systematic studies, it is recommended that plasma triglyceride levels are used to monitor fat utilisation, as the best variable currently available, and that levels no higher than 4–5 mmol/l are aimed for.

Cirrhosis

In the fasting state, the plasma levels of free fatty acids, glycerol, and ketone bodies are increased and free fatty acid and glycerol concentrations do not fully respond to low insulin infusion rates as in healthy subjects. Lipids are oxidised as the preferential substrate and lipolysis is increased with active mobilisation of lipid deposits. There is insulin resistance with regard to the antilipolytic activity.

After a meal, the suppression of lipid oxidation is not uniformly impaired. Plasma clearance and lipid oxidation rates are not reduced and thus the net capacity to utilise exogenous fat does not seem to be impaired. Plasma levels of essential and polyunsaturated fatty acids are decreased in cirrhosis, and this decrement correlates with nutritional status and severity of liver disease.

Surgery and transplantation

In hepatic transplant patients, improved functioning of the reticuloendothelial system was observed when using medium-chain triglyceride (MCT) or long-chain triglyceride (LCT) emulsions with a lower content of *n*-6 unsaturated fatty acids compared to pure soy bean oil emulsions.

Protein and amino acid metabolism

Acute liver failure

The plasma levels of amino acids are raised three- to fourfold in ALF. The plasma amino acid pattern is characterised by a decrease in branched-chain amino acids (BCAAs) and an increase in tryptophan, aromatic, and sulphur-containing amino acids. In ALF, the splanchnic organs do not take up amino acids, in contrast to the situation in healthy humans or in septic patients, where there is net uptake. Ammonia released from the intestine can no longer be extracted sufficiently by the failing liver, and, despite ammonia detoxification by skeletal muscle, hyperammonaemia ensues. Since elevated arterial ammonia levels have been recognised as an independent predictor of poor outcome in ALF patients, it seems prudent to adjust the provision of amino acids according to the ammonia levels (target: <100 µmol/l) monitored.

Cirrhosis

Protein turnover in cirrhotic patients has been found to be normal or increased. Some authors put the focus on the presence of increased protein break-down, while others suggest that a reduced protein synthesis plays the main role. Albumin but not fibrinogen synthesis rates correlate with quantitative liver-function tests and clinical stages of cirrhosis. Nevertheless, stable cirrhotics are apparently capable of efficient nitrogen retention and significant formation of lean body mass from increased protein intake during oral nutritional therapy. Protein catabolism influences the plasma and muscle amino acid imbalance of cirrhosis and indirectly causes nitrogen overload to the liver, leading to hyperammonaemia. In cirrhosis, after an overnight fast glycogen stores are depleted and metabolic conditions are similar to prolonged starvation in healthy individuals. It has been shown that a late-evening carbohydrate snack has the potential to improve protein metabolism in cirrhotic patients. Insulin resistance is apparently without effect on amino acid disposal.

There are only limited data from explicit and systematic determinations of the protein requirement of patients with liver cirrhosis. Patients with stable cirrhosis were found to have an increased protein requirement, leading to the recommendation of 1.2 g/kg BW/day, in contrast to the recommended minimal intake of 0.8 g/kg BW/day in healthy, well-nourished adults.

Table 12.2 Amino acid pattern in acute liver failure (ALF) (plasma) and liver cirrhosis (plasma and skeletal muscle). Fischer's ratio is >3.0 in healthy individuals and <1.5 in patients with cirrhosis and encephalopathy.

Amino acid (AA)	Plasma	Skeletal muscle
Phenylalanine	↑	↑
Tyrosine	↑	↑
Methionine	↑	
Tryptophane	↑	
Leucine	↓	
Isoleucine	↓	
Valine	↓	↓
Aromatic AA (AAA)	↑	↑
Branched-chain AA (BCAA)	↓	↓
BCAA/AAA (Fischer's ratio)	↓	↓

As in ALF, the plasma amino acid pattern is altered in cirrhosis. It is characterised by an elevation of aromatic (phenylalanine, tyrosine) and sulphur-containing amino acids (methionine) and tryptophane on the one hand, and a decrease in BCAA (leucine, isoleucine, valine) on the other (Table 12.2). Decreased metabolic clearance by the failing liver leads to the accumulation of aromatic and sulphurous amino acids in plasma and skeletal muscle, whereas the increased consumption for gluconeogenesis and ammonia detoxification, as well as portal systemic shunting, contributes to the diminution of BCAA in plasma and skeletal muscle.

Recently, it has been pointed out that, due to the absence of isoleucine from haemoglobin, blood is the source of protein of low biological value, leading to BCAA antagonism after upper-gastrointestinal haemorrhage. This BCAA antagonism readily explains the long-known clinical observation that blood and vegetable protein represent the two extremes in the hierarchy of food proteins regarding comagenic potential. Moreover, it can be shown that this antagonism leading to hyperammonaemia can be overcome by the infusion of isoleucine alone, resulting in improved protein synthesis rates in liver, muscle, and other tissues.

Surgery and transplantation

Preoperatively, the majority of transplant patients are already protein depleted, and the metabolic trauma of surgery adds considerable obligatory protein loss on top of this pre-existing nutritional risk. The extent of surgery-related protein loss is obviously of the

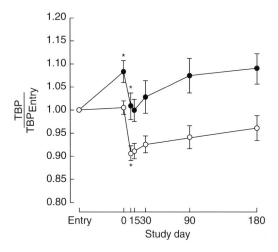

Figure 12.3 Impact of surgery-related protein catabolism in cirrhotics undergoing liver transplantation on total body protein (TBP, mean ± SEM). Graphs show changes in TBP relative to that measured at study entry in patients who received oral nutritional supplements according to a formal protocol (liquid diet, n = 7, closed circles) compared to historic controls, some of whom did not receive nutritional intervention (n = 13, open circles). * indicates significant difference from preceding measurement. Reprinted from Clinical Nutrition, 24: Plank L *et al*. Pre- and postoperative immunonutrition in patients undergoing liver transplantation: a pilot study of safety and efficacy, pp. 288–296, Copyright 2005, with permission from Elsevier.

same magnitude irrespective of the preoperative nutritional regimen, but the loss starts from a higher level in patients receiving formal preoperative nutritional intervention (Figure 12.3). After transplantation, patients remain in negative nitrogen balance for up to 28 days, necessitating an increase in the provision of protein or amino acids. Protein or amino acid intakes of 1.0–1.5 g/kg BW/day have been reported. The determination of postoperative urea nitrogen excretion has proved helpful in the assessment of individual nitrogen requirements.

Vitamins and minerals

No recommendation regarding the requirement for micronutrients can be made on the basis of controlled studies. As in other diseases, the administration of micronutrients has no proven therapeutic effect, apart from the prevention or correction of deficiency states.

Body composition of cirrhotics is altered profoundly and characterised by protein depletion and accumulation of total body water, even in Child–Pugh class A patients. This goes hand in

hand with sodium retention, which therefore does not usually lead to hypernatraemia. On the contrary, depletion of potassium, magnesium, phosphate, and other intracellular minerals is frequent. In an early study comparing parenteral nutrition with oral diet in cirrhotic patients with ascites, the response to diuretics was poorer in those receiving parenteral nutrition.

Zinc and selenium deficiencies have been observed in alcoholic and nonalcoholic liver disease. An impressive association between HE and zinc deficiency has been described in case reports. A deficiency in water-soluble vitamins, mainly group-B vitamins, is common in cirrhosis, especially that of alcoholic origin. Deficiency in fat-soluble vitamins has been observed in cholestasis-related steatorrhoea and bile salt deficiency, and in alcoholics.

Patients with hypophosphataemia after acetaminophen-induced liver damage have a better prognosis. Severe hypophosphataemia, however, results in respiratory insufficiency and dysfunction of the nervous system and erythrocytes, and thus serum phosphate levels should be monitored and corrected in order to support liver regeneration.

12.6 Disease-specific nutrition therapy

Acute liver disease

Acute hepatitis

Acute viral hepatitis is often associated with a varying degree of anorexia and the sensation of abdominal fullness leading to reduced food intake and weight loss. Depending on the magnitude of cholestasis, there may be an impairment of fat malabsorption. Nutrition therapy is warranted in malnourished subjects and when inadequate food intake persists. Since no data from formal trials are available, nutritional management should adopt the strategies outlined for ASH.

Acute liver failure

Without treatment, ALF is fatal within days. In the treatment of ALF, measures to stabilise the metabolism and vital functions and the treatment of brain oedema are of utmost importance. Hypoglycaemia is a clinically relevant and common problem in ALF, resulting from a loss of hepatic gluconeogenetic capacity, lack of glycogen, and hyperinsulinism. As a standard procedure, hypoglycaemia is treated by infusing glucose at a rate of 1.5–2 g/kg BW/day. In ALF, nutritional therapy has two objectives:

(1) Ensuring the adequate provision of energy, and especially ensuring euglycaemia by giving glucose, lipid, vitamins, and trace elements.
(2) Ensuring optimal rates of protein synthesis by providing an adequate intake of protein or amino acids.

In the absence of data from clinical trials, it is difficult to give recommendations. In recognition of this deficit, a survey on issues of parenteral nutrition in patients with ALF was carried out in European hepatology centres. One important result was that centres with a high caseload favour nasojejunal tube feeding, which can be carried out successfully in the majority of cases. It is therefore recommended that patients with ALF receive enteral nutrition via nasojejunal tube. No recommendations concerning a disease-specific composition of enteral formulas can currently be given. The recommended amount of enteral formula is based on the dosage used in critically ill patients with other disease entities.

Also, when using parenteral nutrition, sufficient glucose provision (2–3 g/kg BW/day) is mandatory for the prophylaxis and treatment of hypoglycaemia. Xylitol or sorbitol in exchange for glucose is of no proven benefit in acute ALF; moreover, both have to be metabolised by the liver before they can be utilised. Ensuring euglycaemia has been shown to confer a survival and morbidity benefit to critically ill patients regardless of aetiology. Great care must be taken to avoid hypoglycaemia, however.

There are no systematic data on the role of lipid as a nutrient in this condition. Exogenously applied lipid seems to be well tolerated by most patients. According to the European survey, two-thirds of participating hepatology centres give parenteral lipid in patients with ALF, the majority opting for an MCT/LCT emulsion. In clinical practice, glucose and lipid (0.8–1.2 g/kg BW/day) are given simultaneously; the use of lipid may be especially advantageous in the presence of insulin resistance.

Amino acid administration is not mandatory in hyperacute liver failure. In acute or subacute liver failure, however, amino acids (0.8–1.2 g/kg BW/day in parenteral nutrition) or protein (0.8–1.2 g/kg BW/

Table 12.3 Nutrition plans in acute liver failure (ALF).

Mode	Substrate	Rate
Enteral nutrition	Standard liquid diet (1.0 kcal/ml)	1.4 ml/kg BW/hour
	Liquid diet with high caloric density (1.5 kcal/ml)	1.0 ml/kg BW/hour
Parenteral nutrition	Glucose	2–3 g/kg BW/day
	Fat	0.8–1.2 g/kg BW/day
	Amino acids	0.8–1.2 g/kgBW/day

day in enteral nutrition) should be used in order to support protein synthesis (Table 12.3). The use of amino acid infusions has often been omitted for fear of aggravating existing hyperammonaemia and hyperaminoacidaemia and causing cerebral oedema and HE. In the survey, however, most centres reported giving IV amino acids. Since elevated arterial ammonia levels have been recognised as an independent predictor of poor outcome in ALF patients, it seems prudent to adjust the provision of amino acids according to the ammonia levels monitored. Some clinicians reported use of standard amino acid solutions, while the majority prescribed BCAA-enriched solutions, aiming for a correction of the deranged plasma amino acid pattern. While pathophysiological considerations provide a rationale for the use of liver-adapted solutions rich in BCAA, no clinical trial in acute ALF has shown an outcome benefit in comparison to standard solutions. Adequate metabolic monitoring is necessary in order to adapt nutrient provision to substrate utilisation so as to prevent substrate overload due to inappropriate intake. Strict control of the plasma levels of glucose (target: 5–8 mmol/l), lactate (target: <5.0 mmol/l), triglycerides (target: <3.0 mmol/l) and ammonia (target: <100 μmol/l) is necessary for this purpose (Table 12.4).

Chronic liver disease

Alcoholic steatohepatitis

In ASH patients, survival is poorer in those who do not consume enough food to meet requirements, while those who consume adequate amounts have a better survival. Thus, supplementary enteral nutrition is indicated when ASH patients cannot meet their caloric requirements through normal food and when there are no contraindications, such as ileus.

Table 12.4 Recommended target values for the monitoring of nutritional therapy in acute liver failure (ALF).

Variable	Target value
Blood glucose	5–8 mmol/ml
Serum triglycerides	<5.0 mmol/ml
Blood ammonia	<100 μmol/ml

Clinical trials in ASH patients show that supplementary enteral nutrition by either oral nutritional supplement or tube feeding ensures adequate energy and protein intake without the risk of complications such as HE. Enteral nutrition appears preferable to parenteral nutrition but there has been no large randomised trial comparing the feeding regimens in ASH patients.

In a controlled trial, enteral nutrition was as effective as glucocorticoids in patients with severe alcoholic hepatitis. Survivors of the 28-day treatment period who had been treated with enteral nutrition showed a lower mortality rate in the following year. Severely malnourished ASH patients who achieve an adequate intake of oral nutrition supplements have an improved survival, regardless of whether additional anabolic steroids are used. Malnourished ASH patients are at great risk of developing refeeding syndrome, and additional phosphate, potassium, and magnesium will be required, together with water-soluble vitamins.

In general, oral nutritional supplements are recommended, but if patients are not able to maintain adequate oral intake, tube feeding should be used. There is no evidence that the use of fine-bore nasogastric tubes poses an undue risk in patients with oesophageal varices. Use of percutaneous endoscopic gastrostomy (PEG) is associated with a higher risk of complications (due to ascites or varices) and is not recommended.

As a standard approach, standard whole protein formulas should be used, aiming for a total energy intake of 35 kcal/kg BW/day and a protein intake of 1.2–1.5 g/kg BW/day. Formulas with high energy density (1.5–2.4 kcal/ml) are preferable in patients with ascites, in order to avoid an unduly positive fluid balance (Table 12.5). When patients develop HE during enteral nutrition, BCAA-enriched formulas should be used. A direct comparison between a standard formula and a BCAA-enriched formula has not yet been made in ASH patients. It should be kept

Table 12.5 Nutrition plans in alcoholic steatohepatitis (ASH) or liver cirrhosis without encephalopathy. Note that, in general, 2000 kcal of liquid diet for enteral nutrition provides micronutrients to cover minimum daily requirements, while in parenteral nutrition micronutrients have to be added to the IV nutrition solution.

Mode	Substrate	Rate
Enteral nutrition	Liquid diet with high caloric density (1.5 kcal/ml)	1.0 ml/kg BW/hour
	Liquid diet with high caloric density (2.0 kcal/ml)	0.7 ml/kg BW/hour
Parenteral nutrition	Glucose	4.0 g/kg BW/day
	Fat	1.0 g/kg BW/day
	Amino acids	1.2–1.5 g/kg BW/day

in mind that in ASH patients, as in cirrhotics, a low protein intake can worsen HE.

Parenteral nutrition should be commenced immediately in ASH patients with moderate or severe malnutrition who cannot be fed sufficiently either orally or enterally. Parenteral nutrition supplemental to oral nutrition *ad libitum* failed to improve survival but had no adverse effect on mental state. ASH patients, like cirrhotics, who need to be managed nil by mouth for more than 12 hours (including nocturnal fasting!) should be given IV glucose at 2–3 g/kg BW/day (as discussed later in this section). When this fasting period lasts longer than 72 hours, total parenteral nutrition should be implemented.

Parenteral nutrition should be formulated and administered as in liver cirrhosis patients. All water-soluble vitamins, in particular thiamine, pyridoxine, nicotinamide, and folic acid, as well as fat-soluble vitamins, should be administered daily in a standard TPN dosage. Due to the high risk of Wernicke's encephalopathy, thiamine must be administered prior to starting IV glucose in alcoholic patients. Recently, high doses in both prophylaxis (250 mg intramuscular (IM) daily for 3–5 days) and treatment (500 mg IV t.i.d. for 2–3 days) of Wernicke's encephalopathy have been advocated. In jaundiced patients, vitamin K deficiency due to cholestasis-induced fat malabsorption may require IV vitamin K for the correction of coagulopathy.

Nonalcoholic steatohepatitis

In overweight individuals with NASH, weight reduction is the key to successful treatment. The histopathological changes of NASH can be ameliorated or even fully regressed by weight reduction, regardless of whether it is achieved by dietary counselling, bariatric surgery, or inhibition of intestinal fat absorption by orlistat. Likewise, insulin resistance and lipid metabolism can be improved. Currently no further recommendations can be made regarding the nutrient composition of a diet aimed at the treatment of NASH. Vitamin E 800 IU per day conferred beneficial effects on liver biochemistry and some aspects of liver histology, but not on fibrosis.

Targeting insulin resistance by use of insulin-sensitising drugs like pioglitazone or rosiglitazone, the beneficial effects on liver histology seem to be offset by a considerable gain in body weight and body fat mass.

Taken together, overweight NASH patients benefit from effective long-term weight reduction, regardless of the therapeutic strategy implemented.

Liver cirrhosis

In patients with cirrhosis, the primary goal is to ensure a quantitatively adequate nutrient intake. Increasing protein intake by nutrition therapy can decrease mortality. Adequate nutrition after successful treatment of portal hypertension by transjugular intrahepatic portosystemic stent-shunt has the potential to improve body composition (Figure 12.4). These observations demonstrate that poor nutritional status of cirrhotics must not be too readily accepted and viewed as an unchangeable and progressively deteriorating facet of this disease. Nutritional therapy can improve body composition, physical functioning, and survival in cirrhosis.

Regarding the method of nutritional intervention, nutritional counselling alone or combined with oral nutritional supplements will often prove successful. Supplemental enteral nutrition should be given when patients with liver cirrhosis cannot meet their nutritional requirements from normal food despite adequate individualised nutritional counselling. Patients should be instructed to take the nutritional supplement late in the evening or at bedtime. Nocturnal supplemental feeding improves total body protein status better than daytime feeding, most likely because of the shortening of the interval between a normal evening meal and breakfast. Very often, the spontaneous food intake of cirrhotic patients is overestimated and the therapeutic gain by the timely use of tube feeding

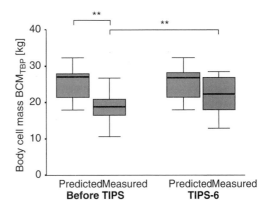

Figure 12.4 Reduced body cell mass (BCM_{TBP}) assessed by total body potassium counting in cirrhotic patients before TIPS (transjugular intrahepatic portalsystemic stent-shunt). Patient values are compared to predicted normal values. Six months after TIPS and advice to follow the ESPEN dietary recommendations, BCM_{TBP} has increased significantly and is no longer different from predicted values. ** indicates $p < 0.01$. Reprinted from J Hepatol, 40: Plauth M et al. Weight gain after transjugular intrahepatic portosystemic shunt is associated with improvement in body composition in malnourished patients with cirrhosis and hypermetabolism, pp. 228–233, Copyright 2004, with permission from Elsevier.

is missed. Due to somnolence and psychomotor dysfunction, oral nutrition is often insufficient, already in subclinical, or grade I HE. Therefore, tube feeding may be required to ensure adequate nutrient provision. The risk of aspiration in uncooperative patients and those with advanced HE should be considered when deciding on whether to feed by the enteral or the parenteral route. As already discussed for ASH patients, tube feeding is not contraindicated in the presence of oesophageal varices, but the use of PEGs in cirrhotics is discouraged. Ascites, impairment of the coagulation system, and portosystemic collateral circulation due to portal hypertension have been reported as contraindications to PEG placement.

On enteral nutrition, cirrhotic patients should achieve a total energy intake of 35 kcal/kg BW/day and a protein intake of 1.2–1.5 g/kg BW/day using a standard whole-protein formula. It was shown that diets containing 1.2 g/kg BW/day protein could safely be administered to patients with cirrhosis suffering from episodic HE, and (even transient) protein restriction did not confer any benefit to patients during an episode of encephalopathy. In stable cirrhotics, formulas enriched in BCAA are not necessary. Such formulas are helpful in the very select subgroup of protein-intolerant patients with HE and when patients develop HE on a standard enteral nutrition diet. In stable cirrhotics, long-term (12- and 24-month) nutritional supplementation with oral BCAA granulate as an oral nutritional supplement has the potential to slow the progression of hepatic failure and prolong event-free survival, but this treatment is not reimbursed in many countries.

Regarding trace elements and vitamins, in a pragmatic approach, liberal supplementation is recommended in the first 2 weeks of nutritional support, because the laboratory diagnosis of a specific deficiency may be more costly and would delay the provision of micronutrients. Oral zinc supplementation as a treatment of HE has been disappointing in controlled trials, despite encouraging case reports. Urea production capacity increased after oral zinc application when previously subnormal plasma levels were normalised. Supplementing zinc and vitamin A may indirectly improve food intake and nutritional state by improving dysgeusia. Supplementation with calcium and vitamin D is recommended for patients with osteopenia, although this did not result in any improvement in bone density in patients with primary biliary cirrhosis; in female patients, oestrogen substitution proved to be much more effective. Vitamin B_1 must be provided to all patients with alcoholic liver disease before providing glucose, as outlined earlier in this section.

Parenteral nutrition is a valuable second-line option and must be implemented immediately when moderately or severely malnourished cirrhotics cannot be nourished sufficiently by either the oral or the enteral route. Parenteral nutrition should be considered in patients with unprotected airways and advanced HE when swallow and cough reflexes are compromised.

Patients with liver cirrhosis suffer from a depletion of hepatic glycogen stores and are thus less prepared to adequately master periods of even short-term food deprivation. A late-evening carbohydrate snack can improve protein metabolism in cirrhotics and thus every patient with cirrhosis who needs to be managed nil by mouth for more than 12 hours (including nocturnal fasting) should be given IV glucose at 2–3 g/kg BW/day as the minimum metabolic intervention. When this fasting period lasts longer than 72 hours, TPN should be implemented; as an intermediary measure, hypocaloric peripheral parenteral nutrition may be used when fasting periods are expected to last for less than 72 hours.

If parenteral nutrition is used as the exclusive form of nutrition, the IV provision of all macro- and micronutrients must be ensured from the beginning of TPN. Carbohydrate should be given as glucose to cover 50–60% of non-protein energy requirements. Ensuring euglycaemia has been shown to confer a survival and morbidity benefit to critically ill patients regardless of aetiology. Great care, however, must be taken to avoid hypoglycaemia. In case of hyperglycaemia, glucose infusion should be reduced to 2–3 g/kg BW/day, and IV insulin infusion should be used.

The simultaneous infusion of lipid and glucose provides a better metabolic profile than glucose alone. Plasma clearance and oxidation of infused lipids are normal in cirrhosis patients. Regarding the optimal composition of IV oxidative fuels, only limited information is available. European guidelines recommend fat provision to cover 40–50% of non-protein energy requirements using emulsions with a content of n-6 unsaturated fatty acids lower than in traditional pure soy bean oil emulsions. Compared to the traditional soy bean-based LCT emulsions (n-6:n-3 = 8:1), new fat emulsions have a lower content of n-6 unsaturated fatty acids due to the admixture of MCTs and/or olive oil and/or fish oil, rendering them less suppressive to leukocyte and immune function and less stimulant of pro-inflammatory modulators.

The infusion of amino acids should provide 1.2 g/kg BW/day in compensated cirrhosis without malnutrition and 1.5 g/kg BW/day in decompensated cirrhosis with severe malnutrition. In clinical trials, studying patients with liver cirrhosis and severe HE, the provision of protein or amino acids ranged from 0.6 to 1.2 g/kg BW/day. In patients with alcoholic hepatitis or alcoholic cirrhosis with or without low-grade HE, the provision ranged from 0.5 to 1.6 g/kg BW/day. For parenteral nutrition in compensated cirrhosis, amino acid solutions with a special BCAA-enriched 'hepatic formula' composition are not required.

For parenteral nutrition of cirrhotics with overt HE amino acid solutions with a special 'hepatic formula' high in BCAA (35–45%) but low in tryptophan, aromatic and sulphur-containing amino acids have been developed (Table 12.6). Such solutions

Table 12.6 Nutrition plan in liver cirrhosis and encephalopathy (III°–IV°), particularly after gastrointestinal haemorrhage.

Mode	Substrate	Rate
Enteral nutrition	Liquid diet of high caloric density (1.2 kcal/ml) enriched in BCAA	1.2 ml/kg BW/hour
Parenteral nutrition	Glucose	4.0 g/kg BW/day
	Fat	1.0 g/kg BW/day
	BCAA-enriched amino acid solution	1.0–1.2 g/kg BW/day

help to correct the amino acid imbalance in liver cirrhosis. The efficacy of BCAA-enriched IV solutions in the treatment of HE has been studied and a meta-analysis showed an improvement in mental state by the BCAA-enriched IV solutions, but no definite benefit in survival. HE of cirrhotic patients, however, is precipitated by serious and life-threatening complications such as infection or haemorrhage, which are more potent determinants of survival than HE. It is therefore not surprising that BCAA-enriched parenteral nutrition regimens failed to improve short-term survival. Likewise, in a Cochrane analysis of seven randomised controlled trials studying patients with acute HE, the parenteral BCAA administration had a significant positive effect on the course of HE but not on survival. A BCAA-enriched complete amino acid solution should be given in more severe HE (III°–IV°). Blood from gastrointestinal haemorrhage is a protein source of low biological value, leading to BCAA antagonism. This antagonism leads to hyperammonaemia, but HE can be overcome by the infusion of isoleucine alone. Isoleucine solutions for IV infusions are not commercially available, however. Special hepatic-formula amino acid solutions contain high amounts of isoleucine and of the other BCAAs, leucine and valine.

For parenteral nutrition, water, electrolytes, water- and fat-soluble vitamins, and trace elements should be given daily in order to cover daily requirements. Trace elements should be administered daily in a standard TPN dose. In a pragmatic approach, routine administration of twice the normal daily requirement of zinc (= 2×5 mg/day) is recommended. Malnourished cirrhotic patients are in danger of developing refeeding syndrome, and additional phosphate, potassium, and magnesium may be required.

Perioperative nutrition

Nutrition therapy prior to elective surgery should be managed according to the recommendations given for the underlying disease, which most likely is liver cirrhosis in the majority of cases. Cirrhotic patients have a reduced rate of complications and an improved nitrogen economy after abdominal surgery if they receive nutritional support instead of just fluid and electrolytes. It may safely be assumed that enteral nutrition in the early postoperative period yields even better results; however, no studies have compared the two regimens in liver cirrhosis. A beneficial effect on gut permeability of sequential parenteral/enteral nutrition (via jejunostomy) as compared to parenteral nutrition alone or no postoperative nutrition has been reported.

Cirrhotic patients should receive early postoperative (additional) parenteral nutrition after surgery if they cannot be nourished sufficiently by the oral/enteral route. In cirrhotic patients undergoing liver resection, oesophageal transection, and splenectomy or splenorenal shunt, the rate of HE was not increased when a conventional rather than a BCAA-enriched amino acid solution was used.

Liver transplantation

Although the prognostic relevance of under-nutrition in transplant candidates is well recognised, it has not yet been shown that preoperative nutritional intervention improves clinically relevant outcomes. However, nutritional therapy in undernourished cirrhotic patients is clearly indicated, as outlined above. In the only randomised trial addressing this question, there was no advantage of oral nutrition supplements over nutritional counselling and normal food in adults. Since normal food and nutritional counselling lead to the same adequate intake as when oral nutrition supplements are added, both regimens are considered similarly effective. Paediatric transplant patients with predominantly cholestatic liver disease show a better increase in BCM if they receive BCAA-enriched formula.

After liver transplantation, normal food and/or enteral nutrition should be initiated within 12–24 hours postoperatively in order to achieve lower rates of morbidity, complications, and cost than on parenteral nutrition. Whole-protein formulas with or without pre- and probiotics or peptide-based formulas via catheter jejunostomy have been used for early enteral nutrition of adult liver-transplant recipients. Nasogastric or nasojejunal tubes after endoscopic placement or via catheter jejunostomy placed during laparotomy are used.

In hepatic transplant patients, the principles of parenteral nutrition are not different from those in major abdominal surgery. In the early postoperative phase, hyperglycaemia due to disturbed glucose metabolism and insulin resistance should be managed by reducing glucose intake because higher insulin doses are unable to increase glucose oxidation. The diabetogenic potential of the immunosuppressant tacrolimus can be lowered by reducing its dose without undue risk of rejection. Regarding lipid emulsions, an improved functioning of the reticuloendothelial system was observed when using MCT/LCT emulsions with a lower content of *n*-6 unsaturated fatty acids compared to pure soy bean oil emulsions.

After transplantation, there is a considerable nitrogen loss, and patients remain in negative nitrogen balance for up to 4 weeks, necessitating an increase in the provision of protein or amino acids. Protein or amino acid intakes of 1.0–1.5 g/kg BW/day have been reported. There is no need to use a BCAA-enriched amino acid solution after liver transplantation.

In transplanted patients, the often pre-existing chronic dilutional hyponatraemia should be corrected carefully in order to avoid central pontine myelinolysis. Magnesium levels need to be monitored in order to detect and treat ciclosporin- or tacrolimus-induced hypomagnesaemia. Postoperative hypophosphataemia and its possible relation to parenteral nutrition following right hemihepatectomy in living donors has been reported by some but not all study groups.

At present, no specific recommendations can be made with regard to optimal organ-donor conditioning. Fatty liver is known to be a risk factor for primary graft malfunction. No data are available addressing the role of nutritional management of the organ donor. Animal data indicate that the balanced nutrition of a brain-dead liver donor, using moderate amounts of carbohydrate, lipid (long-chain fatty acids and possibly fish oil), and amino acids, is associated with improved function of the transplanted organ. The value of donor or organ conditioning that aims to reduce ischaemia/reperfusion damage in humans by provision of high doses of arginine or glutamine is unclear.

Acknowledgements

This chapter has been revised and updated by Mathias Plauth and Tatjana Schütz, based on the original chapter by Marietjie G Herselman, Demetre Labadarios, Christo J Van Rensburg, and Aref A Haffejee.

References and further reading

Cabré E, González-Huix F, Abad A, Esteve M, Acero D, Fernández Bañares F, et al. Effect of total enteral nutrition on the short-term outcome of severely malnourished cirrhotics: a randomized controlled trial. Gastroenterology 1990; 98: 715–720.

Cabré E, Rodriguez-Iglesias, Caballeria J, Quer JC, Sanchez-Lombrana JL, Pares A, et al. Short- and long-term outcome of severe alcohol-induced hepatitis treated with steroids or enteral nutrition: a multicenter randomized trial. Hepatology 2000; 32: 36–42.

Clemmesen JO, Kondrup J, Ott P. Splanchnic and leg exchange of amino acids and ammonia in acute liver failure. Gastroenterology 2000; 118: 1131–1139.

Córdoba J, López-Hellín J, Planas M, Sabín P, Sanpedro F, Castro F, et al. Normal protein for episodic hepatic encephalopathy: results of a randomized trial. J Hepatol 2004; 41: 38–43.

Dharancy S, Lemyze M, Boleslawski E, Neviere R, Declerck N, Canva V, et al. Impact of impaired aerobic capacity on liver transplant candidates. Transplantation 2008; 86: 1077–1083.

Kearns PJ, Young H, Garcia G, Blaschke T, O'Hanlon G, Rinki M, et al. Accelerated improvement of alcoholic liver disease with enteral nutrition. Gastroenterology 1992; 102: 200–205.

Kondrup J, Müller MJ. Energy and protein requirements of patients with chronic liver disease. J Hepatol 1997; 27: 239–247.

Marchesini G, Bianchi G, Merli M, Amodio P, Panella C, Loguercio C, et al. Nutritional supplementation with branched-chain amino acids in advanced cirrhosis: a double-blind, randomized trial. Gastroenterology 2003; 124: 1792–1801.

Merli M, Riggio O, Dally L; PINC. What is the impact of malnutrition on survival in liver cirrhosis Does malnutrition affect survival in cirrhosis? Hepatology 1996; 23: 1041–1046.

Müller MJ, Lautz HU, Plogmann B, Burger M, Korber J, Schmidt FW. Energy expenditure and substrate oxidation in patients with cirrhosis: the impact of cause, clinical staging and nutritional state. Hepatology 1992; 15: 782–794.

Olde Damink SWM, Jalan R, Deutz NEP, de Jong CHC, Redhead DN, Hynd P, et al. Isoleucine infusion during 'simulated' upper gastrointestinal bleeding improves liver and muscle protein synthesis in cirrhotic patients. Hepatology 2007; 45: 560–568.

Peng S, Plank LD, McCall JL, Gillanders LK, McIlroy K, Gane EJ. Body composition, muscle function, and energy expenditure in patients with liver cirrhosis: a comprehensive study. Am J Clin Nutr 2007; 85: 1257–1266.

Plank LD, Metzger DJ, McCall JL, Barclay KL, Gane EJ, Streat SJ, et al. Sequential changes in the metabolic response to orthotopic liver transplantation during the first year after surgery. Ann Surg 2001; 234: 245–255.

Plank LD, McCall JL, Gane EJ, Rafique M, Gillanders LK, McIlroy K, et al. Pre- and postoperative immunonutrition in patients undergoing liver transplantation: a pilot study of safety and efficacy. Clin Nutr 2005; 24: 288–296

Plank LD, Gane EJ, Peng S, Muthu C, Mathur S, Gillanders L, et al. Nocturnal nutritional supplementation improves total body protein status of patients with liver cirrhosis: a randomized 12-month trial. Hepatology 2008; 48: 557–566.

Plauth M, Schütz T, Buckendahl DP, Kryemann G, Pirlich M, Grüngrieff S, et al. Weight gain after transjugular intrahepatic portosystemic shunt is associated with improvement in body composition in malnourished patients with cirrhosis and hypermetabolism. J Hepatol 2004; 40: 228–233.

Schütz T, Bechstein WO, Neuhaus P, Lochs H, Plauth M. Clinical practice of nutrition in acute liver failure – a European survey. Clin Nutr 2004; 23: 975–982.

Schütz T, Hudjetz H, Roske A-E, Katzorke C, Kreymann G, Budde K, et al. Weight gain in long-term survivors of kidney or liver transplantation – another paradigm of sarcopenic obesity? Nutrition 2012; DOI: 10.1016/j.nut.2011.09.019.

Sechi G, Serra A. Wernicke's encephalopathy: new clinical settings and recent advances in diagnosis and management. Lancet Neurol 2007; 6: 442–455.

Selberg O, Böttcher J, Tusch G, Pichlmayr R, Henkel E, Müller MJ. Identification of high- and low-risk patients before liver transplantation: a prospective cohort study of nutritional and metabolic parameters in 150 patients. Hepatology 1997; 25: 652–657.

European guidelines

Plauth M, Cabré E, Riggio O, Assis-Camilo M, Pirlich M, Kondrup J, et al. ESPEN guidelines on enteral nutrition: liver disease. Clin Nutr 2006; 25: 285–294.

Plauth M, Cabré E, Campillo B, Kondrup J, Marchesini G, Schütz T, et al. ESPEN guidelines on parenteral nutrition: hepatology. Clin Nutr 2009; 28: 436–444.

13
Nutrition and the Pancreas

Paula McGurk,[1] Marinos Elia,[2] and Jean-Fabien Zazzo[3]

[1] University Hospital Southampton NHS Foundation Trust, UK
[2] University Hospital Southampton, UK
[3] Hôpital Antoine-Béclère (Assistance Publique-Hôpitaux de Paris), France

13A   DIABETES MELLITUS

Paula McGurk and Marinos Elia

Key messages

- The recent increase in the prevalence of diabetes, which currently affects about 5% or more of the populations of many countries and which is expected to continue to increase in the future, is largely attributable to the rapid growth of obesity. Prevention and treatment of obesity can prevent and treat diabetes or make its management easier.
- Poor metabolic control in those with diabetes increases the risk of short-tem complications (e.g. hypoglycaemia and hyperglycaemia, both of which can produce coma) and long-term complications, such as retinopathy, nephropathy and neuropathy. Good metabolic control, which intimately involves diet, can prevent or delay the appearance of these complications.
- Establishing good metabolic control involves balancing dietary intake, which elevates the blood glucose concentration, with physical activity and insulin/oral hypoglycaemic agents, both of which lower the blood glucose concentration. The diet recom-

mended for diabetes is generally similar to the healthy diet recommended for the general population, but the temporal pattern of food ingestion is more important in those with diabetes than those without.
- Special dietary regimens are required when metabolic instability has developed, for example in diabetic ketoacidosis, or when major changes in dietary intake, physical activity, and insulin sensitivity are expected to occur (e.g. after elective or accidental injury or severe infection).
- In women of child-bearing age with diabetes, poor glycaemic control at the time of conception and early pregnancy are associated with a several-fold increased risk of developing malformations in the offspring. Good glycaemic control during this period can prevent the malformations. The infant of the diabetic mother is prone to neonatal hypoglycaemia, which can be prevented by precautionary regimens.

13A.1 Introduction

Prevalence

Diabetes mellitus is a chronic condition caused by inherited and/or acquired deficiency in the production of insulin by the pancreas or by the ineffectiveness of the insulin produced. The consequent hyperglycaemia and associated metabolic disturbance cause damage to the body systems, in particular the blood vessels and nerves.

Diabetes is a major clinical and public health problem, with important nutritional implications with respect to both its causes and its consequences. The estimated prevalence of diabetes worldwide in 2011 was 366 million, and by 2030 it is expected to rise to 552 million. This projected increase is largely due to the obesity 'epidemic', which is affecting both low- and high-income countries, but especially low-income countries, where the propensity to obesity-induced diabetes is greater. Indeed, obesity can increase the

Clinical Nutrition, Second Edition. Edited by Marinos Elia, Olle Ljungqvist, Rebecca J Stratton and Susan A Lanham-New.
© 2013 The Nutrition Society. Published 2013 by Blackwell Publishing Ltd.

risk of type 2 diabetes by as much as 50–100 times, which helps explain the distribution of diabetes both within countries and between countries. The International Diabetes Federation estimates that in 2011, the five countries with the largest number of people with diabetes were China, India, the United States of America, Russia, and Brazil. In the UK, it is estimated that more than 1 in 20 people have diabetes (diagnosed or undiagnosed). In 2011, those with diagnosed diabetes in the UK amounted to 2.9 million people, and by 2025 it is estimated that this will increase to 5 million people. Low-birth-weight babies are more likely to develop type 2 diabetes in adult life (in both developed and developing countries), implying that early nutritional influences *in utero* programme individuals to develop maturity-onset diabetes (and cardiovascular problems) several decades later.

Pathogenesis and types of diabetes

Two distinct pathways for the pathogenesis of the condition have been identified. Diabetes mellitus caused by the absolute or near-absolute deficiency of insulin is known as type 1 diabetes, which usually presents in childhood. Diabetes mellitus associated with insulin resistance is known as type 2 diabetes, which usually presents in adults. However, the distinction between the two types is not absolute, since patients with type 2 diabetes may require insulin, and those with type 1 diabetes may present in adulthood, although not usually beyond 30 years of age. While the nomenclature of diabetes continues to change, it is reasonable to regard types 1 and 2 diabetes as being at the extreme ends of a spectrum, in which there is an overlap in the middle. Monogenetic causes of diabetes account for a small proportion of the total. One of the genetic causes is maturity-onset diabetes of the young (MODY), which arises from mutations of an autosomal dominant gene, and is associated with presentation of diabetes before the age of 25 years.

Type 1 diabetes occurs because the beta cells of the pancreas, which produce insulin, are destroyed by the body's own immune system. Type 1 sufferers are therefore dependent on exogenous administration of insulin for survival. It is less common than type 2 diabetes and accounts for around 10% of all people with the condition.

Type 2 diabetes, formerly known as non-insulin-dependent diabetes, develops when the beta cells are able to produce insulin but there is resistance to the action of insulin, so that hyperglycaemia occurs, often in association with an elevated circulating insulin concentration. Unlike in type 1 diabetes, in which the pancreas cannot be stimulated to produce insulin, in type 2 diabetes the pancreas can be stimulated to produce more insulin.

Other forms of diabetes also exist, including gestational diabetes mellitus (GDM; also called type 3 diabetes). GDM is largely attributed to insulin resistance, which typically presents in the second trimester of pregnancy and progresses into the third, when insulin sensitivity can be reduced by as much as 80%. The incidence of GDM may range from 1 to 14%, and it accounts for 90% of all diabetes in pregnancy, the remainder being due almost exclusively to type 1 and type 2 diabetes.

Glycaemic control, nutrition, and insulin

In healthy people, the circulating glucose concentration is tightly controlled within the range of 3.4–7.8 mmol/l, despite intermittent ingestion of food containing varying amounts of carbohydrate, episodes of fasting – which may be prolonged for 14 hours or more – and episodes of exercise of varying intensity. Between meals, most of the circulating glucose is largely derived from glycogen that has previously been deposited in the liver and muscle following meal ingestion. After an overnight fast, glucose is released into the circulation at a rate of about 200 g per day, the majority of which arises from glycogen, and the remainder from gluconeogenesis, mainly in the liver and to a lesser extent the kidney. Under normal circumstances, the brain uses glucose (about 120 g per day) as its major energy source, although it can also use ketone bodies during starvation. Hypoglycaemia in the absence of hyperkeonaemia implies that the brain is deprived of nutritional fuel, which can rapidly cause confusion and unconsciousness. Prolonged hypoglycaemia can cause permanent brain damage. Acute hyperglycaemia also has adverse effects, including fluid shifts, dehydration, and even coma and death.

Insulin has a key role in glucose homeostasis in both health and disease. The so-called 'diabetes of injury' arises from systemic stress or inflammation and is generally associated with insulin resistance. As a major regulatory hormone, insulin is normally released from the pancreas in response to dietary nutrients (mainly glucose), so that its concentration increases many times above fasting values, facilitating, along with other regulatory hormones or signals, glucose homeostasis. In diabetes, this regulation is disturbed. Key aspects of glucose transport into cells, insulin-signalling pathways, and insulin resistance are briefly summarised in this section.

Glucose transporters

Due to the presence of the lipid bilayer, water-soluble molecules such as glucose do not directly cross cell membranes. Glucose transport is facilitated by a group of proteins (GLUT transporters), of which more than a dozen have been identified. The first four have been well characterised. GLUT-1 and GLUT-3 are found in most cells. They have a high affinity for glucose, which means that glucose uptake can be maintained even at low circulating concentrations, and so account for basal non-insulin-mediated glucose uptake (GLUT-3 is the main glucose transporter for the brain). GLUT-2 transporters are found on the beta cells of the pancreas (and hypothalamus and other cells) and are involved in glucose sensing. Unlike GLUT-1 and GLUT-3, which show little or no increase in transport at higher ambient glucose concentrations, GLUT-2 transporters have a low affinity for glucose (high Michaelis constant (Km) – that concentration of a substrate that gives half-maximal activity), which means that transport increases as glucose concentration rises to high levels, so that the concentration in the beta cell reflects that in the circulating, especially since the transport is bidirectional. Although GLUT-3-mediated transport is not stimulated by insulin, it triggers release of insulin from beta cells, which has multiple effects on insulin-sensitive tissues. GLUT-4, which is found in skeletal muscle, cardiac muscle, and adipose tissue, is insulin-sensitive and is involved in insulin-regulated glucose storage. Insulin stimulates the movement of cytoplasmic vesicles containing GLUT-4 (which is synthesised by ribosomes and sequestered into vesicles by the Golgi apparatus) so that they fuse with the cell membrane to increase the density of GLUT-4 transporters on the cell membrane and facilitate increased glucose uptake into cells.

Insulin-signalling pathways

To exert metabolic effects, insulin has first to bind to the insulin receptor. This receptor, which consists of four subunits, has a molecular weight of ~320 kDa and is encoded by a single gene, located on chromosome 19. The activation of the insulin transmembrane receptor leads to phosphorylation of the amino acid tyrosine in specific proteins within the cell, which in turn initiate a cascade of three major intracellular signalling pathways. One of these ultimately leads to the translocation of GLUT-4 from within the cell to the outer part of the membrane of insulin-sensitive tissues (see above), such as muscle and adipose, with resulting facilitation of glucose uptake into cells. Another signalling pathway involves phophatidylinositol 3-kinase (PI3K), which mediates many of the metabolic functions of insulin. The third major pathway, the MAP kinase (mitogen-activated protein kinase) pathway, is linked to enhanced cell growth. Control of these insulin-signalling pathways is complex and not entirely understood, although they can be viewed as being partly autoregulatory, with a negative feedback from downstream changes produced by the cascade(s), and partly non-autoregulatory, involving signals from unrelated pathways (e.g. those associated with inflammation). A better understanding of these pathways may provide deeper insights into insulin resistance and new drug therapies for treating diabetes.

Insulin resistance

Despite extensive research to elucidate the mechanism of glucose intolerance and insulin resistance in type 2 diabetes, the processes involved are still not fully understood. It seems that altered insulin-receptor density on cell membranes is not the major cause of the common variety of insulin resistance in type 2 diabetes or obesity. At least part of it is related to disturbances in signals generated in the PI3K pathway. Signals involved in inflammatory pathways are also involved. Triglycerides and fatty acids, both of which are elevated in obesity and type 2 diabetes, are also thought to play a key role, especially since fatty acids compete with glucose for oxidation. Although there are still aspects of these competitive interactions that are not fully elucidated, part of the fatty acid effect appears to involve GLUT-4 receptors, which can be rate-limiting to glucose uptake in at least some circumstances. The exact nature of the lipid moiety responsible for insulin resistance caused by fatty acids is unclear. Exercise can reduce insulin resistance, and part of this process involves insulin-induced GLUT-4 translocation (see earlier in this section). However, muscle activity can stimulate glucose uptake in the absence of increasing insulin levels. Insulin sensitivity to glucose does not necessarily mirror insulin sensitivity to fatty acid and amino acid metabolism, which emphasises further the complexity of the processes involved.

Consequences of poor metabolic control

In the short term, poor metabolic control of diabetes may lead to confusion and collapse, and in the long term it may lead to the development of comorbidities, such as cardiovascular disease and debilitating complications that affect the nerves, eyes, kidneys, and other organs. Some of the long-term complications of diabetes are considered to be due to damage caused to large vessels (macrovascular damage, producing atherosclerosis, which predisposes to common conditions such as myocardial infarction, stroke, and hypertension) and small vessels (microvascular complications, which are much more specific to diabetes, and which can affect the retina, leading to blindness, renal glomeruli, leading to renal failure, and nerves, leading to neuropathy). At least some of this damage is mediated by the presence of an abnormal lipid profile: elevated cholesterol, low-density lipoprotein (LDL), and triacylglycerol concentrations, and reduced HDL concentrations.

Good metabolic control can help prevent both short-term problems and long-term complications, which may appear decades later.

13A.2 Presentation and diagnosis

Presentation

Type 1 diabetes usually presents with a 2–8 week history of polyuria (induced by glycosuria, which develops as a consequence of hyperglycaemia), thirst (due to dehydration), and weight loss. Ketone bodies, formed from the breakdown of fat as a result of insulin deficiency, can cause a 'pear drop'-like smell from the breath. Ketone bodies can be readily detected in urine.

Type 2 diabetes can present with a diverse range of complications, such as repeated skin and urine infections (associated with hyperglycaemia), retinopathy,

tingling and numbness of the feet (neuropathy), cardiovascular disease, and erectile dysfunction. Subacute presentations over months or longer can also occur, with a mixture of polyuria and thirst on the one hand and other complications, such as infections, on the other.

Diagnosis

The diagnosis of diabetes is based on history and examination, and on biochemical tests involving measurement of glucose (see Table 13A.1).

Alternative laboratory criteria for diagnosing diabetes mellitus are also available. One of these concerns haemoglobin, which is glycated with glucose. If the circulating glucose concentration has been high in recent weeks, the extent of glycation (typically reported as % HbA1c or mmol/mol Hb) is increased. Since red cells survive for about 120 days, the % HbA1c is influenced by the circulating glucose concentration over this period. In normal subjects, the values range from 4 to 6% (20 to 42 mmol/mol), and in diabetics it is desirable for HbA1c levels to be less than 6.5% (48 mmol/mol), although they may be considerably higher.

According to a World Health Organization (WHO) report published in 2011, HbA1c can be used as a diagnostic test for diabetes, providing that:

- stringent quality assurance tests are in place;
- assays are standardised to criteria aligned to international reference values;
- there are no conditions present that preclude its accurate measurement.

Table 13A.1 Diagnostic criteria of diabetes mellitus based on glucose concentration (WHO, 2006).

1. Diabetes symptoms (i.e. polyuria, polydipsia and unexplained weight loss) plus:
   - a random venous plasma glucose concentration > 11.1 mmol/l
   or
   - a fasting plasma glucose concentration > 7.0 mmol/l (whole blood > 6.1 mmol/l)
   or
   - 2-hour plasma glucose concentration > 11.1 mmol/l 2 hours after 75 g anhydrous glucose in an oral glucose tolerance test (OGTT)
2. With no symptoms, diagnosis should not be based on a single glucose determination but requires confirmatory plasma venous determination. At least one additional glucose test result on another day with a value in the diabetic range is essential: either fasting, from a random sample, or from the 2-hour post-glucose load. If the fasting or random values are not diagnostic, the 2-hour value should be used.

An HbA1c cut-off point of 6.5% is recommended for the diagnosis of diabetes. A value of less than 6.5% does not necessarily exclude diabetes diagnosed using a glucose tolerance test.

The diagnostic use of HbA1c needs to be interpreted with caution in some situations, such as recent onset of type 1 diabetes or recent onset of diabetes due to acute illness or drugs such as steroids or antipsychotic agents (included in the mixed category of type 4 diabetes). In these situations there has been insufficient time for HbA1c to increase. Vitamin supplements, such as vitamin C and E, and high cholesterol concentration may also influence the results.

HbA1c is often used to monitor long-term control of glucose in those with established diabetes

13A.3 Principles of diabetic management and the role of diet

The management of diabetes is underpinned by observations that good metabolic control can not only prevent short-term problems, such as those associated with hypo- and hyperglycaemia, but also long-term complications. However, it is recognised that beyond a certain stage of structural damage, for example beyond a certain stage of proliferative retinopathy, it may be difficult or impossible to attenuate the progression of diabetes through good metabolic control. This means that early preventive measures need to be implemented, and nutrition has a key role to play in this respect.

The sophisticated mechanisms associated with metabolic regulation of glucose and other nutrients in healthy subjects cannot be easily replicated in those with diabetes. These regulatory mechanisms are complex and are adapted to take into account variations in dietary intake and physical activity (and interactions between them), as well as variations in physical and psychological stresses associated with activities of daily living. Nevertheless, in diabetes attempts are made to balance an appropriate dietary intake (amount and composition of food) with an appropriate type and amount of insulin and physical activity. An increase in dietary intake, particularly of carbohydrate, while physical activity and drug therapy remain unaltered can cause hyperglycaemia, while a decrease in dietary intake can cause hypoglycaemia. An increase in physical activity can produce hypoglycaemia, while a decrease can produce hyperglycaemia. The individual components of a triad comprising drug therapy, physical activity, and dietary intake play a key role in glycaemic control (Figure 13A.1). Although they are individually considered later, it should be remembered that they operate simultaneously in an interactive manner.

In addition to these three factors, other variables can influence glycaemic control, including psychological stress and acute disease. For example, not only can gastroenteritis with vomiting reduce dietary intake, which tends to decrease the circulating glucose concentration, but it may also be associated with insulin resistance, which increases the glucose concentration, making glucose control difficult. Major elective surgery and accidental injury are also typically associated with a decrease in dietary intake and insulin resistance, and careful management is necessary in some circumstances. Following surgery (see Chapter 20 of *Surgery and Trauma* in this series), there is insulin resistance, and several of the postoperative complications are similar to those that occur in diabetes. Insulin resistance is also associated with low-grade inflammatory disease, for example in renal failure. Special nutritional problems, including those involving nasogastric and intravenous feeding, are discussed later. Guidelines for the effective management of both type 1 and type 2 diabetes have been issued by various national and international organisations, including the National Institute for Health and Clinical Excellence (NICE) in the UK.

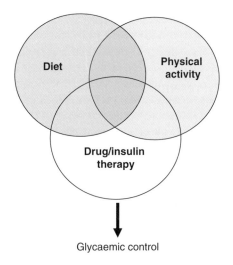

Figure 13A.1 Diet, physical activity, and drug/insulin therapy interact in regulating the circulating glucose concentration.

13A.4 Insulin/drugs

Insulin regimens

There are several different types of insulin, which vary in their speed of action and duration of activity.

- *Rapidly-acting analogues* (e.g. NovoRapid, Humalog) can be injected just before, during, or after food ingestion, and have a peak action at between 0 and 3 hours. They tend to last between 2 and 5 hours – only long enough to cover the effects of individual meals.
- *Long-acting analogues* (e.g. Lantus, Levemir) tend to be injected once daily in order to provide background insulin lasting approximately 24 hours. They can be administered independently of food as they do not have an obvious peak action.
- *Short-acting insulins* (e.g. Actrapid, Humulin S) should be injected 15–30 minutes before a meal to cover the rise in blood glucose levels that occurs after eating. Their peak action is between 2 and 6 hours and can last for up to 8 hours.
- *Medium- and longer-acting insulins* (e.g. Insulatard, Humulin I) are injected once or twice daily to provide background insulin or in combination with short-acting insulin/rapid-acting analogue. Their peak activity is between 4 and 12 hours and they can last up to 30 hours.
- *Mixed insulin* (e.g Humulin M3, Insuman Comb 50) is a combination of medium- and short-acting insulin.
- *Mixed analogue* (e.g. NovoMix 30, Humalog Mix 25) is a combination of medium-acting insulin and a rapid-acting analogue.

These insulin types may be given alone or in combination according to lifestyle, including mealtime routine. The 'basal bolus' regimen consists of combining a long-acting insulin, to provide lasting background cover, with a rapid-acting insulin, to cover the effects of carbohydrate meals/snacks, which are usually eaten three times daily (breakfast, lunch, and evening meal). This popular regimen can be modified to suit individuals according to lifestyle. For example, the dose of a rapidly-acting insulin can be increased before the large meal is taken. Another regimen involves the continuous subcutaneous administration of insulin, often rapid-acting insulin, using an insulin pump; 'boluses' are given by the patient at meal times. The pump attempts to imitate the healthy pancreas, although it delivers insulin into the peripheral circulation, whereas the pancreas delivers it into the portal circulation (where the insulin concentration is much higher than in peripheral blood), which produces important 'first-pass' metabolic effects in the liver. The main advantage of using insulin-pump therapy is that it allows flexibility in coping with different patterns of dietary intake and physical activity, both of which can vary from day to day. However, the pump is expensive, its use requires training, and local skin infections can occur. An alternative but less flexible option is the 'twice-daily fixed-dose insulin regimen', which involves a combination of a short- and an intermediate/longer-acting insulin injected twice daily, typically 20–30 minutes before breakfast and before the evening meal. This regimen is suitable for individuals who have a fairly fixed routine, in which physical activity and meals occur at similar times and in similar amounts each day.

Oral drugs

There are three main groups of oral drugs that are commonly used in the treatment of type 2 diabetes: biguanides, sulphonylureas, and thiazolidinediones (often referred to as 'glitazones'). The properties of some of these drugs are shown in Table 13A.2. The biguanide metformin, which increases insulin sensitivity, at least partly because it suppresses hepatic gluconeogenesis, is often used as the initial oral hypoglycaemic agent (in conjunction with an appropriate lifestyle change). This is partly because weight loss in overweight or obese individuals is more likely to be facilitated by metformin, which does not stimulate insulin secretion, than sulphonylureas, which do stimulate insulin secretion. Metformin has also been shown to have clear cardioprotective properties, to be as effective as sulphonylurea or insulin in reducing microvascular risk, and to have some beneficial effects independent of its hypoglycaemic actions. If metformin is inadequate in controlling the blood glucose concentration, another class of drug, such as a sulphonylurea or a glitazone, can be added; if these are insufficient, insulin may be used either alone or in combination with oral hypoglycaemic agents, which allows a lower dose of insulin to be administered.

Other drugs

New drugs (intravenous and oral) for the treatment of diabetes continue to be developed. Among these

Table 13A.2 Examples and properties of some oral drugs commonly used for the treatment of type 2 diabetes.

Generic name (trade name)	Min./max. dose	When taken	Mode of action	Comments
Biguanides				
Metformin (Glucophage)	500–3000 mg	With or after food	Reduced hepatic output	Drug of choice for overweight patients
Metformin prolonged-release (Glucopahge SR)	500–2000 mg	With or after evening meal, if once	Improved peripheral insulin sensitivity	Gastrointestinal side effects are initially common
		Breakfast and evening meal, if twice		Should be used cautiously in renal impairment
Sulphonylureas				
Glibenclamide (Glibenclamide)	2.5–15 mg	With or immediately after breakfast or first main meal of the day	Increased insulin secretion	Due to longer half life and risk of hypoglycaemia, use should generally be avoided in the elderly
Gliclazide (Diamicron)	40–320 mg	Before a meal		Intermediate half life
Gliclazide MR (Diamicron MR)	30–120 mg	With breakfast		Largely metabolised in the liver, but can be used in renal impairment
Glimepiride (Amaryl)	1–6 mg	Shortly before or with first main meal		Active metabolites excreted by the kidney and should be avoided in renal impairment
Glipizide (Minodiab)	2.5–20 mg	Before food		
Tolbutamide (Tolbutamide)	500–2000 mg	With or immediately after food		Lower maximal efficacy than other sulphonylureas
				Shorter half-life
Thiazolidinediones ('glitazones')				
Pioglitazone (Actos)	15–45 mg alone or in dual or triple therapy, or with insulin	With or without food	Increased peripheral sensitivity to insulin	Increased risk of bone fractures in women
				Contraindicated in liver impairment or heart failure

are the postprandial regulators, such as nateglinide and repaglinide, which are oral hypoglycaemic agents with predominant effects in the postprandial period. Another group of drugs of particular nutritional interest was developed from physiological observations that orally administered glucose produces greater insulin response than intravenous glucose. This is believed to be largely due to the release of two gastrointestinal peptides (glucose-dependent insulinotropic peptide (GIP) and glucagon-like-peptide-1 (GLP1)) which are clearly stimulated by oral and not intravenous administration of glucose. This so-called incretin effect appears to be attenuated in type 2 diabetes, and therefore injectable incretin analogues have been developed, with the aim of achieving better glycaemic control in type 2 diabetes (GIP and GLP1 are also putative physiological signals that suppress appetite). Inhibitors of the enzyme dipeptidyl peptide 4 (DPP4), which rapidly destroys GLP-1 (e.g. linagliptin and saxagliptin), are also available. The

thiazolinediones are another group of agents that reduce insulin resistance. They are commonly used in some centres, but they have a tendency to cause weight gain, and one of them (rosiglitazone) has been withdrawn from formularies because it was suspected of increasing risk of cardiovascular disease.

13A.5 Physical activity

Physical activity has clear beneficial effects on cardiovascular risk and can improve glycaemic control in diabetes, especially in the postprandial period. Physical activity has been shown to reduce mortality in diabetes and can be safely used in patients with type 2 diabetes treated by diet alone or in conjunction with oral hypoglycaemic agents. In those treated with insulin or drugs that stimulate insulin secretion, precautionary measures must be taken to prevent exercise-induced hypoglycaemia. Such precautionary measures may involve consuming additional carbohydrate in amounts that depend on the duration and intensity of the activity and on the blood glucose reading before the activity begins, or reducing the amount of insulin administered before activity. The blood glucose concentration should optimally be in the normal range before the activity is undertaken.

13A.6 Diet

Dietary intake has a special role to play in the management of diabetes, not only because it is one of the three main components influencing glycaemic control and metabolic function, but because it is the only one of the three components illustrated in Figure 13A.1 that can be used to treat hypoglycaemia (by taking a snack or drink containing a rapidly absorbed sugar). The other two components, physical activity and drug/insulin therapy, tend to reduce the blood glucose concentration and may predispose to hypoglycaemia.

Dietary advice for diabetes should be broadly based on the healthy eating principles that apply to the general population. However, there are specific considerations for diabetes, which relate to the timing of food intake. In a patient with a good 24-hour profile of glucose concentration, changes in the timing and distribution of the same diet during the day can cause hypoglycaemia and/or hyperglycaemia, which are not seen in healthy people. Personal preferences and willingness to change lifestyle, including dietary habits, need to be considered carefully when devising a care plan for patients with diabetes.

Dietary advice has tended to encourage a similar dietary intake from day to day, and a similar timing of meals. Such advice is simple and practical, and can result in good glycaemic control, especially when there is little or no day-to-day variation in drug/insulin therapy and physical activity. However, this approach demands a rather fixed lifestyle, which some patients find rather restrictive. Therefore, a variety of carbohydrate-counting regimes, such as the DAFNE regime (Dose Adjustment for Normal Eating), have been developed to allow greater versatility in lifestyle. Such regimens can be of considerable value to motivated subjects with type 1 diabetes who understand the principles of diabetic care. The

regimens involves self-management of diabetes through experience in undertaking regular blood glucose measurements and making appropriate adjustments in insulin infusion rates to match the carbohydrate ingested and physical activity undertaken or about to be undertaken. With appropriate training and supervision, such regimens improve glucose control without risk of hypoglycaemic episodes, and improve treatment satisfaction and quality of life. For individuals with type 2 diabetes, the effectiveness of 'carbohydrate counting' is largely unknown, although it appears to be of considerable value to some individuals. For those on a twice-daily fixed-insulin regimen there is less flexibility. Consistency in the quantity of carbohydrate and glycaemic index of foods on a daily basis is associated with improved HbA1c levels.

Since many individuals with type 2 diabetes are overweight, diet and lifestyle changes that promote weight loss are key aspects of the management of the condition. Glucose control can improve considerably after substantial weight loss, and the dose of drugs can be reduced or even stopped. The same has been observed after weight loss produced by bariatric surgery.

In summary, while the healthy diet for healthy people is also generally appropriate for people with diabetes, there are also specific considerations associated with the timing of food ingestion Further specific features of diabetic management in special circumstances are discussed in the rest of this section, after a consideration of the composition and properties of food ingested by subjects with diabetes.

Composition and properties of the diet
Carbohydrate
Advice about the composition of dietary intake in people with diabetes has varied substantially through recorded history, sometimes favouring high-fat diets and sometimes high-carbohydrate diets. In recent decades, high-carbohydrate diets have been in favour, especially those containing complex carbohydrates, for example starches rather than simple sugars. Therefore, it has been generally recommended that total carbohydrate should account for about 40–60% of total energy intake, and simple sugars such as sucrose less than 10% of total energy intake (but see next paragraph).

Sucrose

Although ingestion of sucrose has traditionally been regarded as having detrimental effects on glycaemic control, recent studies suggest that it does not affect glycaemic control differently from other carbohydrates, if the total amount of carbohydrate ingested is similar. However, the glycaemic response will depend on other food items ingested with the sucrose. Sucrose taken with a meal (e.g. with a breakfast that includes cereal) may have different effects from those produced when sucrose is taken alone. This is because the amount of sugar released into the small intestine for absorption depends on the gastric emptying rate, which is influenced by other dietary constituents, including fat.

Glycaemic index

The concept of the glycaemic index of foods, originally developed by Jenkins *et al.* (1981), was based on the overall glycaemic response to oral ingestion of food items containing carbohydrate. The aim was to provide clear guidance on food choice for those with diabetes. Although the glycaemic index of foods has been established following ingestion of individual food items, the glycaemic response can change substantially when other foods are taken simultaneously with the test food item. For example, a food with a high glycaemic index may exhibit an attenuated glycaemic response when ingested with fatty foods, which slow down gastric emptying. Nevertheless, a recent review demonstrated a 0.5% reduction in HbA1c (a marker of long-term glucose concentration in people with diabetes) in those who adopted a diet consisting of low-glycaemic foods, although only one of the studies was conducted specifically in adults with type 1 diabetes.

Dietary fibre

Dietary fibre has several beneficial effects, although there are no specific recommendations for those with diabetes. Amongst the putative beneficial effects of fibre are earlier satiation, which may be due to slowing of gastric emptying, and lower postprandial glucose changes, which may be partly due to slowing down of gastric-emptying effects and partly due to small-intestinal effects. Subjects ingesting high-fibre diets tend to show attenuated postprandial hyperglycaemic response, although some studies do not show significant effects, possibly because of differences in the type and amount of fibre used and differences in study design. The effect of fibre in weight reduction has generally been unimpressive.

Fat

Saturated fat should be limited and replaced by unsaturated fats, predominantly monounsaturated fats (MUFAs) within the range recommended in healthy guidelines for the population. Recommendations about the proportion of energy derived from fat are not etched in stone, but a fat intake of 35% or less of total energy intake is commonly advocated because of its demonstrable beneficial effects on lipid profiles, weight, and blood pressure.

Alcohol

For the general population, a moderate consumption of alcohol has been associated with a reduction in cardiovascular risk; this also generally applies to those with diabetes. However, alcohol poses several additional risks. In those receiving insulin or drugs that increase insulin production, alcohol tends to cause hypoglycaemia, which can be severe and last for up to 12 hours. Alcohol can also exacerbate hypertriglyceridaemia, which is common in many individuals with type 2 diabetes. Furthermore, since many people with type 2 diabetes tend to be overweight, the contribution of alcohol to total energy intake also needs to be considered.

Diet in special circumstances

Diabetes and pregnancy

A particular problem in women of childbearing age with diabetes is that poor glucose control in the early stages of pregnancy can produce a three- to eightfold increase in foetal malformations, which affect up to about 2% of pregnancies in those without diabetes. Clinical trials to achieve tight blood glucose control in the preconception period and the first trimester of pregnancy have demonstrated major reductions in malformations. Therefore, it is particularly important to emphasise the benefits of good glucose control in the preconception period and to reinforce this later. Appropriate dietary advice during this early period can help prevent distressing problems that manifest themselves later on in pregnancy or after delivery.

Newborn infant of the diabetic mother

A specific nutritional complication in the newborn infant of the diabetic mother is hypoglycaemia. This arises because maternal glucose crosses the placenta but insulin does not. The result is that the foetal pancreas hypersecretes insulin in response to the elevated glucose concentration, but when the supply of maternal glucose stops at delivery, rebound hypoglycaemia results. Therefore, it is important to measure the blood glucose concentration in the baby immediately after delivery and at regular intervals thereafter while an infusion of glucose infusion is provided to guard against hypoglycaemia. If by 12 hours glucose stability is established, the infusion can be weaned. The mother is encouraged to feed the baby as quickly as possible after delivery.

Artificial nutrition

A change from normal intermittent food ingestion to continuous administration of nutrients using parenteral nutrition or enteral tube feeding may occur in a patient with diabetes, for example when a swallowing problem develops following a stroke. This change in the pattern of nutrient delivery into the gut can destabilise glucose control, particularly in those receiving large bolus injections of short-acting insulin. Hypoglycaemic coma can occur, and this may be difficult to recognise if the patient is already confused or unconscious as a result of the underlying condition. Apart from changes in feeding schedule, which may be continuous 24-hour feeding, cyclic nocturnal feeding, or bolus feeding, changes in the amount of feed prescribed and weaning off these regimens while oral feeding is reintroduced can also destabilise glycaemic control, as can disease complications, such as acute infections. In unstable patients, regular glucose monitoring linked to a sliding-scale insulin regime is typically undertaken to establish control, although subcutaneous insulin injections may be used once such control is established.

Intensive care

Most patients in intensive care receive artificial nutritional support and insulin infusions. Inadvertently stopping nutritional support in such patients can result in hypoglycaemia, especially in those in whom the insulin is used to achieve tight glucose control (4.4–6.1 mmol/l). A study in the intensive-care unit suggested that glucose control is better achieved when a diabetes-specific feed is used instead of a standard feed. One of the constituents of such feeds is fructose, which does not require insulin for its initial metabolism in the liver. However, fructose also increases the risk of lactic acidosis, which is common in intensive-care units.

Surgery

Elective surgery often requires the patient to be fasted preoperatively. In addition, dietary intake is often reduced after major surgery, sometimes for many days, and this tends to reduce the blood glucose concentration. In contrast, the stress of surgery, which causes insulin resistance, tends to produce hyperglycaemia. The following is a typical management plan for insulin-dependent patients undergoing elective surgical operations; while there are several approaches to the management of patients with diabetes undergoing surgery, the following is a pragmatic and safe approach. Management may be easier if the patient is first on the morning operating list, although this may not be possible. The day before surgery, any long- or intermediate-acting insulin is substituted for short-acting insulin. An infusion of insulin (and potassium) is given during surgery and postoperatively. Glucose is monitored frequently and the dose of insulin and/or the glucose infusion is adjusted according to needs, which often change as oral food intake is reintroduced and increased towards normal intake. Studies exploring preoperative carbohydrate intake in conjunction with oral drugs or insulin suggest that gastric emptying is no different from healthy subjects. This may increase postoperative insulin sensitivity, as in healthy subjects.

A similar approach is used for emergency surgery, although an insulin infusion is often used before surgery to control the blood glucose concentration, which is often elevated.

Complications of diabetes

The risk of developing many of the complications of type 1 and type 2 diabetes is related to poor long-term glycaemic control and its duration. Trials suggest that the risk of developing complications can be reduced by better control, although little effect can be expected to occur in the advanced stages of the conditions.

Retinopathy

Retinopathy is caused by damage to the small blood vessels in the retina and is a common cause of partial-sightedness or blindness in diabetes. It can affect those with type 1 and type 2 diabetes and is correlated with the duration and extent of hyperglycaemia. Although no robust evidence has specifically emerged from investigations into the role of diet in the management of retinopathy, given that glycaemic control is of paramount general importance, dietary advice should not be overlooked.

There has been an interest in the link between eye disease and the antioxidant carotenoids lutein, which is widely distributed in the retina, and xeaxanthin, which is concentrated in the macula. The damage caused to the eye during the development of diabetic retinopathy and cataracts is associated with free-radical formation. Boosting antioxidant defences by administering carotenoids might attenuate or delay the appearance or progression of these conditions, but at present there is insufficient evidence to recommend routine use of xeaxanthine and lutein in the prevention and treatment of these conditions.

Nephropathy
Kidney damage is common in long-standing diabetes, but this can range from asymptomatic proteinurea to end-stage renal failure requiring dialysis. In the absence of a urinary-tract infection, nephropathy is characterised by persistent proteinuria of >500 mg of total protein per 24 hours or 300 mg albumen per 24 hours. There appear to be no randomised controlled trials investigating the efficacy of dietary interventions in the management of diabetes in kidney disease. A review examining the role of protein restriction in the management of diabetic nephropathy concluded that the evidence was not robust enough to justify routine use of protein restriction. However, the authors suggested that some people may respond favourably to low-protein diets, and therefore recommended a 6-month therapeutic trial, which should be closely monitored. Of course, chronic kidney disease may be associated with a range of altered nutrient requirements, such as a reduction in potassium and phosphate requirements, which need to be taken into account. Dietary treatment during pre- and post-dialysis treatment can vary, as indicated in Chapter 14.

Neuropathy
Diabetic neuropathy is one of the most common long-term complications of diabetes. Its aetiology is not fully understood, although it probably involves damage to the small vessels supplying blood to the nerves (vasa nervosa), as well as direct damage to the nerves. No specific dietary therapy is indicated, other than the application of the standard dietetic principles necessary to maintain good glycaemic control, which can help prevent or delay the onset of neuropathy.

Infections
The infective complications of diabetes are more likely to occur in those with high blood glucose concentrations. Common infections include skin infections (boils, abscesses), urinary infections (especially in those with glycosuria), chest infections, and oral infections, sometimes in association with gingivitis and xerostomia, both of which can reduce oral food intake. While acute infections reduce appetite and food intake, which tends to decrease the blood glucose concentration, the insulin resistance associated with the infections causes elevated glucose concentrations. More regular blood glucose checks are necessary during such episodes in order for appropriate changes to be made to the dose of insulin or oral hypoglycaemic agents. In difficult cases, especially those in which diabetic ketoacidosis has been precipitated by acute infections, hospital admission may be necessary to re-establish glycaemic control using an appropriate diet and a sliding-dose insulin regimen. Correction of fluid and electrolyte disturbances, such as the hypokalaemia which tends to develop during insulin therapy, are guided by a combination of laboratory and clinical assessments.

Good long-term glucose control that involves appropriate dietary advice can prevent infections from developing.

13A.7 Monitoring and follow-up

Like patients with other chronic conditions, it is necessary to follow up those with diabetes in order to monitor metabolic status in the light of drug therapy and lifestyle, especially physical-activity and feeding schedules. Since long-term complications can be a burden to individuals and to healthcare providers, attention to metabolic control can prevent problems from arising many years later. Monitoring of blood glucose concentrations, HbA1c, and lipid profiles can help assess metabolic status. In long-standing diabetes, the complications and comorbidities often require specific and more-detailed attention by specialists, such as ophthalmologists and nephrologists.

13A.8 Concluding remarks

Recent advances in information technology, which have led to the development of 'apps' for mobile phones, have enabled some patients with diabetes to keep better track of blood glucose concentrations, carbohydrate portions, and energy intake, and have thus empowered them to make appropriate decisions for self-care. Developments in information technology can help improve glycaemic control and allow patients to lead a more varied life. However, with the proliferation of information technology and diabetes-related apps, it is important to ensure that individuals choose those designed by authoritative and respected professional bodies.

In patients with type 1 diabetes, pancreatic transplantation has mostly been undertaken in conjunction with kidney transplantation, which is a well-established procedure. Insulin therapy may no longer be needed, which means that lifestyle can become more varied and quality of life can be improved. However, transplanted patients are at risk of tissue rejection, which means that they need to be on lifelong immunosuppressive therapy. In such patients, new problems can arise from rejection and immunosuppression, which, either alone or in combination, can reduce dietary intake. Islet-cell transplantation from human donors also requires immunosuppressive agents, but the use of islet cells derived from stem cells can eliminate the need for these agents, which is why research into this area is active.

Research into type 2 diabetes continues to focus on the development of agents that would allow a more normal life to occur. For example, long-acting drugs that facilitate physiological insulin release in response to dietary intake may simplify drug therapy, reduce the risk of hypo- and hyperglycaemia, and enable individuals to have a less restrictive lifestyle, including less-restrictive dietary schedules. However, such therapy is still a long way from being established.

References and further reading

DAFNE Study Group. Training in flexible, intensive insulin management to enable dietary freedom in people with Type 1 diabetes: dose adjustment for normal eating (DAFNE) randomised controlled trial. British Medical Journal 2002; 325: 746–752.

Dyson PA, Kelly T, Deakin T, Duncan A, Frost G, Harrison Z, *et al.* Diabetes UK evidence-based nutrition guidelines for the prevention and management of diabetes. Diabet Med 2011; 28: 1282–1288.

Elia M, Ceriello A, Laube H, Sinclair AJ, Engfer M, Stratton RJ. Enteral nutritional support and use of diabetes-specific formulas for patients with diabetes: a systematic review and meta-analysis. Diabetes Care 2005; 28(9): 2267–2279.

Jenkins DJ, Wolever TM, Taylor RH, Barker H, Fielden H, Baldwin JM, *et al.* Glycemic index of foods: a physiological basis for carbohydrate exchange. Am J Clin Nutr 1981; 34: 362–336.

NICE. Type 1 Diabetes: Diagnosis and Management of Type 1 Diabetes in Children, Young People and Adults. Clinical Guidance 15 (updated 2009). London: National Institute for Health and Clinical Excellence, 2004.

NICE. Diabetes in Pregnancy. Clinical Guidance 63. Clinical Guidance 10. London: National Institute for Health and Clinical Excellence, 2008.

NICE. Type 2 Diabetes: Newer Agents. Clinical Guidance 87. London: National Institute for Health and Clinical Excellence, 2009.

SIGN. Management of Diabetes. SIGN Publication No. 116. Edinburgh: Scottish Intercollegiate Guidelines Network, 2010.

WHO. Definition and Diagnosis of Diabetes Mellitus and Intermediate Hyperglycaemia: Report of a WHO/IDF Consultation. Geneva: World Health Organization, 2006.

WHO. Use of Glycated Haemoglobin (HbA1c) in the Diagnosis of Diabetes Mellitus. Abbreviated Report of a WHO Consultation. WHO reference number: WHO/NMH/CHP/CPM/11.1 Geneva: World Health Organization, 2011.

13B   PANCREATITIS
Jean-Fabien Zazzo

Key messages

- The pancreas is a dual-function organ, consisting of exocrine and endocrine cells. Ninety-eight per cent of the pancreas is made up of exocrine cells. Disease of the pancreas can result in diabetes, pancreatitis (acute or chronic), or both.
- The dietary management of diabetes has changed radically in the last century in response to increased understanding of the pathophysiology of diabetes and the increased and improved range of available insulins.
- Pancreatitis represents a wide spectrum of clinical disease, involving a diffuse inflammatory process of the pancreas with variable involvement of other regional tissues and/or remote organ systems.

- The metabolism of acute pancreatitis involves a stress state very similar to that seen in sepsis.
- Not all patients suffering from acute pancreatitis need nutritional support, but in severe acute pancreatitis nutritional support is indicated to supply metabolic demands, to prevent wasting, to attempt to modulate the inflammatory response, to protect gut-barrier function, and to prevent bacterial translocation.
- Total parenteral nutrition should only be considered in those patients with severe pancreatitis who are intolerant for enteral feeding or in whom enteral access cannot be obtained.
- Early enteral nutrition improves morbidity, shortens length of stay in hospitals, and probably decreases mortality.

13B.1 Introduction

Pancreatitis represents a wide spectrum of clinical disease, involving a diffuse inflammatory process of the pancreas with variable involvement of other organ systems. Overall, the mortality rate is 7–10%. Patients with mild pancreatitis account for 80% of hospital admissions for pancreatitis. These patients can usually be supported with intravenous-fluid resuscitation and analgesia, and rapidly return to oral diet. Severe pancreatitis is differentiated from mild cases by the presence of severe hypovolaemia and organ failure. Persistent organ failure during the first week is a marker of fatal outcome (Johnson & Abu-Hilal, 2004). This group (20% of hospital admissions for pancreatitis) has a higher mortality (about 10–30%) and is more likely to require nutritional support. Necrotising forms develop in 20% of patients (Banks & Freeman, 2006). Gallstones are the most common cause of acute pancreatitis worldwide. Other risk factors include alcohol, hyperlipidaemia, hypercalcaemia, endoscopic retrograde cholangiopancreatography (ERCP), postoperative trauma, and the side effect of drugs. In 10–25% of the patients with acute pancreatitis, no obvious risk factors are present.

13B.2 Pathogenesis of acute pancreatitis

Early deaths are related to the presence of comorbid conditions and to the development of a systemic inflammatory response syndrome (SIRS) and multi-organ failure (MOF), occurring mainly in the necrotising forms of pancreatitis.

The first phase is characterised by SIRS, during which MOF and death may supervene (Figure 13B.1).

In severe acute pancreatitis, shock induces intestinal ischaemia and loss of gut-barrier function, and then contributes to SIRS, which ultimately leads to MOF. There is increasing evidence that intestinal injury can result in the gut becoming a cytokine-generating organ. Early increased permeability has also been demonstrated in patients suffering from acute pancreatitis. This increased permeability correlates with disease severity, being significantly greater in severe attacks. Similarly, significantly higher levels of endotoxaemia were detected in patients who developed MOF or died. Unless this process is arrested and reversed by natural defences or therapeutic intervention, the second phase ensues.

The second phase is characterised by local complications such as infected pancreatic necrosis, usually becoming apparent in the second week of the illness.

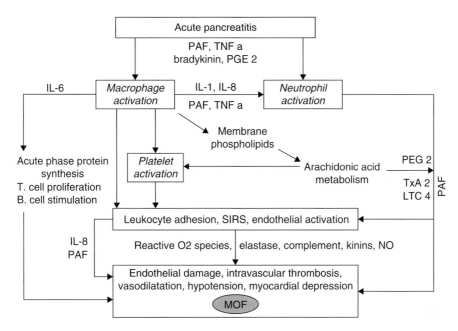

Figure 13B.1 Pathways in acute pancreatitis leading to systemic inflammatory response syndrome (SIRS) and multi-organ failure (MOF). Adapted by permission from BMJ Publishing Group Ltd. Neoptolemos JP *et al*. Acute pancreatitis: the substantial human and financial costs. Gut 1998; 42: 886–891.

The bacterial flora related to the necrotic infection are dominated by enteric bacteria, indicating that the gut may play an important role in the pathogenesis of pancreatitis-related infection. In the early phase after induction of experimental pancreatitis, there is a persistent reduction in intestinal motility, with bacterial overgrowth in the ileum and colon and bacterial translocation to mesenteric lymph nodes.

In acute pancreatitis, the gut may be the primary origin of the bacteria which are present in infected necrosis. Bacterial translocation has been proposed as a mechanism of sepsis in critically ill patients, and especially in pancreatitis. A decrease in intestinal motility and transit causes an increased intraluminal count of bacteria. Intestinal motility may be worsened by morphine administration, which is often used to control pain in these patients. Experimental studies suggest that this is a cause of bacterial translocation. Prognosis is then mainly due to infected necrosis. Suspected infected necrosis is evocated in the presence of clinical deterioration despite fluid challenge, oxygen or mechanical ventilation, and haemodynamic or acute renal failure. Mesenteric ischaemia and acute inflammation induce free-radical overproduction. Infection of necrotic tissue must

be removed by drainage under contrast-enhanced computed tomography (CT) and antibiotics. This minimally invasive approach, as compared with open necrosectomy, has reduced complications, hospital length of stay, and death (van Santvoort *et al.*, 2010).

13B.3 Severity scores

Acute pancreatitis may be a fatal disease, with a reported mortality rate between 20 and 25%. This mortality depends on the severity of the disease, and the severity depends on whether or not pancreatic necrosis is present. Distinction must be made between mild and severe forms, and necrotic and oedematous lesions, since acute pancreatitis in its severe form requires urgent treatment in an intensive-care unit.

At admission, clinical examination is unreliable in predicting the severity of pancreatitis. Authors have tried to develop a combination of criteria to predict severity. Three of these are used in the literature: the Ranson score (1974) (Table 13B.1), the Glasgow Score (1984) (Table 13B.2), and the Acute Physiology and Chronic Health Evaluation (APACHE) II (1989). The Balthazar–Ranson score

Table 13B.1 Prognostic factors in acute pancreatitis by Ranson score. LDH, lactate dehydrogenase; ASAT, aspartate aminotransferase. This article was published in Surg Gynecol Obstet, 139, Ranson JH *et al*. Prognostic signs and the role of operative management in acute pancreatitis, pp. 69–81, Copyright Elsevier 1974.

On admission	
Age	>55 years
White-cell count	>16 000/mm^3
Glucose	>11 mmol/l
LDH	>700 UI or 1.5 N
ASAT	>250 IU/l or 6 N
Within 48 hours of admission	
Haematocrit drop	>10%
Blood urea nitrogen increase	>5 mg/l or 1.8 mmol/l
Serum calcium	<8 mg/l or 2 mmol/l
Pao$_2$	<60 mmHg or 8 kPa
Base deficit	>4 mmol/l
Fluid sequestration	>6 l

Table 13B.2 Prognostic factors in acute pancreatitis by Glasgow Score. LDH, lactate dehydrogenase. Reprinted with permission from Imrie *et al*. (1978), © John Wiley and Sons.

Age	>55 years
White-blood cell count	>15 000/mm^3
Glucose	>10 mmol/l
Blood urea nitrogen increase	>16 mmol/l
Pao$_2$	<8 kPa
Serum calcium	<2 mmol/l
Serum albumin	<32 g/l
LDH	>1.5 N

(1989) established outcome according to necrotic lesions and pancreas vascularisation (Balthazar *et al*., 1990). Single markers of prognosis are continuously published; the most recent are C-reactive protein (CRP) and procalcitonin (Mofidi *et al*., 2009). Monitoring of patients with severe pancreatitis must include a baseline contrast-enhanced CT scan, repeated at least weekly or until improvement. The presence of necrosis increases the morbidity and mortality. Most complications of acute pancreatitis occur in patients in whom the initial diagnosis is based upon peripancreatic fluid collections (grade D or E), and an excellent correlation has been established between the CT depiction of necrosis and the development of complications and death. Patients with pancreatic necrosis have been shown to have a morbidity of about 82% and a mortality of 23%, whereas those without necrosis have a morbidity of 6% and a mortality of 0%.

13B.4 Metabolic consequences of acute pancreatitis

The metabolism of acute pancreatitis involves a stress state very similar to that seen in sepsis, characterised by hyperdynamic changes, hypermetabolism, and hypercatabolism. These changes are important in considering appropriate feeding.

Alterations in carbohydrate metabolism may result from increased cortisol and catecholamine secretion. Gluconeogenesis is increased, while glucose oxidation is diminished. In addition, insulin resistance leads to a glucose intolerance which may necessitate insulin use even in the nondiabetic patient. Alterations in fat metabolism are less frequent. Lipolysis and lipid oxidation are usually increased, but clearance from the blood can be reduced, resulting in hyperlipidaemia and hypertriacylglycerolaemia.

In acute pancreatitis, skeletal muscle proteolysis and amino acid release are associated with an increased consumption of circulating amino acids. This results in amino acid depletion, increased ureagenesis, and nitrogen excretion that can reach more than 30 g per day. Total amino acid concentrations in the plasma of patients with acute pancreatitis have been shown to be lower than those of normal controls. Amino acids involved in gluconeogenesis, such as alanine, threonine, and serine, are particularly low. The concentration of glutamine may fall to levels of only 55% of normal. Depression in glutamine and alanine in plasma occurs despite an increased release of both amino acids from skeletal muscle. These important changes suggest that administration of amino acid solutions may be beneficial to the prevention of wasting by supplying amino acids exogenously.

The most common mineral abnormalities described in acute pancreatitis are hypocalcaemia and hypomagnesaemia, which particularly occur in alcoholic patients.

Reactive oxygen species and related oxidative damage have been implicated in the initiation of acute pancreatitis. A significant correlation between disease severity and endogenous antioxidant status in patients with mild or severe pancreatitis has been shown. Markers of oxidative stress include antioxidant vitamins (alpha-tocopherol, ascorbic acid), lucigenin-amplified chemiluminescence, and thiobarbituric acid-reactive substances.

13B.5 Artificial nutrition

Not all patients suffering from acute pancreatitis need nutritional support. In mild pancreatitis, the majority of patients (80%) are likely to return to oral diet within 7 days. Early refeeding is usually well tolerated and leads to exacerbation of the disease process in only a very small percentage of patients. In a recent randomised clinical study, patients with a mild pancreatitis were allowed to eat immediately. The number of complications was not different between groups and the length of stay was significantly shorter – by one-third – in the oral feeding group (Eckerwall *et al.*, 2007).

In severe acute pancreatitis, as in other critical situations, nutritional support is indicated in order to supply metabolic demands, to prevent wasting, to modulate (if possible) the inflammatory response, to protect gut-barrier function, and to prevent bacterial translocation. Recently, the Guidelines Committee of the Society of Critical Care Medicine (SCCM) and the American Society for Parenteral and Enteral Nutrition (ASPEN) expressed that lack of nutrition support therapy beyond 7 days is deleterious for nutritional status and has an adverse effect on clinical outcome (McClave *et al.*, 2009).

Experimental data suggest that the function of the gut as a barrier against sepsis may be impaired in pancreatitis. Nutritional therapy may influence this barrier function.

In a rat model of acute pancreatitis, jejunal administration of enteral nutrition maintains immune responsiveness and gut integrity, which reduces bacterial and/or endotoxin translocation when compared with total parenteral nutrition (TPN), but without improving outcome. In animals, chow and complex enteral diet maintain a normal balance between immunoglobulin A (IgA)-stimulating and IgA-inhibiting cytokines while preserving normal antibacterial and antiviral immunity. These data are consistent with severely impaired mucosal immunity with intravenous TPN and partial impairment with intragastric TPN, and provide a cytokine-mediated explanation for the reduction in diet-induced mucosal immunity. A few data suggest that maintaining gut-barrier and local immune function by nutritional intervention could potentially improve outcome in pancreatitis, as has been suggested in other critical situations.

Parenteral nutrition

In some experimental studies, glucose given parenterally appeared to be shown to suppress pancreatic function, whereas amino acid solutions did not. A series of controlled studies have refuted these early reports, demonstrating that parenteral infusion of fatty acids does not stimulate pancreatic exocrine secretion in humans.

The results of animal studies and some case reports in humans suffering from external pancreatic fistulae suggest that intravenous infusion of amino acids, glucose, or fat emulsion alone or in combination does not stimulate exocrine pancreatic secretion, and sometimes decreases pancreatic enzyme secretory capacity. Pancreatic secretion has never been prospectively studied in severe necrotic pancreatitis.

Clinical experience with parenteral nutrition

The only available randomised study included only mild acute pancreatitis. Patients were randomised within 24 hours of admission to receive TPN or intravenous fluid (crystalloids or colloids). Compared with the control group, the patients receiving early TPN had a longer, but not significantly longer, length of stay (16 versus 10 days), and the same complication rate. There was no difference in days to clear liquid diet, return of amylase to normal, or overall complications. All other studies are retrospective or case reports (Table 13B.3). In the absence of properly conducted prospective randomised clinical trials, it remains to be shown whether TPN has any clinical benefit on the outcome of the disease, other than the ability to meet patients' nutritional needs in severe forms.

In order to meet increased metabolic demands and to 'rest' the pancreas, TPN through a central venous catheter was the first route used in patients with acute necrotising pancreatitis.

Numerous clinical trials or reports have demonstrated the safety of administering intravenous lipids to patients with severe acute pancreatitis and in whom hypertriacylglycerolaemia is not an aetiological factor (Table 13B.3). Fat-emulsion tolerance should be evaluated twice a week by measuring triacylglycerolaemia 4 hours after the infusion has been stopped. Plasma level must be under 2 g/l.

Table 13B.3 Trials of intravenous nutrition with or without lipids in patients with acute pancreatitis. PR, prospective randomised; PNR, prospective nonrandomised; R, retrospective; NPO, nothing per os; RS, Ranson score; TPN, total parenteral nutrition; IV, intravenous; WT, well-tolerated; NA, not available; AA, amino acid.

Study	Number of patients	Type of study	Severity	Type of nutrition	Observations
Hyde & Floch (1984)	21	PR	NA	Glucose or glucose + AA or glucose + AA + 10% lipid	WT, lipid safe
Durr et al. (1985)	31	PR	Mild	IV lipids (1.5 g/kg/day) versus NPO	WT, lipid safe
Sax et al. (1987)	54	PR	Mild	Glucose + AA + 10% lipid 2/week versus crystalloids	WT, lipid safe
Silberman et al. (1982)	11	PNR	NA	Glucose + AA + Intralipid	WT, lipid safe
Grant et al. (1984)	73	PNR	38% RS > 3	Glucose + AA + 10% lipid	WT, lipid safe
Van Gossum et al. (1988)	18	R	Mean RS = 5.6	30 kcal/kg/day non-protein energy–lipid = 55%	Triglyceride + glucose intolerance predicted poor outcome
Sitzmann et al. (1989)	73	PNR	50% RS > 3	Glucose + lipid 2/week or lipid daily or glucose	WR, lipid safe Mortality × 10 if negative N balance
Steininger et al. (1989)	4	PNR	NA	Glucose + dipeptide + lipid	WT, lipid safe
Robin et al. (1990)	156	R	29% RS > 3	Glucose + lipid 1/week	WT, lipid safe
Kalfarentzos et al. (1991)	67	PNR	Mean RS = 3.8	Glucose + AA + lipid (20–30% of calories as fat)	WT, lipid safe

Enteral nutrition

The debate over the use of enteral feeds in pancreatitis has occurred because of the potential risks of stimulating the inflamed pancreas. Bypassing the stomach is one way to prevent this from happening. There is a paucity of human studies on the effects of enteral nutrition on pancreatic secretion. In healthy volunteers fed either an elemental diet or a food homogenate via a nasojejunal tube, studies indicate that the latter has a greater stimulatory effect on the secretion of pancreatic lipase and chymotrypsin. The osmolality of the infused solutions does not appear to be important. Infusion of a high caloric load into the jejunum has an inhibitory effect on pancreatic secretions. Nutrients entering the duodenum do not stop cycles of enzyme secretion.

Clinical experience with enteral nutrition

The first report of enteral nutrition via a surgical jejunostomy goes back to 1967. Subsequent case studies suggest some benefit from early enteral nutrition, but only one small study has compared enteral nutrition (n = 13) versus no nutritional support (n = 14) in severe acute pancreatitis. Since 2004, meta-analysis and reviews have collected more than 11 randomised studies comparing enteral and parenteral nutrition on mortality, morbidity, and length of stay. All analysis have shown a significant reduction of infectious complications in patients nourished by

enteral route (Marik & Zaloga, 2004; Olah & Romics, 2010; Petrov et al., 2009; Quan et al., 2011). European consensus on nutrition and the pancreas claims that enteral nutrition is the best route for nutrition in this disease, and may be supplemented by the parenteral vein until the nutritional needs are met (Meier et al., 2006).

In a recent Cochrane review comparing enteral nutrition with parenteral nutrition, the relative risk (RR) for death was 0.50, for multiple organ failure was 0.55, for systemic infection was 0.39, and for operative intervention was 0.44 (Al-Omran et al., 2010). In a subgroup of patients with severe acute pancreatitis, the RR for death was 0.18 and for MOF was 0.46. Enteral nutrition has then to be considered the standard of care for patients requiring nutritional support.

Recommendations in most up-to-date guidelines with high-quality scores state that the enteral route is superior to parenteral nutrition in severe pancreatitis and must be used whenever possible (Loveday et al., 2010).

In Petrov's study, analysing 20 randomised controlled trials, the authors concluded that the use of polymeric versus semi-elemental formulation has no impact on feeding intolerance, complications, or mortality; neither supplementation with probiotics nor the use of pharmaconutrients significantly improves the clinical outcomes (Petrov et al., 2009).

If efforts to provide more than 50–65% of goal calories within the first week of hospitalisation by the enteral route are unsuccessful, the addition of supplemental parenteral nutriton should be considered (McClave *et al.*, 2009).

Early nutritional support

Clinical reports and the three randomised studies suggest that contrary to the conventional wisdom, early enteral feeding is both feasible and desirable in the management of patients with acute pancreatitis. The benefits relate primarily to reduced infections, overall complication rates, and reduced costs. However, the benefit of early nutritional support (either parenteral or enteral nutrition) on severe pancreatitis outcome has not yet been established in a randomised prospective study. The latest meta-analyses suggest that early enteral nutrition reduces the incidence of infectious complications, length of stay in hospital, and probably mortality (Olah & Romics, 2010). A recent retrospective study performed on all patients with severe acute pancreatitis during a 1-year period showed that early initiation of distal jejunal feeding was associated with reduced mortality and shorter intensive-care unit length of stay (Hegazi *et al.*, 2011). The role of enteral nutrition deserves further prospective evaluation, particularly in the subgroup of patients with severe acute pancreatitis.

Enteral nutrition may not be feasible either, because of gastrointestinal stasis, high gastric aspirates, or complications of pancreatitis. Enteral intakes are often lower than prescribed due to vomiting, diarrhoea, interruption for procedures, or tube problems. In these cases, parenteral nutrition is indicated in order to improve provision of calories and protein, but early parenteral nutrition is not associated with better clinical outcomes compared with late enteral or parenteral nutrition (Cahill *et al.*, 2011).

Even if TPN is required, it is probably useful to give a small amount of enteral feeding to prevent bacterial translocation and improve host immune function.

Enteral route: jejunal or gastric?

Nasojejunal feeding cannot be achieved in all patients in the intensive-care unit: less than 20% of feeding tubes pass spontaneously through the pylorus, even with prokinetic drugs. A self-propelling nasojejunal tube has been placed successfully in a recent study, but the placement is directly correlated with severity (92% in Balthazar score B/C, 61% in D, and only 48% in E) (Joubert *et al.*, 2008). Placement involves endoscopists or radioscopy delaying early nutrition. Nutrition in the gastric position has therefore been proposed. Several studies support the efficiency and simplicity of gastric nutrition, without any adverse effects on pancreatitis severity and therefore no more regurgitations (Eatock *et al.*, 2005; Eckerwall *et al.*, 2006). In a systematic review, Petrov *et al.* (2008) concluded that nasogastric feeding was safe and tolerated in 79% of patients.

Substrates

Energy requirements

Patients with pancreatitis have a wide distribution of resting energy expenditure (REE). It has been shown that 10% of patients are hypometabolic, 38% are normometabolic, and only 52% are hypermetabolic. The energy needs of patients with acute pancreatitis are variable with the severity of the disease, the presence of infection, and the use of treatment (pain control, sedation, myorelaxants). Although basal energy expenditure (BEE) is most often estimated by using the Harris–Benedict formula modified by stress factors to account for the severity of the disease, the most accurate way of assessing caloric requirements is by measuring the REE by indirect calorimetry. In a critically ill population, it has been demonstrated that the Harris–Benedict formula overestimates energy needs when compared with REE measured by calorimetry. However, since equipment for measuring indirect calorimetry is expensive and may not always be available, predictive formulas for calculating BEE are more often used to help in preventing over- or under-feeding in this group of patients (see Chapter 9).

Glucose should provide 60–70% of the total non-protein caloric needs, but never in excess of the maximal endogenous capacity to oxidise glucose (4–5 mg/kg/min). If the serum triacylglycerol is normal, 30% of non-protein energy can be provided as fat, but never in excess of 1 g/kg/day, in order to prevent cholestasis. In pancreatitis, all studies have been performed using long-chain triacylglycerol. The theoretical advantages of new emulsions (medium-chain triacylglycerol, structured lipids, olive oil, *n*-3) have not been tested in pancreatitis.

Protein requirements

Protein needs are not different from the needs of critically ill patients. In parenteral studies, authors provided 0.25–0.30 g/kg/day nitrogen. In severe illnesses there may be a relative deficiency of glutamine, but the role of glutamine supplementation in human acute severe pancreatitis has yet to be confirmed.

Micronutrients

Multivitamin and trace-elements solution must be administered early when nutritional support is ordered. Recommended dietary allowances do not cover needs during acute pancreatitis due to previous deficiency (alcoholic pancreatitis), SIRS, or infection (oxidative stress). A supplementation could be useful for zinc, selenium, and vitamins C, A, and E.

Pharmaconutriments and probiotics

Pharmaconutrients (glutamine) have not demonstrated any benefits on morbidity (Olah & Romics, 2010). Probiotics and synbiotics have not demonstrated a clear effect in a recent review of 15 clinical studies (Rayes *et al.*, 2009). In one study in severe acute pancreatitis, probiotics were associated with a higher mortality (Besselink *et al.*, 2008).

Practical guidelines

An algorithm showing the decision-making process with regard to feeding in acute pancreatitis is shown in Figure 13B.2. If the goal is to improve clinical outcome, it is still not clear whether enteral feeding is better than no nutritional therapy. Recent reviews, or consensus statements, propose a number of recommendations for nutritional support with pancreatitis (Kreyman *et al.*, 2006; McClave

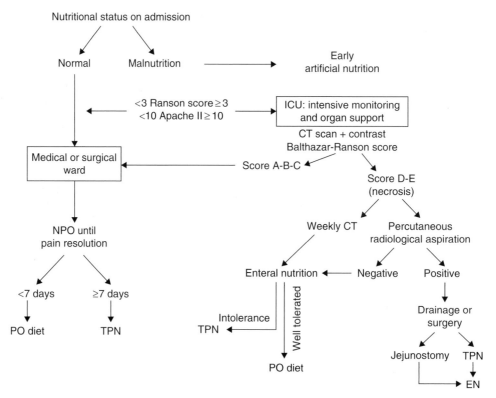

Balthazar-Ranson Score: Grade A = normal pancreas, Grade B = Pancreatic enlargement, Grade C = Pancreatic inflammation and/or peri-pancreatic fat, Grade D = Single peri-pancreatic fluid collection, Grade E = Two or more fluid collection and/or retroperitoneal air

Figure 13B.2 Guidelines for nutritional support.

et al., 2009; Singer *et al.*, 2009). They can be summarised as follows:

- Patients with mild pancreatitis can eat normally and do not benefit from artificial nutritional support.
- Patients with severe acute pancreatitis (Ranson score ≥3 or APACHE II ≥8) are critically ill and must be nourished in order to prevent wasting and to promote metabolic response to stress.
- The exact timing for initiating feeding is still not established, but based on available information, early enteral feeding is recommended.
- Patients requiring surgical intervention should have jejunal tubes placed in theatre.
- The optimal composition of the nutrition formula is not yet known.
- Early enteral feeding by the jejunal route is the preferred form of nutritional support. When enteral nutrition is not possible, TPN should be considered.

13B.6 Chronic pancreatitis

Patients with chronic pancreatitis are usually undernourished. The main reasons are chronic pain exacerbated by eating, pancreatic insufficiency resulting in maldigestion (particularly of fat), glucose intolerance (from 40 to 90%, with insulin-requiring diabetes developing in 20–30%), and alcohol-induced relapse of acute pancreatitis. Patients may also have liver disease secondary to alcohol abuse, which can contribute to further malnutrition.

Nutritional status and deficiencies

Patients with chronic pancreatitis are at risk for many nutrient deficiencies. Low levels of antioxidants have been found in chronic pancreatitis patients compared with healthy controls. Significant decreases are seen in vitamin E, vitamin A, selenium, and glutathione, the carotenoids (beta-carotene, xanthine, beta-cryptoxanthine, and lycopene), but not in zinc or copper. These deficiencies occur despite adequate dietary intake and are thought to be related to malabsorption or increased oxidant stress from the disease. Deficiency may place patients with chronic pancreatitis at risk for greater pancreatic injury from relapses or for progression to carcinogenesis.

Conclusions from a randomised controlled trial have suggested that antioxidant supplementation in patients with chronic pancreatitis may reduce demand for opiate analgesia, frequency of hospital admissions for painful exacerbations, and the requirement for pancreatic surgery. Vitamin B_{12} deficiency may also occur because of the absence of a proteolytic enzyme that normally cleaves a protein-binding competitor for intrinsic factor.

Artificial nutrition in chronic pancreatitis

Most of the time, patients with chronic pancreatitis do not require nutritional support, but it is sometimes required in situations where patients need surgery or develop chronic pancreatitis-related complications.

The main goals of nutritional therapy are to attain and maintain ideal body weight by improving fat and protein absorption with the administration of pancreatic enzymes. Dietary counselling may help patients to improve their nutritional status. Fat is a strong stimulant of pancreatic secretion and may worsen abdominal pain. If this is the case, fat should not exceed 30–40% of total calories. The degree of fat loss (steatorrhea) depends on the degree of exocrine dysfunction and the amount of fat in the patient's diet. Ingestion of pancreatic enzymes can correct protein and fat malabsorptions. The minimal required dose of lipase is 28 000 IU per meal.

Malabsorption of protein may result in hypoalbuminaemia and clinically evident protein-energy malnutrition. It is often difficult for patients with chronic pancreatitis to compensate for protein loss because increased calorie intake often results in aggravation of abdominal pain and the pain itself can lead to anorexia and worsen weight loss. In this case, nutritional support is indicated. Medium-chain triacylglycerol should be used as the major fat source in enteral feeds.

In a study to determine the REE of patients with uncomplicated alcohol-related chronic pancreatitis, REE measured by indirect calorimetry was significantly higher than the predicted energy expenditure calculated with the Harris–Benedict equation. Hypermetabolism was observed in 48.5% of patients with chronic pancreatitis. The percentage rose to 65% in the subgroup of undernourished chronic pancreatitis patients. In undernourished patients, there is a higher energy expenditure per kilogram of fat-free mass. These data suggest that weight loss during chronic pancreatitis is accompanied by hypermetabolism. This hypermetabolism may contribute to wasting and should be taken into consideration when calculating caloric load during nutritional support.

Protein intake should be 1.0–1.5 g/kg/day. Water- and fat-soluble vitamins should also be replaced, as should micronutrients.

Artificial nutrition, if indicated, is rarely ordered by the parenteral route but may be indicated in patients with gastric or duodenal outlet obstruction and in those with fistulating disease. In other patients, the enteral route is the best option until the patient is able to eat oral food with nutritional supplements and pancreatic enzymes (Gianotti *et al.*, 2009; Meier *et al.*, 2006).

Nutrition management of chronic pancreatitis-related complications

Pancreatic ascites

Pancreatic ascites results from either a rupture of the pancreatic duct or leakage of a pancreatic pseudocyst into the peritoneal cavity. The recommendation is to treat with somatostatin analogues, either alone or in combination with parenteral nutrition. Parenteral nutrition is the most frequently used mode of nutritional support, but enteral nutrition is possible if feeds are provided via the jejunum to prevent pancreatic secretion stimulation.

Pancreatic fistulas

Pancreatic fistulas are usually treated either with somatostatin alone or with somatostatin in combination with parenteral nutrition. The only multicentre, controlled, prospective trial randomised 40 patients with digestive fistulas to receive either parenteral nutrition alone or parenteral nutrition in combination with somatostatin. No significant differences between these treatments were observed in the percentage of closure of fistulas, but in those patients receiving parenteral nutrition in combination with somatostatin the fistulas closed within a significantly shorter period of time. Furthermore, this treatment was associated with a significantly lower morbidity.

Pseudocysts

Large pseudocysts usually require surgery and percutaneous or endoscopic drainage, but up to 80% of pseudocysts can be successfully treated by parenteral nutrition or enteral nutrition.

13B.7 Concluding remarks

As has been shown in this chapter, there is still a need for larger randomised controlled trials in acute pancreatitis to study the effects of:

- nutritional support versus no nutritional support;
- enteral feeding versus parenteral feeding;
- early versus very early enteral nutrition;
- the optimal composition of enteral and parenteral feeds, especially the choice of lipid emulsions, pharmaconutrition with a focus on antioxidants.

These studies should be particularly directed towards patients with more severe forms of the disease. However, in order to demonstrate significant reductions in mortality, trials would require large numbers of patients, which is often unrealistic and impractical.

The incidence of acute pancreatitis is increasing in the USA and Europe. Despite this increase, in-hospital mortality has decreased, but this depends on the hospital volume, staff expertise, and surgical and medical resources (Singla *et al.*, 2009). Identification of best practices will induce better outcomes for patients with severe pancreatitis. The key is probably the availability of numerous speciality services and a better efficiency in coordinating multidisciplinary care. Aggressive fluid resuscitation, a minimally invasive step-up approach, innovative endoscopic techniques, and enteral nutrition support have impacted outcome. Nutrition requires further evaluation in order to identify the best procedures in a homogeneous population with the same severity score, demographic, and comorbidities.

References and further reading

Al-Omran M, Al-Balawi Z, Tashkandi M, Al-Ansary L. Enteral versus parenteral nutrition for acute pancreatitis. Cochrane Database of Systematic Reviews 2010; 1: 1–56.

Balthazar EJ, Robinson DL, Megibow AJ, Ranson JH. Acute pancreatitis: value of CT in establishing prognosis. Radiology 1990; 174: 331–336.

Banks P, Freeman M. Practice guidelines in acute pancreatitis. Am J Gastroenterol 2006; 101: 2379–2400.

Besselink MG, van Santvoort HC, Buskens E, Boermeester MA, van Goor H, Timmerman HM, et al. Probiotic prophylaxis in predicted severe acute pancreatitis: a randomised, double-blind, placebo-controlled trial. Lancet 2008; 371: 651–659.

Cahill NE, Murch L, Jeejeebhoy K, McClave SA, Day AG, Wang M, et al. When early enteral feeding is not possible in critically ill patients: results of a multicenter observbational study. JPEN 2011; 35: 160–168.

Durr GH, Schaffers A, Maroske D, *et al.* A controlled study of the use of intravenous fat in patients suffering from acute attacks of pancreatitis. Infusionther Klin Ernahr 1985; 12: 128–133.

Eatock FC, Chong P, Menezes N, Murray L, McKay CJ, Carter CR, *et al.* A randomized study of early nasogastric versus nasojejunal feeding in severe acute pancreatitis. Am J Gastroenterol 2005; 100: 432–439.

Eckerwall G, Axelsson J, Andersson R. Early nasogastric feeding in predicted severe acute pancreatitis – a clinical, randomized study. Annals of Surgery 2006; 244: 959–967.

Eckerwall G, Tingstedt B, Bergenzaun P, Andersson R. Immediate oral feeding in patients with mild acute pancreatitis is safe and may accelerate recovery – a randomized clinical study. Clin Nutr 2007; 26: 758–763.

Gianotti L, Meier R, Lobo DN, Bassi C, Dejong C, Ockenga J, *et al.* ESPEN guidelines on parenteral nutrition: pancreas. Clin Nutr 2009; 28: 428–435.

Grant JP, James S, Grabowski V, Trexler KM. Total parenteral nutrition in pancreatic disease. Ann Surg 1984; 200: 627–631.

Hegazi R, Raina A, Graham T, Rolniak S, Centa P, Kandil H, *et al.* JPEN 2011; 35: 91–96.

Hyde D, Floch M. The effect of peripheral nutritional support and nitrogen balance in acute pancreatitis. Gastroenterology 1984; 86: 119–123.

Imrie CW, Benjamin IS, Ferguson JC, McKay AJ, Mackenzie I, O'Neill J, *et al.* A single centre double blind trial of trasylol therapy in primary acute pancreatitis. Br J Surg 1978; 65: 337–341.

Johnson CD, Abu-Hilal M; Members of the British Acute Pancreatitis Study Group. Persistent organ failure during the first week as a marker of fatal outcome in acute pancreatitis. Gut 2004; 53: 1340–1344.

Joubert C, Tiengou L, Hourmand-Ollivier I, Piquet M. Feasibility of self-propelling nasojejunal feeding tube in patients with acute pancreatitis. JPEN 2008; 32: 622–624.

Kalfarentzos FE, Karavias DD, Karatzas TM, Alevizatos BA, Androulakis JA. Total parenteral nutrition in severe acute pancreatitis. J Am Coll Nutr 1991; 10: 156–162.

Kreyman G, Berger M, Deutz N, Hiesmayr M, Jolliet P, Karandjiev G, *et al.* ESPEN guidelines on enteral nutrition: intensive care. Clin Nutr 2006; 25: 210–223.

Loveday B, Srinivasa S, Vather R, Mittal A, Petrov M, Philips A, *et al.* High quality and variable quality of guidelines for acute pancreatitis: a systematic review. Am J Gastroenterol 2010; 105: 1466–1476.

Marik PE, Zaloga GP. Meta-analysis of parenteral nutrition versus enteral nutrition in patients with acute pancreatitis. BMJ 2004; 328: 1407–1412.

McClave S, Martindale R, Vanek V, McCarthy M, Roberts P, Taylor B, *et al.* Guidelines for the provision and assessment of nutrition support therapy in the adult critically ill patient: Society of Critical Care Medicine and American Society for Parenteral and Enteral Nutrition. JPEN 2009; 33: 277–316.

Meier R, Ockenga J, Pertkiewicz M, Pap A, Milinic M, MacFie J, *et al.* ESPEN Guidelines enteral nutrition: pancreas. Clin Nutr 2006; 25: 275–284.

Mofidi R, Suttie S, Patil P, Ogston S, Parks R. The value of procalcitonin at predicting the severity of acute pancreatitis and development of infected pancreatic necrosis: systematic review. Surgery 2009; 146: 72–81.

Neoptolemos JP, Raraty M, Finch M, Sutton R. Acute pancreatitis: the substantial human and financial costs. Gut 1998; 42: 886–891.

Olah A, Romics L. Evidence-based use of enteral nutrition in acute pancreatitis. Langenbecks Arch Surg 2010; 395: 309–316.

Petrov M, Correia M, Windsor J. Nasogastric tube feeding in predicted severe acute pancreatitis. A systematic review of the literature to determine safety and tolerance. JOP 2008; 9: 440–448.

Petrov M, Loveday B, Pylypchuk R, McIlroy K, Phillips A, Windsor J. Systematic review and meta-analysis of enteral nutriton formulations in acute pancreatitis. Br J Surg 2009; 96: 1243–1252.

Quan H, Wang X, Guo C. A meta-analysis of enteral nutrition and total parenteral nutrition in patients with acute pancreatitis. Gastroenterology Research and Practice 2011; 2011: 1–9.

Ranson JH, Rifkind KM, Roses DF, Fink SD, Eng K, Spencer FC. Prognostic signs and the role of operative management in acute pancreatitis. Surg Gynecol Obstet 1974; 139: 69–81.

Rayes N, Seehofer D, Neuhaus P. Prebiotics, probiotics, synbiotics in surgery – are they only trend, truly effective or even dangerous? Langenbecks Arch Surg 2009; 394: 547–555.

Robin AP, Campbell R, Palani CK. Total parenteral nutrition during acute pancreatitis: clinical experience with 156 patients. World J Surg 1990; 14: 572–579.

Sax HC, Warner BW, Talamini LA, *et al.* Early total parenteral nutrition in acute pancreatitis: lack of beneficial effect. Am J Surg 1987; 153: 117–124.

Silberman H, Dixon NP, Eisenberg D. The safety and efficacy of a lipid-based system of parenteral nutrition in acute pancreatitis. Am J Gastroenterol 1982; 77: 494–497.

Singer P, Berger M, Van den Berghe G, Biolo G, Calder P, Forbes A, *et al.* ESPEN guidelines on parenteral nutrition: intensive care. Clin Nutr 2009; 28: 387–400.

Singla A, Simons J, Li Y, Csikesz N, NG S, Tseng J, *et al.* Admission volume determines outcome for patients with acute pancreatitis. Gastroenterology 2009; 137: 1995–2001.

Sitzmann JV, Steinborn PA, Zinner MJ, Cameron JL. Total parenteral nutrition and alternate sustrates in treatment of severe acute pancreatitis. Surg Gynecol Obstet 1989; 168: 311–317.

Steininger R, Karner J, Roth E, Langer K. Infusion of dipeptides as nutritional substrates for glutamine, tyrosine, and branched-chain amino acids in patients with pancreatitis. Metabolism 1989; 38: 78–81.

Van Gossum A, Lemoyne M, Greig PD, *et al.* Lipid-associated total parenteral nutrition in patients with severe acute pancreatitis. J Parenter Enteral Nutr 1988; 12: 250–255.

van Santvoort H, Besselink M, Bakker O, Hofker H, Boermeester M, *et al.* A step-up approach or open necrosectomy for necrotizing pancreatitis. N Engl J Med 2010; 362: 1491–1502.

14
The Kidney

Roberta Situlin and Gianfranco Guarnieri

University of Trieste, Italy

Key messages

- The functions of the kidney are to eliminate waste products, control body fluid volume and composition, produce erythropoietin, renin, and prostaglandins, and regulate vitamin D metabolism.
- In renal disease, these functions are impaired, leading to the development of uraemic syndrome.
- There is evidence that nutritional treatment can prevent or delay the progression of chronic kidney disease (CKD), control symptoms, and prevent or reduce the development of complications such as protein energy malnutrition (PEM) and cardiovascular disease (CVD).

- PEM is a common clinical finding in renal disease and has a negative bearing on quality of life, morbidity, and mortality, and therefore it should be adequately prevented, diagnosed, and treated.
- Nutritional prescriptions in renal patients are complex because nutritional goals are multiple, and at times conflicting, yet the prescribed diets should be as realistic and practical as possible.
- Nutritional support is needed when spontaneous food intake is inadequate to cover nutrient requirements.

14.1 Introduction

Medical nutrition therapy plays an essential role in the management of renal disease. To appreciate the interaction between nutritional and renal dysfunction, it is important to have an understanding of the normal physiology of the kidney. The kidney is essentially an excretory organ, but it is also involved in the regulation of the volume and composition of body fluids, and has specific endocrine and metabolic functions. The functional unit is the nephron, of which there are approximately 1 million in each kidney. The function and action of a nephron are shown in Figure 14.1. A large volume of blood – about 1.3 l – passes through the nephrons every minute. The rate of ultrafiltration is referred to as the glomerular filtration rate (GFR) and is approximately 125 ml/minute. This value varies with age and sex. The filtrate formed in the glomerulus passes first into the proximal convoluted tubule, then into the loop of Henle, and finally

through the distal convoluted tubule to the collecting ducts. During this process, the filtrate is modified according to the needs of the body through reabsorption and secretion by the tubules (Figure 14.1b).

Renal disease impairs excretory and other kidney functions. Therefore, the serum levels of urea, electrolytes, and other metabolites increase, the metabolism of nutrient changes, and the patient becomes symptomatic. When renal failure reaches its final stages, renal replacement therapy (RRT) is started. This restores most kidney functions, but dialysis is not able to correct all the metabolic changes induced by renal failure.

Dietary modifications have important roles in kidney disease. Interventions in protein, fluid, sodium, potassium, and phosphate intake can counteract the changes induced by loss of kidney function, whether acute or chronic. Another goal is to slow the evolution of kidney disease to renal failure. Chronic kidney disease (CKD) is characterised

---

Clinical Nutrition, Second Edition. Edited by Marinos Elia, Olle Ljungqvist, Rebecca J Stratton and Susan A Lanham-New.
© 2013 The Nutrition Society. Published 2013 by Blackwell Publishing Ltd.

(a)

(b)

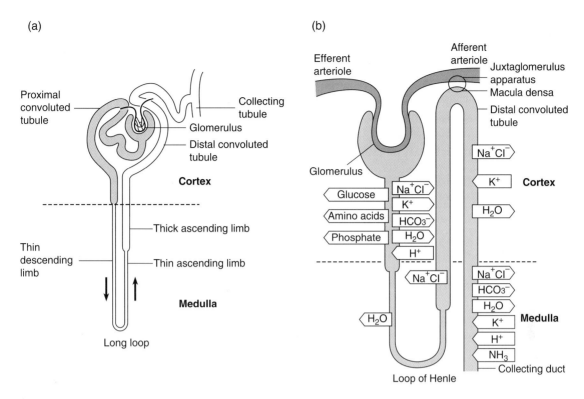

Figure 14.1 The function and action of a nephron. Redrawn from Kumar and Clark (1998), with permission from Elsevier.

by a progressive nature, which leads to a relentless loss of renal mass and function, even when the pathogenic factors of the original damage have been successfully treated. At first the loss of function is compensated for by an adaptive hypertrophy of the remaining functional nephrons (remnant nephrons), associated with increased glomerular plasma flow and transcapillary glomerular hydraulic pressure. These haemodynamic changes allow an increase of total kidney GFR in spite of a reduced kidney mass. In the long term, however, the glomeruli become sclerotic and renal function progressively declines. Much effort has been put into identifying the best nutritional interventions to control the factors involved in the progression of the kidney disease and to delay the need for RRT. Another fundamental role of nutrition is the prevention or control of protein–energy malnutrition (PEM) and cardiovascular disease (CVD), commonly seen in kidney patients, with the aim of improving outcome and survival.

Box 14.1 Types of renal disease

Acute kidney injury (AKI) – the onset of renal failure is rapid.
Chronic kidney disease (CKD) – the onset of renal failure develops over a longer period of time.
Diabetic kidney disease (DKD) – chronic kidney disease in patients with diabetes mellitus.
End-stage renal failure (ESRF) – patients require some form of RRT (haemodialysis or continuous ambulatory peritoneal dialysis, CAPD) or kidney transplantation.

This chapter will be organised according to the type of renal disease, as the role of nutritional management in each situation is different (Box 14.1).

14.2 Assessment of nutritional status in kidney patients

Nutritional assessment needs to be performed regularly in kidney patients in order to identify those at risk of malnutrition, or those who are malnourished, and provide adequate nutritional intervention. Standard multiple methods of assessment are used, including clinical examination, dietary intake evaluation, anthropometry, and measurement of biochemical, functional, and body-composition indices, in order to obtain data about different body components (fat mass, lean body mass, and visceral proteins). All nutritional status indices have prognostic value, with an impact on morbidity and mortality (see Chapter 2).

Methods of nutritional assessment

Food and nutrient intake

The assessment of dietary intake is important in defining the adequacy of the diet and compliance with prescriptions. Evaluation is done by 24-hour recall and through dietary interviews over 3–7 days, carried out by a well-trained dietitian, or by food diaries over 3–7 days. The National Kidney Foundation Kidney Disease Outcomes Quality Initiative (NKF KDOQI) guidelines, for patients on dialysis, suggest a 3-day food diary, covering a dialysis day, a non-dialysis day, and a weekend day. To help the patient quantify portion sizes and household measures, three-dimensional models or pictures of food – printed or on a digital display – can be helpful.

In stable CKD patients with neutral nitrogen balance (nitrogen intake = nitrogen loss) – excluding therefore conditions of weight loss, active catabolism, worsening of renal failure (in pre-dialysis patients), and inadequacy of dialysis in haemodialysis or continuous ambulatory peritoneal dialysis (CAPD) – protein intake can be assessed indirectly through the protein equivalent of total nitrogen appearance, calculated from the urea nitrogen appearance in the urine or dialysate via equations specific to the treatment modality (conservative or RRT).

Anthropometric measurements

Body weight and height, used to calculate the body mass index (BMI), should always be measured and recorded at the first visit in order to obtain a basal reference value, which is useful in monitoring any change at follow-up. In patients on conservative treatment, patients with oedema, or dialysed patients, it is important to consider the *dry weight* or oedema-free body weight, based on clinical estimation or defined

as the weight measured after haemodialysis – or after empting the peritoneal cavity in CAPD patients – in order to exclude the effect of fluid retention. In haemodialysis patients, mortality is higher for subjects with a post-dialysis $BMI < 23 \, kg/m^2$, or $< 20 \, kg/m^2$ in elderly subjects. Therefore, the European Renal Best Practice (ERBP) guidelines recommend that dialysis subjects should maintain a $BMI > 23 \, kg/m^2$. Being overweight, on the other hand, both in haemodialysis and CAPD subjects, seems to be protective even at levels equivalent to obesity ($BMI > 30 \, kg/m^2$) or severe obesity ($BMI > 35 \, kg/m^2$).

Unintentional weight loss over time is important information to add to absolute weight when assessing the risk of PEM. Percentage weight loss in the previous 3–6 months is used to define PEM.

According to the ERBP guidelines for haemodialysis, the percentage change in body weight should be calculated from the difference between the averaged, over 1 month, post-dialysis weight and the averaged post-dialysis weight of the previous month.

Body weight gives only a rough estimate of body-composition changes. Skeletal or fat mass should therefore be assessed by other anthropometric measurements (limb circumferences and areas and skinfold thickness, taken at multiple sites) or by body-composition methods (BIA, bioelectrical impedance analysis; dual-emission X-ray absorptiometry, DXA). It is important to note that water retention in end-stage renal disease (ESRD) or on RRT may limit the reliability of anthropometric indices.

Biochemical indices

In RRT patients, laboratory data should be measured before the haemodialysis session or after the equilibration phase in CAPD. Urea nitrogen appearance is calculated during the interdialytic interval.

Creatinine excretion reflects muscle mass, but creatinine kinetics is altered in CKD, and therefore the creatinine/height ratio should not be used. With RRT, in the absence of renal excretion, pre-dialysis serum creatinine can be used again.

Serum proteins synthesised by the liver, such as albumin, pre-albumin, and transferrin, are indicators of the visceral protein pool. The differences in the protein half lives modify their sensitivities in detecting nutritional changes, but multiple non-nutritional factors, such as plasma volume, urinary excretion, and inflammation, can modify serum-protein concentration.

Albumin has a long half life of 21 days and its synthesis decreases with the liver production of positive acute-phase proteins, such as C-reactive protein (CRP). Hypoalbuminaemia (cut-off value 3.8–4.0 g/dl) is associated with both higher mortality and cardiac disease risk and is considered more a negative prognostic than a PEM indicator.

Transferrin has a shorter half life of 9 days, which makes it a more sensitive index of malnutrition; however, the protein concentration is also influenced by iron status, infections, and inflammation.

Pre-albumin is a protein with a very short half life that can detect short-term changes in visceral protein status. In pre-dialysis patients, however, the serum concentration of the protein is influenced by renal function. Pre-albumin levels may therefore rise as GFR declines, independent of the nutritional status of the patient. In dialysed patients pre-albumin can instead be used as a nutritional marker. Values < 30 mg/dl are generally indicative of PEM and are associated with an increased mortality risk.

Low or declining values of total cholesterol serum levels may indicate malnutrition, but this change may also be the consequence of inflammation or comorbid conditions. Values less than 150 mg/dl are associated with a higher mortality risk.

CRP serum-level measurement is useful in detecting inflammation and an increased risk of atherosclerosis and cardiovascular mortality. A rise in the plasma levels of this protein is associated with malnutrition and reduced albumin levels. There is no consensus about including CRP as a diagnostic index of PEM.

Functional indices

Functional indices are useful as they may detect early changes in nutritional status. The most common indices in clinical practice are lymphocyte count (to measure immune response) and hand grip strength (to measure skeletal muscle function).

Subjective global assessment

Subjective global assessment is a clinical tool which integrates history about gastrointestinal symptoms and weight loss in the last 6 months with a physical examination of fat and muscle mass. Subjective global assessment gives a quick assessment of nutritional status, without the need for complex anthropometric or laboratory data. In CKD, the modified CANUSA (Canada-USA) study version should be used. Other

tools based on subjective global assessment modifications include the patient-generated subjective global assessment, the Malnutrition and Inflammation Score, and the Dialysis Malnutrition Score, which include laboratory or body-composition measurements in order to overcome the limitations of subjective judgement.

14.3 Acute kidney injury

Introduction

'Acute kidney injury' (AKI) is the newest term introduced by the Kidney Disease: Improving Global Outcomes guidelines, in place of the previous 'acute renal failure' (ARF). AKI indicates the spectrum of injuries which may affect the kidney: from the mildest uncomplicated forms, treated with medical interventions, to the most severe, associated with trauma, sepsis, or other organ failure, and requiring RRT. AKI is characterised by a rapid loss of kidney function and an accumulation of metabolic end products normally excreted by the kidneys. Fluid, electrolyte, and acid–base balance are altered and plasma levels of urea, creatinine, hydrogen ions, potassium, and uric acid become elevated. Protein catabolism increases, contributing to the higher plasma urea levels. The scientific international societies are working to reach a globally shared definition and diagnostic modalities in staging for AKI. The prevalence of AKI, through time is not well known, due to modifications of its definition. AKI may involve between 5 and 20% of critically ill patients. The overall mortality is between 40 and 90%, despite many recent improvements in treatment. Patients with shock, sepsis, or multiple organ failure have the worst prognosis. Relevant determinants of outcome are the degree of protein hypercatabolism induced by AKI and its associated conditions, and the need for RRT. In the last 2 decades, the options for dialysis treatment have increased to include not only intermittent haemodialysis (IHD) and peritoneal dialysis but also different forms of continuous renal replacement therapy (CRRT), such as continuous veno–venous haemofiltration, continuous veno–venous haemodialysis, and continuous venous–venous haemodiafiltration, or the latest so-called 'hybrid' modalities of RRT, such as extended-duration dialysis, sustained low-efficiency dialysis, and the Genius system. While the efficacy of the different treatments is not yet defined by the literature, all of them have an impact on the nutritional status of the patient, which must be taken into account.

Nutritional treatment in AKI

The presence of PEM with hypercatabolism has a strong prognostic value, being a predictor of in-hospital mortality independent of other complications and comorbidities. On the other hand, it is yet to be clearly demonstrated that nutritional intervention can improve outcome, but clinical experience indicates that treatment may have important benefits. The markedly negative nitrogen balance often seen in the most severe patients and the poor prognosis suggest the importance of a well-planned nutritional treatment, with optimal amounts of energy, nitrogen, and other nutrients.

Nutritional support for patients with AKI must take into account not only the metabolic disturbances associated with the kidney injury, but also the underlying disease process and the associated complications, as well as the treatment modalities (conservative or RRT). RRT causes loss of both macro- and micronutrients, which must therefore be supplemented. The impact of RRT depends on the method utilised and its intensity. CRRT causes significant loss of water-soluble, low-molecular-weight substances. A total daily loss of 10–15 g amino acids and 5–10 g protein has been reported.

Metabolic changes

Protein metabolism

Severe protein catabolism with a highly negative nitrogen balance and the release of amino acids from skeletal muscle is characteristic of AKI. Hypercatabolism is defined on the basis of daily increases in blood urea nitrogen (>11 mmol/l), blood urea nitrogen-to-creatinine ratio (>10), or urea nitrogen appearance (>10 g/day).

Increased hepatic gluconeogenesis and ureagenesis occur in response to this protein hypercatabolism, and nitrogen losses can be as high as 150–200 g/day. Box 14.2 shows the main causes of hypercatabolism in AKI. Injury to the kidney is associated with the development of an intense proinflammatory state, with increased levels of cytokines. Endocrine abnormalities can be partly responsible for the increased gluconeogenesis, proteolysis, and accelerated protein turnover seen in AKI. The secretion of

Box 14.2 Factors responsible for hypercatabolism in acute kidney injury

- endocrine abnormalities:
  - raised glucagon;
  - raised cortisol;
  - raised catecholamines;
  - insulin resistance;
- uraemic toxins;
- metabolic acidaemia;
- associated events (sepsis, shock, SIRS, MOF, trauma, burns, etc.);
- inflammation (increased cytokine activity);
- resistance to growth factors;
- reduced nutrient intake;
- immobilisation;
- loss of nutrients;
- renal replacement therapy.

counter-regulatory hormones, such as catecholamines, glucagon, and cortisol, is increased, leading to insulin resistance. Protein breakdown is also induced by metabolic acidosis. RRT, which is often necessary in AKI, is a strong catabolic stimulus, due to the loss of nutrients (amino acids, peptides, and vitamins) during the dialytic procedure and the production and release of protein catabolism-inducing cytokines and proteases during the blood contact with the dialysis membranes. Imbalances of plasma and intracellular amino acids have been described in AKI, due to metabolic abnormalities, decreased renal function, loss through the dialysis membranes, and altered plasma clearance. As a consequence, amino acids such as histidine, arginine, tyrosine, serine, and cysteine, which are non-essential in healthy subjects, may become conditionally essential in AKI. The levels of amino acids such as phenylalanine and methionine are increased, while the concentration of non-essential amino acids involved in the urea cycle (arginine and ornitine) is reduced.

Lipid and carbohydrate metabolism

Lipid metabolism is severely affected by AKI. Plasma concentrations of triglycerides, very low-density lipoproteins (VLDLs) and low-density lipoproteins (LDLs) are usually elevated in renal patients, while cholesterol and high-density lipoprotein (HDL) levels may be low. Impaired lipolysis is the main reason for these changes, as the activities of key enzymes of lipid metabolism (post-heparinic lipoprotein-lipase, hepatic triglyceride lipase, and peripheral lipoprotein lipase) are altered, both at peripheral and at hepatic levels. Plasma lipid clearances are altered and the ability to utilise exogenous lipids may be reduced; therefore, the amount of lipids given in AKI should be lower than in non-uraemic patients.

Vitamins and minerals

RRT causes major losses of water-soluble vitamins, which must be supplemented. The intake of vitamin C should be 30–50 mg/day, in order to avoid secondary oxalosis, but the requirement may be double with CRRT. Plasma levels of fat-soluble vitamins A and E, involved in the body antioxidant defence system, are reduced. The risk of supplemented vitamin A accumulation and toxicity over time requires monitoring of the vitamin levels. Vitamin K levels are normal or even elevated. Magnesium, calcium, and selenium may need supplementation.

Nutritional requirements

Guidelines on enteral and parenteral nutrition in patients with AKI have been developed and recently reviewed by the European Society for Clinical Nutrition and Metabolism (ESPEN) (Table 14.1).

Patients with AKI derived from primary renal involvement (most often drug or contrast media-induced) with a low degree of catabolism (urea nitrogen appearance <6 g/day) and a short expected duration of renal insufficiency can be treated with oral low-protein diet (LPD) (0.6–0.8 g/kg/day, max. 1) in order to maintain blood urea nitrogen lower than 100 mg/dl (~36 mmol/l). This intake, which is lower than or equal to the 0.8 g/kg/day for healthy adults set by the Recommended Dietary Allowances (RDAs) in order to meet the needs of almost all (97–98%) individuals in a group, allows reduction of the nitrogen toxic load. However, because of the associated protein hypercatabolism, lower amounts should be avoided. In acutely ill patients on RRT, protein requirements are higher (1–1.5), and they are even higher on CRRT (up to a maximum of 1.7 g/kg/day).

AKI is not a cause of increased energy demand *per se*. On the contrary, patients with uncomplicated AKI may have a lower energy expenditure compared to healthy controls. Energy need is influenced more by the coexisting disease (e.g. sepsis, surgery, or trauma). An amount of energy not exceeding 1.3 times the basal metabolic rate (i.e. 25–35 kcal/kg/day) is generally

Table 14.1 Nutritional guidelines for AKI patients. IBW, ideal body weight (Metropolitan Life Insurance tables). ESPEN, 2006 and 2009: www.espen.org.

Protein, g/kg IBW/day	0.6–0.8, max. 1
conservative treatment	0.8–1.2, max. 1.5
extracorporeal treatment	Up to 1.7
CRRT	
Energy, kcal/kg IBW/day, as non-protein calories	20–30 (adapted according to the weight of the patients)

suggested in these patients, the higher amount being reserved for hypercatabolic patients with higher urea plasma levels and very negative nitrogen balance. Energy >35 kcal/kg/day is seldom needed. Measuring or calculating energy expenditure, on the basis of estimated dry weight, is useful to avoid overfeeding.

Carbohydrate and fat intake should be maintained within 3–5 g/kg/day (max. 7) and 0.8–1.2 g/kg/day, respectively. These indications take into account the presence of insulin resistance and the impaired ability to metabolise exogenous lipids.

Nutritional support

Nutritional support can be implemented through enteral nutrition, oral nutritional supplementation (ONS) or tube feeding, or parenteral nutrition.

Available formulas for enteral nutrition are either standard or kidney disease-specific, for patients on conservative treatment (low-protein, high-energy, and reduced electrolyte concentration) or on RRT (high-protein, high-energy – 1.5 g and 2 kcal/ml – and reduced content of potassium and phosphate). Uncomplicated AKI patients, with low–moderate catabolism, unable to achieve full nutritional requirements with food, can be treated with ONS to increase nutrient intake. With severe hypercatabolism, nutritional support by enteral nutrition should be initiated within 24 hours. Standard formulas are generally adequate, but dialysis-specific formulas may be used when electrolyte control is a problem. Enteral nutrition, even though preferable to parenteral nutrition, is not always possible, especially in some sicker patients; furthermore, nutrition requirements, especially for protein, may not be reached. Total parenteral nutrition (TPN) should be considered in those patients without a functioning gut or to supplement inadequate feeding by the enteral route. ESPEN guidelines suggest the use of standard parenteral nutrition formulas, which are considered adequate for most patients. In cases of electrolyte problems, three-in-one electrolyte-free or customised formulas can be used. Products enriched with glutamine, arginine, nucleotides, or omega-3 fatty acids (immune-modulating formulas) are not recommended, since clear benefits have not been confirmed.

14.4 Chronic kidney disease and diabetic kidney disease

Rationale and goals of nutritional therapy

The goals of medical nutrition therapy in CKD and diabetic kidney disease (DKD) are multiple and at times conflicting (Box 14.3). Medical nutrition therapy requires knowledge of: factors involved in renal failure progression, causes of malnutrition, the presence of PEM, other risk factors and complications, and nutrient requirements, according to the disease type and stage. Dietary prescription may be difficult to understand and follow for many patients. The motivation and education of patients and their families are key factors in fostering dietary compliance.

Definition of CKD

CKD in the pre-dialysis phase of conservative treatment is characterised by a progressive decline in renal function and is defined and classified in stages, according to the NKF KDOQI guidelines (Box 14.4). Stages 3–5 are identified by GFR alone, whereas the definition of stages 1 and 2 additionally requires the presence of structural abnormalities or of persistent proteinuria, albuminuria, or haematuria.

The UK national service framework for renal services has adopted the KDOQI classification of CKD, but stage 3 has been divided in two subgroups: 3A and 3B, with GFR of 45–59 and 30–44 ml/min/1.73 m^2, respectively.

The GFR is calculated from the creatinine clearance according to different formulas, such as, for example, the Cockcroft–Gault formula or the Modification of Diet in Renal Disease formula.

Progression of CKD is defined as a decline in GFR of more than 5 ml/min/1.73 m^2 within 1 year, or more than 10 ml/min/1.73 m^2 within 5 years.

Definition of DKD

Diabetes mellitus is at present the greatest single cause of CKD worldwide. DKD can develop in subjects

---

Box 14.3 Goals of medical nutritional therapy in CKD

- Delay the progression of CKD or DKD.
- Reduce uraemic symptoms.
- Prevent/control PEM.
- Prevent or treat other nutritionally related complications (cardiovascular diseases; mineral and bone disorders).

Box 14.4 Definition of CKD

CKD is present with:

- Kidney damage for a period > 3 months, with or without decreased GFR, manifested by either structural abnormalities of the kidneys (shown by ultrasound scanning or other radiological tests, or kidney biopsy) or blood or urine markers of kidney damage, such as persistent microalbuminuria, proteinuria, or haematuria.
- GFR < 60 ml/min/1.73 m^2 for a period > 3 months, with or without kidney damage, irrespective of diagnosis.

Stages of progression to ESRF (according to the level of kidney function decline, irrespective of the CKD diagnosis):

- Stage 1: normal or increased GFR (>90 ml/min/1.73 m^2) with evidence of kidney damage.
- Stage 2: mild GFR reduction (60–89 ml/min/1.73 m^2) with evidence of kidney damage.
- Stage 3: moderate GFR reduction (30–59 ml/min/1.73 m^2).
- Stage 4: severe GFR reduction (15–29 ml/min/1.73 m^2).
- Stage 5: ESRF, established renal failure (GFR < 15 ml/min/1.73 m^2) or dialysis.

---

with either type 1 or type 2 diabetes and involves 20–30 % of diabetic patients. The criteria for DKD, according to the KDOQI guidelines and clinical practice recommendations for diabetes and CKD, are shown in Box 14.5.

It is recommended that patients are screened for DKD 5 years after the diagnosis of type 1 diabetes mellitus, and from the time of first diagnosis in type 2 diabetes.

Nutritional factors involved in the progression of CKD or DKD

Protein intake

Dietary proteins induce haemodynamic and structural changes in the kidney, mediated by mechanisms such as increased secretion of hormones (glucagon,

Box 14.5 Definition of DKD

CKD in diabetic patients can be attributed to diabetes mellitus in the presence of:

- Microalbuminuria: albumin/creatinine ratio (ACR) between 30 and 300 mg/g in a spot urine sample or 30 and 300 mg/24 hours in a 24-hour urine collection, associated with diabetic retinopathy or type 1 diabetes of at least 10 years' duration.
- Macroalbuminuria: ACR > 300 mg/g or > 300 mg/24 hours.

growth hormone, corticosteroids, insulin-like growth factor (IGF)), increased synthesis of angiotensin II, prostaglandins, and nitric oxide, activation of growth factors and complement fractions, induction of cytokine synthesis, and higher production of reactive oxygen species. Protein intake restriction may delay progression to ESRD. Before RRT became widely available, protein-restricted diets (so called 'nephro diets', such as the Giordano–Giovannetti diet) were life-prolonging and able to reduce some ESRF symptoms.

The effectiveness of an LPD in slowing the progression of kidney disease was first shown in animal models. It was then extensively investigated in CKD patients using either an LPD of about 0.6 g/kg ideal body weight (IBW)/day, in earlier stages of failure, or an LPD or a very low-protein diet (VLPD) of about 0.3 g/kg/day, supplemented with essential amino acids or their ketoanalogues, in later stages.

The role of protein restriction in reducing the rate of loss of renal function in progressive renal failure however is not fully defined. Furthermore, protein restriction may increase the risk of PEM. Compliance may be poor and the regimens may interfere with the patient's quality of life. Some randomised studies, including the large Modification of Diet in Renal Disease (MDRD) study, reported a small or moderate beneficial effect on GFR slowing in patients with advanced renal failure. In patients with early renal failure on an LPD, a 28% reduction of GFR worsening was found, in comparison with patients maintained on a normal protein diet. Vegetable protein has been shown to be more effective in slowing the progression of kidney disease than animal protein, suggesting a possible role for the protein quality. Beneficial effects of protein restriction were reported in diabetic patients with DKD (see later). Present guidelines on the management of CKD suggest a moderate protein restriction in later phases of CKD and an earlier restriction in DKD (see later).

Phosphate intake

Phosphate intake can cause kidney damage independently of protein, most likely through parenchimal deposition of calcium-phosphate precipitates, in the presence of hyperphosphataemia, and changes in intracellular calcium metabolism, which may modify renal haemodynamics and mesangial growth factors. A low phosphate intake may delay progression of renal damage (but this role is not definitely accepted) and allows an improvement in divalent ion metabolism and parathyroid hormone (PTH) changes. A controlled phosphate intake is suggested in later stages of CKD. Since protein and phosphate are associated in the same types of food, a LPD allows also a lower phosphate intake.

Dyslipidaemia and dietary fat

Dyslipidaemia is a frequent complication of uraemia and a relevant risk factor for CVD, which may have a role in the progression of kidney failure. Hypercholesterolaemia may cause excessive activation of monocytes and macrophages. Both hyperlipidaemia and the intramesangial oxidative modification of LDL may be responsible for glomerular damage. The renoprotective effect of statin treatment seems to confirm the damaging effects of dyslipidaemia. The combination of hypertension and hyperlipidaemia may have a very negative prognostic relevance. The quality of dietary fat may also play a role, through its influence on the synthesis of eicosanoids involved in the inflammatory processes. Diets supplemented with polyunsaturated n-3 fatty acids in experimental conditions showed beneficial effects on proteinuria, the progression of renal failure, and survival. Clinical trial results were, however, inconsistent, and omega-3 supplementation to slow kidney-failure progression is not recommended by present guidelines.

Systemic hypertension

The role of hypertension, together with that of proteinuria, in determining the rate of progression of CKD is well established. Hypertension *per se* is a frequent cause of CKD (hypertension-associated kidney disease). Kidney damage results from increased glomerular hypertension and changes in the renin–angiotensin system (RAS). Hypertension is also a

Food groups and daily servings	Serving size
Grains, 6–8	1 slice bread
	1/2 to 1 1/4 cup dry cereal, depending to type
	1/2 cup cooked rice, pasta, or cereal
Vegetables, 4–5	1 cup raw leafy vegetable
	1/2 cup raw or cooked vegetable
	4 oz vegetable juice
Fruits, 4–5	4 oz fruit juice
	1 medium fruit
	1/4 cup dried fruit
	1/2 cup fresh, frozen, or canned fruit
Low-fat or fat-free dairy foods, 2–3	8 oz milk
	1 cup yogurt
	1 1/2 oz cheese
Meats, poultry, and fish, 6 or less	1 oz, cooked
Nuts, seeds, dry beans, 4–5 per week	1/3 cup or 1 1/2 oz nuts
	2 tbsp or 1/2 oz seeds
	1/2 cup cooked dry beans
Fats, oils, 2–3	1 tsp soft margarine
	1 tbsp low-fat mayonnaise
	2 tbsp light salad dressing
	1 tsp vegetable oil
Sweets, 5 or less per week	1 tbsp sugar, or jelly or jam
	1/2 cup sorbet or gelatin
	8 oz lemonade

Table 14.2 DASH diet composition (for a 2000-calorie eating plan). Protein 18%, carbohydrate 55%, fat 27%, saturated fat 6% of total energy; cholesterol 150 mg, fibre 30 g, potassium 4.7 g, sodium 2.3 g, calcium 1.25 g, magnesium 0.5 g. Adapted from NIH (2006).

consequence of CKD, which develops in up to 80% of patients in stages 3–5, and an important risk factor of CVD. A good control of blood pressure should be achieved, both through drugs, such as the angiotensin-converting enzyme inhibitors or angiotensin-2 receptor blockers, and dietary modifications.

Nutritional factors involved in the development of hypertension include excessive energy intake – leading to overweight – and high sodium or alcohol use, while physical activity and higher potassium intake are protective. Diets such as the Dietary Approaches to Stop Hypertension (DASH) lower the systolic and diastolic blood pressure, by 11.4 mmHg and 5.5 mmHg, in subjects with first-stage hypertension not associated with CKD (Table 14.2). For this reason, some guidelines suggest the use of this diet, or modified versions of it, in CKD (see later). The diet is rich in vegetables, fruits, whole grains, pulses, fish, and low-fat dairies and meats, while the intake of red meats, simple sugars, and sodium is low compared with the typical American diet.

Obesity

A number of studies have shown that obesity, besides causing complications such as hypertension, insulin resistance, diabetes mellitus, and dyslipidaemia, is a risk factor for both CKD and DKD. The term 'obesity-related glomerulopathy' (ORG) has been introduced. The risk of developing CKD is increased to 1.87 times by overweight, 3.57 by class I obesity (BMI 30–35 kg/m²), 6.1 by class II obesity (BMI 35–40 kg/m²), and 7.0 by extreme obesity (BMI ≥ 40 kg/m²). Obesity can be responsible for up to 15% of CKD in males and 11% in females. The appearance of microalbuminuria or proteinuria in overweight subjects is indicative of renal damage, the proteinuria level being positively correlated with the entity of visceral fat deposition. Furthermore, overweight and its metabolic complications increase cardiovascular risk. The pathophysiology of ORG is complex. Besides causing hyperinsulinaemia, hypertension, and dyslipidaemia, overweight is associated with inflammation. The adipose tissue synthesises cytokines (tumour necrosis factor alpha (TNFα), interleukin 6 (IL-6) and interleukin 1 (IL-1), resistin, and leptin) with proinflammatory effects. Leptin increases the synthesis of proinflammatory cytokines and the levels of damaging reactive oxygen species and proteinuria. Weight loss could reverse or delay the development of ORG, or of

DKD, in obese subjects. However, evidence is limited.

Diabetes mellitus

The risk for ESRF in DKD depends on the duration of diabetes. In type 1 diabetes, ESRF develops in 50% of subjects within 10 years and in >75% within 20 years. In type 2 diabetes, about 20% of patients reach ESRF after 20 years, mainly because of the higher CVD mortality. Risk factors of developing DKD include: a positive family history for kidney disease or hypertension, maternal gravidic hyperglycaemia, early development of diabetes, smoking, obesity with insulin resistance, high blood pressure, hyperglycaemia, poor glycaemic control with higher levels of glycated haemoglobin, genetic predisposition, and levels of protein intake. Hyperglycaemia increases GFR, leading to glomerular hypertrophy, hyperfiltration, and mesangial cell proliferation. The glucose toxicity is sustained by haemodynamic factors, increased oxidative stress, and the formation of advanced glycation end products with proinflammatory action and tissue-damaging properties. A high protein intake causes haemodynamic and structural changes, and worsens proteinuria in diabetic subjects. The onset and progression of DKD can be prevented or delayed by glycaemic and hypertension control and protein restriction, started in its earlier phases. Intensive glycaemic control in stages 1 and 2 of CKD, in type 1 and 2 diabetes mellitus, is effective in reducing the micro- and macroalbuminuria and slowing GFR decline. The Diabetes Control and Complications Trial showed that an intensive blood glucose control, versus conventional treatment, in the early phases of CKD in type 1 diabetes, reduced, at 6.5 years, the occurrence of microalbuminuria by 34 and 43% in the primary and secondary prevention group, respectively. Fewer data are available about the effects of glycaemic control in later stages of CKD or in dialysis patients. As for protein restriction, an intake in the range of 0.5–0.85 g/kg body weight/day showed beneficial effects in subjects with insulin-dependent diabetes mellitus and late nephropathy. At a follow up of 9–33 months, protein restriction caused a significant reduction of albuminuria levels or of the rate of GFR decline, independently of the use of angiotensin-converting-enzyme (ACE) inhibitors. Positive effects of protein restriction were also observed in stage 2 of CKD. Therefore, dietary protein restriction of around 0.8 g/kg body weight/day is considered to be indicated in DKD from its early stages. Animal, especially red-meat, proteins seem to be more damaging, while vegetable and soy protein sources may be more kidney-sparing.

Protein–energy malnutrition

PEM is frequent in CKD, in both the pre-dialysis and the RRT phases. In CKD on conservative treatment, under-nutrition becomes more evident in established renal failure (stages 4 and 5), involving 30–40% of subjects. Malnutrition has been reported in 10–70% of haemodialysis and 18–51% of CAPD patients, according to the modalities of assessment. The presence of PEM is a poor prognostic factor for patients beginning RRT; thus it is important to preserve the nutritional status of patients with advanced renal insufficiency prior to RRT and to start dialysis at GFR > 20 ml/min, especially if there is evidence of a worsening of the nutritional status.

Nutritional status influences both quality of life and patient outcome. Its assessment should therefore be a priority in CKD patients.

In order to manage malnutrition adequately, its causes should be explored. The multiple factors involved in the aetiology of PEM are illustrated in Figure 14.2.

Reduced food intake

Anorexia, from multiple causes, leading to an inadequate dietary intake, is a common feature in patients with a GFR below 60 ml/min and a frequent cause of PEM in CKD. Energy intake is particularly low in CKD patients. LPD, considered unpleasant or difficult to follow, may contribute to an intake of food and nutrients below the recommended amount. The start of dialysis requires higher protein intake, which may be difficult to achieve in subjects with reduced appetite. Some patients also seem to restrict their nutrient intake on interdialytic days in order to limit excessive weight gain. Some medications, alcohol abuse, zinc deficiency, taste changes, and other social, economical, psychological, gastrointestinal, and hormonal factors may interfere with adequate eating. High levels of plasma leptin have been found in CKD, in both pre-dialysis and haemodialysis patients, and even more in those on peritoneal dialysis. The presence of inflammation decreases

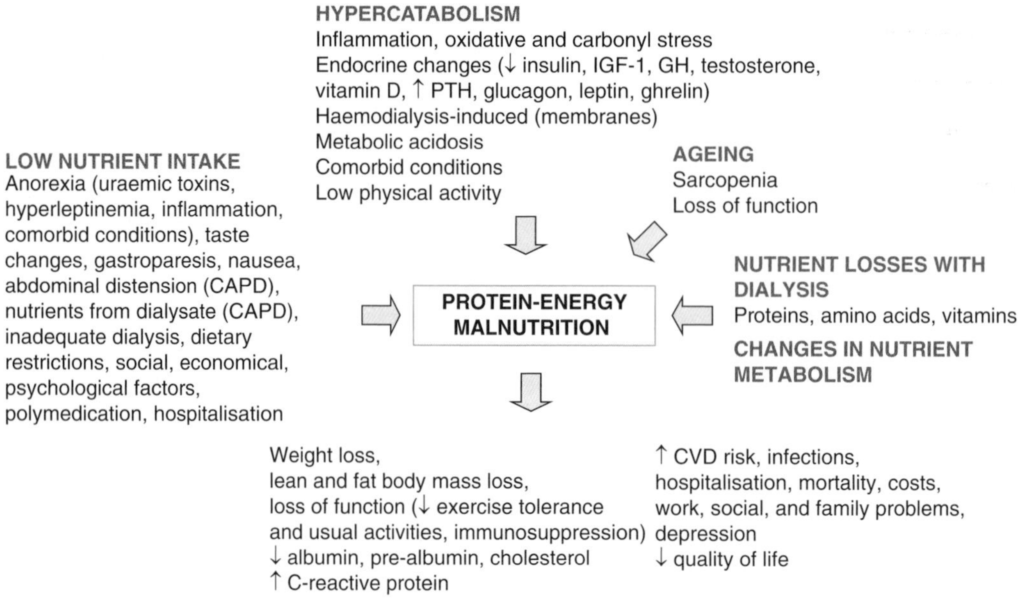

HYPERCATABOLISM
Inflammation, oxidative and carbonyl stress
Endocrine changes (↓ insulin, IGF-1, GH, testosterone,
vitamin D, ↑ PTH, glucagon, leptin, ghrelin)
Haemodialysis-induced (membranes)
Metabolic acidosis
Comorbid conditions
Low physical activity

AGEING
Sarcopenia
Loss of function

LOW NUTRIENT INTAKE
Anorexia (uraemic toxins,
hyperleptinemia, inflammation,
comorbid conditions), taste
changes, gastroparesis, nausea,
abdominal distension (CAPD),
nutrients from dialysate (CAPD),
inadequate dialysis, dietary
restrictions, social, economical,
psychological factors,
polymedication, hospitalisation

**PROTEIN-ENERGY
MALNUTRITION**

**NUTRIENT LOSSES WITH
DIALYSIS**
Proteins, amino acids, vitamins

**CHANGES IN NUTRIENT
METABOLISM**

Weight loss,
lean and fat body mass loss,
loss of function (↓ exercise tolerance
and usual activities, immunosuppression)
↓ albumin, pre-albumin, cholesterol
↑ C-reactive protein

↑ CVD risk, infections,
hospitalisation, mortality, costs,
work, social, and family problems,
depression
↓ quality of life

Figure 14.2 Causes and consequences of malnutrition in chronic uraemia.

appetite through the production of anorexigenic cytokines. In CAPD patients, the abdominal distension caused by fluids in the abdomen can lower food intake, and anorexia can be worsened by the continuous absorption of glucose from the peritoneum. Impaired gastrointestinal function may also be present, with disturbed gastric or intestinal motility.

Increased nutrient losses

In patients on haemodialysis, PEM risk is worsened by nutrient losses (a single haemodialysis session causes a loss of free amino acids and peptides equivalent to 4–9 g and 2–3 g per session, respectively) and increased protein catabolism.

In CAPD patients, the protein losses from the peritoneum are larger than in haemodialysis patients, ranging from 5 to 15 g/day, while the amino acids and peptides lost in dialysis fluid are lower (1.2–3.4 g/24 hours). If mild or severe peritonitis develops, protein loss can be doubled. CAPD patients tend also to be physically inactive, due to the time involved in exchanging dialysis fluid or the abdomen distention.

Metabolic acidosis

Metabolic acidosis induces protein catabolism by increasing branched-chain amino acid oxidation, cortisol secretion, proteolytic enzyme activity, and synthesis of muscle ubiquitin and proteasome. The net effect of metabolic acidosis, especially if associated with a reduced protein intake, is a negative nitrogen balance and muscle wasting. Correction of acidosis can normalise these changes. To avoid the effects of acidosis, arterial bicarbonate should be kept in a normal range (22–26 mmol/l).

Adequacy of dialysis sessions

An inadequate dialysis is associated with lower protein and energy intake in RRT patients, and is thus a causative factor of PEM. Therefore, the prescription of dialysis dose needs to be individualised and monitored by Kt/V assessment, and dialysis quality control should be a priority.

Changes in nutrient metabolism

CKD is associated with insulin resistance, which may be involved in the genesis of accelerated atherosclerosis. Increased plasma concentrations of glucagon and PTH promote gluconeogenesis and protein catabolism. Hypertriglyceridaemia, with high levels of ApoB-rich VLDLs and intermediate-density lipoproteins (IDLs), is frequent in CKD, both on conservative treatment and during RRT. The causes of dyslipidaemia are multiple and involve defects of the enzymes controlling lipid metabolism (lecithin-cholesterol acyltransferase (LCAT), lipoprotein-lipase, and hepatic lipase).

Severe derangement of plasma and intracellular concentrations of amino acids are present in uraemic patients. The ratio of essential to non-essential amino acids in plasma is lower than in normal individuals. The concentration of the branched-chain amino acids, especially valine, and of tyrosine, threonine, and lysine, is reduced. On the other hand, plasma levels of glycine, cystine, methionine, aspartate, and citrulline are increased. In muscle, normal levels of leucine and isoleucine are found, while valine, threonine, taurine, lysine, and histidine are low. Histidine and thyrosine are considered essential in chronic uraemia, due to the specific metabolic impairment.

The protein depletion and muscle wasting observed in uraemic patients are the consequence of increased muscle degradation, associated with a normal or decreased protein synthesis. The latter is an adaptive response which improves tolerance to LPD in CKD, in the short and long term.

Role of inflammation

High levels of TNFα and IL-1 have been found in the plasma of patients with CKD. From our personal observations, CKD patients have increased secretion of TNFα, which is associated with higher circulating levels of soluble TNFα receptors, directly related to serum creatinine. Inflammation influences nutrient intake and metabolism, and increases energy expenditure, thus causing malnutrition. Inflammation in CKD is the result of kidney failure itself, causing retention of glycated or oxidated proteins and lipids, which are normally excreted; and of associated conditions such as CVD and cardiovascular risk factors and low-grade and, at times, occult infections, including nail or urinary infections; leg or foot ulcers in diabetic patients; vascular-access infections, catheter-related infections, or peritonitis in haemodialysis and CAPD patients; hepatitis B and C; and chronic pulmonary or *Helicobacter pylori* infections. Inflammation is also fuelled by factors associated with dialysis procedures, such as blood exposure to bio-incompatible membranes, with liberation of proinflammatory cytokines, or utilisation of non-ultrafiltrated dialysate fluids or unsafe reuse procedures.

The risk of developing atherosclerosis in CKD is related both to PEM and inflammation. Malnutrition, inflammation, and atherosclerosis (MIA) syndrome defines the association of malnutrition, inflammation, and atherosclerosis. An increased oxidative stress, with a reduced antioxidant activity, is also present.

Detection and definition of PEM

CKD patients

According to the KDOQI guidelines, the assessment of nutritional status in CKD subjects with GFR < 20 ml/min should be performed by at least one measurement from each of the following indices (evaluation frequency in parentheses):

(1) serum albumin (every 1–3 months);
(2) oedema-free actual body weight (ABW), or percentage standard (NHANES II) body weight, or subjective global assessment (every 1–3 months);
(3) normalised protein nitrogen appearance (nPNA) (grams per kilogram per day) or dietary interviews and diaries (every 3–4 months).

The UK Renal Association suggests that all patients with stage 4–5 CKD should be screened through the following indices (cut-off values in parentheses), assessed 2–3 times monthly (with GFR < 20), or more often in unstable patients:

- Actual body weight < 85% of IBW;

where IBW (kg) = ideal BMI $(kg/m^2) \times (height (m))^2$. Ideal BMI = 20 with actual BMI < 20; 25 with BMI > 25; and the actual value if BMI lies between 20 and 25 kg/m^2.

- reduction in body weight (of 5% or more in 3 months or 10% or more in 6 months);
- BMI < 20 kg/m^2;
- subjective global assessment (B/C on 3-point scale or 1–5 on 7-point scale).

The UK National Institute of Clinical Excellence (NICE) guidelines give similar indications and define malnutrition as:

- BMI < 18.5 kg/m^2;
- unintentional weight loss > 10% in 3–6 months;
- BMI < 20 kg/m^2 and unintentional weight loss > 5% in 3–6 months.

RRT patients

KDOQI guidelines suggest measuring:

(1) percentage change of usual weight (%UW) (once a month);
(2) serum albumin (once a month);

	Type 1 (marasmus-like)	Type 2 (kwashiorkor-like)
Causes	Low dietary intake	Low or normal dietary intake with inflammation
		Comorbidities
		Dialysis-related factors
Protein catabolism	Decreased	Increased
Resting energy expenditure	Normal	Increased
Oxidative stress	Increased	Markedly increased
Serum albumin	Normal/low	Low
Response to nutritional support	Good	Reduced

Table 14.3 Classification of PEM in CKD. Information from Stenvinkel *et al.* (2000), by permission of Oxford University Press.

(3) subjective global assessment (every 6 months);
(4) nPNA (monthly on haemodialysis, every 3–6 months on CAPD);
(5) dietary intake (every 6 months).

ERBP guidelines suggest the use of the same indices, plus cholesterol levels, and do not include subjective global assessment for routine follow-up. Albumin, cholesterol, and nNPA should be measured every 3 months, but once a month in unstable conditions. Nutrient intake should be evaluated every 6–12 months, but every 3 months in subjects with age > 50 years or on haemodialysis for >5 years.

Assessment should be carried out within 1 month of commencement of dialysis, then again 6–8 weeks later, and every 4–6 monthly in stable haemodialysis and CAPD patients.

PEM nomenclature

There is a need for a new nomenclature of PEM. The International Society of Renal Nutrition and Metabolism (ISRNM) supports the terms 'protein energy wasting' (PEW) and 'kidney disease-PEW', independent of the cause. PEW is defined by: (i) low serum levels of albumin, transthyretin, or cholesterol; (ii) reduced body mass (low or reduced body or fat mass, or weight loss with reduced intake of protein and energy); and (iii) reduced muscle mass (sarcopaenia or muscle wasting, or reduced mid-arm muscle circumference). Indices of inflammation are considered useful but not diagnostic of PEW. A definitive consensus on the nomenclature of PEM has not been reached. Other groups give more relevance to the causes of PEM and suggest classifying chronic PEM into two sub-types (Table 14.3).

Box 14.6 Major risk factors of CVD in CKD

Classical:

- hypertension;
- insulin resistance or diabetes;
- low HDL and elevated LDL and total cholesterol;
- sedentary lifestyle;
- overweight;
- smoking.

Nonclassical:

- proteinuria;
- activation of the renin angiotensin system;
- inflammation;
- malnutrition;
- abnormal calcium/phosphate metabolism, with increased PTH and decreased vitamin D levels (causing metastatic vascular calcification);
- higher oxidative stress;
- low folate levels, elevated homocysteine levels and anaemia.

Risk of cardiovascular disease

Cardiovascular risk factors develop in CKD from the early stages of renal failure. In DKD patients the CVD risk is particularly high. The presence of microalbuminuria with normal renal function doubles the risk of CVD. In subjects with macroalbuminuria, the mortality rate increases above the CKD progression rate. Of all death in ESRF patients, 40–50% are due to CVD. According to the KDOQI guidelines for cardiovascular disease and the American Heart Association (AHA), patients with CKD should be considered in the highest risk category for CVD. Both classical and nonclassical risk factors are involved (Box 14.6). Nonclassical factors are mostly related to the loss of renal function and are observed, on average, at GFR decline $< 60\,ml/min/1.73\,m^2$. Most of these factors are complications of CKD and are also responsible for the progression of renal failure.

Secondary hyperparathyroidism and other complications

The high PTH levels present in CKD may cause renal osteodystrophy and CKD mineral and bone disorder. The Kidney Disease: Improving Global Outcomes guidelines recommend that the term 'renal osteodystrophy' be used only for alterations in bone morphology and the term 'CKD mineral and bone disorder' for the systemic disorder associated with one or more of the following findings: laboratory abnormalities of calcium, phosphorus, PTH, or vitamin D metabolism; changes in bone turnover, mineralisation, volume, linear growth, and strength; and vascular or other soft-tissue calcifications. Mineral and bone disorders are responsible for extraskeletal calcification, associated with respiratory, joint, and cardiovascular complications. Hyperphosphataemia and low vitamin D levels become apparent in the later stages of kidney failure (GFR $< 30\,ml/min$). A low-phosphate diet during the course of renal failure may not only contribute to lowering the progression of renal failure but also prevent and/or control mineral and bone disorder. A lower phosphate intake needs to be continued after the beginning of dialysis, since phosphate removal is insufficient.

Other complications which may require nutritional modification include: fluid and electrolyte unbalance, observed at the end stages of renal failure or during dialysis treatment; anaemia, which is mostly the consequence of erythropoietin and sometimes iron deficiency; peripheral neuropathy; restless leg syndrome; fatigue; failure to thrive; dry skin; pruritus; bleeding tendency from platelet dysfunction; and encephalopathy, pericarditis, and so on from uraemic toxicity. Some of these symptoms may respond, for a short period, to reduced protein intake, or they may require the beginning of dialysis treatment.

Dietary prescription in CKD without diabetes mellitus

Goals

(1) To delay the progression of kidney disease.
(2) To prevent or control complications including PEM, dyslipidaemia, systemic hypertension,

CVD, and secondary hyperparathyroidism or other uraemic symptoms.

Diet characteristics

The prescription of a diet takes into account: (i) the stage of CKD; (ii) the specific requirement for protein and energy; (iii) the need to control the intake of other macronutrients, such as fat, to prevent CVD, or micronutrients, such as phosphate, potassium, or sodium.

With time, there has been an evolution in the definition of the diet composition for CKD patients. Some guidelines (Table 14.4) suggest the implementation of a reduced protein intake in the early stages of CKD, once the diagnosis has been made, starting from GFR levels $< 70\,ml/min$ (corresponding to the middle value of stage 2, used today). However, more recent guidelines, such as the KDOQI guidelines on hypertension and diabetes management in CKD, advise prescribing protein restriction only in stages 3 and 4 of kidney failure. Evidence for the efficacy of LPDs in earlier stages is considered insufficient when possible complications are taken into account. In stages 1 and 2, a protein-rich diet is instead suggested, with 18% of the total energy intake coming from proteins (about 1.4 g of protein/kg IBW/day). Since not only the quantity but also the quality of the diet is considered important, the DASH dietary model is suggested. The diet is characterised by a high intake of vegetable products, including wholegrain cereals, pulses and nuts, fruits and vegetables, a choice of animal products – mainly poultry and fish, low-fat dairies, and a reduced intake of red meat – simple sugars (sweets or beverages), and salt. Because of the emphasis on vegetable proteins and the low intake of red meat, the diet is considered less nephrotoxic. Furthermore, it has a blood pressure-lowering effect, due to its high potassium and low sodium ($< 2.3\,g/day$) content. The fat composition, with a reduced quantity of total and saturated fat (< 30 and 10% of the total energy, respectively) and of cholesterol ($< 200\,mg/day$), is in line with the prevention or control of dyslipidaemia. The high phosphate or potassium intake is not considered negative in the early stages of renal failure.

Dietary protein restriction to 0.6–0.8 g/kg/day is suggested by most guidelines, starting from stages 3 and 4. For this purpose, the DASH diet (Table 14.2) can be modified opportunely to reduce protein

Table 14.4 Nutritional guidelines for patients with CRF or DKD on conservative treatment and under stable clinical conditions. HBV, high biological value; IBW, ideal body weight (Metropolitan Life Insurance tables); SBW, standard body weight (NHANES II); ABW, adjusted body weight = IBW + (IBW − actual body weight) × 0.25. This correction factor is used in underweight or overweight subjects to avoid overfeeding or underfeeding); EAA, essential amino acids; KA, ketoanalogues; ESPEN, European Society for Clinical Nutrition and Metabolism; NKF KDOQI, National Kidney Foundation Kidney Disease Outcomes Quality Initiative; SIGN, Scottish Intercollegiate Guidelines Network.

	ESPEN (Cano *et al.*, 2006, 2009)	NKF KDOQI (2007)	SIGN (2008)	UK Renal Association (2010)
Protein (g/kg IBW, SBW, or ABW/day)				
Stages 1–2 (GFR 60–90 ml/min)	*GFR = 25–70 ml/min* 0.5–0.6 (75% HBV)	1.4 (50–75% HBV) with CKD, as DASH diet 0.8 (50–75% HBV) with DKD, as modified DASH diet	Insufficient evidence for restriction	Not reported
Stages 3 and 4 (GFR, 15–60 ml/min)	*GFR < 25 ml/min* 0.5–0.6 (75%HBV) or 0.28 + EAA or EAA + KA or 0.3–0.4 with KA	0.6–0.8 (50–75% HBV) as modified DASH diet (with or without diabetes)	Stage 3: insufficient evidence for restriction Stage 4: intake > 1 g/ kg IBW, not recommended	0.75 as minimum daily intake to prevent PEM Assess adequacy in single patients
Energy (kcal/kg IBW, SBW, or ABW/day)				
	35, adjusted for under- or overweight	35 30–35 (age > 60 years)	Not indicated	30–35, depending upon age and physical activity Assess adequacy in single patients
Potassium (g/day)				
Stages 1–2	1.5–2 .0	>4		
Stages 3–4		2.4		
Phosphate (g/day)				
Stages 1–2	0.6–1, depending on age, gender, severity of PEM, lean body mass, level of physical activity	1.7	Insufficient evidence on progression of CKD for restriction Phosphate restriction for management of renal bone disease (stages 4 and 5)	
Stages 3–4		0.8–1 .0		

intake. This also allows a reduction of the phosphate and potassium content from 1.7 to 0.8–1.0 g/day and from >4 to 2.4 g/day, respectively. The modifications can be complex, however, because of the need to keep a high level of high-biological-value (HBV) proteins. In patients with GFR values < 25 ml/min, VLPDs of 0.28 g/kg/day, with no limitation on quality, plus essential amino acids (EAAs) or a mixture of EAAs and ketoanalogues of EAAs, have been prescribed. Because EAA supplements are no longer available, VLPDs with 0.3–0.4 g of protein/kg/day, plus ketoanalogues, are used in fewer selected cases, such as patients affected by terminal illness or elderly subjects.

Ketoanalogues, which are transaminated to form their respective amino acids in the body, allow the essential amino acid requirements to be reached at a lower nitrogen intake, causing a reduced formation of nitrogenous waste products and uraemic toxins. This regimen, if prescribed for short periods of time before starting dialysis, can maintain a neutral nitrogen balance, if the energy intake is adequate. The risk of PEM is high, however. Furthermore, the essential amino acids and ketoanalogues are not available in all countries and the compliance is often low. Initiation of dialysis is preferred to VLPDs, which are not recommended by most recent guidelines.

Guidelines are homogenous in suggesting an energy intake of 35 kcal/kg/day in CKD, on modified diets. A high energy intake is important with reduced-protein diets in order to optimise nitrogen utilisation. This amount can be a little lower in the elderly (aged > 60 years) and more sedentary subjects.

Dietary prescription in DKD

Goals

(1) To slow GFR decline and control uraemia through a strict glycaemic and blood-pressure control and a moderate protein restriction.
(2) To control a particularly high risk of CVD: increasing mortality, even before patients reach the end stages of renal failure. This is done through lifestyle modification and pharmacological agents.
(3) To manage multiple factors at once, including hyperglycaemia, hypertension, and dyslipidaemia.

Diet characteristics

In type 1 diabetes, strict glycaemic control requires frequent control of blood glucose levels (three or more times daily, before meals and at bedtime) and adequate insulin treatment, matched to carbohydrate intake and levels of physical activity. In type 2 diabetes, blood glucose measurement can be less frequent, but compliance to the lifestyle and pharmacological prescription needs to be higher. The American Dietetic Association (ADA) recommends a HbA1c target of <7%, or as close to normal as possible. Other groups suggest the same goal or an even lower HbA1c target of <6.5%. Intensive glycaemic control requires particular attention: the risk of hypoglycaemia is increased in DKD by the reduced kidney gluconeogenesis and the lower clearance of insulin by the failing kidney. The diet is characterised by protein restriction to an intake of 0.8 g/kg/day (50–75% HBV), which, according to the KDOQI guidelines, should be started in stages 1 and 2. This amount of protein is equivalent to the RDA for normal subjects, and therefore it is not really a restrictive regimen. Still, the intake is lower than the average. A modified DASH diet is suggested. The abundance of fibre in the regimen may contribute to the glycaemic control. The protein intake is reduced to 0.6–0.8 g/kg/day in stages

3 and 4 of CKD. The ADA guidelines endorse the same kind of regimens. However, a specific model of diet is not reported. The KDOQI guidelines stress the importance of controlling overweight, even though the benefits of the weight control are not clearly defined. In obese subjects, a gradual and modest weight loss may be achieved by regular physical exercise and a moderate reduction in energy intake.

Practical tips for LPD

An LPD may be difficult to follow. Foods, such as meat, which are rich in protein (average 20 g/100 g of raw product), even if HBV, need to be restricted. This can be difficult, especially in countries like northern or western Europe or North America, and others with a tradition for meat dishes. Other subjects are used to a high protein intake because of dieting (Atkins or the Zone diet, among others), body building, or personal preferences. Energy intake may be difficult to achieve with an LPD. Education of patients in selecting appropriate foods to achieve a low-protein and an adequate energy intake is of paramount importance. Meats, for example, provide little energy, at least if lean cuts are chosen, as indicated for dyslipidaemia or overweight control. Cheeses are rich in calories (up to 400 kcal/100 g) but have the highest protein content per gram (up to 30 g/100 g, as for example in parmesan cheese); therefore, their intake needs to be limited. Furthermore, less-caloric, low-fat dairies need to be chosen for CVD prevention. Vegetable foods such as grains (pasta, rice, bread, etc.) are energy-rich (280 kcal/100 g for baked bread; 350 kcal/100 g for uncooked pasta) but contain less protein than meat or cheese (about 8–10 g/100 g for baked white bread and uncooked pasta or rice), and of a lower quality. The need to limit lower-biological-value proteins, while maintaining a high energy intake, may require the use of special commercial low-protein grain products (pasta, bread, pizza, cookies, etc.) made from ingredients such as corn, potato, or rice starches. One hundred grams of uncooked, low-protein pasta contains 0.6 g proteins, 352 kcal energy, and <50 mg phosphate. The poorer texture and taste and higher price (unless cost is subsidised by state programmes) of these foods may interfere with an adequate intake. The protein content of vegetables is generally low (e.g. <2 g in half a cup of cooked vegetables), but this amount should also be included in the total quota of the daily protein allowance, making the protein restriction still harder. At times, compliance to the reduced dietary protein is adequate but the energy intake is too low. A practical solution to some of these problems may be to prepare 'all-in-one' dishes, such as pasta with ragout or tuna sauce, oriental-style dishes prepared with diced meat or fish mixed with grains and greens, or vegetables stuffed with meat or small quantities of dairy product.

Dietary prescription in RRT patients

Goals

(1) To prevent or control complications, including PEM, dyslipidaemia, systemic hypertension, CVD, secondary hyperparathyroidism, and other uraemic symptoms not corrected by dialysis.

Diet characteristics

RRT changes requirements for protein, energy, minerals, and vitamins (Table 14.5).

The available data suggest that a protein intake of 1.0–1.2 g/kg/day (at least 50% HBV) is adequate to maintain a neutral nitrogen balance in most haemodialysis patients. ESPEN guidelines recommend a protein intake of 1.2–1.4 g/kg IBW/day (50% HBV).

The KDOQI and UK Renal Association guidelines suggest an intake of 1.2 g/kg/day.

In CAPD patients, the protein requirement is 1.2–1.5 g/kg/day (at least 50% HBV), according to nutritional status and the amount of protein lost in the dialysate. An additional 0.1–0.2 g/kg/day may be needed if peritoneal inflammation occurs. According to the KDOQI and UK Renal Association indications, the daily protein intake should be at least 1.2 g/kg IBW/day.

The energy intake for patients with a normal BMI, both on haemodialysis and on CAPD, should be 30–35 kcal/kg/day, depending on the age and the level of daily activities. The total energy intake in CAPD patients must take into account the contribution of energy from the glucose absorbed from the dialysate. This can be in the order of 100–200 g/day. According to the KDOQI guidelines, from the age of 60 years energy intake should be kept in the lower range.

Control of cardiovascular risk factors

Dyslipidaemia

The KDOQI Work Group suggests, for patients with CRF in stages 1–4, following the guidelines of the National Cholesterol Education Task Force, Adult Treatment Panel III (ATP III), with a target for LDL cholesterol levels of <100 mg/dl (or <70 mg/dl in very

Table 14.5 Nutritional guidelines for patients on RRT. HBV, high biological value; IBW, ideal body weight (Metropolitan Life Insurance tables); SBW, standard body weight (NHANES II); ABW, adjusted body weight = IBW + (IBW − actual body weight) × 0.25. This correction factor is used in underweight or overweight subjects and is introduced to avoid overfeeding or underfeeding); ESPEN, European Society for Clinical Nutrition and Metabolism; NKF KDOQI, National Kidney Foundation Kidney Disease Outcomes Quality Initiative; ERBP, European Renal Best Practice guidelines; nPNA, normalised protein nitrogen appearance.

	ESPEN (Cano et al., 2006, 2009)	NKF KDOQI (2007)	ERBP (Foque et al., 2007)	UK Renal Association (2010)
Haemodialysis				
Protein (g/kg IBW, SBW, or ABW/day)	1.2–1.4 (>50% HBV)	1.2 (≥50% HBV)	At least 1.1 (nPNA at least 1)	1.2
Energy (kcal/kg IBW, SBW, or ABW/day)	35	35, <60 years 30–35, >60 years	30–40, adjusted to age, gender, and level of physical activity	30–35, depending upon age and physical activity Assess adequacy in single patients
CAPD				
Protein (g/kg IBW, SBW, or ABW/day)	1.2–1.5 (> 50% HBV) Higher if peritonitis	1.2–1.3 (≥50% HBV)		1.2
Energy (kcal/kg IBW, SBW, or ABW/day, including energy from dialysate)	35, adjusted for over- or underweight	35, <60 years 30–35, >60 years		30–35, depending upon age and physical activity Assess adequacy in single patients

high-risk patients). The dietary prescription should be aimed at maintaining total dietary fat intake at between 25 and 35% of total calories, saturated fatty acids at <7%, and cholesterol at <200 mg/day. An adequate intake of fibre should also be implemented, especially through soluble fibre-rich foods (such as vegetables, fruits, and pulses, supplements of viscous fibre such as psyllium, and other products containing mixtures of insoluble and soluble fibres). Plant sterols increase cholesterol excretion by interfering with the intestinal absorption. A daily intake of 2–3 g sterols (reachable through supplements) can reduce LDL levels by 6–15% without affecting HDL cholesterol or triglycerides. In subjects with elevated serum triglycerides, the total intake of carbohydrate, especially simple sugars, and alcohol, should be limited. Physical activity is also useful, since it increases HDL cholesterol levels and decreases triglycerides. Of course, drug treatment for dyslipidaemia may be needed. CKD patients may have low serum cholesterol levels, which in any case are associated with an increased CVD risk and a worse outcome (a paradoxical inverse association). This relationship may be a consequence of the presence of an MIA syndrome, mostly seen in haemodialysis patients.

Overweight

Some CRF patients are overweight at the time of diagnosis, and even though malnutrition is frequent, some may gain weight afterwards. Contributing factors include reduced energy expenditure from lower physical activity, excessive eating as a response to psychological stress, smoking cessation, use of drugs that cause weight gain, and, in the case of peritoneal dialysis, absorption of glucose from the dialysate fluid, contributing to a positive energy balance. Obesity in haemodialysis and CAPD patients shows a paradoxical association with a lower CVD morbidity and mortality, even in cases of severe obesity, and after correction for other factors, such as age, diabetes, and dialysis characteristics. The reason for this relationship is not clear, but it may be due to a higher negative prognostic impact of the nonclassical risk factors in CKD. The value of weight loss in overweight patients is therefore controversial. In CKD patients, as in the general population, central obesity is associated with a higher CVD risk. Therefore, the Scottish Intercollegiate Guidelines Network (SIGN) guidelines suggest weight management in cases of increased abdominal circumferences: above 94 cm in males and 80 cm in females.

Lack of regular physical activity

Considering the benefits of exercise (preservation and increase of lean body mass and function, control of cardiovascular risk factors, and improvement of quality of life scores on well-being), SIGN and UK Renal Association guidelines recommend regular exercise programmes in CKD patients. Progressive resistance training and aerobic exercise should be included.

Mineral, fluid, and vitamin intake

Phosphate and calcium

Calcium and phosphate levels require careful and frequent monitoring.

Phosphate intake generally needs to be limited only in advanced stages of CKD, to control BMD and to reduce the formation in kidney and vessels of damaging calcium-phosphate precipitate with negative effects on CKD progression and CVD risk. The KDOQI Clinical Practice Guidelines for Bone Metabolism and Disease recommend restricting phosphate intake to 800–1000 mg/day (in relation to the levels of protein intake) when serum phosphorus levels are increased above 4.6 mg/dl or 1.49 mmol/l in CKD stages 3 and 4, or above 5.5 mg/dl or 1.78 mmol/l in stage 5, or when total plasma PTH is increased above the levels expected for each renal failure stage. The phosphorus content of food is directly related to that of proteins. LPDs therefore limit dietary phosphate. On RRT, the removal of phosphate is insufficient (a session clears between 500 and 700 mg of the mineral), while the diet needs to be protein-rich. Phosphate intake therefore still needs to be kept low, around 800–1000 mg/day (8–17 mg/kg/day). A further restriction is not feasible, because of the higher protein requirements of these patients. Patients need to be educated about food best choices, without compromising their protein intake. Phosphate is present mainly in animal food, and especially in dairy products (milk, yogurt, and cheese). In whole-grain cereals or pulses, the presence of phytate interferes with phosphate absorption. Other phosphate-rich foods are baking powder, chocolate, cola-like soft drinks, beer or ale, coffee or tea, and phosphate additive present in processed and convenience foods (cold cuts, cheeses, dressings, beverages, bakery products, etc.). These sources are often poorly recognised. Phosphate binders, taken at the beginning of or during meals, in addition to the dietary modification, are generally required to reduce phosphate absorption from the gut. Calcium intake may also be inadequate due to the exclusion or limitation of dairy foods, required to control phosphate, energy, or cholesterol levels, and supplementation may be required. To avoid any excess, a calcium intake equivalent to 2 g/day, including food and supplements, is suggested. With the use of phosphate binders containing calcium, dietary intake should be maintained within 1 g/day. A dialysate with lower calcium content may be necessary. Recently, it has been suggested that total intake of calcium be reduced to 1200 mg/day, avoiding supplementation greater than 500 mg/day.

Sodium and fluids

Since sodium intake may favour hypertension, the KDOQI guidelines suggest a limited intake of less than 2.3 g/day in CKD in all stages, from 1 to 4, with the exception of 'salt-losing' conditions such as polycystic kidney disease. In the pre-dialysis phase, an adequate water and sodium excretion is generally maintained until GFR declines to 10–15 ml/minute: at this point, sodium and fluid restriction may be necessary to control extracellular volume expansion, hypertension, or oedema. In RRT patients, liquid and sodium intake must be limited to avoid excess interdialytic weight gain, hypertension, and the need for high fluid removal during the dialysis session. In RRT, in order to keep the interdialytic weight gain within acceptable values (2.0–2.5 kg), sodium intake should be maintained at between 2.0 and 2.3 g/day or 5 and 6 g of salt, and fluid intake at around 1000 ml, including water in food, plus the equivalent of any residual urine volume.

Potassium

The control of potassium levels in CKD may be needed in stages 3 and 4 (recommended intake: 2.4 g/day) and on dialysis (recommended intake: 1.9–2.7 g/day, 50–70 mmol, about 1 mmol/kg). Causes of hyperkalaemia, independent of CKD, need to be considered, such as metabolic acidosis, drugs (ACE inhibitors, angiotensin-2 receptor blockers, spironolactone, beta-blockers, nonsteroidal anti-inflammatory drugs (NSAID) products), salt-substitute abuse, inadequate

dialysis, fasting, and hypercatabolism, due to acute illnesses. High-potassium foods include many fruits and vegetables. The potassium content in vegetables can be reduced by boiling them in plenty of water, to be discarded after cooking.

Zinc and selenium

Deficiencies may develop from long-term LPD, but supplements are not usually recommended.

Vitamins

Vitamin depletion in CKD may result from low dietary intake, reduced gastrointestinal absorption, abnormal kidney metabolism (as for example with vitamin D), and losses with dialysis. The risk of deficiency involves mainly the water-soluble vitamins. The suggested vitamin intake in CKD is reported in Box 14.7. Vitamin supplements are taken regularly by many patients, with dosages that may be higher than recommended. In some countries, specific renal multivitamin formulas are available. Products for the general public may have a

> ### Box 14.7 Recommended intake of vitamins in CKD patients
>
> - Pyridoxine: 10–15 mg (dietary recommended intake (DRI) in healthy adults: 1.3 in women (1.5 >50 years), 1.3 in males (1.7 >50 years). In haemodialysis, the requirement may be increased from erythropoietin-induced erythropoiesis.
> - Folic acid: 1 mg/day (DRI in healthy adults: 400 µg). The requirement is increased from reduced intestinal absorption and dialysis-induced losses. Supraphysiological replacement to modify serum homocysteine levels and vascular risk is not recommended. Folate intake of 5 mg/day, plus 50 mg pyridoxine and 0.4 mg B_{12}, is suggested by the National Kidney Foundation Task Force on Cardiovascular Disease.
> - B12: 24 µg/day (same as the DRI for normal subjects), but supplementation may be needed.
> - Riboflavin: 1.1–1.3 mg (same as the DRI for normal subjects).
> - Vitamin C: 30–60 mg on conservative treatment, 75–90 mg in RRT (because of the high losses during the dialysis sessions and the role of the vitamin in folic-acid metabolism, response to erythropoietin, and prevention of muscle cramps). Higher intake may cause oxalosis and should be avoided.
> - Vitamin D: the dosage needs to be determined according to the serum calcium and PTH levels.
> - Vitamin A: supplementation is not recommended, since it may lead to toxicity.
> - Carnitine: current guidelines do not recommend a general supplementation, but it can be useful in selected patients on dialysis who do not adequately respond to standard therapy.

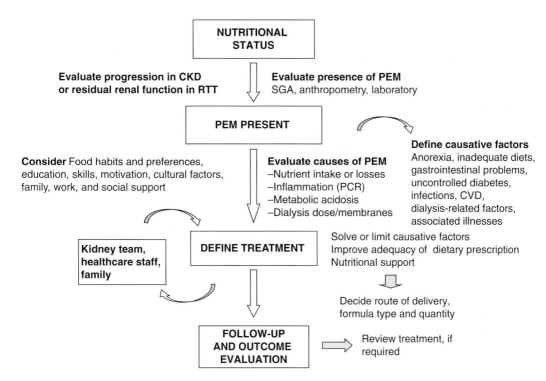

Figure 14.3 Flow chart for the treatment of PEM in CKD.

composition inadequate for CKD patients. In haemodialysis patients, water-soluble vitamin supplements can be given intravenously, at the end of the dialysis sessions. Carnitine, a metabolite which allows fatty acid transport to sites of beta-oxidation in the mitochondria, is also involved in the regulation of energy metabolism and in the prevention of organic acid accumulation in the mitochondria. In haemodialysis, losses through the dialytic membranes may cause depletion. Carnitine supplementation in haemodialysis is associated with clinical benefits including enhanced response to erythropoietin, improved exercise tolerance, and reduced intradialytic or postdialytic symptoms (hypotension, arrhythmias, muscle cramps, and fatigue); furthermore, it may improve insulin resistance, protein balance, lipid profile, and cardiac function.

Nutritional support in CKD and RRT malnourished patients

A flow chart on how to address PEM is shown in Figure 14.3; see also Chapter 9.

The stages of CKD and the nutritional status should be evaluated together with the assessment of the causal factors responsible for PEM. To manage malnutrition, first of all reversible factors (infections, inflammation, gastrointestinal problems, dialysis management, low education, understanding, or skills) should be addressed. In patients at ESRF and malnutrition, the beginning of dialysis should not be delayed. In haemodialysis patients, treatment should be optimised through increased dialysis dose, use of biocompatible membranes, and ultrapure water. Normalisation of serum bicarbonate may have a role. Nutritional education, supportive nutritional counselling by an expert dietitian, encouragement, motivational techniques, empowerment, and follow-up are the first-line strategies in preventing PEM or improving the nutritional status. If an acute condition has developed, causing increased protein and energy requirements, the same guidelines should be followed as for AKI. In patients in stable clinical conditions, but gradually losing weight, fat, or muscle mass after controlling for other factors, guidelines for nutritional support in CKD, by oral supplements, or by enteral or parenteral nutrition, should be followed. The modalities of nutritional support are guided by the level of the gap between the spontaneous intake and nutrient requirements, the severity of malnutrition, the type of treatment (conservative or RRT), and the general clinical conditions of the patient.

Special nutritional formulas (so-called kidney formulas), specifically designed for patients with CKD on conservative treatment or on dialysis, are commercially available, for both enteral and parenteral nutrition support. For enteral nutrition, the most recently available products are 'ready-to-use' liquid, polymeric formulas, characterised by a reduced (for CKD patients on conservative treatment) or a high (for dialysis patients) protein content, lower electrolyte concentration (potassium and phosphate), and high energy (1.5–2.0 kcal/ml). The high nutrient density of these products may also be useful in controlling fluid balance. The *nitrogen-sparing formulas*, containing only essential amino acids, are no longer employed, since both essential and non-essential amino acids are required to ensure nitrogen balance. Some products, however, are enriched with histidine and tyrosine, which are essential amino acids in renal failure.

Oral nutritional supplementation

ONS, with palatable and easy-to-drink formulas, is the easiest form of nutritional support. It should be prescribed only to integrate regular, but insufficient, food intake; ONS allows energy and protein intake to be increased by about 500 kcal/day (or 5–10 kcal/kg/day) and 0.4–0.6 g/kg/day, respectively. Some patients have poor compliance to ONS because of anorexia, dysgeusia, and taste aversion or fatigue. To improve ONS intake, the formulas may be taken in between meals or as late-evening snack. In CKD on conservative treatment, ONS improves the intake of energy, as required for better nitrogen utilisation, and, at times, of proteins – total and HBV – which may be difficult for some subjects to achieve. In haemodialysis patients, ONS can be taken during or at the end of the dialysis session in order to minimise the catabolic effect of the RRT. For ONS, the use of standard formulas is suggested. The cost of such supplements is not always covered by health systems, and patients often complain about the low palatability of the products.

Intradialytic parenteral nutrition

In haemodialysis patients noncompliant to oral supplementation, nutrient intake can be improved by a form of intermittent parenteral nutrition, infused through the dialysis line, which allows a supply of nutrients during dialysis sessions, for a total of 10–15 hours a week. About 800–1200 kcal and 30–60 g of amino acids can be infused per haemodialysis session. The intervention is, as in the case of ONS, effective if the spontaneous energy and protein intake is ≥ 20 kcal and ≥ 0.8 g/kg/day. In CAPD patients, intraperitoneal amino acid supplementation may be used.

Total enteral or parenteral nutrition

Nutrient prescription for malnourished, but not acutely ill, patients should follow the same indications as for non-malnourished subjects. For enteral nutrition lasting longer than 5 days, disease-specific formulas are suggested. Overnight tube feeding can be a way of incrementing intake without disrupting the patient's daily routine.

Pharmacological therapies to improve the nutritional status

Anabolic agents such as subcutaneous growth hormone, insulin-like growth factor, and androgens, as well as antioxidant vitamins and anti-inflammatory drugs, including statins, can improve the nutritional status, body composition, and efficacy of nutritional support. Guidelines taking into account the potentiality of severe side effects, the limited evidence of benefits, and the costs, do not recommend the use of anabolic agents to treat under-nutrition.

14.5 Kidney transplantation

Transplant patients need to be followed carefully from the nutritional point of view, before and in the early weeks after surgery, and in the long term. Renal transplantation either largely or partially restores renal function, and dietary prescription may be more liberalised. However, dietary modifications are needed to maintain graft survival or to treat chronic graft rejection or metabolic, cardiovascular, and bone complications.

Pre-transplant nutritional assessment

In the pre-transplant phase it is very important to evaluate the patient in order to identify risk factors which might reduce survival or the chances of a successful transplant. In particular, diabetic, obese, and elderly patients should be adequately assessed and monitored. Severe malnutrition should be corrected, if necessary, by nutritional support. Particular attention should be paid to the treatment of hypertension and dyslipidaemia. In diabetic patients, the glycaemic control must be optimal. Patients must be determined to stop smoking. Control of energy intake should be encouraged in obese patients, since obesity is associated with a higher rate of complications, especially at higher levels of overweight. Bone metabolism, which may be rapidly impaired by post-transplant steroid therapy, should be assessed by bone mineral-density measurement, and measurement of the serum levels of calcium, phosphorus, and PTH.

Nutritional management

Post-transplant early phases

The first 4–6 weeks after renal transplantation are characterised by higher protein requirements from the increased skeletal muscle catabolism, induced by the surgical stress, and by pharmacological treatment with corticosteroid, at high dosage. Protein intake should therefore be in the range of 1.3–1.4 g/kg IBW/day. This amount is also prescribed if immediate post-transplant dialysis is necessary. Energy intake should be in the range of 30–35 kcal/kg/day, adjusted for malnourished or obese patients. To limit the risk of corticosteroid-induced hyperglycaemia, energy from carbohydrates should be limited to 50%, with higher lipid intake (30–35%). Fluid and electrolyte intake needs to be adjusted according to the clinical conditions. In case of post-transplant phosphaturia, a normal to high phosphate dietary intake is prescribed.

Post-transplant later phases

Treatment is defined by the need to control graft dysfunction or failure and any complications which might develop in long-term immunosuppressive therapy (Box 14.8).

Cardiovascular risk factors, besides increasing mortality, may also enhance the rate of graft failure.

> **Box 14.8 Major complications in later phases of kidney transplantation**
>
> - sustained protein catabolism, with loss of lean body mass;
> - weight gain up to 35%, mostly in the first 12 months, with abdominal fat deposition;
> - glucose intolerance or new-onset diabetes after transplantation (NODAT);
> - dyslipidaemia;
> - hypertension;
> - increased risk of CVD;
> - increased risk of mineral and bone disorders.

On average, the recommended protein intake in stable patients on maintenance immunosuppression is around 0.8–1.0 g/kg IBW/day, with energy intake in the range of 25–30 kcal/kg/day. If required, this will be lower for overweight patients. Calcium intake should be around 1000 mg/day (1300 in post-menopausal women), achieved through the diet with supplements, if necessary, and phosphate intake around 1200–1500 mg/day. Vitamin D supplementation is recommended at about 0.5 μg on alternate days. In cases of graft-rejection risk, with an adequate energy intake and a low prednisone dosage, a lower protein (0.6–0.8 g/kg/day) and phosphate (800 mg/day, associated with binders, if necessary) intake should be prescribed. This regimen can however only be applied in cases with a low catabolic stimulus. The increased CVD risk is managed by lifestyle modification, including increased physical activity, lower energy intake to reduce overweight, control of fat type and quantity, lower dietary sodium to lower hypertension, and adequate fibre (25–30 g/day) and drug prescription. Many compounds may interfere with electrolyte balance. Cyclosporine, beta-blocker agents, or ACE inhibitors may increase potassium levels, while diuretics may reduce them. Cyclosporine may cause hypomagnesaemia.

14.6 Concluding remarks

Nutritional management of CKD patients has gone through many changes as new evidence on causative factors of progression of kidney disease has been explored. Obesity-related problems and the role of weight control or of fatty-acid manipulations in modifying inflammation or immune responses require further study. The nomenclature of PEM and tools for screening and assessing nutritional status, for early identification of malnutrition should be better defined in order to improve treatment strategies and outcome.

More focus should be put on the definition of whole dietary patterns, to prevent or treat kidney disorders, and on effective educational tools, to modify lifestyle. Vitamin requirements still pose many open questions, especially for vitamins such as folate and vitamins B_{12}, B_6, and D, which are characterised by complex and partially unexplored functions.

Acknowledgements

This chapter has been revised and updated by Roberta Situlin and Gianfranco Guarnieri, based on the original chapter by Gianfranco Guarnieri, Roberta Situlin, and Gabriele Toigo.

References and further reading

Cano N, Fiaccadori E, Tesinsky P, Toigo G, Druml W; DGEM (German Society for Nutritional Medicine), *et al*. ESPEN guidelines on enteral nutrition: adult renal failure. Clin Nutr 2006; 25: 295–310.

Cano NJM, Aparicio M, Brunori G, Carrero JJ, Cianciaruso B, Fiaccadori E, *et al*. ESPEN guidelines on parenteral nutrition: adult renal failure. Clin Nutr 2009; 28: 401–414.

Dukkipati R, Noori N, Feroze U, Kopple JD. Dietary protein intake in patients with advanced chronic kidney disease and on dialysis. Semin Dial 2010; 23(4): 365–372.

Fouque D, Vennegoor M, ter Wee P, Wanner C, Basci A, Canaud B, *et al*. EBPG guideline on nutrition. Nephrol Dial Transplant 2007; 22(Suppl. 2): 45–87.

Fouque D, Kalantar-Zadeh K, Kopple J, Cano N, Chauveau P, Cuppari L, *et al*. A proposed nomenclature and diagnostic criteria for protein-energy wasting in acute and chronic kidney disease. Kidney Int 2008; 73(4): 391–398.

Guarnieri G, Situlin R, Biolo G. Carnitine metabolism in uremia. Am J Kidney Dis 2001; 38(Suppl. 1): S63–67.

Guarnieri G, Antonione R, Biolo G. Mechanisms of malnutrition in uremia. J Ren Nutr 2003; 13(2): 153–157.

Kalantar-Zadeh K, Ikizler TA, Block G, Avram MM, Kopple JD. Malnutrition-inflammation complex syndrome in dialysis patients: causes and consequences. Am J Kidney Dis 2003; 42(5): 864–881.

Kidney Disease: Improving Global Outcomes (KDIGO). Clinical practice guidelines. 2008, 2009. http://www.kdigo.org/clinical_practice_guidelines/index.php.

Kopple JD, Feroze U. The effect of obesity on chronic kidney disease. J Ren Nutr 2011: 21(1): 66–71.

Kumar P, Clark M (eds). Renal disease. In: Clinical Medicine, pp. 519–595. Edinburgh: Saunders, 1998.

Modification of Diet in Renal Disease Study Group. Short term effects of protein intake, blood pressure, and antihypertensive therapy on glomerular filtration rate in the Modification of Diet in Renal Disease Study. J Am Soc Nephrol 1996; 7: 2097–2109.

Monk RD, Bushinsky DA. Making sense of the latest advice on vitamin D therapy. J Am Soc Nephrol 201; 22(6): 994–998.

NIH. Your guide to lowering your blood pressure with DASH. Washington, DC: National Institutes of Health, 2006.

National Institute for Health and Clinical Excellence (NICE). Chronic kidney disease 2008. http://www.nice.org.uk/CG073fullguideline.

NKF KDOQI. Guidelines and commentaries. 2007. http://www.kidney.org/professionals/KDOQI/guidelines_commentaries.cfm.

Renal Service Network, Australia. Evidence-based guidelines for the nutritional management of adult kidney transplant recipients. 2009. http://www.healthnetworks.health.wa.gov.au/network/renal_links.cfm.

SIGN (Scottish Intercollegiate Guidelines Network). Diagnosis and management of chronic kidney disease. A national clinical guideline. 2008. http://www.sign.ac.uk/pdf/sign103.pdf.

Stenvinkel P, Heimburger O, Lindholm B, Kaysen GA, Bergstrom J. Are there two types of malnutrition in chronic renal failure? Evidence for relationships between malnutrition, inflammation and atherosclerosis (MIA syndrome). Nephrol Dial Transplant 2000; 15(7): 953–960.

Stratton RJ, Bircher G, Fouque D, Stenvinkel P, de Mutsert R, Engfer M, Elia M. Multinutrient oral supplements and tube feeding in maintenance dialysis: a systematic review and meta-analysis. Am J Kidney Dis 2005; 46: 387–405.

UK Renal Association. Clinical practice guidelines. 2010. http://www.renal.org/Clinical/GuidelinesSection/Guidelines.aspx.

15

Nutritional and Metabolic Support in Haematological Malignancies and Haematopoietic Stem-cell Transplantation

Maurizio Muscaritoli, Saveria Capria, Anna Paola Iori, and Filippo Rossi Fanelli

La Sapienza University of Rome, Italy

Key messages

- Patients with haematological malignancies are at increased risk of malnutrition, so it is important that all patients are nutritionally assessed and receive nutritional counselling at diagnosis and during the course of treatment.
- To prevent the negative impact on nutritional status of high-dose radio- and chemotherapy, artificial nutrition is frequently indicated in haematological malignancy.
- Mucositis of the gastrointestinal tract represents the main indication for artificial nutrition in haematological malignancy.

- Haematopoietic stem-cell transplantation (HSCT) may negatively affect oral food intake and nutrient absorption, and increase nutrient and energy needs. Nutritional and metabolic intervention should be considered an integral part of supportive care of HSCT patients.
- Parenteral nutrition still represents the main tool by which to provide nutritional support to patients undergoing HSCT. Enteral nutrition is also feasible, and should be attempted as soon as gastrointestinal impairment resolves.

15.1 Introduction

The impact of haematological malignancies on nutritional status is extremely variable and is essentially a function of disease- and treatment-related impairment in nutrient absorption, nutrient losses, and altered energy and protein metabolism. Until recently, however, little attention has been paid to the nutritional implications of haematological malignancies. Unlike solid tumours, which have a dramatic impact on a person's metabolic homeostasis and nutritional status, haematological malignancies are, at least initially, rarely associated with a significant deterioration of nutritional status. The advent of aggressive antineoplastic regimens involving the use of high-dose combination chemotherapy, followed or not by haematopoietic stem-cell transplantation (HSCT) in order to achieve high disease remission rate and longer disease-free

survival, has created a new scenario wherein nutritional and metabolic impairment occur as a consequence not of the underlying disease, but rather of the deleterious side effects of antineoplastic treatments. Therefore, patients who are initially well nourished (as most haematological patients are) may become acutely at risk of malnutrition or overtly malnourished, making nutritional intervention necessary (Table 15.1).

This chapter will mainly focus on the nutritional sequelae of the therapeutic regimens for haematological diseases, including HSCT.

15.2 Haematological malignancies

Haematological malignancies represent a heterogeneous group of diseases, including leukaemia, lymphoma, and other lympho-myeloproliferative disorders.

Clinical Nutrition, Second Edition. Edited by Marinos Elia, Olle Ljungqvist, Rebecca J Stratton and Susan A Lanham-New.
© 2013 The Nutrition Society. Published 2013 by Blackwell Publishing Ltd.

Table 15.1 Disease-dependent and treatment-dependent nutritional risks in haematological malignancies.

Disease	Disease-dependent nutritional risks	Treatment-dependent nutritional risks
Myelodysplastic syndromes		×
Acute myeloid leukaemia		×
Chronic myeloid leukaemia	×	×
Acute lymphocytic leukaemia		×
Chronic lymphocytic leukaemia		×
Hodgkin's lymphoma	×	×
Non-Hodgkin's lymphoma	×[a]	×

[a]Weight loss is more frequent in high-grade lymphomas.

Myeloproliferative disorders

Myeloproliferative disorders are caused by acquired clonal abnormalities of the haematopoietic stem cells. They produce characteristic syndromes with a well-defined clinical and biological picture, which can show either a more indolent behaviour, like chronic myeloid leukaemia (CML), polycythemia vera, essential thrombocytemia, and myelofibrosis, or more aggressive features, like acute myeloid leukaemia (AML) and high-risk myelodysplastic syndrome (MDS). These conditions require an intensive treatment, but in a proportion of cases they fail to respond or relapse after an initial response to therapy.

Nutritional intervention is most frequently indicated for patients with MDS and AML.

Myelodysplastic syndrome

MDS is characterised clinically by a hyperproliferative bone marrow, reflective of ineffective haematopoiesis, and is accompanied by one or more peripheral blood cytopaenias. Bone-marrow failure results, leading to death from bleeding and infection in the majority, while transformation to acute leukaemia occurs in up to 40% of patients. Supportive therapy with transfusions and growth factors (erythropoietin, granulocyte colony-stimulating factor) and hormonal therapy (androgens, danazol) have a limited indication for the forms at low risk of trasformation in acute leukaemia. In high-risk MDS, long-term results with conventional chemotherapy are disappointing. In recent years, the introduction of demethylating and differentiating agents has seemed promising. In young patients with high-risk MDS, the use of high-dose chemotherapy followed by allogeneic bone-marrow or peripheral blood stem-cell (PBSC) infusion is also utilised as first-line therapy.

Acute myeloid leukaemia

AML is the most common variant of acute leukaemia occurring in adults, making up approximately 80–85% of cases of acute leukaemia diagnosed in individuals over 20 years of age. Currently, between 60 and 80% of young adults can achieve complete remission. The possibility of obtaining a durable complete remission decreases with age, and the chance of long-term survival in a patient more than 60 years old doesn't exceed 30%. The French–American–British (FAB) morphological classification named the AML according to the normal marrow elements that it most closely resembled (M0–M7 and hybrid leukaemias), and was widely employed until 1998, when it was replaced by the World Health Organization (WHO) classification, which takes into account current knowledge about the diagnostic prognostic role of clonal cytogenetic and molecular aberrations.

Most patients with AML present with anaemia, thrombocytopaenia, and leukocytosis (median white blood cell count 10 000–20 000/μl). Patients with AML generally present initially with symptoms related to complications of pancytopaenia, including weakness, easy fatigability, infections of variable severity, and haemorrhagic findings such as gingival bleeding, ecchymoses, epistaxis, and menorrhagia. Combinations of these symptoms are common. Although increased resting energy expenditure has been described in paediatric and adult patients with AML, nutritional status is usually good upon diagnosis. Protein turnover is also increased.

Changes in plasma free amino acid concentration have been described in AML that only partially resemble those observed in solid tumours. In a study performed in 40 AML patients upon diagnosis, a significant increase in glutamic acid, ornithine, free tryptophan, and glycine plasma concentrations was reported, while serine, methionine, and taurine were significantly reduced with respect to control subjects. When patients were stratified according to their response to chemotherapy and their status at 18 months after chemotherapy, it was shown that taurine, its precursor serine, and methionine tended to be even lower in patients who had not responded to or had relapsed after high-dose chemotherapy.

Thus, it would appear that taurine deficiency may have some relevance in the clinical outcome of AML, since it has been previously demonstrated that taurine is the most abundant intracellular free amino acid in AML, and that its plasma concentrations drop after chemotherapy, while its intracellular content correlates to the chemosensitivity of a leukaemia cell line.

Therapy for AML has traditionally been divided into stages: induction, post-remission therapy of varying intensity and duration, and post-relapse therapy.

- Induction therapy is designed to produce rapid clearing of leukaemic cells from the peripheral blood with subsequent marrow aplasia, and is achieved with combined therapy including an anthracycline in association with ara-C, causing severe mucosal damage.
- Post-remission therapy includes intensive consolidation with intermediate/high-dose cytarabine with or without anthracycline, followed in most cases by a stem-cell transplant; both allogeneic and autologous HSCT have been advocated for selected patients in first remission, depending upon the patients' age, clinical and biological risk factors, and donor availability.
- Relapsed and refractory AML are usually treated with non-cross-resistant combining chemotherapy.

A transient reduction of energy expenditure may be induced by chemotherapy. However, fever, immunosuppression, and consequent opportunistic infections may again increase metabolic rate and protein wasting, particularly in the neutropaenic period.

Chronic myeloid leukaemia

CML is a clonal myeloproliferative disorder of a pluripotent stem cell with a specific cytogenetic abnormality, the Philadelphia (Ph) chromosome, which is responsible for the generation of a pathologic fusion protein (p210) with tyrosine-kinase activity. The proein induces a dysregulation in the control mechanisms of white blood cell proliferation and death. The first phase of the disease, the chronic phase, terminates in a second, more acute or abrupt course, called the blast phase. Symptoms and signs usually develop insidiously and include fatigue, anaemia, progressive splenomegaly, and leukocytosis. In the chronic phase, the myeloid cells in the peripheral blood show all stages of differentiation, but the myelocyte predominates. The therapeutic approach of CML has radically changed in the last 10 years. Until 2000, the best therapeutic options for young CML patients were recombinant interferon-gamma (rIFN-γ) and allogeneic stem-cell transplant; but since then the first treatment choice has become the use of tyrosine-kinase inhibitors (TKIs) (imatinib, dasatinib, nilotinib). These compounds, orally administered, target the pathologic fusion protein responsible for the proliferation and apoptosis impairment, and are capable of inducing cytogenetic remissions in a high proportion of patients. Currently the indication for stem-cell transplant in CML is limited to those patients not responding to TKI and to those in accelerated/blastic phase.

Lymphoproliferative disorders

Acute lymphocytic leukaemia

Acute lymphocytic leukaemia (ALL) makes up 80% of the acute leukaemias of childhood. The peak incidence is between 3 and 7 years of age. It also occurs in adults, causing approximately 20% of acute adult leukaemias. Adults with ALL are treated with combination chemotherapy, including daunorubicin, vincristine, prednisone, and asparaginase. This treatment produces complete remission in 80–90% of patients. After complete remission, central nervous system prophylaxis is performed.

Post-remission consolidation is achieved with variably myelosuppressive doses of cytarabine and other chemotherapeutic agents in varied combinations, while no standard approach has been devised for relapsed or refractory ALL.

High-dose chemotherapy plus bone-marrow transplantation represents a therapeutic option in selected categories of high-risk patients in first complete remission and in most patients after relapse.

Chronic lymphocytic leukaemia (CLL)

Chronic lymphocytic leukaemia (CLL) is characterised by a progressive accumulation of monoclonal B lymphocytes. During the initial asymptomatic phase, patients are able to maintain their usual lifestyle, but during the terminal phase, the performance status is poor, with recurring need for hospitalisation. The most frequent causes of death are severe systemic infections (especially pneumonia and septicaemia), bleeding, and malnutrition with cachexia.

Most cases of early CLL require no specific therapy. Standard treatment with chlorambucil is well tolerated and usually effective, and does not cause any nutritional impairment, but in young patients (<60 years) with biological features associated with a poor prognosis and a significant reduction of life expectancy with standard therapy, the indication to perform an allogeneic stem-cell transplant is increasing.

Malignant lymphoma

The malignant lymphomas are neoplastic transformations of cells that reside predominantly within lymphoid tissues. Although Hodgkin's and non-Hodgkin's lymphomas (NHLs) are among the most sensitive malignant neoplasms to radiation and cytotoxic therapy, their response rates are markedly different (nearly 75% for Hodgkin's lymphomas and 35% for NHLs).

Hodgkin's lymphoma

Hodgkin disease is a group of lymphoproliferative disorders characterised by the pathognomonic finding of Reed–Sternberg cells, with varying degrees of normal reactive and inflammatory cells and fibrosis within involved lymph nodes.

The disease has a bimodal age distribution, with one peak in the 20s and a second over age 50. Presenting symptoms include fever, weight loss, night sweats, generalised pruritus, and the occurrence of a painless mass, generally in the neck. Patients with stage I–II Hodgkin's disease with favourable prognostic factors are candidates for radiotherapy alone or for modified radiotherapy and chemotherapy. Patients with unfavourable prognostic factors should receive chemotherapy (adriamycin, bleomycin, vincristin, and daunorubicin; ABVD) and radiotherapy as initial treatment. ABVD is also the treatment of choice in advanced disease. For patients who fail to achieve remission with primary chemotherapy, and for those who relapse after initial treatment, the best therapeutic option is autologous stem-cell transplantation. Allogeneic bone-marrow transplantation has been performed in patients with advanced Hodgkin's disease, but results are controversial due to the high toxicity.

Non-Hodgkin's lymphoma

NHLs are a heterogeneous group of neoplasms of lymphocytes. The pathogenesis of these disorders has been widely clarified with the aid of molecular biology. Although classification of the lymphoma is a controversial area in continuous evolution, lymphoma classification schemas are mainly based on lymph-node architecture, cytological classification of the neoplastic cells, and lymphoid cell immunophenotype (WHO classification of lymphoid neoplasms).

Unlike patients with Hodgkin's disease, who present with weight loss, fever, or night sweats, patients with NHL generally do not present with systemic complaints, but mainly with painless peripheral lymphadenopathy.

The appropriate therapeutic regimen is strictly dependent upon the histology and extent of disease. The patient's age and the presence of comorbid diseases also influence the treatment choice. Patients with early-stage NHL usually undergo involved field irradiation, while those with advanced-stage NHL are treated by systemic combination chemotherapy. In CD20-positive lymphomas, the use of the anti-CD20 monoclonal antibody (rituximab) in association with chemotherapy has become the standard therapeutic approach. High-dose therapy and autologous HSCT has a standard indication in patients after relapse, while during first-line treatment the indication is still controversial.

The treatment of high-grade lymphomas (such as lymphoblastic, Burkitt's, and Burkitt's-like lymphomas) involves the use of high-dose combined chemotherapy regimens. Disease relapse is treated by supralethal doses of chemotherapy, often in combination with radiation therapy, and syngeneic, allogeneic, or autologous stem-cell transplantation in order to circumvent myelosuppression.

Multiple myeloma

Multiple myeloma is a haematological malignancy defined by the proliferation of a single plasma-cell clone capable of producing a large amount of a specific immunoglobulin, known as 'monoclonal component'. Main symptoms are renal impairment, anaemia, hypercalcaemia, and lytic bone lesions, which are often responsible for vertebral collapse and other bone fractures. Standard treatment for symptomatic myeloma includes antiangiogenetic agents (thalidomide) and proteasome inhibitors (bortezomib), followed, in patients younger than 65, by autologous stem-cell transplantation, which is currently the best therapeutic choice in patients responding to first-line treatment.

15.3 Rationale for nutritional intervention in haematological malignancies

As stated previously, patients with haematological malignancies should be considered at high risk of developing malnutrition despite their good initial nutritional status. In fact, nutritional impairment in this heterogeneous group of clinical conditions is essentially a consequence of therapeutic intervention; that is, of radiotherapy, chemotherapy, and HSCT. The rationale for nutritional and metabolic support in haematological malignancies is illustrated in Figure 15.1.

Mucositis of the gastrointestinal tract

This condition represents one of the main indications for artificial nutrition in patients undergoing chemotherapy for haematological malignancies. The rapidly proliferating cells of the oropharyngeal and gastrointestinal mucosa are particularly vulnerable to the cytotoxic effects of both chemotherapy and radiotherapy (Figure 15.2). Combined aggressive chemotherapy favours serious gut impairment enhanced by concomitant myelosuppression, particularly if methotrexate is used. Within 7–10 days following remission-induction regimens, patients almost invariably develop oro-oesophageal mucositis and gastrointestinal impairment. These two conditions may cause decreased oral intake, nausea, vomiting, diarrhoea, decreased nutrient absorption, and loss of nutrients from the gut (especially amino acids) secondary to the altered transmembrane transport of nutrients.

Although both the severity and the duration of gastrointestinal impairment may greatly differ among individuals, food intake and absorption are significantly reduced for up to 2–3 weeks following chemotherapy or radiotherapy initiation. Diarrhoea is common after total-body irradiation (TBI) or bowel irradiation, or after chemotherapy administration with cisplatin, carboplatin, and other chemotherapy agents. Adequate hydration must be maintained, and antiemetics that do not have diarrhoea as a side effect may be indicated. Mild diarrhoea is controlled with opioid drugs such as loperamide and diphenoxylate atropine and by lowering the fibre content of food.

When immunosuppression is present, infectious pathogenesis should also be considered. Neutropaenic enterocolitis is a serious complication of chemotherapeutic regimens administered in the treatment of both acute leukaemias and lymphomas (Figure 15.2). This acute inflammatory disease may involve the terminal part of the ileum, cecum, and colon. Although the precise aetiology of this seldom-fatal condition is still unknown, neutropaenia, infections, and drug-induced alterations of the bowel mucosal surface have been proposed to have a role. Ileotyphlitis is a life-threatening complication of neutropaenic enterocolitis frequently occurring in neutropaenic patients receiving high-dose idarubicin-containing chemotherapy. Its clinical picture is characterised by fever, diarrhoea, abdominal pain, and ileus.

The diagnosis of ileotyphlitis may be delayed because the presenting clinical features (fever, diarrhoea, and/or abdominal pain) are not specific and may suggest other abdominal diseases, such as chemotherapy-induced mucositis, antibiotic-related colitis, cytomegalovirus colitis, *Salmonella* spp.

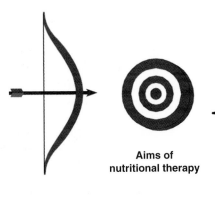

Nutritional:
–Maintenance of nutritional status
Metanutritional:
–Improved tolerance to chemotherapy and radiotherapy;
–Maintenance of immuncompetence;
–Reduction of infective complications;
–Prevention or reduction of mucositis

Aims of nutritional therapy

Figure 15.1 Rationale for nutritional therapy.

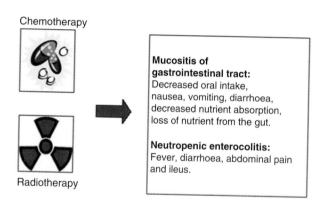

Chemotherapy

Radiotherapy

Mucositis of gastrointestinal tract:
Decreased oral intake, nausea, vomiting, diarrhoea, decreased nutrient absorption, loss of nutrient from the gut.

Neutropenic enterocolitis:
Fever, diarrhoea, abdominal pain and ileus.

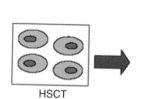

HSCT

GVDH: Large fluid and protein loss (for skin involvement); cholestasis, steatorrhoea, diarrhoea, nausea, vomiting, abdominal pain, ileus, abnormal mucosal absorptive capacity.
Altered metabolism:
Decrease in body cell mass,negative nitrogen balance, impaired glucose tolerance (related to steroids and/or cyclosporin administration), abnormalities in lipid metabolism, malabsorption of water and lipid-soluble vitamins, trace elements deficiency.
Veno-occlusive liver disease (VOD)

Figure 15.2 Treatment-related nutritional problems.

gastroenteritis, or cryptosporidiosis. Computed tomography or ultrasonography of the abdomen yields characteristic findings, such as dilated bowel loops and thickening of the bowel wall >8 mm, reflecting the pathology of the disease, which consists of transmural inflammation, mucosal ulceration, wall oedema, necrosis, teleangectasia, and formation of intramural haematomas.

Although most patients with ileotyphlitis undergo surgical observation, abdominal surgery has no therapeutic role in this syndrome, which is routinely treated with bowel rest, achieved by total parenteral nutrition, and antibiotic therapy.

Haematopoietic stem-cell transplantation

HSCT is a therapeutic procedure consisting of the administration of high-dose chemo-radiotherapy followed by intravenous infusion of haematopoietic stem cells, aimed at restoring lymphohaematopoiesis in patients with damaged or defective bone marrow, reconstituting marrow function after marrow ablating chemo- or radiotherapy, and treating a number of genetic and nonmalignant disorders.

HSCT is a well-established therapy, administered to thousands of patients every year across the world (Box 15.1). The source of haematopoietic stem cells may be bone marrow (by bone-marrow transplantation), peripheral blood, or umbilical cord blood. For this reason, the term 'bone marrow transplantation' is currently being replaced by 'haematopoietic stem cell transplantation'.

Types of HSCT

Two types of HSCT can be performed: allogeneic HSCT (allo-HSCT) and autologous HSCT (a-HSCT).

Box 15.1 Diseases treated by bone-marrow transplantation

Haematological malignancies

- acute myelogenous leukaemia;
- acute lymphocytic leukaemia;
- chronic lymphocytic leukaemia;
- myeloproliferative disorders;
- multiple myeloma;
- non-Hodgkin's lymphoma;
- Hodgkin's disease.

Solid tumours

- breast cancer;
- testicular cancer;
- ovarian cancer;
- glioma;
- neuroblastoma;
- small-cell lung cancer;
- non-small-cell lung cancer.

Other pathological conditions

- severe aplastic anaemia;
- beta-thalassaemia;
- severe combined immunodeficiency;
- autoimmune disorders;
- amyloidosis;
- hereditary metabolic disorders.

Allogeneic bone-marrow transplantation (allo-HSCT)

Allo-HSCT involves the transfer of marrow from a donor to another person (the recipient). Best results are seen after BMT from HLA-genotypically matching sibling donors, but only 30% of patients have such a donor. Therefore, in 1989 an international registry of volunteer donors of haematopoietic stem cells (Bone Marrow Donors Worlwide, BMDW) was founded to allow the transplant procedure in patients who lack a family donor. However, since the probability of finding an unrelated donor is only about 40%, 30% of patients who could benefit from a transplant procedure lack a stem-cell source (both in the family and in BMDW). Fortunately, in the late 1970s a new source of stem cells was been identified in the cord blood, and in 1989 the first allogenic bone transplantation (allo-BMT) was performed from a related cord-blood unit. Thanks to the creation of Cord Blood Banks, in 1995 the first experience of allo-HSCT from unrelated cord blood in patients with haematological diseases was published.

Once a donor has been identified and found suitable for donation, the patient undergoes chemotherapy with or without radiotherapy in order to:

- Induce immunosuppression, which is necessary to avoid rejection due to immunologically active host cells.
- Destroy the residual leukaemic cells and provide space for the new marrow to grow, in the case of myeloablative conditioning regimens.

In recent years there has been an increasing use of conditioning regimens with a reduced dosage of chemo- and radiotherapy (reduced-intensity conditioning regimen, RIC) and non- myeloablative conditioning regimens (NMA). In these cases, the curative role of transplant relies on the antileukaemic long-term effect of the donor immunocompetent cells (graft versus leukaemia effect, GVL), rather than on the citotoxic effect of the conditioning regimen based just on the high dose of the therapy. The low toxicity of the RIC and NMA conditiong regimens has allowed allo-HSCT to be employed in elderly and unfit patients.

Preparative (or conditioning) regimens for allo-HSCT usually consist of radiotherapy combined with alkylating agents. The major advantages of an allogeneic graft include the absence of malignant cells, the antileukaemic effect of the graft (the graft-versus-leukaemia effect), and the ability to treat both malignant and nonmalignant diseases. The major disadvantages of allo-HSCT include the difficulty of finding an appropriate HLA-matched donor and the occurrence of graft-versus-host disease (GVHD).

GVHD is one of the most important causes of morbidity and mortality after allo-HSCT, occurring when immunocompetent cells in the graft target antigens on the cells in the recipient. For historical rather than clinical or pathophysiological reasons, GVHD has been categorised as acute GVHD (a-GVHD), arising before day 100 after transplantation, and chronic GVHD (c-GVHD), arising later than day 100. Today, this strict differentiation has been overcome. A condition which arises after day 100 post-HSCT and shows the clinical features of the classical a-GVHD is regarded as a late-onset a-GVHD. a-GVHD affects mainly the skin, the liver, and the gastrointestinal tract. Leading symptoms are rash or erythema, jaundice, diarrhoea, and nausea. c-GVHD can affect one or more of the following organs: skin, lung, muscle, eyes, liver, mouth, and gastrointestinal mucosa. The clinical features of c-GVHD are similar to those of autoimmune diseases.

The gold standard for diagnosis is the histology, and there are long-established criteria for GVHD's histological diagnosis and grading.

Autologous bone-marrow transplantation (a-HSCT)

Autologous BMT (a-BMT) involves the use of the patient's own marrow to re-establish haematopoietic cell function after the administration of high-dose chemotherapy. The major advantages of autologous transplantation include the ready availability of a stem-cell product and the absence of GVHD, which translate into lower morbidity, mortality, and cost. The major disadvantages of a-BMT include the potential for tumour-cell contamination within the graft, with a higher risk of relapse, and the lack of a graft-versus-tumour disease.

Peripheral blood-progenitor cell transplant

Peripheral blood-progenitor cell transplant (PBPCT) consists of autologous or allogeneic infusion of haematopoietic stem cells collected from peripheral blood. The cells are collected after the administration of haematopoietic growth factors, associated or not with chemotherapy.

In the allogeneic transplant setting, the health donor receives granulocyte growth factors (G-CSF) 3–5 days before collection. In an autologous, setting the potential advantages of PBPCT over a-BMT include stem-cell collection without the need for general anaesthesia or repeated painful bone-marrow aspirations, more rapid engraftment, particularly for platelets, and decreased tumour contamination. For these reasons, PBPCT can also be safely performed older patients. PBPCT has recently been proposed as a possible treatment for severe intractable autoimmune diseases such as multiple sclerosis, systemic lupus erythematosus, rheumatoid arthritis, and others.

In the PBSC allogeneic transplant, the donor avoids general anaesthesia and repeated painful bone marrow aspirations, but other possible side effects have been observed, such as thrombotic events and spleen rupture. In patients receiving PBSCT, the engraftment is faster than with BMT, but there is evidence of an increased risk of chronic GVHD; there-fore, the choise of stem-cell source depends on various factors relating to both the donor and the recipient.

Cord-blood transplantation

In cord-blood transplantation (CBT), the haematopoietic stem cells are collected from cordal and placental blood immediately after delivery. Umbilical cord-blood cells are phenotypically different, functionally more immature, and have a higher proliferative potential with respect to bone-marrow progenitor cells.

In the past, CBT was mainly employed in children; there is more likely to be a cord-blood unit with a suitable cell dose in a patient with a lower body weight compared to an adult patient. With the introduction of two cord-blood units, an increased cell dose, and an RIC regimen, however, the procedure has increasingly been used in adults with haematological disease, and it can even be used in elderly or unfit patients. New approaches are being investigated in order to improve clinical results, such as co-infusion with mesenchimal cells, expansion of cord-blood cells, and the intrabone injection of a single unit.

Nutritional and metabolic support in HSCT

Irrespective of the type of HSCT employed, conditioning regimens, particularly myeloablative conditioning regimens, have tremendous and deleterious consequences for the anatomical and functional integrity of the gastrointestinal tract (Figure 15.2). However, relevant differences exist in the impact on nutritional status exerted by autologous and allogeneic transplantation. In fact, although patients receive high-dose chemotherapy prior to autologous transplant, the employment of PBSC and the use of growth factors has significantly reduced the time to engraftment, the duration of profound neutropaenia (<7 days), and, consequently, the duration of neutropaenic mucositis.

Indeed, in these patients, sufficient oral food intake is achieved rather often, which may significantly reduce the need for parenteral nutrition, unless severe complications occur.

Conversely, allo-HSCT patients undergoing a myeloablative conditioning regimen show a severe and prolonged mucositis. Moreover, the occurrence of a-GVHD, involving the gut, may increase intestinal problems with abdominal pain and severe diarrhoea. The use of high-dose steroid drugs for the management of GVHD, as well as of antimicrobial drugs used to prevent infectious complications, further contributes to the onset of malnutrition.

The main complications of HSCT and their nutritional implications are detailed in the following sections.

Acute and chronic graft-versus-host disease

a-GVHD affects mainly the skin, the liver, and the gastrointestinal tract When the involvement of the skin is severe, and extensive skin areas are involved, large fluid and protein losses may occur. When the liver is involved, severe cholestasis occurs, as a result of small-bile-duct destruction. Serum bilirubin concentrations are frequently elevated, with concomitant impairment of other liver-function tests. Intestinal GVHD is characterised by diarrhoea with or without nausea, vomiting, and abdominal pain. Occasionally ileus occurs, resulting from the destruction of intestinal crypts. As a consequence, mild to severe gastrointestinal impairment may develop, ranging from profuse secretory mucous diarrhoea, with severe nitrogen loss, to mucosal ulcers, with possible perforations and need for emergency surgical treatment.

Hepatic GVHD-induced steatorrhea, secondary to bile-salt synthesis and enterohepatic circulation derangements, may further worsen diarrhoea. Interestingly, mucosal absorptive capacity may remain abnormal even after apparent healing of the intestinal mucosa.

Chronic GVHD also has deleterious consequences for nutritional status or normal growth if it occurs in paediatric patients. Oral (mucositis, sicca syndrome), oesophageal (strictures, dysphagia), hepatic (cholestasis, hyperbilirubinaemia), and intestinal (mucositis, malabsorption) involvement may impair both nutrient oral intake and intestinal nutrient absorption.

Altered metabolism

HSCT may have a dramatic impact on the recipient, affecting protein, energy, micronutrient, and vitamin metabolism. An overall decrease in body cell mass with no changes in body fat or lean body mass has been described in allo-HSCT recipients, with these patients showing an increase in extracellular fluid and a significant decrease in intracellular fluid. Negative nitrogen balance is a common feature in HSCT patients, as a consequence of both intestinal losses with diarrhoea and the catabolic effects on skeletal muscle initially exerted by the underlying disease, then by conditioning regimens, and subsequently by possible HSCT complications such as sepsis and GVHD. Although data on energy expenditure following HSCT are not conclusive, it is generally assumed that HSCT patients have increased energy needs.

Steroid and/or cyclosporine administration or the occurrence of septic complications may negatively affect carbohydrate metabolism and induce impaired glucose tolerance. HSCT *per se* might negatively affect pancreatic beta-cell function and induce glucose intolerance or overt diabetes.

Abnormalities in lipid metabolism are uncommon in the initial phases following HSCT, while elevated serum-cholesterol and triacylglycerol concentrations frequently occur in patients maintained on long-term cyclosporine therapy for chronic GVHD.

Vitamin status may be altered in HSCT patients due to poor intake and malabsorption of both water- and lipid-soluble vitamins secondary to intestinal mucositis or hepatic GVHD. The use of cyclophosphamide and radiation has been reported to increase the need for antioxidant vitamins such as tocopherol and beta-carotene.

Malabsorption and an increased need for bone-marrow reconstitution may induce trace-element deficiency. In particular, zinc deficiency has been shown to correlate with mortality after BMT. Trace-element deficiency may be prevented in some patients receiving plasma and/or blood-derivative transfusions.

Veno-occlusive disease of the liver

This is a serious and often fatal event which may complicate both a-HSCT and allo-HSCT, occurring in about 20% of cases. Veno-occlusive disease (VOD) is, however, not exclusive to HSCT patients, since it may also complicate high-dose cyclophosphamide and busulfan, without TBI. VOD is histologically characterised by narrowing and occlusion of hepatic venules and injury to hepatocytes, due to the toxic effects of chemotherapy. The clinical manifestations of VOD usually appear within 2–4 weeks after high-dose conditioning regimens, often during the phase of profound pancytopaenia, before bone-marrow recovery, and include right upper-quadrant abdominal pain, hepatomegaly, jaundice, and elevation of serum transaminase activities, often followed by oliguria, sodium and water retention and ascites, liver failure, and hepatic encephalopathy. The pathogenesis of this severe clinical picture is yet to be fully elucidated, although a possible role might be played by the obstruction of the hepatic venules by endothelial cell injury and thrombosis, the shift of albumin- and electrolyte-rich fluid to the extravascular space, and the consequent reduction in renal blood flow, with activation of the renin–angiotensin axis and retention of sodium and fluid.

Assessment of nutritional status in patients receiving HSCT

Nutritional assessment and evaluation of nutritional risk is mandatory in all patients undergoing HSCT. Evaluation of nutritional status does not represent a problem prior to HSCT, particularly in haematological patients, but the evaluation of the effect of nutritional support on nutritional status is more difficult. Immunological indices are not of great value because of the underlying disease or the effects of chemotherapy. Biochemical indices do not accurately reflect changes in the nutritional status of HSCT recipients. In fact, HSCT patients frequently develop acute complications (sepsis, GVHD, etc.) that may influence *per se* the concentrations of plasma proteins. Anthropometric measurements may be influenced by fluid and electrolyte disturbances.

Nitrogen balance is considered the most accurate way to perform nutritional assessment in HSCT patients, since it is the direct expression of the imbalance existing between protein breakdown and synthesis. However, in the clinical setting of HSCT patients, urine collection may be difficult, while vomiting and diarrhoea may make calculations of nitrogen losses less accurate.

15.4 Nutritional and metabolic support following HSCT

HSCT is largely used in the treatment of both solid tumours and haematological malignancies, including leukaemia and lymphomas. The impact on nutritional status varies depending on the indication for HSCT. Haematological patients are usually well nourished at the time of HSCT, while patients with solid tumours exhibit malnutrition more frequently. Impaired nutritional status before transplantation represents a negative prognostic factor for outcome after HSCT. Irrespective of nutritional status prior to HSCT, it is well recognised that patients undergoing high-dose chemotherapy are at risk of developing malnutrition. Therefore, nutritional support is frequently given routinely following HSCT, in order to prevent malnutrition secondary to either drug-induced side effects or increased nutritional requirements.

Energy and nutrient demands are increased because of the induced catabolic state due to the cytoreductive therapy, the presence of sepsis, or, in allo-HSCT, GVHD. Optimal blood-cell reconstitution is also thought to increase nutritional requirements.

In recent years, indications for parenteral nutrition have markedly decreased in favour of enteral nutrition. However, high-dose chemotherapy, followed or not by HSCT, represents a major field for parenteral-nutrition utilisation, mainly because of the gastrointestinal sequelae of the preparative cytoreductive chemotherapy, TBI, infections, or GVHD. High-dose chemotherapy-induced gastrointestinal impairment precludes optimal nutrient intake and absorption. Nausea, vomiting, and oro-oesophageal mucositis make placement of nasogastric tubes difficult. Furthermore, the majority of patients undergoing HSCT have a central venous catheter placed, through which parenteral nutrition can be given (via a dedicated lumen). Finally, parenteral nutrition allows more accurate modulation and provision of fluids, electrolytes, and macronutrients, which has pivotal importance, especially when complications of HSCT occur, such as a-GVHD or VOD. However, it is possible to insert feeding tubes safely with up to grade 2 mucositis, and this is progressively becoming a common practice in HSCT.

HSCT patients should be assessed and monitored, and nutritional support should be prescribed on an individual basis. This prescription may change during the course of the post-HSCT period.

For all these reasons, controlled trials on the effects of enteral nutrition in HSCT patients are to date still rare.

Energy expenditure may differ between a-HSCT and allo-HSCT patients, but consensus exists that energy requirements in HSCT recipients may reach 130–150% of the predicted basal energy expenditure. Therefore, 30–35 kcal/kg body weight per day is usually administered. Lipids should provide 30–40% of non-protein energy. Lipids may be particularly useful in achieving the energy target if hyperglycaemia develops as a consequence of steroid treatment or infection, or when fluid restriction is warranted. Increased protein needs may be satisfied by provision of 1.4–1.5 g/kg body weight per day of a standard amino acid solution. What still remains less well defined is when artificial nutrition should be started in these patients. Despite the increasingly successful use of nasogastric or nasojejunal enteral nutrition during HSCT, feeding-tube placement and tolerance can be difficult or impossible once mucositis has developed, and enteral feeding may be poorly tolerated. However, as mentioned above, the use of enteral feeding in HSCT recipients has increased significantly during recent years. Parenteral nutrition is often considered to be an expensive procedure and is therefore started only 'when it becomes necessary'; that is, after severe mucositis develops, significantly affecting oral nutrient intake, and oral feeding falls below 60–70% of requirements for three days. This may occur variably after transplantation, depending on the underlying disease, type of HSCT, and conditioning regimen. As a general rule, artificial-nutrition withdrawal should be considered when patients are able to tolerate approximately 50% of their requirements enterally, but there are no data specific to this context.

Although benefits of parenteral-nutrition administration have been reported, including a decrease in disease relapse rate, increase in disease-free survival, and improved survival rate, when the prevalence of malnutrition is considered the only indication for parenteral-nutrition administration, up to 37% of a-HSCT recipients without whole-body irradiation, up to 50% of a-HSCT recipients undergoing full-intensity conditioning, up to 58% of allo-HSCT recipients undergoing full-intensity conditioning, and up to 92% of allo-HSCT recipients with irradiation and HLA-incompatible donors may have indications for parenteral nutrition.

15.5 Concluding remarks

The first evidence that prophylactic standard parenteral nutrition could significantly improve outcome of HSCT patients was provided by Weisdorf, who showed that the 3-year survival rate of parenteral nutrition-treated patients was improved with respect to those who did not receive any nutritional support.

Since then, artificial nutrition has rapidly moved from simple supportive care (mainly aimed at the maintenance of nutritional status) to adjunctive therapy, on the basis of the potential 'metanutritional' benefits deriving from a specialised nutritional intervention. Several effects not directly derived from the maintenance or improvement of nutritional status could, at least theoretically, be obtained through an optimal specialised nutritional approach to patients undergoing HSCT (Figure 15.3).

Artificial nutrition support is in fact provided following HSCT, during the delicate phase of engraftment and haemopoietic reconstitution; it is therefore conceivable that metabolically active substrates administered during this period may influence biological responses, such as time to and success of engraftment itself, occurrence and severity of mucositis, GVHD, and VOD, thus potentially affecting the outcome of HSCT patients.

It is known that some nutritional substrates may interfere with certain physiological and pathophysiological mechanisms or otherwise protect the gastrointestinal tract from radio- and chemotherapy-induced mucosal injuries.

In this respect, lipid substrates and glutamine would appear the more promising nutrients for optimal nutritional and metabolic support to HSCT patients.

Exogenously administered essential fatty acids have been shown to interfere with the synthesis of biological effectors of immunity and inflammation, such as prostaglandins and leukotrienes, via their incorporation into cell membranes, and might therefore play an additional role in affecting the outcome of HSCT patients. The provision of lipid-based parenteral nutrition was associated with a lower incidence of lethal a-GVHD in allo-BMT patients. To explain these findings, it could be hypothesised that the increased availability of arachidonic acid and of its metabolite prostaglandin E2 (PGE2), secondary to exogenous long-chain n-6 triacylglycerol administration, will lead to decreased interleukin 1 (IL-1) and tumour necrosis factor (TNF) macrophage production, reduced expression of major histocompatibility-complex antigens, increased T-suppressor activity, and decreased peripheral blood lymphocyte IL-2 production.

The role of fish oil-derived n-3 fatty acids in the metabolic support of HSCT is yet to be entirely

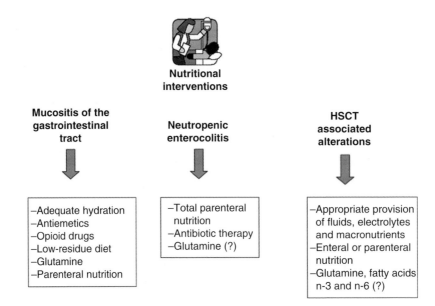

Figure 15.3 Strategy for nutritional interventions. HSCT, haematopoietic stem-cell transplantation.

explored. The ability of these lipid compounds to modulate inflammatory and immune responses could have a role in improving the outcome of HSCT recipients, at least on a theoretical ground; *n*-3 fatty acid administration has in fact been shown to reduce vasoconstriction and platelet aggregation, and to have a profound influence on cell–cell signalling during immunological events, by inhibiting cytokine secretion, as well as lymphocyte activation and differentiation. It could therefore be hypothesised that *n*-3 fatty acid supplementation following HSCT might prove beneficial in the prophylaxis and management of BMT-related complications such as GVHD and VOD. Clinical trials aimed at verifying this hypothesis are still lacking.

The rationale for administering glutamine-supplemented nutrition to HSCT patients was initially based on the concept that glutamine represents a primary fuel for the enterocytes and for gut-associated lymphoid tissue, and that its administration by the enteral or parenteral route could prevent or mitigate treatment-induced gastrointestinal impairment. In HSCT patients, glutamine administration has been reported to minimise the intestinal mucosal atrophy associated with exclusive parenteral nutrition, as well as to reduce liver damage caused by chemotherapy or radiotherapy. Some evidence exists that glutamine supplementation may also ameliorate a number of other clinical and biological parameters, such as nitrogen balance and immune-system function, infection risk, length of hospital stay, financial costs, and survival. A recent study by da Gama Torres *et al.* (2008) showed a positive effect on short-term mortality in allo-HSCT of glutamine-supplemented parenteral nutrition, but other studies have failed to demonstrate such positive outcomes. Overall, the available evidence suggests that HSCT patients may benefit from glutamine-supplemented parenteral nutrition. Although the optimal dose of glutamine to be used in HSCT is not established, studies have suggested that a dose of around 0.6 g/kg/day may be appropriate. Further studies are warranted, including of homogeneous patients and of possible differences exerted by the route of administration of glutamine.

The potential for the use of glutamine in the prevention or treatment of VOD still deserves particular attention. Preliminary data would indeed suggest that glutamine infusion during HSCT preserves hepatic function. The likely mechanism of such action is the maintenance of hepatic glutathione concentrations, which would protect hepatocytes from the oxidant stress of high-dose conditioning regimens. Glutamine supplementation may have a beneficial role in hepatic protection from VOD, both as a prophylactic agent and as a possible treatment.

References and further reading

Bozzetti F, Arends J, Lundholm K, Micklewright A, Zurcher G, Muscaritoli M; ESPEN. ESPEN guidelines on parenteral nutrition: non-surgical oncology. Clin Nutr 2009; 28: 445–454.

Coghlin Dickson TM, Wong RM, Offrin RS, Shizuru JA, Johnston LJ, et al. Effect of oral glutamine supplementation during bone marrow transplantation. JPEN J Parenter Enteral Nutr 2000; 24: 61–66.

da Gama Torres HO, Vilela EG, da Cunha AS, Goulart EM, Souza MH, Aguirre AC, et al. Efficacy of glutamine supplemented parenteral nutrition on short-term survival following allo-HSCT: a randomized study. Bone Marrow Transplant 2008; 41(12): 1021–1027.

Eghbali H, Soubeyran P, Tchen N, de Mascarel I, Soubeyran I, Richaud P. Current treatment of Hodgkin's lymphoma. Crit Rev Oncol Hematol 2000; 35: 49–73.

Garcia-Manero G. Myelodisplastic syndromes: 2011 update on diagnosis, risk stratification and management. Am J Hematol 2011; 86: 490–498.

Gyurkocza B, Rezvani A, Storb RF. Allogeneic hematopoietic cell transplantation: the state of the art. Expert Rev Hematol 2010 ; 3(3): 285–299.

Herrmann VM, Petruska PJ. Nutrition support in bone marrow transplant recipients. Nutr Clin Pract 1993; 8: 19–27.

Isaacson PG. The current status of lymphoma classification. Br J Haematol 2000; 109: 258–266.

Mahadean D, Fisher RI. Novel therapeutics for aggressive non Hodgkin's lymphoma. J Clin Oncol 2011; 29: 1876–1884.

Miller KB. Myelodysplastic syndromes. Curr Treat Options Oncol 2000; 1: 63–69.

Multani P, White CA, Grillo-Lopez A. Non Hodgkin's lymphoma: review of conventional treatments. Curr Pharm Biotechnol 2001; 2: 279–291.

Muscaritoli M, Conversano L, Petti MC, Torelli GF, Cascino A, Mecarocci S, et al. Plasma amino acid concentrations in patients with acute myelogenous leukemia. Nutrition 1999; 15: 195–199.

Muscaritoli M, Grieco G, Capria S, Iori AP, Fanelli FR. Nutritional and metabolic support in patients undergoing bone marrow transplantation. Am J Clin Nutr 2002; 75: 183–190.

Okimoto RA, Van Etten RA. Navigating the road toward optimal initial therapy for chronic myeloid leukemia. Curr Opin Hematol 2011; 18: 89–97.

Passweg J, Gratwohl A, Tyndall A. Hematopoietic stem cell transplantation for autoimmune disorders. Curr Opin Hematol 1999; 6: 400–405.

Pileri SA, Agostinelli C, Sabattini E, Bacci F, Sagramoso C, Pileri A Jr, et al. Lymphoma classification: the quiet after the storm. Semin Diagn Pathol 2011; 28(2): 113–123.

Schulte C, Reinhardt W, Beelen D, Mann K, Schaefer U. Low T3-syndrome and nutritional status as prognostic factors in patients undergoing bone marrow transplantation. Bone Marrow Transplant 1998; 22: 1171–1178.

Weisdorf SA, Lysne J, Wind D, Haake RJ, Sharp HL, Goldman A, et al. Positive effect of prophylactic total parenteral nutrition on long-term outcome of bone marrow transplantation. Transplantation 1987; 43(6): 833–838.

16
The Lung

Peter Collins[1] and Marinos Elia[2]

[1] Queensland University of Technology, Australia
[2] University of Southampton, UK

Key messages

- Chronic obstructive pulmonary disease (COPD) contains a number of phenotypes that affect not only the respiratory manifestations of disease but also the nutritional status of individuals. Subgroups can be classified as having a greater prevalence of underweight, fat-free mass depletion, and obesity. A low body mass, unintentional weight loss, and a decrease in fat-free body mass have been associated with impaired functional status and increased risk of mortality.
- Compromised nutritional status has multiple negative effects on respiratory function in disease. These include weakened respiratory muscles, reduced ventilatory drive, and impaired immune function. Malnutrition may be both the cause and the consequence of respiratory problems, for example predisposing to infections that exacerbate disease progression.
- A low body mass index (BMI) and recent weight loss are associated with poor clinical outcomes in COPD, increasing the frequency of

- infective exacerbations, hospitalisations, and readmission rates, as well as mortality. Patients with poorer nutritional status also have prolonged hospital admissions and need increased ventilator support, which it may be difficult to wean them off.
- In the majority of COPD patients with unintentional weight loss and muscle wasting, it is possible to at least partly reverse or attenuate these changes with nutritional support.
- The association between malnutrition and cytokine-induced inflammatory markers in COPD suggests the need to not only address the underlying inflammatory cause whenever possible, but also to increase nutritional intake at the same time as providing an anabolic stimulus by undertaking physical activity. A multimodal approach is likely to be more effective than individual interventions in the accrual of lean tissue and subsequent improvements in functional capacity and quality of life.

16.1 Introduction

Diseases of the respiratory system can often cause malnutrition, but it is also known that malnutrition has a negative effect on the respiratory system. Malnutrition causes loss of lung tissue and a reduction in the size and contractility of the muscles associated with breathing, such as the diaphragm. In the presence of malnutrition, the respiratory muscles become weaker and suffer from fatigue earlier than the muscles of nourished individuals. Weak respiratory muscles are unable to generate sufficient cough pressure to effectively expectorate and clear the lung of secretions, which may be infected. In patients with borderline respiratory function, the combination of reduced strength and early fatigue can precipitate

respiratory failure or delay weaning from mechanical ventilation.

It is possible that the effects of malnutrition on the respiratory system are even more subtle. For example, starvation can reduce the sensitivity of the respiratory centre to hypoxic stimuli, and this too may delay the weaning of patients off ventilation. It is difficult to establish the exact causality of malnutrition in respiratory disease, as malnutrition may develop as a consequence of increased disease severity, which detrimentally affects nutritional intake. Conversely, it may accelerate disease progression, predisposing to infections of a longer duration due to the effects of malnutrition on the immune system.

The spectrum of respiratory disease is large and the clinical problems are disease-specific. The conditions may be acute, such as asthma and pneumonia, or more chronic, such as chronic obstructive pulmonary disease (COPD), pulmonary fibrosis, and tuberculosis. Some patients may require artificial ventilation either because their respiratory muscles fail or because lung function is inadequate. In those with CO_2 retention, an increase in tidal volume and/or respiratory rate with artificial ventilation may aid CO_2 expiration. In those who are hypoxic, an increase in the inspired oxygen concentration may also help, although there is a risk that high oxygen concentrations may suppress ventilation, which is stimulated by hypoxia. In those who are artificially ventilated, it is possible to use special modes of ventilation that help prevent collapse of airways, especially in the presence of viscous secretions, and aid weaning from artificial ventilators. Respiratory diseases can place considerable demands on the respiratory muscles. Although in healthy subjects the energy cost of breathing is only about 2% of basal metabolic rate (BMR), it may rise to 15–20% in those with acute respiratory distress syndrome, precipitating respiratory muscle fatigue. The lungs can also be affected by diseases of other organs and systems. For example, heart failure may lead to pulmonary oedema, which can impair gaseous exchange across the lungs, with consequent respiratory failure. In contrast, chronic lung disease may cause right-sided heart failure (cor pulmonale) due to the increased workload of the right heart, which has to operate against an elevated pulmonary artery blood pressure.

The focus of this chapter is on COPD, which encompasses both chronic bronchitis and emphysema. COPD is a common condition, frequently associated with malnutrition, and allows the illustration of key clinical and nutritional principles of care. Interest in the nutritional management of chronic respiratory disease, in particular COPD, has changed remarkably over the past two decades. COPD is a disease state characterised by the presence of airflow obstruction or intrinsic airway disease classically typified as chronic bronchitis. The airflow limitation is generally progressive and largely irreversible. Emphysema is defined pathologically as an abnormal permanent enlargement of the air spaces distal to the terminal bronchioles, accompanied by destruction of their walls, without fibrosis. Chronic bronchitis is defined clinically as the presence of a chronic productive cough for 3 months in each of 2 successive years in patients in whom the other causes of chronic cough have been excluded.

Weight loss has long been recognised as a symptom of chronic lung disease. The association between weight loss and emphysema was first described in the late nineteenth century. Interestingly, attempts to describe different COPD classifications found that body weight might be an important discriminating factor. This led to the classical description of the pink puffer (emphysematous type) and the blue bloater (bronchitic type). The pink-puffing patient is characteristically thin and breathless, with marked hyperinflation of the chest. The blue and bloated patient may not be particularly breathless, at least when at rest, but has severe central cyanosis, a bluish-purple discolouration of the skin and mucous membranes resulting from a deficiency of oxygen in the blood. Although these extreme types can indeed be seen, most patients present a mixed picture.

Traditionally, weight loss was considered to be an inevitable and irreversible terminal progression of the disease process. It was thought that nutritional support might even adversely influence the disease by inducing an additional metabolic and ventilatory stress on the pulmonary system. However, studies into the disturbed energy balance during weight loss in COPD have challenged this approach. Furthermore, the concept of COPD as a systemic disorder (Figure 16.1) gave further insights into the role of nutrition in the

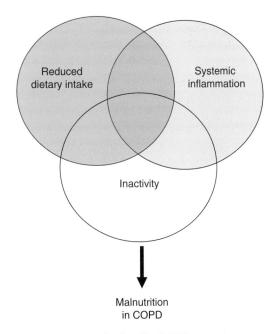

Figure 16.1 Aetiology of malnutrition in COPD.

disease. Nutritional depletion contributes to disability (increased dyspnoea, reduced exercise capacity) and handicap (reduced health status and quality of life), independent of the impaired lung function. In the majority of patients, these adverse consequences of weight loss, and in particular muscle wasting, are partly treatable by appropriate oral nutritional support containing energy, protein, and a balanced mixture of other nutrients. Figure 16.1 provides an overview of both the causes of nutritional depletion in COPD and potential therapeutic targets. For malnutrition to be successfully treated, each of these factors should be addressed.

16.2 Prevalence and consequences of weight loss and muscle wasting

To understand the role of nutritional support in respiratory disease, it is necessary to briefly consider the underlying mechanisms by which nutritional abnormalities in COPD develop. Much of the weight loss is specifically related to the decrease in body cell mass (BCM), the cellular components of tissues such as muscle and organs. Independent of the underlying disease state or condition, a loss of more than 40% of BCM is almost inevitably associated with death.

Muscle function and exercise performance

The prominent symptoms of COPD are dyspnoea (shortness of breath) and exercise intolerance. Besides airflow obstruction and loss of alveolar structure, skeletal muscle weakness is an important determinant of these symptoms, which are predominantly determined by skeletal muscle mass. Muscle mass is the single largest tissue of BCM and can be assessed indirectly in clinically stable COPD patients by measurement of fat-free mass (FFM), using dual-energy-X-ray absorptiometry or bioelectrical-impedance analysis. While relatively easy to perform, both of these methods are confounded by the presence of oedema, which is a common complication in COPD (see Chapter 2 of *Introduction to Human Nutrition* in this series). Besides its effects on muscle strength, FFM is also a significant determinant of exercise capacity and exercise response. Patients with a depleted FFM are characterised by lower peak

oxygen consumption, lower peak work rate, and early build-up of lactic acid in the blood compared with nondepleted patients with a similar severity of respiratory disease. The functional consequences of nutritional abnormalities are therefore not only related to muscle wasting *per se*, but also to intrinsic alterations in muscle morphology and energy metabolism, which may be directed towards early anaerobic metabolism. Indeed, the activity of key enzymes involved in oxidative metabolism, such as citrate synthase and succinate dehydrogenase, and the concentration of energy-rich phosphates (ATP, creatine phosphate) are decreased in some patients with COPD. Furthermore, derangement in muscle electrolyte status, such as decreases in potassium, magnesium, and phosphorus and an increase in sodium, may arise; this occurs more profoundly in the presence of nutritional depletion. Some of these changes alone or in combination can influence muscle function.

Autopsy studies have clearly shown that nutritional depletion leads not only to peripheral skeletal muscle wasting, but also to diaphragmatic muscle wasting. In COPD, the effects of nutritional depletion on respiratory muscle function cannot be separated from the mechanical influences on the diaphragm due to hyperinflation. In severely depleted anorexia nervosa patients, free of any other disease, the influence of nutritional depletion on the diaphragm was illustrated by severely depressed diaphragm contractility. However, with the initiation of nutritional support, this increased significantly: by 42% after 30 days, with body weight increasing by 13% and FFM by 9% during this period.

Mortality and morbidity in COPD

The relationship between being underweight and weight loss with mortality in COPD has been studied since the 1960s. In the early years, a significant association was reported between weight loss and survival. Five-year mortality was 50% in weight-losing patients, compared with 20% in weight-stable COPD patients. Several retrospective studies using different COPD populations from the USA, Canada, Denmark, the Netherlands, and the United Kingdom reported a relationship between low body mass index (BMI) and mortality, independent of disease severity. In all these studies, a decreased mortality risk was observed in overweight patients, not only compared with underweight patients but also with normal-weight subjects (Figure 16.2). In patients with severe COPD, the lowest mortality rates have been observed in the obese. This remarkable observation has been termed the 'obesity paradox' or 'reverse epidemiology' and is not limited to COPD but has been reported in other chronic wasting diseases, such as renal and heart failure. In COPD, this paradox might be related to the fact that depletion of FFM is not only a consequence of weight loss but may also occur in normal-weight patients with a relatively high fat mass. Increased mortality risk in patients with COPD has been found to be associated with a depletion of FFM, independent of BMI. In addition, COPD patients with lower body weight tend to have a reduced diffusing capacity of the lungs compared to the overweight or obese. Therefore, it is plausible that the obesity paradox is partially driven by differences in the diffusive capacity of the

emphysematous and chronic bronchitis phenotypes of COPD. Statistical adjustments for the obstructive components of disease may not adequately control for the severity of respiratory disease as a whole, which includes other abnormalities such as impaired diffusing capacity. Importantly, a Dutch study has shown that weight gain in malnourished COPD patients is associated with reduced mortality risk.

Many patients with COPD suffer from acute infective exacerbations, which often require hospitalisation. A low BMI and recent weight loss have been identified as important factors for predicting the outcome of acute exacerbations, as indicated by the frequency of hospital readmissions, the length of hospital stay and readmission rate, the need for mechanical ventilation, and the inability to wean from the ventilator. In 608 COPD patients hospitalised for an infective exacerbation, those with a $BMI < 18.5 \, kg/m^2$ were 2.5 times more likely to die during that admission. Inpatients who had experienced more than 10% unintentional weight loss were almost four times more likely to experience early readmission to hospital. It remains to be established whether nutritional intervention in malnourished individuals with an infective exacerbation of COPD results in subsequent reductions in healthcare use.

Prevalence of malnutrition in COPD

The prevalence of malnutrition in COPD is high, with up to 60% of inpatients and 45% of outpatients reported to be at risk. In clinically stable patients with moderate to severe COPD, depletion of FFM has been reported to occur in 20% of outpatients and in 35% of those eligible for pulmonary rehabilitation. Only limited data are available regarding the prevalence of nutritional depletion in mild COPD. Weight loss and a low BMI are more frequently observed in predominantly emphysematous patients compared with those with predominantly chronic bronchitis. A low BMI is usually associated with loss of fat and FFM, but depletion of FFM, with all its adverse functional consequences, can occur with little or no decrease in fat mass, as in some patients with chronic bronchitis.

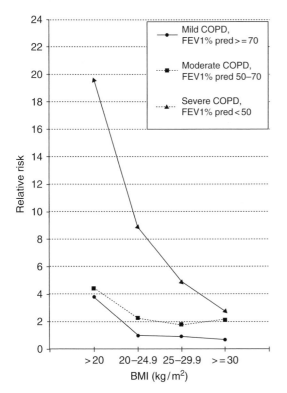

Figure 16.2 COPD-related mortality by BMI in 2132 subjects with mild, moderate, and severe COPD. Reprinted with permission of the American Thoracic Society. Copyright © 2012 American Thoracic Society. Landbo C *et al*, 1999, Prognostic value of nutritional status in chronic obstructive pulmonary disease. Am J Respir Crit Care Med; 160: p1856–1861. Official Journal of the American Thoracic Society.

Health-related quality of life

The functional consequences of underweight and particularly of depletion of FFM are not only reflected at the disability level in exercise tests but also in a decreased health-related quality of life measured by the disease-specific St George's Respiratory Questionnaire (http://www.healthstatus.sgul.ac.uk/).

16.3 Causes of weight loss and muscle wasting

Weight loss producing depletion of fat mass occurs when energy expenditure exceeds dietary intake. Muscle wasting is a consequence of an imbalance between protein synthesis and protein breakdown. Weight loss producing loss of lean tissue occurs when protein (N) loss exceeds protein (N) intake. Since weight loss is typically associated with a loss of both fat and lean tissue, a negative energy balance is normally associated with a negative N balance. Catabolic conditions producing loss of lean tissue also cause loss of appetite and reduced energy intake, which largely explains why negative N and energy balances coexist. In unusual situations, such as when a patient with a catabolic condition receives excess energy, perhaps using artificial nutrition support, a negative N balance may coexist with a positive energy balance. Furthermore, immobility leads to loss of body protein, mainly from muscle, which can be difficult to replete even in the presence of excess energy intake.

Energy metabolism

Daily total energy expenditure (TEE) is often divided into two components:

(1) BMR;
(2) physical activity and thermogenesis (e.g. dietary- or cold-induced thermogenesis).

Given that resting energy expenditure (REE) is the major component of TEE in healthy individuals, and even more so in sedentary individuals, the extent to which it might be elevated in COPD is an important consideration. Several studies have reported an increase in REE in COPD of approximately 10–20%, after adjustment for the size of FFM. Some of this resting hypermetabolism is due to the increased work of breathing, particularly in emphysematous patients. During infective exacerbations of chronic lung disease, hypermetabolism may increase further due to the effects of the underlying infection, which is partly

due to inflammatory cytokines such as tumour necrosis factor alpha (TNFα). TNFα is often elevated in those individuals who are losing weight, and it is also associated with a suppression of appetite and a reduction of dietary intake. Despite the increased REE seen in COPD and other chronic inflammatory diseases, TEE often remains unaltered, and in some cases even reduced, mainly as a result of a decrease in physical activity.

Altered substrate metabolism

Studies examining various aspects of substrate-energy metabolism have revealed a variety of abnormalities in patients with COPD – including those affecting lipolytic rates, amino acid metabolism, and protein kinetics – but it has proved difficult to integrate all of them into a single overarching mechanism that explains the changes in lean tissue mass and its associated functions. Focus is now turning towards an examination of the requirements of certain amino acids, which appear to be increased, especially during infective episodes. Provision of specific nutritional formulations, which include particular amino acid profiles, may help preserve FFM, but investigations so far have yet to provide definitive answers. In addition, a limited number of data exist to suggest that altered fatty acid profiles of nutritional formulations may also have a potential positive immunomodulatory effect during the acute phase of respiratory disease, and this is an area of active research.

Reduced dietary intake

Dietary intake in weight-losing patients is lower than in weight-stable patients, both in absolute terms and in relation to measured REE. The reasons for the relatively low dietary intake seen in COPD are not completely understood, but it is often compounded during times of infection and increased dyspnoea. Patients with COPD may eat suboptimally due to changes in both breathing patterns and oxygen-saturation levels, which may be exacerbated further by chewing and swallowing of food. Indeed, in hypoxaemic patients a rapid decrease in SaO_2 (percentage saturation of haemoglobin with oxygen in arterial blood) is seen, which slowly recovers after completion of the meal. The decrease in SaO_2 is related to

Table 16.1 Simple dietary practices that may help patients with COPD. CPAP, continuous positive airway pressure; BiPAP, bi-level positive airway pressure.

Respiratory symptom	Dietary modification
Dyspnoea (shortness of breath)	Eat small, energy-dense, frequent meals and snacks
	Eat soft meals to reduce work of chewing and swallowing
	Sit up for meals, and out of bed if possible
Oxygen therapy	Wear nasal prongs instead of an oxygen mask when eating
Dry mouth	Eat moist meals
	Use artificial saliva
Constipation	Increase fluid and fibre intake encourage activity
Dysphagia	Review by speech and language therapy
Taste alterations	Provide meals and drinks with strong flavours
CPAP/BiPAP	Employ nasogastric feeding
Regurgitation of meals	Employ post-pyloric enteral feeding
Immobility	Undertake social review regarding home help and support with shopping and meal preparation

increased dyspnoea sensation. The severity of the drop may depend on the composition of the meal. The gastric emptying time of a meal may also affect dietary intake, since gastric filling in COPD patients reduces the functional residual capacity of the lungs and leads to an increase in dyspnoea. Simple dietary practices may help to overcome these problems (Table 16.1).

Systemic factors may also affect dietary intake. Recent studies suggest that appetite regulation may be adversely affected by systemic inflammation. The adipocyte-derived hormone leptin represents the afferent hormonal signal to the brain in a feedback mechanism regulating fat mass. Circulating leptin levels are increased in some patients. This increased plasma leptin level is positively related to an increase in some of the markers of systemic inflammation and inversely related to dietary intake adjusted for REE. These clinical data are in line with experimental animal studies showing that administration of endotoxins or cytokines produces a prompt increase in serum leptin levels and a decrease in appetite and dietary intake. However, a large and growing array of appetite signals has been identified, some of which have stimulatory effects, and others inhibitory effects. Most of these are little studied in patients with lung diseases.

16.4 Outcomes of nutritional intervention

The first clinical trials investigating the effectiveness of nutritional intervention consisted of nutritional supplementation by means of liquid oral nutritional supplements (ONS) or enteral tube feeding. A recent review has shown that nutritional support in COPD results in significant improvements in a number of outcomes: body weight, hand grip strength, respiratory muscle strength, quality of life and feelings of breathlessness. The effect of refeeding and weight gain on the immune response is less investigated, but has been associated with a significant increase in total lymphocyte count and an increase in reactivity to skin-test antigens after 21 days of refeeding. The evidence base for nutritional support in COPD is mainly based on ONS, but one study has demonstrated that a 6-month intervention consisting of dietary advice delivered by a dietitian and provision of milk powder is effective in improving body weight and quality of life. Importantly, these improvements continued 6 months beyond the period of intervention. A recent review suggests a gain in weight towards 2 kg to be the threshold at which functional improvements are seen in stable malnourished patients with COPD. However, in studies of subjects suffering from a wide range of acute conditions, improvements in functional and clinical outcomes may occur with little change in body weight relative to the control group. The progressive nature of weight loss in COPD requires appropriate feeding strategies to improve, maintain, or attenuate loss of body weight and associated body function. Studies involving ONS have been reported to produce functional improvements in COPD patients participating in a rehabilitation programme that includes exercise. These functional improvements seen with nutritional supplementation have even been observed in those classified as well nourished, suggesting a potential role for nutritional support beyond simply treating malnutrition. From a nutritional point of view, it is sensible to incorporate nutritional support with some form of exercise therapy, not only because physical activity increases nutritional requirements, but because it creates an anabolic drive that favours lean-tissue deposition, provided an adequate supply of dietary nutrients is available. A daily nutritional supplement as an integrated part of an 8-week pulmonary rehabilitation programme has been reported to produce a significant weight gain (0.4 kg/week), which has been associated with a significant improvement in FFM and respiratory muscle strength. Weight gain and an increase in respiratory muscle strength have also been associated with significantly improved survival rates. In addition, pulmonary rehabilitation programmes that include nutritional support have been shown to improve peripheral skeletal muscle strength, exercise capacity, and general health status.

Composition of nutritional supplements

While nutritional support often focuses on the fat, carbohydrate, and protein content of the diet and supplements, the provision of other nutrients is also important, especially since micronutrient deficiencies may coexist with protein-energy deficiency. Liquid ONS are often used to treat malnutrition in COPD; they are readymade and contain not only macronutrients but the full range of micronutrients to varying levels.

Nutrition and ventilation are intrinsically related, as oxygen is required for optimal energy exchange. Meal-related dyspnoea and limited ventilatory reserves may restrict the quantity and composition of nutritional support in patients with respiratory disease. It was long believed that patients with respiratory disease should consume a fat-rich diet in order to decrease carbon dioxide load, since the respiratory quotient of fat oxidation is 0.7, compared to 0.83 for protein and 1.0 for carbohydrate oxidation. Clinical evidence supporting this theory is scarce, however, and not convincing. More recent reports suggest that patients experience less dyspnoea after a carbohydrate-rich liquid supplement than after an equicaloric fat-rich supplement. This result is not surprising, as gastric emptying time is significantly longer after an equicaloric fat-rich supplement than after a carbohydrate-rich supplement, which may also help

repletion of muscle glycogen reserves and aid rehabilitation. Protein requirements have not yet been specifically investigated in COPD, but evidence of a benefit from administering ONS high in protein (>20% of energy) to patients with a wide range of conditions in hospital and community settings has recently been provided in a systematic review. Based on data in other chronic wasting conditions, it is reasonable to suggest a daily protein intake of 1.5 g/kg body weight or more. Recently there has been increased interest in the effects of both the composition and the dosage of protein on the accrual and function of FFM.

Skeletal muscle serves as an important reserve system in maintaining supplies of amino acids for metabolism and protein synthesis. Alterations in plasma and muscle amino acid profiles have been observed in COPD. Specifically, disturbances in leucine metabolism, which takes place in muscle, have been reported in association with decreased intramuscular concentrations of glutamate. Glutamate is known to be an important precursor for the antioxidant glutathione, as well as for glutamine synthesis in muscle. In COPD muscle, glutamate is strongly associated with glutathione concentration, although not with glutamine. Understanding the mechanisms and significance of such disturbances and the correction of abnormalities using targeted nutritional support could be of value in the prevention of oxidative stress in the skeletal muscle of COPD patients.

Nutritional modulation of muscle metabolism by amino acids or other substrates and co-factors may not only be relevant to tissue repletion of wasted patients, but also in anabolism induced by exercise training. This approach, which has been applied to elite athletes, suggests that improvements can occur independently of nutritional state. However, research also shows that the metabolic response to exercise is altered in COPD patients. In a recent study, 20 minutes of submaximal constant-work-rate exercise caused a reduction in the levels of most amino acids in muscle, while an increase above normal was found in several plasma amino acids. This suggests that circulating concentrations of these amino acids may have arisen from an increased release from muscle, at the expense of depleting the intramuscular pool of amino acids.

The effects of specific amino acid supplementation prior to or immediately after exercise on protein metabolism, protein balance, and exercise performance are unknown.

The effects of nutritional supplementation have mostly been studied in clinically stable patients. In some patients, weight loss follows a stepwise pattern, associated with acute infectious exacerbations. There is often negative energy balance at the time of acute exacerbations, due to the sudden reduction in energy intake. These patients may also have increased protein breakdown. Factors contributing to weight loss and muscle wasting during acute exacerbation include an increase in symptoms, flare-up of the systemic inflammatory response, alterations in the metabolism and the effects of appetite signals, including leptin, and the use of high doses of glucocorticoids. Indeed, a significant inverse association was shown between daily glucocorticoid dose and nitrogen balance during hospitalisation for acute exacerbations. Strategies that aim to attenuate the detrimental loss of tissue and function during acute exacerbations are important, since it may take considerable time to regain function after these exacerbations. A positive effect of nutritional support on well-being and some lung function tests has been reported, but since data are sparse, more research is needed to supplement the larger evidence base in the clinically stable patient.

Identification of malnutrition and the use of nutritional support

In order for nutritional support to be effective, it is necessary to tackle the underlying mechanisms responsible for nutritional depletion (Figure 16.1). The therapeutic triad of controlling the inflammatory process, providing nutritional support, and encouraging appropriate physical activity represents a rational approach to treatment. Although each of these is considered separately in this section, they are usually applied simultaneously.

Disease (inflammatory process)

As with other inflammatory conditions, treatment of the underlying catabolic disease process will allow nutritional support to be more effective. Acute infective exacerbations of COPD require treatment of the underlying infection and inflammation using appropriate medications, which may include antibiotics or corticosteroids. During the more stable chronic phase, there may also be opportunities to treat the chronic inflammatory process or attenuate its progression by stopping smoking and avoiding exposure to pollutants.

Nutritional support

In order for individuals at risk of malnutrition to be identified and to receive prompt appropriate nutritional intervention, simple routine nutritional screening should be performed using a validated nutritional screening tool, linked to a nutritional care pathway that guides treatment. Patients are typically characterised by BMI and the presence or absence of involuntary weight loss. In view of the high mortality risk in malnourished patients with COPD, nutritional supplementation is usually indicated when BMI is less than $20 \, kg/m^2$. Treatment should also be considered in patients with a BMI above $20 \, kg/m^2$ when involuntary weight loss (>5%) is progressive, showing no signs of abating, and approaching 10% or more in the preceding 6 months. Nutritional screening tools such as the 'Malnutrition Universal Screening Tool' ('MUST') (see Chapter 2), which combines BMI and unintentional weight loss, have been validated in COPD. It has been suggested that FFM might be more useful than body weight in identifying individuals who are likely to benefit from nutritional support, but this requires separate assessment of body composition, which may be time-consuming. Some bedside composition techniques, such as skinfold thickness, may be relatively quick to undertake, but there can be substantial inter-observer variability, especially in obese individuals, and training in the technique is required.

Oral nutritional support is the mainstream of treatment of malnourished patients with COPD. This often involves dietary modifications aimed at improving nutrient composition and increasing energy density. When this is insufficient to meet the goals, which may be to increase body weight (or reduce the rate of weight loss) and improve body function and well-being (or attenuate deterioration in these outcomes), ONS are usually prescribed. In individuals with a low BMI ($<20 \, kg/m^2$), the recommendation is to initiate ONS at the start of treatment; this can be done alone or in combination with dietary modification. Since in patients with severe COPD large meals can cause breathlessness and reduced exercise tolerance, supplements are often given in divided doses throughout the day. A large supplemental load, both in volume and in energy, may cause early satiety, abdominal distention, and a reduction in exercise tolerance. A dietitian can advise on the appropriate therapy and monitor the effectiveness of nutritional treatment, in order to ensure the supplementation of a balanced mixture of macro- and micronutrients.

Physical activity

Patients should be encouraged to engage in physical activity, and where possible to attend an exercise rehabilitation programme. For severely disabled patients unable to perform exercise training, even simple strength manoeuvres combined with training of daily activities and energy-conservation techniques may be effective. Exercise is likely to not only improve the effectiveness of nutritional therapy but also stimulate appetite. However, programmes that substantially increase energy expenditure, and which are not accompanied by increased dietary intake, may induce or accelerate weight loss. Therefore, such programmes should routinely consider the role of nutrition and of nutrition–exercise interactions. After approximately 6–12 weeks, response to therapy can be assessed. If weight gain and functional improvement have occurred, the caregiver and the patient can decide whether further improvement can be achieved by continuing therapy. The review process may involve changing the type of exercise training, including its frequency and intensity, as well as the type and/or amount of any nutritional support. If functional improvements and weight gain have not occurred, issues relating to compliance, lack of motivation, lack of knowledge, decreased cognitive functioning, lack of social support, anxiety, and depression may need to be addressed. A multidisciplinary-team approach is likely to be the most effective way of managing COPD patients.

16.5 Acute lung injury

Acute lung injury ranges from simple localised lung infections to the diffuse alveolar damage seen in adult respiratory distress syndrome. Anorexia, fatigue, malaise, cough, dyspnoea, and need for ventilatory support all compromise oral intake. If mechanical ventilation is necessary and is anticipated to be required for long periods of time, artificial nutrition support (tube feeding or parenteral nutrition) should be started. However, it should be remembered that during the acute phase of severe catabolic disease it is a reasonable therapeutic aim to attenuate losses of lean tissues. Repletion during the acute phase of the illness can be difficult even in those with substantial malnutrition. In addition, immobility or the use of muscle relaxants to ensure that the patient complies with the ventilator makes it difficult to replete patients. A negative nitrogen balance reduces respiratory muscle strength and ventilatory drive and compromises immune function, which in turn has long-term effects on outcome and recovery. Repletion is more likely to be achieved once an individual is stabilised during recovery from illness. For more on nutritional support, see Chapter 9.

16.6 Concluding remarks

Further characterisation and understanding of the altered substrate metabolism and underlying molecular mechanisms in COPD may change our perspective on nutritional intervention in the future. Through targeted nutritional modulation of specific problems, at either the physiological or the pharmacological level, it may be possible to improve outcomes. Better understanding of the nutritional phenotypes contained under the umbrella term 'COPD' may also allow for more targeted interventions with specific nutritional goals.

The interaction between nutritional depletion and systemic inflammation raises the possibility of using anticatabolic agents to modulate the systemic inflammatory response. Several agents, such as *n*-3 fatty acids and non-steroid anti-inflammatory agents, have been investigated in other wasting conditions such as HIV, cancer, and sepsis, with encouraging results in the changes in proinflammatory mediators and weight response in at least some circumstances. Their application as a potential therapeutic alternative for some patients with COPD remains to be investigated. In addition to the effects of inflammation on energy balance and protein metabolism, recent experimental *in vitro* studies point towards a direct effect of inflammatory mediators on aspects of the muscle cell cycle, such as differentiation and apoptosis. Unravelling the underlying molecular mechanisms and the interaction between nutritional and pharmacological interventions could help us understand and reverse the wasting process. Within two decades, the role of nutrition in chronic respiratory disease has thus moved from ignorance and mere supportive care to targeted intervention with functional and health consequences, which is now supported by a robust and growing evidence base. Therefore, nutrition should be an integral component of the clinical management of patients with respiratory diseases, particularly COPD.

16.7 Acknowledgements

This chapter has been revised and updated by Peter Collins and Marinos Elia, based on the original chapter by Annemie MWJ Schols and Emiel FM Wouters.

References and further reading

Collins PF, Stratton RJ, Elia M. Nutritional support in chronic obstructive pulmonary disease: a systematic review and meta-analysis. Am J Clin Nutr 2012; 95(6): 1385–1395.

Landbo C, Prescott E, Lange P, Vestbo J, Almdal TP. Prognostic value of nutritional status in chronic obstructive pulmonary disease. Am J Respir Crit Care Med 1999; 160: 1856–1861.

Pison CM, Cano NJ, Cherion C, Caron F, Court-Fortune I, Antonini MT, et al. Multimodal nutritional rehabilitation improves clinical outcomes of malnourished patients with chronic respiratory failure: a randomised controlled trial. Thorax 2011; 66(11): 953–960.

Raguso CA, Luthy C. Nutritional status in chronic obstructive pulmonary disease: role of hypoxia. Nutrition 2011; 27(2): 138–143.

Schols AM, Slangen J, Volovics L, Wouters EF. Weight loss is a reversible factor in the prognosis of chronic obstructive pulmonary disease. Am J Respir Crit Care Med 1998; 157: 1791–1797.

Steer J, Norman E, Gibson GJ, Bourke SC. Comparison of indices of nutritional status in prediction of in-hospital mortality and early readmission of patients with acute exacerbations of COPD. Thorax 2010; 65: A127.

Stratton RJ, Green CJ, Elia M. Disease-related Malnutrition. An Evidence-based Approach to Treatment. Oxford: CABI Publishing (CAB International), 2003.

Weekes CE, Emery PE, Elia M. Dietary counseling and food fortification in stable COPD: a randomized trial. Thorax 2009; 64: 326–331.

17
Nutrition and Immune and Inflammatory Systems

Bruce R Bistrian[1] and Robert F Grimble[2]

[1] Beth Israel Deaconess Medical Center, USA
[2] University of Southampton, UK

Key messages

- The immune system may become activated by microbial invasion, as well as by a wide range of stimuli and conditions. The immune response exerts a high metabolic and nutritional cost upon the body.
- Nutrition has a two-way influence on the immune system. The activities of the immune system exert a deleterious influence on nutritional status and alterations in nutrient intake modulate the intensity of the various activities of the immune system.
- Proinflammatory cytokines have far-reaching metabolic effects throughout the body, including changes in protein, fat, vitamin, and trace-element metabolism, alteration of body temperature and appetite, and changes in liver protein synthesis.
- An individual's nutritional status and intake of specific nutrients can modify cytokine biology in ways which have major implications for health and well-being.

- Antioxidants may suppress inflammatory components of the response to infection and trauma, and enhance components related to cell-mediated immunity.
- The unsaturated fatty acid and cholesterol content of the diet also plays a role in the inflammatory response. While n-6 polyunsaturated fatty acids (PUFAs) and cholesterol exert a proinflammatory influence, n-3 PUFAs and monounsaturated fatty acids exert the opposite effect.
- Single base changes (single-nucleotide polymorphisms, SNPs) in the promotor region of cytokine genes raise, or lower, the amount of cytokines produced during the inflammatory response. This phenomenon has been shown in many studies to increase mortality and morbidity during infection and trauma.
- SNPs interact with nutrient status during the inflammatory response, altering the efficacy of immunonutrients. Further knowledge in this area will pave the way to personalised clinical nutrition.

17.1 Introduction

Humans live in the presence of many types of microorganism, which exert pathological effects if they succeed in penetrating the surface defences of the body. Once entry is gained, rapid multiplication occurs, which, if unchecked, can end in death. However, we possess an immune system that has a great capacity for immobilising invading microbes, creating a hostile environment for them, and bringing about their destruction. Humans and warm-blooded animals have survived because their immune systems have the ability to focus a range of lethal activities upon the invader. This biological property is important because many microbes can multiply at least 50 times faster than the cells of the system. The immune system must therefore become rapidly effective once invasion has occurred. The immune system can also become activated, in a similar way to the response to microbial invasion, by a wide range of stimuli and conditions; these include burns, penetrating and blunt injury, the presence of tumour cells, environmental pollutants, radiation, exposure to allergens, and the presence of chronic inflammatory

Clinical Nutrition, Second Edition. Edited by Marinos Elia, Olle Ljungqvist, Rebecca J Stratton and Susan A Lanham-New.
© 2013 The Nutrition Society. Published 2013 by Blackwell Publishing Ltd.

diseases. This latter group of stimulatory conditions includes such diseases as rheumatoid arthritis, Crohn's disease, asthma, and psoriasis, as well as more common conditions such as atherosclerotic heart disease, obesity, diabetes, and Alzheimer's disease. The strength of the response to this disparate range of stimuli may vary, of course, but it will contain many of the hallmarks of the response to invading pathogens. In the normal response to perturbation, the immune system goes from a state of activation to one of deactivation as the body becomes repaired from the effects of the invasion. However, in chronic inflammatory disease the initial activation continues unabated.

As will be seen later, the immune response exerts a high metabolic and nutritional cost upon the body. Inappropriate prolongation of the response will have a deleterious effect upon the nutritional status of the patient.

17.2 The response of the immune system to activation

The immune system is located throughout the body. It consists of clearly recognised structures, such as the spleen, thymus, and lymph nodes, and diffuse populations of cells. Examples of the latter component of the system are lymphocytes, which circulate around the body via the bloodstream and lymphatic circulation. In addition, macrophages (cells capable of engulfing foreign particles, bacteria, viruses, and fungi) populate the linings of the lungs, and together with lymphocytes occupy areas deep in the walls of the small and large intestine. There is also a network of immune cells (dendritic cells) within the skin, which form an important part of the overall immune defence. Thus virtually every part of the body comes under the vigilance of the immune system.

In general terms, the reaction of the immune system to activation can be divided into two components: an innate response, which is unaffected by whether the subject has encountered a particular pathogen before, but is rapid, nonspecific, and the main mediator of the inflammatory response; and a specific immune response, which 'remembers' a previous encounter with a pathogen and produces a much-enhanced focused response on each subsequent exposure (Figure 17.1).

The specific immune response is further subdivided into a cell-mediated and a humoral response. The former involves T lymphocytes, which originate in the bone marrow and undergo further development in the thymus. The second involves B lymphocytes, which originate in the bone marrow and, when stimulated with molecules that are foreign to the body (antigens), develop into cells capable of producing antibodies (immunoglobulins, Igs). These are highly specific to the antigen and aid in its destruction.

While potentially thousands of discretely different Igs can be produced (one for each antigenic substance/organism that might be encountered by the body), they fall into five main classes, depending upon their gross structure. The classes are labelled G, M, A, D, and E. For example, IgA has the ability to cross cell-epithelial cell layers and is thus found in tears, saliva, gut secretions, and milk. IgE, on the other hand, has the ability to attach to mast cells, and when activated leads to the release of histamine and other chemicals associated with allergy.

B cells also come under the influence of a type of T cell, called the helper T cell. Both these forms of lymphocytes and macrophages secrete a range of proteins called cytokines, which act as the 'hormones of the immune system'. Within this group are the interleukins (ILs), tumour necrosis factors (TNFs), and interferons (IFNs). The cytokines act in an apocrine, paracrine, and endocrine manner and modify many activities of the immune system (Table 17.1).

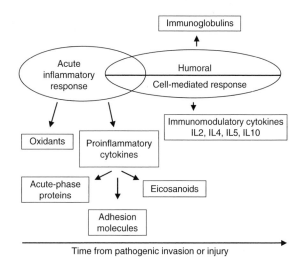

Figure 17.1 The response to infection and injury.

In addition to their direct influence on immune cells, the cytokines IL-1, IL-6, and TNF have widespread metabolic effects upon the body and stimulate the process of inflammation. These cytokines are thus subclassified as proinflammatory cytokines. Key features of the effects of this group of molecules are shown in Figure 17.2.

Nutrition has a two-way influence on the immune system. The activities of the immune system exert a deleterious influence on nutritional status and alterations in nutrient intake modulate the intensity of the various activities of the immune system. Experimental studies and clinical observation have shown that many aspects of the immune response can be modified by alteration in the intake of protein, specific amino acids, lipids, and micronutrients.

Table 17.1 Some examples of cytokines and their effects.

Cytokine	Major effects
Interleukin 1[a]	Fever, muscle protein loss, raised blood glucose, changes in blood trace-element concentration
Tumour necrosis factor-alpha[a]	Fever, appetite loss, muscle protein loss, raised blood lipids, changes in blood trace-element concentration, stimulates oxidant production
Interleukin 6[a]	Stimulates acute-phase protein production by the liver
Interleukin 2	Stimulates T-lymphocyte proliferation
Interleukin 8	Causes attraction of immune cells: chemotaxis
Interleukin 10	Inhibits proinflammatory cytokine production

[a] There are varying degrees of overlap between the actions of these proinflammatory cytokines.

17.3 The effects of proinflammatory cytokines

Many of the signs and symptoms experienced after infection has occurred, such as fever, loss of appetite, weight loss, negative nitrogen and mineral balance, and lethargy, are caused directly and indirectly by proinflammatory cytokines (Figure 17.2). The indirect effects of cytokines are mediated by actions upon the adrenal glands and endocrine pancreas, resulting in increased secretions of the catabolic hormones epinephrine (adrenaline), norepinephrine (noradrenaline), glucococorticoids, and glucagon. Insulin insensitivity occurs in addition to a 'catabolic state'. Reduced insulin sensitivity leads to hyperglycaemia in all but the mildest inflammatory responses. Although increased blood glucose levels do provide greater energy supply to immune cells, fibroblasts, and the brain, which may assist the systemic inflammatory response, hyperglycaemia, particularly if severe, increases morbidity and mortality in the critically ill.

The diverse range of metabolic changes caused by the proinflammatory cytokines can be seen as a coordinated response (Figure 17.3) designed to:

- create a hostile environment for the invading organism;
- provide nutrients, from within the body, to support the actions of the immune system;
- enhance the defence systems of the body to protect healthy tissue from the potent actions of the inflammatory response.

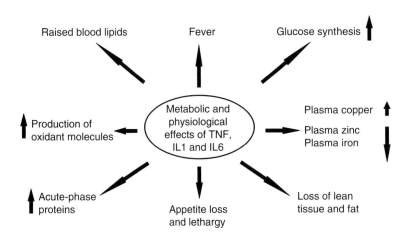

Figure 17.2 General physiological and metabolic effects of proinflammatory cytokines.

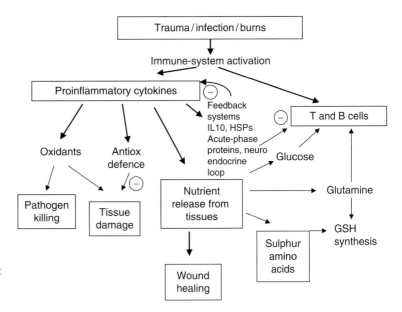

Figure 17.3 The physiological and metabolic consequences of proinflammatory cytokine production.

Changes in protein and fat metabolism

The biochemistry of an infected individual is thus fundamentally changed in a way that will ensure that the immune system receives nutrients from within the body to perform its tasks. Muscle protein is catabolised to provide amino acids for the synthesis of new cells and proteins for the immune response. Furthermore, amino acids are converted to glucose (a preferred fuel for the immune system). The extent of this process is highlighted by the major increase in urinary urea excretion, ranging from 9 g/day in mild infection to 20–30 g/day following major burn or severe traumatic injury. Fat is catabolised at an accelerated rate and the fatty acids released help to satisfy the increased energy needs of the infected person (the resting metabolic rate increases by 13% for every 1 °C rise in body temperature).

Alteration of body temperature and appetite

The rise in temperature is part of the body's attempt to create a hostile environment for the invader. In past centuries, physicians often advocated steam baths for the treatment of infection. It is also interesting to note that when infected, cold-blooded animals, which are unable to raise their body temperature by endogenous means, often move to hotter areas of their immediate environment in an attempt to create hostile conditions for invading organisms.

In mammals, the changes in temperature are mediated by the interaction of proinflammatory cytokines with specialised neurons in the hypothalamus. There is some debate over whether the cytokines gain access directly to the hypothalamus by crossing the blood–brain barrier, or whether circulating cytokines are excluded by the barrier but induce cytokine production within the hypothalamus. The interaction of cytokines with the hypothalamus also brings about a loss of appetite. This may be transient in nature, or prolonged and profound, as is the case in chronic infections such as tuberculosis or during cancer. It is interesting to note that the body-fat regulatory hormone leptin is induced by TNF, but as yet no direct role for leptin in the significant weight loss during infection and cancer has been found.

Changes in trace-element and vitamin metabolism

Major changes occur in plasma cation concentration, such as of iron, copper, zinc, and selenium. These changes in iron and zinc are often misinterpreted as indicating mineral deficiency, but are very likely to be due to a major redistribution of these elements within the body in an attempt to 'starve' bloodborne microbes of nutrients or to foster certain beneficial aspects of the systemic inflammatory response in specific organs. However, micronutrient deficiency can be precipitated by the response to infection, as urinary loss of many micronutrients is accelerated following infection and injury. The resultant deficiencies in zinc, iron, and copper have deleterious effects on general immune function and wound healing. The cytokines also stimulate the synthesis of potent oxidant molecules (hydrogen peroxide, nitric oxide, hydroxyl radical, hypochlorous acid, and superoxide anion), which damage the cellular integrity of the invading organism. A similar lowering of certain vitamin or provitamin levels in the serum or plasma, like fat-soluble vitamins A, D, and E and water-soluble vitamins in the B and C series, also occurs in response to systemic inflammation, which is of uncertain significance but does make the diagnosis of deficiency more difficult and uncertain.

Changes in liver protein synthesis

Specialised proteins, called acute-phase proteins, which focus the actions of the immune system on the invader and help to protect healthy tissue from 'collateral damage' in the 'battle' with pathogens, are synthesised in increased amounts by the liver. Important acute-phase proteins and their respective functions are highlighted in Table 17.2. The liver focuses its activities on acute-phase protein synthesis by slowing the synthesis of its main protein product, serum albumin, and of a number of other secretory proteins, such as prealbumin, retinol-binding protein, and transferrin. This latter group of proteins is termed the 'negative acute-phase reactants'.

Serum albumin concentration is often regarded as an index of protein nutritional status. Thus, the fall in albumin concentration that occurs during infection and inflammatory disease is often misunderstood as a sign of protein deficiency and complicates the assessment of protein status in patients. In virtually every instance, a low serum albumin concentration clinically reflects the presence, or recent occurrence, of a systemic inflammatory response. The response produces malnutrition by inducing anorexia, decreasing voluntary activity, and reducing the metabolic efficiency of endogenous and exogenous protein utilisation. However, low serum albumin concentration is not specifically a measure of nutritional status, since only an unattainably low protein

Table 17.2 Biological functions of major acute-phase proteins.

Function	Acute-phase proteins
Inhibition of proteinase released during the inflammatory response	Alpha-1 proteinase inhibitor Alpha-1 antichymotrypsin Alpha-2 macroglobulin
Removal of antigens from the host	C-reactive protein Serum amyloid A
Activation of the immune response	C-reactive protein C3 complement
Suppression of the immune response	Proteinase inhibitors Alpha-1 glycoprotein
Antioxidant properties	Ceruloplasmin Alpha-1 acid glycoprotein
Binding and transport of metals and biologically active compounds	Ceruloplasmin Haptoglobin Transferrin Alpha-1 acid glycoprotein

intake, in conjunction with an adequate energy intake, will even modestly affect serum albumin concentrations. For instance, patients with very severe anorexia nervosa, with losses of body weight in excess of 30%, will have normal concentrations of serum albumin.

Many of these complex metabolic changes result in the balance being swung from being in favour of the invading organism to being in favour of the infected individual.

17.4 Control systems for cytokines

Proinflammatory cytokines also induce a cascade of production of other cytokines from lymphocytes. The cascade has modulating actions on lymphocyte function (IL-2 stimulates lymphocyte proliferation, IL-8 attracts immune cells to the site of invasion, IL-4 alters the class of antibodies produced). It is of interest to note that cytokines are also capable of autoregulation: IL-10 with IL-4, produced in response to proinflammatory cytokines, suppresses production of further proinflammatory cytokines.

Conceptually, there is evidence that there can be a poor outcome from an excessive systemic inflammatory response. This is referred to as the systemic inflammatory response syndrome (SIRS) and is manifested by increased TNF concentrations in sepsis or following burn injury. However, there is a compensatory anti-inflammatory response syndrome (CARS), reflected in increased production of IL-4 and IL-10, which, if excessive, can also have a deleterious outcome. It has been hypothesised, from a growing body of research data, that the relative balance between SIRS and CARS has an impact on survival. This is probably why attempts to block proinflammatory cytokine production with monoclonal antibodies have met with limited success in reducing mortality.

Nutritional modulation that affects both sides of the SIRS/CARS equation offers a greater promise of success. A class of proteins called heat-shock proteins (HSPs), which were originally identified in heat-stressed cells, are also produced by cells exposed to proinflammatory cytokines. HSPs have a general anti-inflammatory influence and suppress cytokine production. These autoregulatory mechanisms are very important biological phenomena, because, while cytokines are essential for effective operation of the immune system, they exert a high metabolic cost on the body and can exert damaging and lethal effects (Figure 17.3). Conceptually, the systemic inflammatory response should be viewed as a general benefit in most instances, but as having the potential for harm through excessive or prolonged activation of SIRS or CARS. These adverse impacts can result from excessive inflammation, immunodepression, and/or the development of protein-energy malnutrition.

17.5 Damaging and life-threatening effects of cytokines

Although cytokines are essential for the normal operation of the immune system when produced at the right time and in the right amounts, they play a major damaging role in many inflammatory diseases, such as rheumatoid arthritis, inflammatory bowel disease, asthma, psoriasis, and multiple sclerosis, and in cancer. They are also thought to be important in the development of atheromatous plaques in cardiovascular disease. In conditions such as cerebral malaria, meningitis, and sepsis, they are produced in excessive amounts and are an important factor in increased mortality. In these diseases, the cytokines are being produced in the wrong biological context.

The end stages of many chronic conditions have, as a root cause, an ongoing systemic inflammatory response, which is documented by either elevated

plasma cytokines, their soluble receptors, IL-1 receptor antagonist, IL-6, spontaneous or stimulated release of cytokines from peripheral blood mononuclear cells (PBMCs), or elevated acute-phase protein concentrations, particularly C-reactive protein (CRP). These conditions include end-stage liver disease (TNF), end-stage renal disease (IL-6, CRP, soluble cytokine receptors), congestive heart failure (TNF), weight-losing chronic obstructive pulmonary disease (COPD) (IL-6); elevated CRP concentrations are also found in poorly controlled diabetes and obesity. Furthermore, concentrations of this acute-phase protein, when measured by high-sensitivity assay, have been associated with higher risk of coronary or cerebrovascular disease.

Adverse effects of an individual's genotype

It has recently become apparent that single base changes (single-nucleotide polymorphisms, SNPs), usually in the promoter region of genes responsible for producing the molecules involved in the inflammatory process, exert a modulatory effect on the intensity of inflammation. *In vitro* production of TNFα by PBMCs from healthy and diseased subjects stimulated with inflammatory agents shows remarkable individual constancy in men and postmenopausal women. This constancy suggests that genetic factors exert a strong influence. A number of studies have shown that SNPs in the promoter regions for the TNFα and lymphotoxin alpha (LTα) genes are associated with differential TNFα production. The *TNF2(A)* and *TNFB2(A)* alleles (at −308 and +252 for the TNFα and LTα genes, respectively) are linked to high TNF production, particularly in homozygous individuals.

A large body of research has indicated that SNPs occur in the upstream regulatory (promoter) regions of many cytokine genes (e.g. IL-6 −174, IL-1β −511). Many of these genetic variations influence the level of expression of genes and the outcome from the inflammatory response. Both pro- and anti-inflammatory cytokines are influenced by the differences in genotype.

In a study on inflammatory lung disease, caused by exposure to coal dust, the *TNF2* (LTα +252A) allele was almost twice as common in miners with the disease as in those who were healthy. Development of farmer's lung, from exposure to hay dust, was 80% greater in individuals with the *TNF2* allele than in those without the allele. The *TNF2* allele was also twice as common in smokers who developed COPD as in those who remained disease-free.

In addition to disease progression, genetic factors have important effects on mortality and morbidity in infectious and inflammatory disease. In a study on malaria, children who were homozygous for *TNF2* had a sevenfold increase in the risk of death or serious pathology compared to children who were homozygous for the *TNF1* allele. In sepsis, patients possessing the *TNF2* allele had a 3.7-fold greater risk of death than those without the allele, and patients who were homozygous for the LTα +252A allele had twice the mortality rate of and higher peak plasma TNFα concentrations than heterozygotic individuals. The *TNF2* allele has also been found in increased frequencies in systemic lupus erythromatosus, dermatitis herpetiformis, and insulin-dependent and non-insulin-dependent diabetes mellitus.

Genetic factors also influence the propensity of individuals to produce oxidant molecules and thereby influence nuclear transcription factor kappa B (NFκB) activation. Natural resistance-associated macrophage protein 1 (NRAMP1) has effects on macrophage functions, including TNFα production and activation of inducible nitric oxide synthase (iNOS), which occurs through cooperation between the NRAMP1, TNFα, and LTα genes. There are four variations in the NRAMP1 gene, resulting in different basal levels of activity and differential sensitivity to stimulation by inflammatory agents. Alleles 1, 2, and 4 are poor promoters, while allele 3 causes high gene expression. Hyperactivity of macrophages, associated with allele 3, is linked to autoimmune disease susceptibility and high resistance to infection, while allele 2 increases susceptibility to infection and protects against autoimmune disease.

SNPs also occur in genes for anti-inflammatory cytokines. There are at least three polymorphic sites (−1082, −819, −592) in the IL-10 promoter which influence production. In intensive-care patients, the occurrence of the *1082*G* allele, which produces IL-10, was high in those who developed multiorgan failure, with a frequency one-fifth of that of the normal population.

Thus it now appears that each individual possesses combinations of SNPs in their genes, associated with inflammation corresponding to 'inflammatory drives' of differing intensities when microbes or tissue injury are encountered. At an individual level, this may express itself as differing degrees of morbidity and mortality.

In general, men are more sensitive to the genomic influences on the strength of the inflammatory process than women. In a study on LTα genotype and mortality from sepsis, it was found that men possessing a *TNFB22* (LTα +252AA) genotype had a mortality of 72%, compared with men who were *TNFB11* (LTα +252GG), who had a 42% mortality rate. In female patients, the mortalities for the two genotypes were 53 and 33% respectively. In a study on patients undergoing surgery for gastrointestinal cancer, it was found that postoperative CRP and IL-6 concentrations were higher in men than in women. Multivariate analysis showed that men possessing the *TNF2* (TNFα −308A) allele had greater responses than men without it. The genomic influence was not seen in women. Furthermore, possession of the IL-1 −511 T allele was associated with a greater length of stay in hospital in old men admitted for geriatric care. Women were unaffected by these genetic influences.

Many studies have shown a clear link between obesity, oxidant stress, and inflammation. The link may lie in the ability of adipose tissue to produce pro-inflammatory cytokines, particularly TNFα. There is a positive relationship between adiposity and TNF production. Leptin has also been shown to influence proinflammatory cytokine production. Thus plasma triglycerides, body fat mass, and inflammation may be loosely associated because of these endocrine relationships.

In an investigation of cytokine production in healthy men, one of the authors found that, in the study population as a whole, there were no statistically significant relationships between body mass index (BMI), plasma fasting triglycerides, and the ability of PBMCs to produce TNFα. However, individuals with the LTα +252AA genotype (associated with raised TNF production) showed significant relationships between TNF production and BMI and fasting triglycerides. Thus, despite the study population comprising only healthy subjects, within that population were individuals with a genotype that resulted in an 'aged' phenotype as far as plasma lipids, BMI, and inflammation were concerned.

Adverse effects of proinflammatory cytokines on body composition

Experience worldwide shows that infections are a potent inhibitor of growth. The actions of IL-1, IL-6, and TNF exert a high metabolic cost on the body. Substrate released from muscle, skin, and bone under their influence will undoubtedly nourish the immune system and help wound healing; however, in a growing child a conflict of interests occurs and nutrients will be diverted away from growth. The metabolic cost of cytokine action also has potentially deleterious effects in adults. In malaria, tuberculosis, sepsis, cancer, human immunodeficiency virus (HIV) infection, and rheumatoid arthritis, the cytokines bring about a loss of lean tissue, which can seriously debilitate an individual. It is a well-known phenomenon that infection is accompanied by a raised body temperature and an increased output of nitrogenous excretion products in the urine. The loss of nitrogen from the body of an adult during a bacterial infection may be equivalent to 60 g of tissue protein, and in a period of persistent malarial infection, over 500 g of protein.

There are four clinical conditions that cause maximal protein catabolism: (i) major third-degree burns of more than 30% of body surface area; (ii) multiple trauma; (ii) closed head injury with a low Glasgow Coma Score; and (iv) severe sepsis. These result in losses of nitrogen of up to 30 g/day, which is equivalent to 200 g tissue protein. The latter translates into losses of 900 g lean tissue/day, at the usual conversion figure of 30 : 1 for lean tissue to grams of nitrogen.

Important endocrine changes occur during the systemic inflammatory response, which impact upon growth and tissue composition. There is a reduction in anabolic stimuli for growth, including a reduction in testosterone and insulin resistance. Despite increases in growth hormone, which enhances fat mobilisation and gluconeogenesis, production of insulin-like growth factor 1 (IGF-1), which is responsible for the growth-promoting actions of growth hormone, is not promoted. Furthermore, insulin resistance in carbohydrate metabolism fosters an increase in hepatic glucose production and a reduced uptake by skeletal muscle.

These changes, which at first sight appear detrimental, may be beneficial during the systemic inflammatory response, primarily because they result in an increase in blood glucose. Glucose is an ideal metabolic fuel because, having no charge and a small size, it is easily diffusible; further, it can be oxidised to easily excreted products (carbon dioxide and water), or it can uniquely be metabolised to produce ATP without a requirement for oxygen by anaerobic glycolysis. This latter process is particularly important in ischaemic tissues and in macrophages and fibroblasts, which are facultative anaerobes.

Other beneficial results of the systemic inflammatory response are the release of glutamine from muscle, which is important for cells of the immune system and other rapidly dividing cells, and the creation of ammonium ions from deamination of glutamine, which assist in acid–base balance.

Potential damage from the interaction of oxidants with cytokine production

There are further characteristics of cytokine biology which can damage an infected individual indirectly. The oxidant molecules produced by the immune system to kill invading organisms can also activate the important cellular control molecule NFκB. This factor is a control switch for biological processes, not all of which are advantageous to the individual. Activated NFκB migrates to the nucleus, where it switches on genes for cytokine, glutathione, and acute-phase protein production. Unfortunately, however, it also increases HIV replication. This sequence of events accounts for the ability of minor infections to speed the progression of individuals who are infected with HIV towards the acquired immune deficiency syndrome (AIDS) (Figure 17.4).

In the last decade it has become increasingly clear that an individual's nutritional status and intake of specific nutrients can modify cytokine biology in ways that have major implications for health and well-being.

17.6 Influence of malnutrition on key aspects of the cytokine response

Malnutrition has a major effect upon the normal operation of the immune and inflammatory components of the immune system. In a sense, malnutrition was the first-known 'acquired immune deficiency' disease; the effects of malnutrition have much in

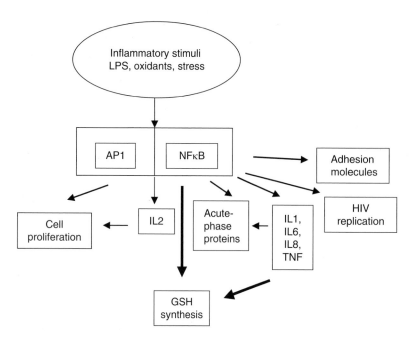

Figure 17.4 The effect of inflammatory stimuli on cell biology via activation of transcription factors. AP1, activator protein 1; NFκB, nuclear transcription factor kappa B; IL, interleukin; GSH, reduced form of glutathione; LPS, lipopolysaccharide; HIV, human immunodeficiency virus; IL, interleukin; TNF, tumour necrosis factor.

common with the later-recognised AIDS due to HIV infection. Malnutrition influences virtually all of the components of the immune response. The most obvious ones are a reduction in the cell number and function of the lymphocytes associated with cell-mediated immunity, shrinkage or impaired development of the organs of the immune system (thymus, spleen, and gut-associated lymphoid tissue), and suppression of some aspects of the inflammatory response.

Influence of protein-energy malnutrition

Children hospitalised with protein-energy malnutrition often show no fever when they are experiencing bacterial, viral, and parasitic invasion. As nutritional rehabilitation proceeds, the children become febrile and may develop an overwhelming inflammatory response marked by oxidant damage and 'shock-like' symptoms. It is unknown whether the afebrile state is due to impaired cytokine production or to changes in the responsiveness of the central nervous system. Studies in rats, rabbits, and guinea pigs have shown that protein-deficient diets reduce the ability of macrophages to produce cytokines. In monkeys, other macrophage functions such as the ability to engulf and kill microorganisms have also been shown to be depressed.

Pure protein deficiency in humans does not exist as a discrete entity, but occurs in combination with deficiencies of other nutrients. However, it was shown in 1982, by studies in Boston, that circulating white blood cells from malnourished elderly patients had an impaired ability to produce inflammatory cytokines and that normal function could be restored by dietary protein and energy supplements. Paradoxically, chronic food deprivation in previously healthy subjects has been reported to enhance TNF production by monocytes stimulated by phytohaemagglutinin (PHA). A similar phenomenon has been found in basal TNF production in patients with anorexia nervosa.

Influence of vitamin A deficiency

Vitamin A intake has a potent effect on immune function in malnourished populations. Supplementation studies have shown reductions of approximately 30% in childhood mortality in many countries where vitamin A deficiency is endemic. The mechanisms for the increased effectiveness of the immune system are not fully understood; however, it seems likely that the effects of the nutrient in improving epithelial barriers and IgA production may play a role. In addition, vitamin A supplements have been shown to enhance IL-1 production in malnourished children. Supplemental zinc has also been shown to have a restorative effect on immune function in malnourished experimental animals and individuals. Further details of the effect of micronutrients on immune function are described in Chapters 9 and 10 of *Introduction to Human Nutrition* in this series.

17.7 Antioxidant defences and their impact on immune and inflammatory systems in patients

The increase in oxidant production which occurs in the presence of cytokines carries the risk that healthy tissues within the body may become damaged alongside invading organisms. When glutathione synthesis was blocked in rats by injection of diethyl maleate, a sublethal dose of TNF became lethal. The onset of sepsis in patients (going on to develop multiple organ failure) leads to a transient decrease in the total antioxidative capacity of blood. The capacity returns to normal values over the following 5 days; this was found not to be the case for patients who died, however, for whom values remained well below the normal range. Oxidants enhance the production of a number of cytokines through the activation of nuclear transcription factors, such as NFκB and activator protein 1 (AP1). A change in cell redox status results in the activation of these factors and migration into the nucleus, where they initiate transcription of a wide range of genes associated with inflammation and cell proliferation (Figure 17.4).

A number of components of antioxidant defence are enhanced by proinflammatory cytokines. Glutathione synthesis and the activities of superoxide dismutase (SOD), catalase, glutathione peroxidase, and reductase are increased. Gamma-glutamyl cysteine synthetase, the rate-limiting enzyme in the biosynthetic pathway for glutathione, has an NFκB-activated domain in the promoter region for its gene.

Normally, the ability of cytokines to raise the level of antioxidant defences offers a measure of protection to host tissues. Nonetheless, there is evidence of oxidative damage in a wide range of clinical conditions in which cytokines are produced. Lipid peroxides and increased thiobarbituric acid-reactive substances (TBARS) are present in the blood of patients with septic shock, asymptomatic HIV infection, chronic hepatitis C, breast cancer, cystic fibrosis,

diabetes mellitus, and alcoholic liver disease. Peroxides also increase following cancer chemotherapy, open heart surgery, bone-marrow transplantation, and haemodialysis.

A pivotal role for glutathione in antioxidant defence

While all antioxidants are important in maintaining robust antioxidant defences, glutathione is a pivotal member of this group of compounds due to its multifunctional role in maintaining other antioxidants (alpha-tocopherol, ascorbate) in a reduced state, by acting as a reservoir of sulphur amino acids for acute-phase protein synthesis, and by functioning as an immunomodulator.

In addition to its important role as a component of antioxidant defence, glutathione can influence aspects of immune function that are related to T lymphocytes. T-cell functions can be potentiated by glutathione administration *in vivo*. However, the relationship between cellular concentrations and cell numbers is complex. In healthy subjects, the numbers of helper (CD4+) and suppressor (CD8+) T lymphocytes increased in parallel with intracellular glutathione concentrations of up to 30 nmol/mg protein. A 7% increase in CD4+ and a 50% increase in CD8+ occurred over the concentration range. However, numbers of both subsets declined at concentrations between 30 and 50 nmol/mg protein. When the subjects of the study engaged in a programme of intensive physical exercise daily for 4 weeks, a fall in glutathione concentrations occurred in liver, muscle, and blood. Individuals with glutathione concentrations in the optimal range before exercise who experienced a fall in concentration after exercise showed a 30% fall in CD4+ T-cell numbers. The decline in T-cell number was prevented by administration of *N*-acetyl cysteine, which did not arrest the decline in glutathione concentration. The studies therefore suggest that immune-cell function may be sensitive to a range of intracellular sulphhydryl compounds, including glutathione and cysteine.

In HIV-positive individuals and patients with AIDS, a reduction in cellular and plasma glutathione has been noted. It is unclear at present whether the depletion in lymphocyte population is related to this phenomenon.

Antioxidant defences are depleted by infection and trauma

As indicated earlier, the enhancement of antioxidant defences that occurs during the inflammatory process may not be able to completely protect the subject from tissue damage. Furthermore, a decrease in some components of antioxidant defence may occur in some diseases. Observations in experimental animals and patients indicate that antioxidant defences become depleted during infection and after injury. In mice infected with the influenza virus, there were 27, 42, and 45% decreases in the blood levels of vitamin C, vitamin E, and glutathione, respectively. In asymptomatic HIV infection, substantial decreases in glutathione in blood and lung epithelial lining fluid have been noted.

In patients undergoing elective abdominal operations, the glutathione content of blood and skeletal muscle fell by over 10 and 42%, respectively, within 24 hours of the operation. While values in blood slowly returned to preoperative levels, concentrations in muscle were still depressed 48 hours postoperatively. Furthermore, reduced tissue glutathione concentrations have been noted in hepatitis C, ulcerative colitis, and cirrhosis. In patients with malignant melanoma, metastatic hypernephroma, and metastatic colon cancer, plasma ascorbic acid concentrations fell from normal to almost undetectable levels within 5 days of commencement of treatment with IL-2. In patients with inflammatory bowel disease, substantial reductions in ascorbic acid concentrations occurred in inflamed gut mucosa.

Risks of oxidant damage posed by parenteral feeding with solutions containing PUFAs

Many lipid sources in total parenteral nutrition (TPN) formulations are rich in polyunsaturated fatty acids (PUFAs). Requirements for the antioxidant vitamin E are related to PUFA intake, as these fatty acids are susceptible to peroxidation. The risk of increased peroxidation is apparent in patients receiving home TPN. When healthy volunteers and home-TPN patients were given a linoleic acid-rich infusion, there was a marked rise in breath pentane, indicating increased lipid peroxidation. The intake of vitamin E was 45 mg/day, which is substantially above estimated daily requirements.

Evidence of depleted antioxidant defences and increased lipid peroxidation in patients receiving home parenteral nutrition has also been shown in a study in which n-6-rich TPN was given. Serum malondialdehyde (an index of lipid peroxidation) was positively correlated with n-6 PUFA given and negatively correlated with plasma alpha-tocopherol. Clinical measures to improve iron status may unwittingly increase oxidant stress. Normally, free-iron concentrations are kept at very low levels in tissues by sequestration with binding proteins during inflammation, since the ion catalyses free-radical production. Thus, provision of iron to patients experiencing a SIRS is often likely to be harmful. This is even more likely in the presence of malnutrition complicating infection or inflammation, since serum transferrin levels are reduced, further increasing free-iron levels in the serum. For this reason, iron is generally not included in the nutritional rehabilitation of severely malnourished children with kwashiorkor, where it has been shown to worsen outcome.

It can be seen that the antioxidant defences of the body do not offer complete protection for host tissues against the oxidative molecules produced by the immune system. There is therefore potential to improve antioxidant defences. The capacity of the host for enhancement of antioxidant defences will depend upon the previous and concomitant intakes of nutrients. Synthesis of acute-phase proteins and glutathione is influenced by protein intake, sulphur amino acid sufficiency, and glutamine supplementation. The intake of micronutrients such as copper, zinc, and selenium influences the activity of antioxidant enzymes. Other components of the antioxidant defences are derived directly from the diet, including ascorbic acid, tocopherols, beta-carotene, and a number of less well-characterised phytochemicals (see Chapter 14 of *Nutrition and Metabolism* in this series).

Immunomodulation by manipulation of antioxidant defences

Without doubt, antioxidant defences provide a potentially effective target for immunomodulation. An impressive number of studies in animal models of infection and trauma in healthy subjects and hospitalised individuals indicate that a wide range of nutrients are able to modulate the functioning of the

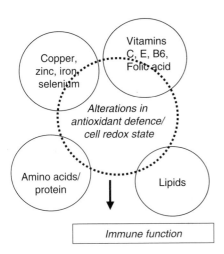

Figure 17.5 Nutrients which modulate immune function by partially influencing antioxidant defences and cellular redox state.

immune system. These include protein, specific amino acids, PUFAs, copper, zinc, iron, vitamins B_6, C, and E, and riboflavin. All of these nutrients are directly or indirectly linked to antioxidant defence or the ability of the patient to produce an oxidative environment within their tissues. As illustrated in Figure 17.5, the mechanisms whereby the nutrient brings about immunomodulation via changes in the antioxidant status vary – from nutrients which clearly operate via this mechanism (vitamins C and E) to nutrients which alter the oxidant/antioxidant environment of the cell to a smaller extent as part of their immunomodulatory influence via changes in this cellular characteristic (PUFAs, vitamin B_6, iron, and zinc).

Antioxidant defences are interlinked and interactive

Many of the components of antioxidant defence interact to maintain the antioxidant capacity of the tissues. For example, when oxidants interact with cell membranes, the oxidised form of vitamin E is restored to the antioxidant form through reduction by ascorbic acid. Dehydroascorbic acid formed in this process is reconverted to ascorbic acid by interaction with the reduced form of glutathione. Subsequently, oxidised glutathione formed in the reaction is reconverted to the glutathione by glutathione reductase. In healthy subjects, a daily dose of 500 mg ascorbic acid for 6 weeks resulted in a 47%

increase in the glutathione content of red blood cells. Vitamins E and C and glutathione are thus intimately linked in antioxidant defence. Vitamin B_6 and riboflavin, which have no antioxidant properties *per se*, also contribute to antioxidant defences indirectly. Vitamin B_6 is a co-factor in the metabolic pathway for the biosynthesis of cysteine. Cellular cysteine concentration is rate-limiting for glutathione synthesis. Riboflavin is a co-factor for glutathione reductase, which maintains the major part of cellular glutathione in the reduced form (Figure 17.6).

Many potentially immunomodulatory nutrients and pronutrients may operate by enhancing glutathione status. In Figure 17.7, it can be seen that glutathione synthesis might be altered by changes in the supply of the three precursor amino acids via an increase in cysteine supply from *N*-acetyl cysteine treatment, or from an increase in metabolic flux through the transmethylation and transulfuration pathway, assisted by vitamin B_6 and folic acid, and provision of L-2-oxothiazolidine-4-carboxylate (pro-cysteine).

The anti-inflammatory and immunoenhancing influence of antioxidants

There is a growing body of evidence to show that antioxidants suppress inflammatory components of the response to infection and trauma and enhance components related to cell-mediated immunity. The reverse situation applies when antioxidant defences become depleted.

Influence of vitamin E intake

Vitamin E exerts modulatory effects on both inflammatory and immune components of immune function. In general, vitamin E deficiency and low tissue vitamin E content enhance components of the inflammatory response and suppress components of the immune response. Dietary vitamin E supplementation brings about the opposite effect. When elderly subjects were supplemented with 800 IU of alpha-tocopherol for 30 days, there was a 50% increase in the delayed-type hypersensitivity response, a 65% increase in IL-2 production, and a decrease in oxidative stress, as indicated by a major decrease in plasma lipid peroxides and increased TBARS.

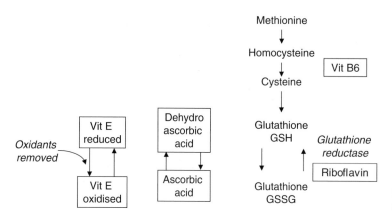

Figure 17.6 Major components of antioxidant defence and their metabolic interrelationships.

Studies in animals have demonstrated that vitamin E deficiency impairs cellular and humoral immunity and is associated with an increased incidence of disease. Supplementation of the diet with vitamin E at levels that are several-fold greater than requirements increases resistance to a number of pathogens. The resistance of chickens and turkeys to *Escherichia coli* and of mice to pneumococci was enhanced by vitamin E supplementation. A similar phenomenon may also occur in humans, since epidemiological evidence shows a lower incidence of infectious disease in subjects with high plasma alpha-tocopherol concentrations. Rats consuming diets that were deficient in vitamin E and given injections of endotoxin showed a greater degree of anorexia and greater concentrations of plasma α_1-acid glycoprotein and IL-6 than animals consuming adequate amounts of the vitamin. In smokers, a low intake of vitamin E was associated with an increased intensity of the inflammatory response to cigarette smoke. Plasma concentrations of α_1-acid glycoprotein were 50% greater in subjects in the lowest tertile of intake than in subjects in the highest tertile.

In healthy subjects and smokers, a 4-week period of supplementation with 600 IU of alpha-tocopherol resulted in a significant reduction in TNFα production from PBMCs stimulated with endotoxin. Intense exercise of healthy young and elderly subjects resulted in the appearance of a mild inflammatory response characterised by raised blood IL-1, IL-6, and acute-phase protein concentrations. A twice-daily supplement of 400 IU of alpha-tocopherol inhibited the response. However, in large, randomised studies of vitamin E supplementation in healthy populations,

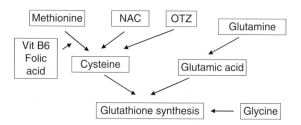

Figure 17.7 Nutrients and pronutrients which contribute to glutathione synthesis. NAC, N-acetyl cysteine; OTZ, L-2-oxothiazolidine-4-carboxylate (procysteine).

or with heart disease, high dose supplementation at similar levels was either not effective or was even harmful in certain instances. On the other hand, multivitamin supplementation of both fat- and water-soluble vitamins at requirement levels or at several multiples of these levels did improve pregnancy outcomes in HIV-positive women.

Influence of vitamin C intake

The effect of vitamin C status on immune function has been studied extensively. High concentrations of the vitamin are found in phagocytic cells. While the role of the vitamin as a key component of antioxidant defence is well established, most studies have shown only minor effects upon a range of immune functions. Unlike deficiencies in vitamins B_6, E, and riboflavin, deficiency of vitamin C does not cause atrophy of lymphoid tissue. Studies in guinea pigs have shown that the humoral response is unaffected by vitamin C deficiency but that cell-mediated responses are reduced. The function of phagocytic cells is influenced by vitamin C status. While the ability of neutrophils from guinea pigs affected by scurvy to produce H_2O_2 and kill staphylococci is similar to that in neutrophils from well-fed animals, peritoneal macrophages from animals with scurvy are smaller and have a decreased ability to migrate. However, no defect in phagocytic ability of the cells has been noted.

The effect of vitamin C status and large doses of ascorbic acid on the response of healthy volunteers to the common cold virus has been studied in great detail. Only minor effects on immune function have been observed, although a reduction in the severity of symptoms has been noted. In a study of ultra marathon runners, dietary supplementation with 600 mg/day reduced the incidence of upper respiratory tract infections following a race by 50%. It is interesting to note that strenuous exercise has been shown to deplete tissue glutathione content. The interrelationship between glutathione and ascorbic acid may therefore play a role in the effect of exercise on immune function.

When immunological parameters and antioxidant status were measured in adult males fed 250 mg/day of vitamin C for 4 days, followed by 5 mg/day for 32 days, plasma ascorbic acid and glutathione decreased and impairment of antioxidant status became evident from a doubling in semen 8-hydroxydeoxyguanosine concentration. A fall in vitamin content in PBMCs was noted and the delayed-type hypersensitivity reactions to seven recall antigens were reduced.

An unconfirmed study has reported that vitamin C supplementation resulted in clinical improvement in AIDS patients. An *in vitro* study also showed that a thymocyte cell line infected with HIV, when incubated with calcium ascorbate, glutathione, and *N*-acetyl cysteine, inhibited HIV replication. The clinical usefulness of this observation is unclear, since intravenous administration of ascorbic acid would be necessary to achieve the intracellular concentrations that were shown to be effective in inhibiting viral replication *in vitro*.

Ascorbic acid may exert its most potent effects upon the inflammatory component of the immune response. In rats that have been made congenitally unable to synthesise ascorbic acid, elevated concentrations of acute-phase proteins occur in the absence of any applied inflammatory stimulus. The inflammatory influence of cigarette smoke is partly modulated by vitamin C intake. Individuals consuming less than 80 mg/day of vitamin C had plasma ceruloplasmin and CRP levels 10 and 59% greater than those in individuals with a higher intake of the vitamin.

Influence of vitamin B$_6$

Although it has no antioxidant properties, vitamin B$_6$ plays an important part in antioxidant defences because of its action in the metabolic pathway for the formation of cysteine, which is the rate-limiting precursor in glutathione synthesis. Vitamin B$_6$ status has widespread effects upon immune function. Animal studies have clearly demonstrated that a deficiency of the vitamin results in large effects on lymphoid tissues. Thymic atrophy occurs and lymphocyte depletion in lymph nodes and spleen has been found in monkeys, dogs, rats, and chickens. Antigen processing was normal, but the ability to make antibodies to sheep red blood cells was depressed. In human studies, the ability to make antibodies to tetanus and typhoid antigens is not seriously affected unless the diet is also deficient in pantothenic acid.

Various aspects of cell-mediated immunity are also influenced by vitamin B$_6$ deficiency. Skin grafts in rats and mice survive longer during deficiency, and guinea pigs exhibit decreased delayed-hypersensitivity reactions to bacille Calmette–Guérin (BCG).

Deficiency of vitamin B$_6$ is rare in humans but can be precipitated by the antituberculosis drug isoniazid. However, experimental deficiency in elderly subjects has been shown to reduce total blood lymphocyte numbers and decrease the proliferative response of lymphocytes to PHA and Concanavalin A (ConA). Likewise, IL-2 production is reduced by vitamin deficiency. Restoration of vitamin B$_6$ intake to normal by dietary supplements restores immune function. However, intakes that are higher than current recommended values are required to normalise all immune functions, suggesting that optimal immune function can only be achieved in this way. It is unclear at present whether a similar situation occurs in younger subjects.

One mechanism for the effect of vitamin B$_6$ on immune function may derive from the importance of the vitamin in cysteine synthesis, as outlined earlier. Deficiency of the vitamin may limit the availability of cysteine for glutathione synthesis. In rats, vitamin B$_6$ deficiency resulted in decreases of 12 and 21% in glutathione concentrations in plasma and spleen, respectively. In healthy young women, large doses of vitamin B_6 (27 mg/day for 2 weeks) resulted in a 50% increase in plasma cysteine content, presumably due to increased flux through the transulfuration pathway of methionine metabolism. As cysteine is a rate-limiting substrate for glutathione synthesis, these findings may have implications for the response to pathogens because of the importance of glutathione in lymphocyte proliferation and antioxidant defence. However, while vitamin B_6 has cellular effects on the immune system, evidence is lacking for any effect upon the inflammatory response.

Mechanisms for the anti-inflammatory immunoenhancing effects of antioxidants

There are a number of candidate mechanisms for the immunoenhancing, anti-inflammatory actions of antioxidants. Oxidant damage to cells will, indirectly, create a proinflammatory effect through the production of lipid peroxides. This situation may lead to upregulation of NFκB activity, since the transcription factor is activated in endothelial cells cultured with the main dietary n-6 PUFA linoleic acid, and the effect is inhibited by vitamin E and N-acetyl cysteine. A change in the redox state of the cell towards more oxidative conditions will directly lead to activation of NFκB. By 'quenching' oxidants, antioxidants will counteract the trend towards NFκB activation.

Differential effects of oxidants and antioxidants on transcription-factor activation

Evidence is emerging that not all transcription factors respond to the effects of antioxidants in the same way. In an in vitro study on HeLa cells and cells from human embryonic kidney, both TNF and hydrogen peroxide resulted in activation of NFκB and AP1. Addition of the antioxidant sorbitol to the medium resulted in suppression of NFκB activation (as expected) but activation of AP1 (Figure 17.8). Thus the antioxidant environment of the cell might exert opposite effects upon transcription factors closely associated with inflammation (e.g. NFκB) and cellular proliferation (AP1).

Further evidence for this biphasic effect was seen when glutathione was incubated in vitro with

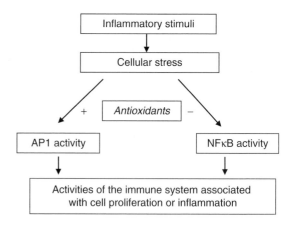

Figure 17.8 A hypothesis to explain the anti-inflammatory and immunoenhancing effects of antioxidants. AP1, activator protein 1; NFκB, nuclear factor kappa B.

immune cells from young adults. A rise in cellular glutathione content was accompanied by an increase in IL-2 production and the mitogenic response to ConA, and a decrease in production of the inflammatory mediators prostaglandin E2 (PGE2) and leukotriene B4 (LTB4). As indicated earlier, supplementation of elderly subjects with large doses of alpha-tocopherol not only improves IL-2 production and cell-mediated immunity but decreases TBARS in plasma, which might have arisen from a proinflammatory state. Indeed, it has been noted that in healthy elderly subjects there is an increase in proinflammatory cytokine production, which may be linked with the loss of lean tissue that occurs during the ageing process.

Modification of the glutathione content of liver, lung, spleen, and thymus in young rats through diets containing a range of casein contents changed immune cell numbers in the lung. It was found that the number of lung neutrophils decreased with dietary protein intake and tissue glutathione content in unstressed animals. However, in animals given lipopolysaccharide (LPS), cell numbers related inversely to tissue glutathione content. Addition of methionine to the protein-deficient diets normalised glutathione content and restored lung neutrophil numbers to those seen in unstressed animals fed a diet of adequate protein content.

Thus it can be hypothesised that antioxidants exert an immunoenhancing effect by activating transcription factors that are strongly associated with cell proliferation (e.g. AP1) and an anti-inflammatory effect by preventing activation of NFκB by oxidants produced during the inflammatory response (Figure 17.8).

17.8 Immunomodulatory effects of lipids

Lipids have been shown to be potent modulators of inflammation – not a surprising fact, given that a large number of the modulatory compounds cited earlier are derived from the hydrolysis of membrane phospholipids by the action of phospholipase A2 (prostaglandins, thromboxanes, and leukotrienes), phospholipase C (diacylglycerol, DAG), phospholipase D (phosphatidic acid), and sphingomyelinases (ceramide). Many of these lipid mediators modulate the activity kinases in the intracellular signalling pathways (e.g. MAP kinases) or transcription factors (e.g. NFκB).

Mode of action of fatty acid composition on cytokine biology

The fats consumed in diets contain widely differing amounts and proportions of unsaturated fatty acids. Many vegetable oils (e.g. corn, safflower, and sunflower oils) are rich in the *n*-6 PUFA linoleic acid (LA). Saturated animal fats, such as those of beef, lamb, and butter, contain low concentrations of linoleic acid, as does coconut oil. All other fats of plant origin are rich in linoleic acid. Maize, palm, and olive oils and butter contain substantial quantities of the monounsaturated fatty acid oleic acid. Oils from fatty fish are rich in the long-chain *n*-3 PUFAs eicosapentaenoic acid (EPA) and docosahexaenoic acid (DHA). The *n*-3 PUFA linolenic acid (LNA) can act as a precursor for EPA and DHA, although the conversion rates of LNA to EPA and DHA are very low. Much higher tissue levels of EPA and DHA result from their feeding directly. LNA is derived from leafy vegetables, although none except linseed oil is particularly rich in this nutrient.

The most likely site in the cell for lipids to modulate inflammation is the cell membrane. Dietary unsaturated fatty acids can alter the composition of the fatty acyl chains of membrane phospholipids. Fatty acids may be incorporated into any of the various classes of phospholipid within the membrane: phosphatidyl choline (PC), phosphatidyl ethanolamine (PE), phosphatidyl serine (PS), phosphatidyl inositol (PI), and sphingomyelin (SPH). Thus the nature of the substrate for PG, LT, DAG, phosphatidic acid, and ceramide production may be changed.

The changes in fatty acid composition may also exert a biophysical influence on membrane structure by altering the fluidity characteristics of the membrane. Theoretically, changes in fluidity may influence the activity of membrane-associated enzymes important to the control of cytokine production. For example, fluidity changes may alter G-protein activity, thereby altering the activity of enzyme systems which are influenced by G proteins (e.g. adenylate cyclase, phospholipase A2 (PLA2), and phospholipase C activity). Alterations in membrane phospholipids will also directly influence the synthesis of lipid-derived mediators such as the eicosanoids, DAG, phosphatidic acid, ceramide, and platelet-activating factor.

The fatty acid composition of all of these mediators will reflect membrane phospholipid composition. The pattern of eicosanoid production will be influenced by the fatty acid incorporated into the *sn*-2 position, as activation of PLA2 will release fatty acid from this location for eicosanoid synthesis. The position is usually occupied by unsaturated fatty acids. Arachidonic acid (AA) is the parent compound of prostanoids and leukotrienes of the 2 and 4 series respectively, whereas EPA is the precursor of the less potent prostanoids and leukotrienes of the 3 and 5 series respectively. Eicosatetraenoic acid (ETA), which is produced under conditions of essential fatty acid deficiency, does not serve as an eicosanoid precursor, and thereby dramatically reduces 2-series prostaglandins, protacyclins, and thromboxanes and 4-series leukotrienes. Dietary fat composition may thus modulate the proportions of all three eicosanoid precursors (Figure 17.9). Furthermore, EPA and DHA are the source of the active anti-inflammatory compounds the resolvins and the neuroprotectins.

Influence of fats on responses to inflammatory agents and diseases

In theory, fats may influence inflammation by altering the production of cytokines and other inflammatory mediators, or by changing the sensitivity of

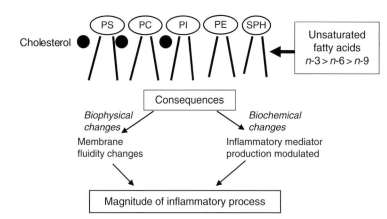

Figure 17.9 The consequences of differential incorporation of unsaturated fatty acids into the membranes of cytokine-producing and cytokine-responsive cells. PS, phosphatidyl serine; PC, phosphatidyl choline; PI, phosphatidyl inositol; PE, phosphatidyl ethanolamine; SPH, sphingomyelin.

target tissues to inflammatory mediators, or by acting at both levels. Lipids also have substantial and profound effects on cellular and humoral aspects of immunity. These aspects are dealt with in detail in Chapter 4 of *Nutrition and Metabolism* in this series.

In general terms, *n*-3 PUFAs downregulate or inhibit T-cell proliferation and function. Monounsaturated fatty acids may have a similar but less potent effect.

Studies have investigated the influence of lipids on the responses of animals to bacteria, bacterial extracts, burns and other forms of injury, and injections of recombinant proinflammatory cytokines. In addition, studies have examined the effects of lipids on *in vivo* and *in vitro* proinflammatory cytokine production from cells of the immune system. The ability of lipids to modify the gross inflammatory process in both animal models and disease states in humans has also been examined.

Influence of fats on responses to proinflammatory cytokines and inflammatory agents

Numerous studies have shown that fats rich in *n*-3 PUFAs exert a generalised anti-inflammatory influence. Guinea pigs fed fish oil for 6 weeks experienced a smaller fever in response to IL-1 than animals fed safflower oil. Likewise, rats fed fish oil exhibited a lesser degree of anorexia in response to IL-1 and TNF than animals fed corn oil.

Olive oil and butter, which, like coconut oil, have a low content of linoleic acid, almost without exception suppress both the effects of inflammatory agents that

are clearly mediated by eicosanoids, such as anorexia and fever, and those that are not, such as elevation of plasma acute-phase protein concentrations and increases in protein synthetic rates in liver, lung, and kidney. Olive oil and butter contain substantial amounts of the monounsaturated fatty acid oleic acid, which may bestow anti-inflammatory properties on these fats.

Addition of olive oil to the diet of rats almost totally suppressed metabolic responses to an endotoxin injection. Conversely, diets rich in linoleic acid had a proinflammatory influence in animal models of inflammation. The inflammatory response to burn injury in guinea pigs was enhanced by safflower oil when it constituted 30–50% of dietary energy. In rats, the degree of anorexia, fall in body temperature, elevation of ceruloplasmin, and liver protein and zinc content in response to endotoxin injections was increased in a stepwise manner when maize oil was included in their diets in amounts of 50, 100, and 200 g/kg.

Although oleic acid is capable of inhibiting incorporation of linoleic acid and AA into membrane phospholipids, it is improbable that it is exerting its influence on visceral protein responses by modulating eicosanoid metabolism. *In vitro* studies have shown that oleic acid is also able to activate protein kinase C, which has been implicated in the downregulation of receptors for TNF.

Cholesterol may exert a proinflammatory effect by enhancing cytokine production. Studies on rabbits showed that IL-1 and TNF synthesis in the aorta wall in response to an LPS injection was enhanced by inclusion of cholesterol (3 g/kg) in diets containing maize oil. Cholesterol may also exert a more generalised proinflammatory effect. *In vitro* studies on monocytes showed that incubation with cholesterol increased expression of HLA-D subregion products. Cholesterol was also shown to increase the proliferative response of human peripheral blood lymphocytes to PHA.

In summary, it would seem that the intensity of many of the metabolic changes that are part of the inflammatory process is influenced by the unsaturated fatty acid and cholesterol content of the diet. While *n*-6 PUFAs and cholesterol exert a proinflammatory influence, *n*-3 PUFAs and monounsaturated fatty acids exert the opposite effect.

Influence of fats on cytokine production

Relatively few studies have examined the modulatory effects of lipids on the ability of cells to produce cytokines. In human volunteers, supplementation of the diet for 6 weeks with 18 g/day of a fish oil concentrate rich in EPA and DHA reduced the ability of monocytes to produce IL-1α and β and TNFα and β by at least a third. The effect was still evident 10 weeks after cessation of dietary supplementation. A similar suppressive effect of dietary supplementation with fish oil was noted on IL-1 production by stimulated monocytes in rheumatoid patients, and on IL-1, IL-6, and TNF production in young and old women. In the study on rheumatoid patients, olive oil supplements were given to the control group. A fall in ability to produce IL-1 was noted in this group also. The effect did not reach statistical significance, but it is interesting in view of the anti-inflammatory nature of olive oil in animal studies and the suggestion that rheumatoid arthritis is less common in Mediterranean regions of Europe than elsewhere.

Studies on rats, in which the ability of a range of fats with differing unsaturated fatty acid contents to alter cytokine production from peritoneal macrophages was examined, indicated that production of IL-1 related positively to *n*-6 PUFA intake and that IL-6 production correlated with the total intake of unsaturated fatty acids. The study in rats was partly paralleled by the results of an investigation into the influence of a cholesterol-lowering diet on the immune function of middle-aged subjects. A change in *n*-6 PUFA intake from 6.6 to 8.8% of dietary energy resulted in a 62 and 47% increase in IL-1 and

TNF production, respectively, from stimulated monocytes. An addition of 0.54% of energy as *n*-3 PUFAs counteracted this effect and resulted in decreases of 40 and 7% in the production of the two cytokines, respectively.

Influence of fats on inflammatory responses in disease in animal models and humans

Inflammatory symptoms in rheumatoid arthritis, psoriasis, asthma, Crohn's disease, and ulcerative colitis are ameliorated by fish oil. The substantial weight loss which occurs in pancreatic cancer can be prevented or ameliorated by a daily nutritional supplement containing fish oil. A 5-day period of administration of TPN containing a mixture of soybean oil, medium-chain triglycerides (MCTs), olive oil, and fish oil (SMOF) to surgical patients was found to lower LTB4/LTB5 ratios and shorten hospital stay by 7 days. Although subsequent study has provided some evidence of improvement of clinical outcome in surgical and other critically ill patients receiving short-term nutritional supplementation with parenteral fish oil, the definitive value of parenteral fish oil has not been established. Fish oil provided enterally as an oral supplement or as a component of a nutritional formula has however clearly demonstrated improved clinical outcomes. Fish oil supplementation has been shown to produce a beneficial outcome following renal transplantation in terms of reduced rejection episodes and improved transplant function. It also improves outcome in the rare and generally fatal condition IgA nephropathy. Fish oil, along with other so-called immune-enhancing nutrients such as arginine, glutamine, and supplemental antioxidants as a complete nutritional formula, has been shown convincingly to improve clinical outcome in various categories of hospitalised patients, including following major surgery on the abdomen or chest, following trauma and burns, and in sepsis.

There are many animal models of acute and chronic inflammation in which fats have been shown to modulate these processes. Fish oil protected pigs, rats, and guinea pigs from the lethal effects of endotoxin. The oil exerted protective effects in experimental colitis in rats. The oil also reduced the metabolic response to burn injury in guinea pigs, the number of polymorphonuclear cells in air pouches of rats challenged with bovine serum albumin, and the degree of anorexia and weight loss in mice given the MAC16 colon adenocarcinoma. Diets rich in MCTs produced similar ameliorative effects in the same cancer cachexia model.

Mechanisms whereby fats modulate immune function: observations from experimental studies

The most likely way in which lipids might modulate proinflammatory cytokine biology is by changing the fatty acid composition of the fatty acyl chains of the phospholipids in cell membranes. The fatty acids compete for incorporation into the phospholipid structure. The affinity for incorporation is in the order linolenic acid > linoleic acid > oleic acid. Furthermore, dietary AA and EPA may be incorporated into phospholipids. EPA is incorporated with the highest affinity of all unsaturated fatty acids. Studies in rats indicate that EPA exerts an anti-inflammatory effect by displacing AA from the membrane. Other *n*-3 PUFAs such as DHA and alpha-linolenic acid are much less effective at exerting an anti-inflammatory influence, although DHA may have unique anti-inflammatory effects in the brain.

The *n*-6 PUFA gamma-linolenic acid also exerts an anti-inflammatory effect by suppressing IL-1β and TNFα from human PBMCs. This effect has shown clinical efficacy in studies on patients with adult respiratory distress syndrome given a fatty acid in an enteral feed which also provides fish oil and a number of antioxidant vitamins or provitamins and minerals.

Conversion of the *n*-3, *n*-6, and *n*-9 fatty acids to precursors of eicosanoids occurs after they have become attached to the *sn*-2 position of membrane phospholipids. As a consequence of the changes in the fatty acid component of membrane phospholipids, two interrelated phenomena may occur, namely alteration in membrane fluidity and alteration in the products which arise from the hydrolysis of membrane phospholipids.

Changes in fluidity may alter the binding of cytokines and cytokine-inducing agonists to receptors. They may also alter components of the signal-transduction process, which leads to alterations in cytokine production and effects.

Changes in membrane fluidity

In theory, a decrease in membrane fluidity would be expected to increase the intensity of the immune/inflammatory response, since in a more rigid membrane, cytokines might be able to make contact and bind with greater affinity to their receptors due to a slower velocity of the receptors within the membrane. Inclusion of cholesterol in the diets of rabbits, which might be expected to reduce membrane fluidity, enhanced IL-1 and TNF expression in aorta. However, both ethanol, which increases fluidity, and sterols, which decrease fluidity, have been shown to inhibit IL-2 production.

When both lateral and rotational fluidity were measured in membranes from peritoneal macrophages and hepatocytes from rats fed a wide range of fats, it was found that in general fluidity assessed by either method is influenced in a similar manner in membranes from both types of cell. There was, however, no consistent relationship between membrane fluidity and the intensity of inflammation. Fish and coconut oils resulted in high lateral fluidity and suppressed proinflammatory cytokine production and responsiveness of tissues to inflammatory agents. However, butter and maize oil resulted in low lateral fluidities but had opposing effects on these parameters of inflammation. Thus, the precise nature and significance of alterations in membrane fluidity induced by fat on cytokine-producing and cytokine-sensitive cells requires further investigation.

Implications of experimental observations on lipids and inflammation for inflammatory disease in human populations

With the major decline in infectious disease in populations in industrialised countries, attention has been focused on other diseases in which inflammation plays a part, such as atherosclerosis, rheumatoid arthritis, asthma, inflammatory bowel diseases, and the end stages of heart, lung, kidney, and liver disease.

In many industrialised countries, such as the UK, the USA, and Australia, large increases in the intake of *n*-6 PUFAs have occurred in the last 30 years. In the UK, the dietary polyunsaturated to saturated fatty acid ratio doubled between 1972 and 1988. The intake of *n*-6 PUFAs has risen from 4% of dietary energy in the early 1970s to 6% at present. It has been suggested that the upsurge of asthma that has been observed in the UK, Australia, and New Zealand is related to these increases in PUFA intake. For example, the incidence of asthma is lower in Scotland and the more industrialised north of England than in the south of England. Intakes of *n*-6 PUFAs are highest in the south of England. Likewise, the incidence of asthma is lower in the eastern part of Germany (where intakes of *n*-6 PUFA are lower and atmospheric pollution is higher) than in the western parts of the country (where larger quantities of *n*-6 PUFA are consumed).

In southern Finland, the incidence of asthma in rural children is over three times higher than in children from the more industrialised east of the country. The levels of *n*-6 PUFAs in plasma cholesterol esters are significantly greater in the former region, thus confirming a higher intake of *n*-6 PUFAs. In Japan, where a steady increase in fat intake from 16 to 24% of dietary energy, and a change in the relative amount of *n*-6 to *n*-3 PUFAS in the diet, has occurred as a result of 'Westernisation of the diet' between 1966 and 1985, major rises in the incidence of Crohn's disease have been observed. An epidemiological study reported that an increase in *n*-6/*n*-3 PUFA ratio from 3.3 to 3.8 was associated with a doubling in the number of newly diagnosed cases of the disease. The unexplained increase in the incidence of eczema and allergic rhinitis, and regional differences in inflammatory disease within countries, may relate to *n*-6 PUFA intake.

While the impact of changes in dietary fat intake on the incidence of inflammatory disease in populations has played little part in the recommendations of governmental committees, recommendations from a Committee on Medical Aspects of Food Policy (COMA) report (1994), although targeted at coronary heart disease, may have a beneficial influence on the burden of inflammatory disease in the population. The document recommends that 'no further increase in the average intakes of *n*-6 PUFAs occur' and that 'the proportion of the population consuming in excess of about 10% of energy (as *n*-6 PUFAs) should not increase'. For *n*-3 PUFAs, it is recommended that 'the population average consumption of long chain *n*-3 PUFAs [should increase] from 0.1 g/d to about 0.2 g/d'.

The incidence of atherosclerotic heart disease is reduced by about 30% in individuals consuming two fish meals per week, which provides about 0.5 g EPA + DHA/day, reflecting these modest intakes. In the USA, this level of intake is recommended by the American Heart Association (AHA) for all adults, and a level of 1 g EPA + DHA/day is recommended for those with heart disease. However, achieving the dramatic effects in altering disease outcomes in the studies previously quoted generally takes at least 1 g of *n*-3 PUFA intake daily. This amount would be present in approximately 3 g of cold-water fish oil, in four meals per week of fatty cold-water fish, or in an appropriate number of fish oil capsules.

Possible role of conjugated linoleic acid as an anti-inflammatory and immunoenhancing agent

Conjugated linoleic acid (CLA) appears particularly in milk fat as a result of the hydrogenisation of linoleic acid by bacteria in the rumen, resulting in the formation of a number of isomers. CLA enters the bloodstream and is extracted by the mammary gland and incorporated into milk fat. The amount of CLA varies according to the diet of the milk-producing animal. A number of animal-feeding studies have shown that CLA has widespread effects upon the actions of the immune system. CLA increases phagocytosis of rat and chicken lymphocytes, increases IL-2 production by lymphocytes from mice, and suppresses TNF and IL-6 production from rat macrophages. The effect on IL-2 may indicate that CLA could be used as an immunoenhancing agent in patients. The effect on TNF and IL-6 may indicate that it could be used in patients to suppress inflammation. Research still remains to be done in this area.

17.9 Route and content of nutritional provision and immune function and patient outcome

The massive wasting of lean tissue and immunosuppression which can follow trauma and sepsis continues to be a matter of concern in those caring for hospitalised patients. Individuals with these characteristics have an increased risk of serious infection and mortality. It is generally thought that a normally nourished individual can manifest an optimal systemic inflammatory response of moderate severity for 7–10 days, with accompanying semi-starvation. Beyond this period, and earlier in those with pre-existing malnutrition, exogenous nutritional support to meet energy, protein, and other essential nutrient needs is necessary in avoiding the consequences of developing malnutrition.

The pioneering work of Dudrick, Rhoads, and co-workers in the USA in the late 1960s and early 1970s showed that these outcomes could be influenced by intravenous administration of nutrients through the process of parenteral nutrition. Although enteral nutrition is preferred over parenteral nutrition due to the greater complication rates of the latter in less-expert hands and its lower expense, available evidence suggests it is the early nature and adequacy of feeding that improves outcome, and not the route of feeding. There are many choices to be made in the administration of nutrients by the parenteral route:

- Continuous or discontinuous feeding for 10–12 hours/day, with continuous feeding used almost exclusively in the critically ill and discontinuous feeding for those in the recuperative phase or with chronic illnesses requiring home parenteral nutrition.
- Complete profiles of nutrients administered in 'all-in-one bags' or as separately infused components.
- Various lipid emulsions based on natural vegetable oils or fish oil – provided solely or as physical mixtures of these oils, or with MCTs derived from tropical vegetable oils – or on reconstructed triglycerides which chemically combine fatty acids from several of these oils.
- Pure amino acid solutions of various compositions, including essential amino acids only designed for use in renal failure but now rarely used; branched-chain amino acid-enriched solutions, designed for the more critically ill; branched-chain amino acid-enriched solutions with low aromatic amino acids, designed for those with hepatic insufficiency but now uncommonly used; and glutamine-enriched complete nutrient mixes, which may improve outcome through immune enhancement.
- Mixtures enriched with nutrients that have potential 'nutriceutical' properties, such as antioxidant mixtures and dipeptides of glutamine.

These developments have arisen from observations in experimental studies which indicate that immune function can be enhanced, or at least preserved; the rate of tissue wasting can be arrested, or at least slowed; and the number of postoperative complications can be reduced by specific nutrient provision.

Comparative risks and benefits of enteral and parenteral feeding

There is much debate over whether enteral or parenteral feeding is the more effective in feeding patients. A number of studies have suggested that enteral nutrition produces a better patient outcome in terms of lower rates of infection and shorter hospital stays. An often-cited reason for this difference in outcome is the difference in nutritional status of the gut epithelia. In animal models, atrophy of the mucosa occurs in animals fed by TPN. However, evidence for a similar phenomenon in humans is weak. Also in animals, increased bacterial translocation across the gut wall and survival in gut-associated lymph nodes has been noted. Again, evidence for a similar phenomenon in patients is lacking.

A more careful review of comparisons of parenteral versus enteral nutrition in randomised clinical trials in trauma patients reveals a serious flaw in study execution. In each study, substantially and significantly more energy was provided in the parenteral arm, and substantial hyperglycaemia was noted. Given the effect of blood glucose >220 mg/dl on the risk of nosocomial infection, it is reasonable to conclude that this was the likely reason for the differences seen. When similar amounts of energy were provided enterally and parenterally in multiple trauma or severe head injury, as well as in routine postoperative care following major abdominal surgery in malnourished patients, there was no difference in outcome. However, given the relative cost differences and the perhaps greater risk of complications with parenteral nutrition in less-skilled hands, enteral nutrition, if possible, is preferred.

There is no doubt that TPN is a life-saving therapy in patients who cannot be fed by the enteral route, but its effects on patients may be less than ideal in certain circumstances.

Adverse effects of total parenteral nutrition

In the early days of TPN, it was recognised that reticulo-endothelial cells might become engorged with fat during TPN and that this condition impaired immune function. Most of the evidence was based on animal models, with a small amount of data from studies on patients. This phenomenon requires careful consideration, since there are data from studies in patients to both support and refute it. In a prospective crossover study on 23 surgical patients in which two iso-nitrogenous TPN regimens were used (one containing soybean oil, the other lipid-free), *in vitro* IL-2 production and lymphocyte cytotoxicity were increased by inclusion of lipid in the regimen. There was no effect of lipid inclusion on patient outcome. However, a report on a prospective randomised study on the effects of the inclusion of lipid in TPN on outcome in 60 trauma patients indicates that inclusion of lipid in TPN resulted in increased length of hospitalisation (39 days vs. 27 days). Length of stay in intensive care also increased (29 days vs. 18 days), more days were spent on ventilation, and suppression of T-cell function occurred. Twice as many infections were experienced in the group receiving TPN containing lipid as in the group receiving lipid-free TPN. However, the group receiving lipid were overfed compared to those fed lipid-free TPN.

The mechanisms for the immunosuppression in this study are unclear. The immunosuppressive effects of PGE2 were not responsible, as PGE2 production by both stimulated and unstimulated peripheral blood lymphocytes was similar in the two dietary groups.

Overcoming the problems associated with total parenteral feeding

A study in nonsurgical patients with HIV infection compared the effects of long-chain triglycerides (LCTs) and a mixture of LCTs and MCTs on immune function. While the LCT infusion decreased the response of lymphocytes to PHA, the LCT/MCT mixture had no effect and resulted in a small but statistically nonsignificant rise in CD4+/CD8+ ratio. A study on bone-marrow transplant patients examined the effect of TPN containing high (25–30%) or low (6–8%) concentrations of lipid on bacteraemia and fungaemia. The incidence was almost identical in each dietary group: 54 and 55%, respectively. A review of many of these studies has suggested that it is the rate of LCT administration that is the likely cause of adverse outcomes. As long as the infusion rates are below 0.11 g/kg/hour, adverse effects are not seen. That is equivalent to 1 l of 10% fat (100 g) over 12 hours.

In many comparative studies in patients, as suggested earlier, significantly more calories were provided to the parenteral groups, which may have resulted in overfeeding, thereby increasing complication rates. Certainly, overzealous provision of nutrients by the parenteral route to critically ill patients is associated with substantial metabolic problems:

- Infusion of glucose at rates greater than 5 mg/kg/min is associated with hyperglycaemia, hyperinsulinaemia, and increased CO_2 production.
- Administration of more than 2 g lipid/kg body weight/day results in fatty deposition in liver, hepatomegaly, elevated serum transaminase concentrations, impaired phagocytosis, and neutrophil chemotaxis. In some studies, it exaggerated proinflammatory and vasoconstrictive eicosanoid production.
- Administration of more than 2 g protein/kg body weight/day results in increased ureagenesis and ammoniagenesis and does not improve net protein balance. However, when energy intake is limited, improved protein utilisation occurs if protein intake is increased towards the desirable level of 1.5 g/kg.

At least one of the complications, hyperglycaemia, increases the risk of nosocomial infections and has recently been closely linked to increased mortality in critically ill patients. Hyperglycaemia is common in critical illness, but its incidence is greatly increased during feeding, with a greater impact of parenteral feeding. This increase with both types of feeding results from the failure of exogenous carbohydrate to reduce glucose production by the liver or to foster glucose uptake by skeletal muscle due to insulin resistance. Following severe injury or inflammation, glucose production is increased from a normal postabsorptive rate of 2 mg/kg/min or about 200 g glucose/24 hours by about 50% to 300 g/24 hours. Unlike in nonstressed man, exogenous carbohydrate does not slow gluconeogenesis at all in critical illness, so that exogenous glucose totalling up to as much as 400 g/24 hours is added to the endogenous glucose production to present a very high rate of glucose appearance. Coupled with insulin resistance to glucose uptake by skeletal muscle, this leads to a greatly increased risk of hyperglycaemia. Although hyperglycaemia is known to be immunosuppressive, it is not certain what the root cause is for increased morbidity and mortality – that is, the hyperglycaemia itself or the hyperglycaemia as a marker for the intensity of the systemic inflammatory response – since this differential effect of hyperglycaemia is not found in patients with diabetes. However, lowering blood glucose with intensive insulin-therapy glucose to a strictly normal range of 80–110 mg/dl in surgical patients improves morbidity and mortality, whereas this level may be too low for medical patients, who fare better if their blood glucose levels are only lowered to below 150 mg/dl. Thus, intensive insulin therapy with very strict target levels for blood glucose, which was once widely employed worldwide in the critically ill, is now reserved for surgical patients, with less-intense control recommended in medical patients.

Furthermore, while it was initially thought that both parenteral and enteral feeding would only show beneficial effects if patients were malnourished when feeding started, this is now most relevant to the less-severely stressed, such as routine postoperative patients or those less-severe medical conditions such as pneumonia, inflammatory bowel disease, pancreatitis, and less-severe infections generally that can be managed on general medical and surgical wards. This is not an altogether surprising finding, since the metabolic processes which follow trauma and infection, outlined in Section 17.3, result in the release of substrate from endogenous sources to supply the immune system. In a well-fed individual, these resources would be plentiful, but this would not be the case in a malnourished subject. However, overfeeding is not helpful in this setting, and can be harmful. In the most severely ill, including those with severe sepsis, severe traumatic brain injury, major third-degree burns, multiple trauma, and those with high clinical severity scores (APACHE 2, SOFA, Injury Severity Score, etc.) generally, all requiring intensive-care unit (ICU) admission, early and adequate feeding within the first 24 hours can improve outcome. The definition of adequate is still uncertain, but it does appear that something less than the actual energy requirements is more beneficial in the most critically ill, presumably due to the greater risk of hyperglycaemia. However, protein intakes should be maintained at at least 1 g/kg and up to 1.5 g/kg if possible. Since many such patients will be adequately nourished initially, and significant malnutrition would not be expected to develop in the first week, it is hypothesised that the effect of nutrition in this setting is to reduce the intensity of the systemic inflammatory response and thereby ameliorate some of its adverse impacts. The definition of adequate feeding is not definitively known, but it probably requires at least 50% of energy needs, usually estimated at 25–30 kcal/kg, and recommended protein needs, 1.5 g protein/kg, for the critically ill: about 10–20 kcal/kg and at least 1.0 g protein/kg. However, the level of adequate feeding is still not convincingly established, and nor is the role of supplemental parenteral feeding if early and adequate feeding by these criteria is not achieved. Thus parenteral nutrition can be looked upon as an effective form of nutrition when used appropriately, but one which carries with it a higher risk of error than feeding by the enteral route.

Finally in these studies, two important variables must be considered: the presence of malnutrition and the severity of the systemic inflammatory response. Where malnutrition existed, nutritional support was more likely to be efficacious, and the sicker the patient, the more likely that nutritional benefit could be achieved. Parenteral and enteral nutrition can be about equally effective if one or both of these conditions is met.

17.10 Concluding remarks

Evidence to date strongly supports the effectiveness of parenteral or enteral nutrition in improving outcome in the malnourished and/or the seriously stressed patient. Given that nutritional repletion is not possible in the stressed patient and that overfeeding can be harmful, strong evidence is developing that modest energy intakes of 75–100% of energy expenditure and protein intakes of 1.2–1.5 g/kg will optimally support the systemic inflammatory response while limiting the risk of adverse consequences related to overfeeding. It has been shown that 1 l of 7% amino acids and 20% dextrose, providing 70 g protein and about 1000 kcal, is as effective clinically in critically ill patients for the first 10 days of hospitalisation as energy provided to meet estimated energy needs, with somewhat less risk of feeding-related complications. More recent retrospective analysis has shown that the outcome in medical patients seems best in those receiving about half of their estimated protein and energy requirements. Definitive studies of the goals of feeding, beyond the dictum not to overfeed and to provide at least 1 g protein/kg, have not been established, and these goals are likely to be different based on the type of patient – whether medical or surgical – and the severity of illness. There remains considerable room for improvement, since it is estimated that about half of critically ill patients are not fed at all for the first 48 hours in the ICU. Beyond this period, or after 2 weeks, it is likely that full feeding is more appropriate.

A second major development is the commercial availability of immune-enhancing diets containing various mixtures of *n*-3 PUFAs, arginine, glutamine, and ribonucleic acids. These enteral formulas have demonstrated efficacy in postoperative feeding of malnourished cancer patients and in the more seriously stressed trauma patients. In a meta-analysis of more than 1000 patients, the use of these diets was shown to reduce the length of stay in hospital by 2.9 days, reduce the time spent on support on a ventilator by 2.6 days, and result in a reduction in infection rates. These results are clearly encouraging. Other formulas containing fish oil and an oil containing a high gamma linolenic acid content have been shown to improve outcome in adult respiratory-distress syndrome and sepsis. Given the limited efficacy demonstrated so far by a variety of pharmacological agents in adult respiratory-distress syndrome or sepsis in the critically ill, these positive benefits of simple nutritional therapy confirm the importance of nutritional support in the critically ill.

For the future, two strategies that may bear fruit in improving the efficacy of immunonutrients are, first, to develop other active nutrients that influence patient outcome and, second, to understand the precise relationship between the genetic characteristics of patients and their responsiveness (or not) to immunonutrients.

References and further reading

Bistrian BR, McCowen KC. Nutritional and metabolic support in the adult intensive care unit: key controversies. Crit Care Med 2006; 34(5): 1525–1531.

Blackburn GL, Wollner S, Bistrian BR. Nutrition support in the intensive care unit: an evolving science. Arch Surg 2010; 145(6): 533–538.

Burke PA, Young LS, Bistrian BR. Metabolic vs nutrition support: a hypothesis. JPEN J Parenter Enteral Nutr 2010; 34: 546–548.

COMA (Committee on Medical Aspects of Food Policy). Nutritional aspects of cardiovascular disease. Report of the Cardiovascular Review Group. Rep Health Soc Subj (Lond) 1994; 46: 1–186.

Doig F, Simpson F. Parenteral vs. enteral nutrition in the critically ill patient: a meta-analysis of trials using the intention to treat principle. Intensive Care Med 2005; 31: 12–23.

Doig GS, Heighes PT, Simpson F, Sweetman EA, Davies AR. Early enteral nutrition, provided within 24 h of injury of intensive care unit admission, significantly reduces mortality in critically ill patients: a meta-analysis of randomized controlled trials. Intensive Care Med 2009; 35; 2018–2027.

Gadek JE, DeMichele SJ, Karlstad MD, Pacht ER, Donahoe M, Albertson TE, et al. Effect of enteral feeding with eicosapentaenoic acid, gamma-linolenic acid and antioxidants in patients with acute respiratory distress syndrome. Crit Care Med 1999; 27: 1409–1420.

Grimble RF. Interaction between nutrients, pro-inflammatory cytokines and inflammation. Clin Sci 1996; 91: 121–130.

Grimble RF. Effect of antioxidative vitamins on immune function with clinical applications. Int J Vitamin Nutr Res 1997; 67: 312–320.

Grimble RF. Dietary lipids and the inflammatory response. Proc Nutr Soc 1998; 57: 1–8.

Grimble RF. The true cost of in-patient obesity: impact of obesity on inflammatory stress and morbidity. Proc Nutr Soc 2010; 69: 511–517.

Paoloni-Giacobino A, Grimble R, Pichard C. Genomic interactions with disease and nutrition. Clin Nutr 2003; 22: 507–514.

Soeters PB, Grimble RF. Dangers, and benefits of the cytokine mediated response to injury and infection. Clin Nutr 2009; 28: 583–596.

18
The Heart and Blood Vessels

Kate Gatenby, Stephen Wheatcroft, and Mark Kearney

University of Leeds, UK

Key messages

- Nutrition and diet play a key role in the development of athero-sclerosis, hypertension, and heart failure.
- These diseases are currently the leading cause of death in developed countries and are set to become the most common cause of death worldwide in the next 2 decades.
- The amount and the type of dietary fat consumed in the diet play a fundamental role in the development and management of atherosclerosis.
- An increased plasma concentration of low-density lipoprotein (LDL) cholesterol is a key risk factor for the development of coronary heart disease, and reducing LDL levels, by diet or by drugs, is a fundamental goal of disease prevention.

- Lifestyle changes such as dietary modification are useful adjuncts to antihypertensive drug therapy in individuals with hypertension and, if adopted on a large scale, may reduce the incidence of coronary heart disease and stroke in the population.
- Malnutrition (cancer cachexia) can be seen in up to 30% of patients with severe chronic heart failure.
- Although the results of trials using vitamin and mineral supplements have been disappointing, achieving a high intake of beneficial micronutrients through diets rich in fruit and vegetables, such as the 'Mediterranean-style diet', may contribute to the reduced incidence of coronary heart disease.

18.1 Introduction

Diseases of the heart and blood vessels are the most common causes of death in developed countries and over the next 20 years will become the most important cause of death worldwide. The evidence that nutritional factors are central to the aetiology of cardiovascular disorders such as atherosclerosis, hypertension, and cardiac failure is compelling. Diet therefore plays a key role in their management.

Atherosclerosis underlies the majority of vascular disorders, as illustrated in Figure 18.1. Atherosclerotic diseases, and in particular coronary heart disease, form the focus of this chapter. Knowledge of the pathobiology of atherosclerosis is vital to understanding the ways in which nutrients may be implicated in its development, and the chapter begins with a review of the processes involved.

Dietary fats are the most important nutritional determinants of coronary heart disease and the evidence for the principal role of saturated fat is discussed in depth. The evolving roles of monounsaturated and polyunsaturated fatty acids are also explored. Plasma lipoproteins are thought to be integral to the link between dietary fats and vascular disease, and a summary is provided of lipoprotein types, lipoprotein metabolism, and the common dyslipidaemias. An overview of lipid-lowering drugs is accompanied by a summary of the landmark clinical trials that support the benefits of these agents.

Recent studies highlight the importance of factors other than dietary saturated fats and plasma lipids in the prevention of coronary heart disease. The roles of antioxidants, proteins, and alcohol are discussed. In particular, the evidence for a protective effect of

Clinical Nutrition, Second Edition. Edited by Marinos Elia, Olle Ljungqvist, Rebecca J Stratton and Susan A Lanham-New.
© 2013 The Nutrition Society. Published 2013 by Blackwell Publishing Ltd.

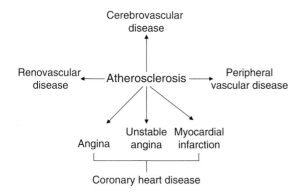

Figure 18.1 The central role of atherosclerosis in cardiovascular disorders.

a Mediterranean-style diet and a diet high in fish oils is discussed.

This chapter also summarises the role of dietary factors in the aetiology of hypertension, stroke, and peripheral vascular disease and discusses the nutritional aspects of chronic heart failure, one of the most frequent sequelae of coronary heart disease. The chapter concludes with an outline of the contribution of micronutrients to cardiovascular disorders.

18.2 Atherosclerosis

Atherosclerosis is the pathological process that underlies the majority of vascular diseases. The atherosclerotic plaque is a collection of lipid, inflammatory cells, smooth-muscle cells, and fibrous tissue within the vessel wall. Atherosclerotic plaques may lead to clinical problems by two principal mechanisms. First, bulky plaques encroach upon the vessel lumen, restricting blood flow by reducing the vessel internal diameter, and lead to ischaemia in organs and tissues supplied by that vessel. Second, plaques may rupture and stimulate localised platelet aggregation and clot formation, which cause symptoms either by embolising and occluding smaller vessels downstream or by occluding the vessel at the site of the plaque and causing ischaemia or infarction of the target organ.

The arterial wall consists of three layers: the intima, media, and adventitia (see Figure 18.2). Atherosclerosis is primarily a disease of the innermost layer, the intima, which comprises smooth-muscle cells

lined by a single layer of endothelial cells. The endothelium provides a barrier between the constituents of circulating blood and the remainder of the vessel wall. The importance of the endothelium, however, far exceeds its role as a physical barrier. Endothelial cells maintain vascular homeostasis by secreting a number of locally acting substances, which exert effects on neighbouring cells in the vessel wall and cells within the vessel lumen. Endothelial production of substances such as nitric oxide, which promote vasodilatation and inhibit platelet aggregation, is of vital importance in maintaining vessel health.

The presence of coronary-heart-disease risk factors leads to the loss of the protective actions of the endothelium, triggering the development of atherosclerosis. One of the earliest events in this process is the adhesion of circulating leukocytes (monocytes) to dysfunctional/damaged endothelium. This process is facilitated by the expression of binding proteins known as adhesion molecules on the surface of dysfunctional endothelial cells. Once bound, adherent monocytes migrate into the intima and transform into macrophages, and are joined by other leukocytes, such as T lymphocytes, in mediating a complex inflammatory response. The macrophages within the intima avidly take up lipid and change into lipid-laden foam cells, giving rise to a lesion known as the fatty streak. Fatty streaks are the earliest visible manifestation of atherosclerosis and are detectable in the aorta and coronary arteries in humans from a very young age.

Inflammatory cells within fatty streaks secrete cytokines and growth factors, whcih fuel the gradual progression of the fatty streak to a mature atherosclerotic plaque. Platelets adhering to adjacent endothelium provide another source of cytokines and growth factors. Smooth-muscle cells migrate from the media to the intima in response to growth factors and form the bulk of the plaque. Macrophages continue to accumulate lipid, principally in the form of cholesterol esters. The cholesterol is taken up into the vessel wall from the circulation, where it is carried by specialised proteins known as lipoproteins.

Low-density lipoprotein (LDL) is the most atherogenic circulating lipoprotein. This is most avidly taken up by macrophages in the plaque after it has been oxidised. LDL oxidation, therefore, is a crucial step in atherosclerosis, and increased 'oxidant

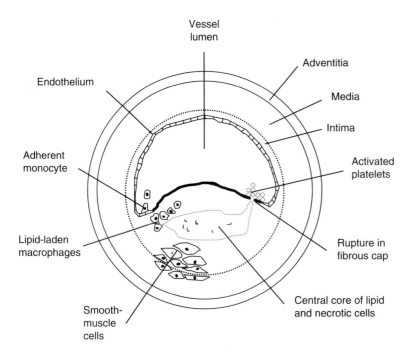

Figure 18.2 The atherosclerotic plaque.

stress' in the vascular wall is a feature of many pro-atherosclerotic states (such as diabetes mellitus, smoking, and hypertension).

A mature atherosclerotic plaque consists of a connective tissue cap, smooth-muscle cells, macrophages, and other inflammatory cells, and a central core of lipid-rich, necrotic debris (see Figure 18.2).

Two main types of plaque are described. 'Stable' plaques have a thick (often calcified) fibrous cap, which has a low propensity to rupture, and they form a chronic obstruction to blood flow. 'Unstable' plaques have a thin, friable cap, which is prone to rupture, exposing the potent thrombogenic lipid core to blood within the vascular lumen. When these plaques rupture, platelet aggregation and subsequent initiation of the clotting cascade leads to thrombus formation. Unstable plaques are typically less bulky and encroach less upon the vessel lumen than stable plaques, and they may be asymptomatic until plaque rupture occurs. Following rupture, however, thrombus may completely occlude the vessel and lead to infarction in the territory supplied by that vessel.

Figure 18.3 illustrates the way in which nutritional factors may interact with the multiple biological processes involved in the development of atherosclerosis.

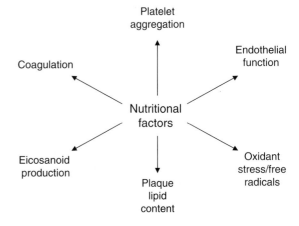

Figure 18.3 The role of nutritional factors in atherosclerosis.

18.3 Dietary lipids and coronary heart disease

There is compelling evidence that dietary lipids play a fundamental role in the development of atherosclerosis. These data have accrued over many years from a combination of epidemiological studies revealing an association between dietary fat consumption and the incidence of coronary heart

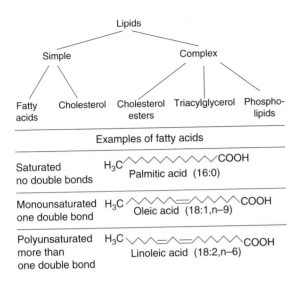

Figure 18.4 Types of lipid.

Table 18.1 Food sources of types of dietary fat.

Type of fat	Food source
Saturated fats	Dairy products
	Beef
	Lamb
	Poultry
	Pork
Monounsaturated fats	Olive oil
	Canola oil
Polyunsaturated fats	Margarines
	Vegetable oils (corn, sunflower, safflower, soy)
	Fatty fish and fish oils
Cholesterol	Egg yolks
	Meats
	Dairy products

disease, experimental studies showing that feeding lipids to animals causes atherosclerosis, and studies in which changing lipid consumption in humans reduces the risk of disease.

Before these are discussed, it is necessary to review the principal types of dietary fat and how they are classified.

Types of dietary lipid

Lipids are hydrocarbon-based organic molecules that are insoluble in water. Figure 18.4 illustrates the way in which lipids are classified as 'simple' or 'complex' depending on whether they are unmodi-fied or have been esterified by the addition of a molecule containing an alcohol group. Simple lipids are further divided into saturated, monounsatu-rated, and polyunsaturated forms, depending upon the number of double bonds within their structure (see Figure 18.4). Table 18.1 shows the main dietary sources of these fats.

Biochemically, fatty acids are described by a numerical code, which defines the following:

- the number of carbon atoms within the molecule;
- the number of double bonds;
- the position of the first double bond, as counted from the terminal carbon atom.

For example, oleic acid is described as $(18:1,n-9)$ because it contains 18 carbon atoms and 1 double

bond, with the double bond situated 9 carbon atoms from the terminal end.

The link between saturated fat consumption and coronary heart disease

Epidemiology

Cross-population studies allow the identification of factors which may predispose to coronary heart dis-ease in groups with substantially different diets and rates of coronary heart disease. The Seven Countries Study, which began in 1958, was a classic cross-population study in which the relationship between dietary composition and coronary-heart-disease mortality was assessed in more than 12 000 men (aged 40–59 years) living in Japan, Italy, Greece, the Netherlands, the former Yugoslavia, Finland, and the USA. The study demonstrated that mortality from coronary heart disease is strongly related to the mean serum cholesterol level in a population, which in turn is strongly associated with the average intake of satu-rated fat (Figure 18.5).

Comparison of coronary-heart-disease rates between populations suffers from a number of poten-tial confounding effects, including genetic differ-ences between the populations studied. This was addressed by the Ni Hon San Study, which followed migrants from Japan (Nippon) to Hawaii (Honolulu) and California (San Francisco). Japanese migrants living in Honolulu and San Francisco consumed sig-nificantly greater proportions of total fat in the diet, and had higher mean total cholesterol levels, than

(a)

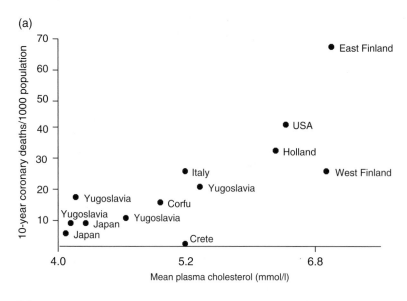

(b)

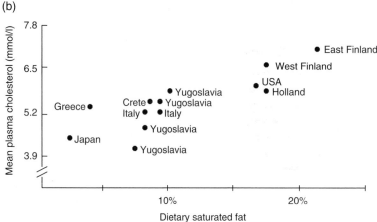

Figure 18.5 The Seven Countries Study. From Keys (1980). Copyright © 1980 Harvard University Press.

Japanese natives. This was associated with a significant increase in coronary-heart-disease mortality rates in the migrants (Figure 18.6).

Further studies performed within populations are consistent with cross-population studies in showing a significant correlation between consumption of total lamb and saturated fat and coronary-heart-disease mortality. Within-population studies have also been instrumental in determining which individual risk factors predispose to coronary heart disease. For example, long-term follow-up of residents of Framingham, a small town in the USA, has identified several important predictors of increased coronary-heart-disease risk. These include total cholesterol, LDL cholesterol, high-density lipoprotein (HDL)

cholesterol (inversely related to coronary heart disease), hypertension, smoking, and diabetes. Framingham data have been used to construct risk-factor charts and scoring systems to predict the risk of coronary heart disease in a given individual. While caution must be employed in extrapolating data from a single population to other, potentially different populations, such tools have proved extremely useful in clinical practice.

A number of other within-population studies have strengthened the evidence of an association between plasma cholesterol levels and coronary heart disease. The Multiple Risk Factor Intervention Trial (MRFIT) is of particular relevance, as it studied over 360 000 men. The data demonstrate convincingly that there is

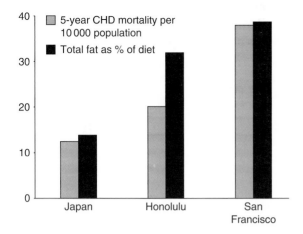

Figure 18.6 The Ni Hon San Study. Data from Kato *et al.* (1973) and Worth *et al.* (1975).

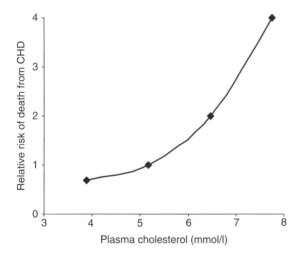

Figure 18.7 The relationship between plasma cholesterol and death from coronary heart disease (the MRFIT Study). Adapted from Martin *et al.* (1986), copyright 1986, with permission from Elsevier.

a continuous and graded relationship between serum total cholesterol and coronary-heart-disease mortality (Figure 18.7).

The British Regional Heart Study followed 7735 men chosen at random from general practices in 24 towns in England, Scotland, and Wales to assess the impact of variations in personal, economic, and social factors on coronary heart disease. Again, there was strong, graded association between total cholesterol and the risk of a major coronary event, even after adjustment for other risk factors.

Experimental evidence

Further support for the idea that dietary fats play a role in the development of atherosclerosis comes from studies in animals, which demonstrate a direct link between consumption of saturated fat, increased plasma cholesterol levels, and atherosclerosis. Feeding animals such as rabbits and non-human primates a diet high in saturated fat leads to predictable elevations of total and LDL cholesterol and subsequent development of vascular intimal lesions characteristic of human atherosclerosis. Furthermore, reduction of blood cholesterol levels by dietary modification leads to regression of established atherosclerosis in these animals.

Animal studies also show that certain fats, particularly the long-chain saturated fatty acid stearic acid, are able to induce platelet aggregation and thrombus formation. In contrast, diets rich in (*n*-3) polyunsaturated fatty acids reduce the incidence of arterial thrombosis in animals and lower the predisposition to fatal cardiac-rhythm disturbances in models of coronary artery occlusion.

The effect of reducing saturated-fat consumption on the risk of coronary heart disease

Although epidemiological and experimental studies provide persuasive evidence for a major role of saturated fat in the development of coronary heart disease, proof of its involvement requires that dietary modification, such as a reduction in the consumption of saturated fat, leads to a decrease in the incidence of coronary heart disease.

In fact, a large number of clinical trials performed over the last half century have demonstrated that diets low in saturated fat reduce the incidence of coronary events. As it is difficult in clinical trials to precisely regulate the food intake of free-living subjects in the community, many diet-intervention studies have been centred on residents living in institutions or hospitals.

In the first large-scale trial of an experimental diet, the Finnish Mental Hospital Study, over 10 000 patients in psychiatric hospitals were given a diet low in saturated fat. This led to a significant reduction in plasma cholesterol and coronary-heart-disease mortality.

The Los Angeles Veterans Administration Study randomly assigned men living in a war veterans' home to an experimental diet low in saturated fat or to a control diet. Subjects consuming the experimental diet experienced a 31% decrease in cardiovascular events.

The Oslo Trial investigated the effects of dietary and smoking advice in 1232 healthy men aged 40–49 years. These men, who were at high risk of cardiovascular disease due to a high prevalence of hypercholesterolaemia and cigarette smoking, were randomly allocated either to an intervention group, who received dietary and antismoking advice, or to a control group, who did not receive any advice. The recommended diet was low in saturated fat and high in fibre. During the course of the study, there was a 47% reduction in the incidence of myocardial infarction and sudden death in the intervention group.

Not all intervention studies of a diet in saturated fat have yielded positive results. For example, the Minnesota Coronary Survey involved feeding 9057 men and women living in psychiatric hospitals and nursing homes in Minnesota a low-saturated fat diet. Despite a reduction of 14% in mean serum cholesterol, there were no significant differences in the rates of myocardial infarction and sudden cardiac death. It is possible that the negative results reflect a low baseline cholesterol and young age of the study population.

Moreover, saturated-fat intake in this study was replaced by n-6 polyunsaturated fatty acids. It is now recognised that increasing consumption of n-6 fatty acids without increasing n-3 fatty acids may unfavourably disrupt the balance of eicosanoid production and offset the benefits of LDL reduction (see later). Such a diet is no longer recommended.

Analysis of pooled data strongly suggests that the magnitude of benefit gained by reducing saturated fat intake is strongly dependent on the replacement nutrition. For example, while replacing saturated fat with polyunsaturated fat (preferably of both n-6 and n-3 varieties, as discussed earlier) appears to correlate with a significant reduction in the risk of developing cardiovascular disease, replacing saturated fat with a carbohydrate appears to have no impact on the same end point. Whether this effect encompasses refined carbohydrates and those deemed to have a low glycaemic index is less clear. The effect of replacing saturated fat with monounsaturated fat is unclear.

The effect of saturated fats on plasma cholesterol and atherosclerosis

The principal way in which saturated fats contribute to atherosclerosis is likely to be by increasing plasma concentrations of LDL cholesterol. This is mediated, at least in part, by a decrease in LDL-cholesterol catabolism, possibly by saturated fats inducing a reduction in LDL receptor numbers or causing decreased cell-membrane fluidity. LDL is taken up from the circulation into the vessel wall, where it makes up an important part of the atherosclerotic plaque. Macrophages within the plaque become activated after acquiring oxidised LDL and secrete a number of substances, which may further promote atherosclerosis progression.

Saturated fats vary in their ability to raise plasma LDL cholesterol. Myristic and palmitic acids have been reported to possess the greatest cholesterol-raising potential, whereas stearic acid has little effect on plasma cholesterol levels (although interestingly, it may still be atherogenic).

Dietary cholesterol and coronary heart disease

Cholesterol is a component of a normal diet and is present at high levels in foods such as eggs, dairy products, and red meats. Cholesterol esters form a fundamental part of the atherosclerotic plaque and it has been known for many years that feeding animals with a diet high in cholesterol leads to atherosclerosis. Moreover, epidemiological studies reveal a strong positive relationship between the intake of dietary cholesterol and the incidence of coronary heart disease in humans. Interpretation of these data, however, is complicated by the fact that cholesterol-rich foods are often also high in saturated fats. The strong association between dietary saturated fats and coronary heart disease has been discussed. In fact, dietary cholesterol appears to be a less potent determinant of plasma cholesterol levels than are the dietary fatty acids, particularly saturated fatty acids. The effect of lowering dietary cholesterol intake independently of changes in saturated-fat consumption on coronary-heart-disease incidence has not been studied.

Nonetheless, most dietary strategies for protection from coronary heart disease recommend a reduction in intake of both saturated fat and dietary cholesterol.

It is important, however, to be aware of the distinction between a 'cholesterol-lowering' diet and a 'low-cholesterol' diet.

Dietary polyunsaturated fats and coronary heart disease

Dietary polyunsaturated fats are divided into two main families – n-6 and n-3 – according to the position of the double bond in their molecular structure. Linoleic acid (n-6) and alpha-linolenic acid (n-3) are found in plants and vegetable oils and are termed 'essential fatty acids' as they are not synthesised by humans. Once ingested, however, these essential fatty acids are biochemically processed (by desaturation and elongation) to form long-chain fatty acids (Figure 18.8). Long-chain polyunsaturated fatty acids are also contained in the diet, for example in fish oils.

Long-chain polyunsaturated fatty acids are important in the synthesis of eicosanoids: potent biologically active substances which act locally within cells and tissues to regulate processes such as vessel tone, inflammation, and platelet aggregation. n-6 and n-3 fatty acids compete for enzymes in each other's metabolic pathways, so that high levels of linoleic acid, for example, may inhibit the conversion of linolenic acid to its longer-chain forms. The relative abundance of n-6 and n-3 polyunsaturated fatty acids in the diet, therefore, may determine the relative production of

pro- and anti-atherosclerotic eicosanoids. The balance between dietary n-6 and n-3 fatty acids is also important, as the two families compete for incorporation into cell membranes. n-3 fatty acids exert beneficial effects on membrane fluidity and ion transport, and may lead to clinically relevant cardioprotective effects (see Section 18.6).

Polyunsaturated fatty acids have traditionally been used as substitutes for saturated fatty acids in low-saturated fat diets. When the potential health implications of reducing saturated-fat intake first became apparent, the food industry replaced many traditional sources of fat (such as lard and butter) with vegetable oils and margarines. These were principally derived from sunflower, safflower, and corn oils, which are high in linoleic acid. The n-6 fatty acid content of the UK diet, therefore, has risen substantially over the last 20 years, without a corresponding increase in n-3 fatty acids. Although such a pattern is effective in reducing plasma LDL cholesterol, there are concerns that a high ratio of dietary n-6 to n-3 fatty acids may not reduce cardiovascular risk where the overall intake of n-3 fats is low. The benefits of increasing the intake of n-3 fatty acids have become apparent in the light of recent clinical trials (see Section 18.6).

Foods rich in n-3 fatty acids include seed oils (e.g. linseed oil, rapeseed oil, soya oil, walnut oil), nuts (e.g. walnuts, peanuts), meat (e.g. beef), green leafy vegetables (e.g. spinach), and oily fish (e.g. tuna, salmon, mackerel, sardines, herring).

Dietary monounsaturated fats and coronary heart disease

Monounsaturated fatty acids contain one double bond in their molecular structure and are found in all animal products and vegetables. Rich dietary sources include olives, rapeseed, avocado, nuts, meat, and peanut oil. Early studies suggested that dietary monounsaturated fatty acids had a neutral effect on plasma lipoprotein levels. More recently, however, it has become apparent that monounsaturates, when substituted for dietary saturated fatty acids, lead to reductions in LDL cholesterol and triacylglycerols (TAGs) and small increases in HDL cholesterol.

Oleic acid is present in large amounts in olive oil, an important source of dietary lipid in Mediterranean countries. The long life expectancy and low risk of

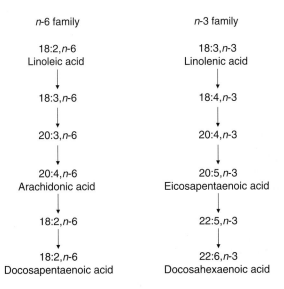

n-6 family	n-3 family
18:2,n-6 Linoleic acid	18:3,n-3 Linolenic acid
↓	↓
18:3,n-6	18:4,n-3
↓	↓
20:3,n-6	20:4,n-3
↓	↓
20:4,n-6 Arachidonic acid	20:5,n-3 Eicosapentaenoic acid
↓	↓
18:2,n-6	22:5,n-3
↓	↓
18:2,n-6 Docosapentaenoic acid	22:6,n-3 Docosahexaenoic acid

Figure 18.8 Families of polyunsaturated fatty acids.

coronary heart disease in some Mediterranean countries, such as Greece, has led to the promotion of a Mediterranean-style diet as being cardioprotective. The Mediterranean-style diet is dealt with in detail in Section 18.6.

Dietary trans-fatty acids and coronary heart disease

Fatty acids exist in two molecular configurations, known as *cis-* and *trans-*isomers. Vegetable oils largely consist of *cis-*fatty acids, in which the hydrogen groups are on the same side of the carbon chain (Figure 18.9). In contrast, *trans-*isomers contain hydrogen moieties on opposite sides of the carbon chain. *Trans-*fatty acids are present naturally at low levels in the diet, but the majority are formed artificially by the hydrogenation of vegetable oils. Hydrogenation converts liquid vegetable oils to a semi-solid state and is widely used in the manufacture of hard margarines and other processed foods. Diets high in *trans-*fatty acids do not have a beneficial effect on the lipoprotein profile and may, in fact, lead to elevation of LDL- and reduction of HDL-cholesterol levels.

There is now significant evidence that *trans-*fatty acid consumption is linked to the development of coronary heart disease. Analysis of data obtained from the Nurses' Health Study suggests that for every 2% increase in calories obtained from *trans-*fats as opposed to carbohydrates, the risk of developing coronary heart disease roughly doubles. An extrapolation of these data would suggest that *trans-*fats could account for between 30 000 and 100 000 excess deaths from coronary heart disease in the USA per annum.

As a result of this overwhelming evidence, many Western countries have set up guidelines suggesting significant restriction on the use of *trans-*fats in products. In 2003, for example, Denmark set an upper limit for artificial *trans-*fat levels of 2 g per 100 g of oil or fat, which has led to the virtual elimination of *trans-*fats in Denmark. Irrespective of guidelines placed upon them by nations, many large manufacturers and retailers have banned the use of *trans-*fats in their products.

It should be mentioned that while the evidence strongly supports a restriction on the use of artificially manufactured *trans-*fats, there is some evidence that consumption of naturally occurring *trans-*fats, such as those found in the meat of ruminant animals, may not have the same adverse effects and in fact may have a beneficial effect on lipid profile.

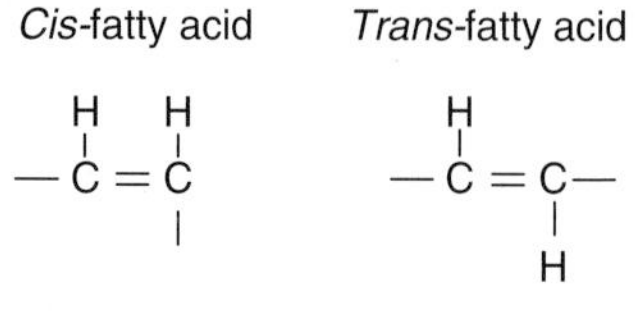

18.4 Plasma lipoproteins

An increased plasma concentration of LDL cholesterol is a key risk factor for the development of coronary heart disease, and reducing LDL levels, by diet or drugs, is a fundamental goal of disease prevention. In recent years, the importance of more subtle changes in the plasma lipid profile has emerged. Although a detailed description of plasma lipoproteins is beyond the scope of this chapter, a basic knowledge of their structure and metabolism is integral to understanding the mechanisms of cardiovascular risk reduction.

The two major lipids in plasma, cholesterol and TAG, are insoluble in an aqueous environment and therefore circulate in association with specialised proteins (apoproteins) in complexes known as lipoproteins. Lipoproteins consist of a central lipid core of cholesterol esters and TAGs, surrounded by an outer layer comprising phospholipids, free cholesterol, and apoproteins (Figure 18.10). Apoproteins play an important role in lipoprotein metabolism by interacting with cellular receptors and enzymes.

Cis-fatty acid   Trans-fatty acid

Figure 18.9 *Cis-* and *trans-*fatty acids.

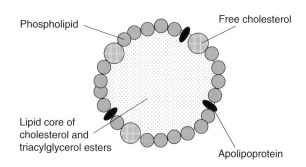

Figure 18.10 Lipoprotein structure.

Table 18.2 Composition of plasma lipoproteins. TAG, triacylglycerol; VLDL, very low-density lipoprotein; IDL, intermediate-density lipoprotein; LDL, low-density lipoprotein; HDL, high-density lipoprotein.

	Composition (%)					
	Cholesterol (free)	Cholesterol (esters)	TAG	Phospholipid	Protein	Major apolipoproteins
Chylomicrons	1	3	85	9	2	B_{48}, E, C-II
VLDL	7	13	50	20	10	B_{100}, E, C-II
IDL	12	22	26	22	18	B_{100}, E
LDL	8	37	10	20	25	B_{100}
HDL	2	15	4	24	55	A-I, A-II

Plasma lipoproteins are classified into five groups according to their density, which determines the way the lipoproteins separate when subjected to ultracentrifugation. Table 18.2 shows the ways in which lipid distribution and apoprotein composition vary between the lipoprotein classes.

- *LDL cholesterol* makes up approximately 70% of total serum cholesterol. It contains a single apoprotein, apo B. LDL is the major atherogenic lipoprotein, and delivers cholesterol to the vessel wall, where it is incorporated into atherosclerotic plaque. Oxidation of LDL significantly increases its atherogenicity.
- *HDL cholesterol* normally makes up 20–30% of the total serum cholesterol. HDL levels are inversely correlated with the risk of coronary heart disease. HDL helps to protect against atherosclerosis, mainly by carrying cholesterol away from the vessel wall to the liver, in a process known as reverse cholesterol transport.
- *Very low-density lipoproteins* (VLDLs) are TAG-rich lipoproteins, but contain 10–15% of serum cholesterol. VLDLs are produced by the liver and are precursors of LDLs. VLDLs may be degraded in the circulation to form VLDL remnants, which are rich in cholesterol and may contribute to atherosclerosis.
- *Intermediate-density lipoproteins* (IDLs) are produced by the catabolism of VLDLs. Their role in atherosclerosis is not well defined. In clinical practice, IDL is measured as part of the LDL fraction.
- *Chylomicrons* are TAG-rich lipoproteins. They are formed in the intestine from dietary fat and pass into the bloodstream. When partially degraded, chylomicrons (then known as chylomicron remnants) may carry some atherogenic potential.

18.5 Lipoprotein metabolism

The plasma lipoproteins transport fats within the circulation, which are either absorbed from the intestine or manufactured endogenously. Lipoprotein metabolism is characterised by complex interactions between lipoproteins of different classes, regulatory enzymes, and cellular receptors. These interactions may be simplified by considering three main areas: the exogenous pathway, the endogenous pathway, and reverse cholesterol transport. These are illustrated in schematic form in Figure 18.11.

Exogenous pathways

After digestion, dietary cholesterol and fatty acids are absorbed within the intestine and re-esterified to form TAGs and cholesterol esters in intestinal mucosal cells. Here they are packaged with apoproteins, phospholipids, and cholesterol to form chylomicrons. Apolipoprotein B-48, essential for chylomicron formation, is added by the action of microsomal transfer protein. Chylomicrons are secreted into intestinal lymphatics and carried by the thoracic duct into the bloodstream.

Once in the bloodstream, TAGs within chylomicrons are rapidly hydrolysed to free fatty acids and glycerol by lipoprotein lipase, an enzyme bound to vascular endothelial cells within muscle and adipose tissue. The resulting fatty acids are either delivered to muscle as fuel or re-esterified and stored as TAGs in adipose tissue. During the process of TAG hydrolysis, chylomicrons acquire cholesterol ester from other lipoproteins, such as mature HDLs, in exchange for TAGs by the action of cholesterol ester transfer protein. The particles become progressively depleted in TAGs and enriched in cholesterol esters, and acquire

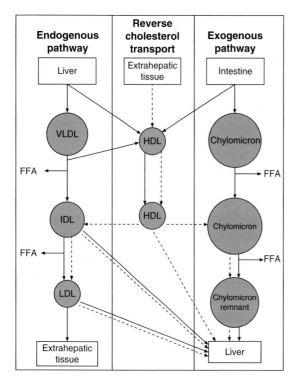

Figure 18.11 Overview of lipoprotein metabolism. VLDL, very low-density lipoprotein; IDL, intermediate-density lipoprotein; LDL, low-density lipoprotein; HDL, high-density lipoprotein; FFA, free fatty acids.

apoprotein E from HDL to become chylomicron remnants. These remnants are rapidly cleared from the circulation by the liver, after binding to hepatocyte receptors which recognise apoprotein E.

Endogenous pathway

Cholesterol and TAGs are synthesised by the liver and secreted in VLDL particles for transport to peripheral tissues. Cholesterol is manufactured by a complex synthetic pathway using acetyl conenzyme A (CoA) derived from fatty acid oxidation and carbohydrate metabolism. The rate of cholesterol synthesis is determined by the enzyme hydroxymethyl glutaryl (HMG) CoA reductase. Hepatic TAGs are produced from fatty acids originating in adipose tissue or by lipogenesis from carbohydrates. Newly synthesised TAGs combine with those acquired by chylomicron remnant uptake to be secreted in VLDL. VLDL particles, like chylomicrons, are formed by the packaging together of TAGs, cholesterol esters, cholesterol, phospholipids, and apolipoproteins. Apolipoprotein B-100, the major apolipoprotein of VLDL, is added by microsomal transfer protein.

After release into the bloodstream, TAGs in VLDL are rapidly hydrolysed by lipoprotein lipase to release free fatty acids. During this process, VLDL particles exchange lipids with HDL to form cholesterol-rich IDL particles. IDL particles are either taken up by LDL receptors on the liver, or further metabolised by hepatic lipase to form LDL.

LDL constitutes the major cholesterol-carrying lipoprotein, serving to deliver cholesterol to peripheral cells and remaining in the circulation for 2–3 days. LDL is taken up from the circulation by the interaction of its B-100 apolipoprotein with cell-surface LDL receptors. Around 75% of LDL is cleared by the liver and 25% by peripheral tissues. Receptor-mediated LDL uptake is of crucial importance in regulating plasma cholesterol concentrations. After binding, the receptor/LDL complex is delivered to the cytoplasm, where cholesterol esters are hydrolysed to form free cholesterol. The LDL receptor recycles to the cell membrane, whereas the increased intracellular cholesterol concentration maintains cholesterol homeostasis by a number of mechanisms. HMG CoA reductase is inhibited, reducing *de novo* cholesterol synthesis; the enzyme acyl CoA:cholesterol acyl transferase is activated, promoting re-esterification of cholesterol to cholesterol esters; and, in addition, LDL receptor expression is downregulated.

Reverse cholesterol transport

Cholesterol surplus to cellular requirements is returned from peripheral tissues to the liver by HDL in a process called reverse cholesterol transport. HDL particles are the smallest of the lipoproteins and are synthesised in the liver and intestine as bilayer discs containing apoprotein A and phospholipids. Newly formed HDL avidly takes up cholesterol from cell membranes and other lipoproteins to become a cholesterol-rich spherical particle. Free cholesterol within HDL particles is rapidly esterified to cholesterol esters by the enzyme lecithin cholesterol acyl transferase, which circulates along with HDL. Mature HDL particles are heterogeneous and interact with lipoproteins of other classes. In doing so, cholesterol esters within HDL particles are transferred to

Box 18.1 Secondary causes of dyslipidaemia

- diabetes;
- insulin-resistance syndrome;
- hypothyroidism;
- obesity;
- alcohol excess;
- renal failure;
- liver disease;
- gout;
- eating disorders (anorexia nervosa and bulimia nervosa);
- pregnancy;
- drugs (cyclosporin, antiretroviral drugs for HIV, anticonvulsant drugs, etc.).

particles such as IDLs and chylomicrons, in exchange for TAGs, by cholesterol ester transfer protein.

A minority of cholesterol-rich HDL is taken up directly by the liver. The majority of cholesterol within HDL particles, however, returns to the liver indirectly after transfer to lipoproteins of lower density.

Types of dyslipidaemia

Abnormalities of the plasma lipid profile may arise as a primary defect or may occur secondary to an underlying condition or drug therapy. Primary dyslipidaemias include both rare inherited lipid disorders, often arising as a consequence of single gene mutations, and the common type of dyslipidaemia, frequently seen in clinical practice, which has a polygenetic background.

Secondary causes of dyslipidaemia are summarised in Box 18.1.

Lipid-modifying drugs and coronary heart disease

Coronary-heart-disease prevention has been revolutionised in recent years with the widespread availability of safe, effective drugs that modify the lipid profile. Large, well-designed studies have conclusively shown that the addition of lipid-modifying drugs to diets low in saturated fat leads to substantial reductions in coronary-heart-disease events and mortality.

The main classes of lipid-modifying drugs, and their effects on plasma lipoproteins, are summarised in Table 18.3.

Table 18.3 Lipid-modifying drugs and their effects on plasma lipids. LDL, low-density lipoprotein; HDL, high-density lipoprotein; TAG, triacylglycerol.

	LDL cholesterol	HDL cholesterol	TAG
Resins	↓↓	↑	↑↓
Nicotinic acid	↓	↑	↓↓
Fibrates	↓	↑↑	↓↓
Statins	↓↓	↑	↓
Ezetimibe	↓↓	↑↓	↓

Resins

Resins (such as cholestyramine) bind bile acids in the intestine and prevent their reabsorption. An increased amount of cholesterol is therefore diverted to bile-acid synthesis in the liver, and hepatic LDL receptors are upregulated, thus lowering plasma LDL. There is limited evidence from clinical trials of a reduced incidence of coronary-heart-disease events with cholestyramine.

Resins, which are administered as powders, are not generally used in the prevention of coronary heart disease, due to the inconvenience of administration and gastrointestinal side effects.

Nicotinic acid derivatives

Nicotinic acid (niacin) is a vitamin which at high doses causes reductions in LDL and TAGs. It is particularly effective in hypertriglyceridaemia, where large falls in TAG levels are accompanied by elevations of HDL. Nicotinic acid reduces the flux of fatty acids from adipose tissue to liver. This action inhibits hepatic output of VLDL and reduces hepatic TAG synthesis. The use of nicotinic acid is limited due to side effects such as flushing, pruritus, nausea, and glucose intolerance. These are less troublesome with the nicotinic acid derivative acipimox, though this compound is far less potent. There are currently no robust data to suggest that adding niacin to a statin as combination therapy improves cardiovascular outcome, but trials are ongoing to assess this further.

Fibrates

The fibrates (or fibric acid derivatives) have complex actions, including an enhanced clearance of TAGs from the circulation by stimulation of lipoprotein lipase. Their main effect is to reduce TAG levels, although consistent increases in HDL and variable reductions in LDL are also clinically relevant. They are first-line drugs for the treatment of hypertriglyc-eridaemia. Their role in the prevention of coronary heart disease had been eclipsed by the statins, although there has been recent interest in their potential to increase HDL.

Early trials of fibrates (using clofibrate) were complicated by drug-induced gallstone formation and an unexplained increase in non-cardiac deaths. In a secondary prevention trial, bezafibrate failed to reduce coronary events, although there was a significant reduction in events in patients with high TAG levels.

Two recent studies using gemfibrozil produced more encouraging results. In the Helsinki Heart Study (HHS), a major primary-prevention trial, 4082 men were randomised to a lipid-lowering diet alone or diet plus gemfibrozil. After 5 years' follow-up there was a 35% reduction in the primary end point of combined nonfatal and fatal myocardial infarction in the gemfibrozil group.

The potentially beneficial effect of using fibrates to raise HDL was explored in the Veterans Affairs High-Density Lipoprotein Intervention Trial (VA-HIT). In this secondary-prevention trial, subjects with low HDL levels were randomised to receive gemfibrozil or placebo. After 5 years there was a significant 22% reduction in the combined end point of nonfatal myocardial infarction and death from coronary heart disease in the fibrate-treated group. Statistical analysis suggested that the majority of the beneficial effect was mediated by an increase in HDL.

In current clinical practice, the focus with respect to lipids and the prevention of coronary heart disease is on achieving target levels of total cholesterol or LDL by the use of diet and statin drugs. With increasing recognition of HDL as an important cardiovascular risk factor, however, fibrates and other interventions designed to increase HDL are likely to receive greater prominence in future.

Statins

The statins are potent, specific inhibitors of the enzyme HMG CoA reductase, which catalyses the rate-determining state in hepatic cholesterol synthesis. By inhibiting cholesterol synthesis, statins increase hepatic LDL-receptor activity and increase the uptake of LDL with a consequent reduction in plasma LDL levels. Statins also lead to a small increase in HDL and modest reduction in TAGs. They are first-line treatment for familial hypercholesterolaemia but are mostly used as an adjunct to diet in the prevention of coronary heart disease. Their widespread use in this capacity follows the demonstration of their efficacy and excellent safety record in a series of large, well-designed, randomised controlled clinical trials.

In the primary-prevention setting, significant reductions in coronary events were observed in the West of Scotland Coronary Prevention Study (WOSCOPS). This showed that a combination of dietary advice and statin therapy in a high-risk population with moderately elevated cholesterol levels reduced the risk of fatal and nonfatal myocardial infarction, cardiovascular mortality, and total mortality.

In another primary-prevention trial, the Air Force/Texas Coronary Atherosclerosis Prevention Study (AFCAPS/TexCAPS), the population studied was at much lower baseline risk, with average LDL levels but low HDL. Even in this group, diet and statins significantly reduced the incidence of first major coronary events.

Extrapolation of AFCAPS/TexCAPS findings to the general population suggests that large numbers of people might benefit from statin therapy. The widespread adoption of such a policy, however, has huge cost implications and is unlikely to be financially tenable. Current primary-prevention strategies, therefore, take into account other risk factors, such as age, sex, smoking status, hypertension, and diabetes, and recommend statin therapy only if the calculated risk exceeds a threshold level. This is in accordance with the conclusions drawn in the latest Cochrane Collaboration review of the use of statins for the primary prevention of cardiovascular disease (Taylor et al., 2011a).

The important role of statins in the secondary prevention of coronary heart disease is now established unequivocally. Three large randomised trials have revealed significant reductions in coronary events with the combination of diet and statins in patients with established coronary heart disease.

The Scandinavian Simvastatin Survival Study (4S) showed a 44% reduction in major coronary events and a 30% reduction in total mortality with diet and statin treatment in high-risk patients with prior myocardial infarction or angina and elevated cholesterol levels.

The Cholesterol and Recurrent Events (CARE) study went on to assess whether lowering plasma cholesterol reduces the risk of recurrent coronary events in patients with average baseline cholesterol levels. Treatment with dietary measures and pravastatin in survivors of myocardial infarction with LDL levels of 3–4.5 mmol/l reduced the primary end point of fatal coronary events and nonfatal myocardial infarction by 24%. The subjects in the CARE study were typical of the majority of survivors of myocardial infarction.

The Long-term Intervention with Pravastatin in Ischemic Disease (LIPID) study also enrolled patients with a broad range of cholesterol levels (4.0–7.0 mmol/l), but, in contrast to CARE, both unstable angina and myocardial infarction were included as entry criteria. Diet and statin treatment in the LIPID study led to a significant 24% reduction in mortality from coronary heart disease and reduced all-cause mortality by 22%.

The Heart Protection Study enrolled over 20 000 men and women who were at increased risk due to established cardiovascular disease, peripheral vascular disease, diabetes, or hypertension. Regardless of plasma cholesterol levels, dietary advice and statin treatment reduced the risk of death from coronary heart disease by 18%.

Given the impressive reductions in coronary event rates in these landmark trials, there is a strong argument for recommending a combination of dietary modification and a statin in virtually all patients at increased risk of coronary heart disease, regardless of their plasma cholesterol levels.

Although a reduction in LDL cholesterol is integral to the cardioprotection mediated by statins, it is likely that other properties also contribute to their beneficial effects. These include inhibition of smooth-muscle proliferation and platelet aggregation, enhancement of endothelial function, and anti-inflammatory effects.

Ezetimibe

Ezetimibe lowers cholesterol by inhibiting the absorption of dietary cholesterol from the gastrointestinal tract. There is good evidence that the use of ezetimibe leads to a reduction in the level of LDL cholesterol and exerts a favourable effect on triaglycerol levels. It also causes a very modest increase in HDL cholesterol. Despite the undoubtedly advantageous effects on lipid profile, there are currently no outcome data to show that ezetimibe montherapy reduces the risk

of developing cardiovascular disease. It does, however, currently have a role in the treatment of dyslipidaemia when used as part of combination therapy, or in cases where stains cannot be tolerated.

Summary of the evidence supporting a positive relationship between dietary saturated fats, plasma cholesterol levels, and coronary heart disease

Epidemiological studies reveal a strong association between intake of saturated fat, plasma cholesterol levels, and incidence of coronary heart disease.

Experimental studies in animals and in humans show that consumption of saturated fats leads to increased plasma cholesterol levels and promotes the development of atherosclerosis.

Clinical trials show that lowering cholesterol levels through a diet low in saturated fat and/or through use of drugs leads to a reduction in the incidence of coronary events.

Other lipid risk factors and coronary heart disease

High-density lipoprotein

It has been recognised for many years that HDL cholesterol is inversely associated with the risk of coronary heart disease. The Framingham Heart Study, for example, convincingly showed that HDL is inversely related to coronary-heart-disease incidence in men and women – an effect that is independent of LDL. The Prospective Cardiovascular Münster (PROCAM) study, which recorded major coronary events in almost 20 000 individuals aged 16–65 years, found that after 8 years of follow-up the incidence of major coronary events was significantly higher in individuals with an HDL < 0.9 mmol/l than in those with HDL > 0.9 mmol/l.

The magnitude of protection predicted by HDL levels is substantial. Analysis of pooled data from four large prospective studies shows that for every 0.3 mmol/l increase in HDL, the predicted incidence of coronary events decreases by 20% in men and 30% in women.

HDL protects against atherosclerosis by carrying out reverse cholesterol transport and, perhaps, by delivering endogenous antioxidant enzymes, such as paroxonase, to the vessel wall.

Low HDL levels are associated with type 2 diabetes, obesity, cigarette smoking, and lack of regular exercise. Weight loss may increase HDL levels, as there is a linear inverse relationship between body mass index (BMI) and HDL. This should be achieved by a combination of reduced energy diet and increased physical exertion, as exercise increases HDL in its own right. Smoking cessation also increases HDL by a modest amount.

The role of drugs such as fibrates and statins has been discussed.

HDL may be increased by:

- weight loss;
- increase in physical activity;
- smoking cessation;
- fibrates.

Triacylglycerols

Many, though not all, prospective epidemiological studies have reported a positive relationship between serum TAG levels and the incidence of coronary heart disease. Early multivariate analyses, however, failed to identify TAG as an independent risk factor, probably because of the close interrelationship between TAG and other lipid risk factors.

Large studies have helped to clarify matters and have established TAG levels as an independent risk factor for coronary heart disease. For example, multivariate analysis after 8 years' follow-up in the PROCAM study, discussed above, demonstrated that TAGs are an independent risk factor for major coronary events, even after adjustment for LDL, HDL, and other classical cardiovascular risk factors.

Furthermore, recent meta-analyses of this and other studies have confirmed that TAGs are an independent risk and that each 1 mmol/l increase in serum TAG levels increases the relative risk of cardiovascular disease by 14% in men and 37% in women.

It remains unclear whether the observed association between TAGs and coronary heart disease represents a direct atherogenic effect of TAGs themselves or an indirect effect mediated by changes in other lipoproteins.

Four potential ways in which TAGs might promote atherosclerosis are:

(1) Reduction in HDL levels.
(2) Formation of atherogenic chylomicron remnants.

> **Box 18.2 Causes of elevated TAGs**
>
> - obesity;
> - alcohol excess;
> - physical inactivity;
> - very high-carbohydrate diets;
> - diabetes;
> - renal failure;
> - nephrotic syndrome;
> - bulimia;
> - pregnancy;
> - drugs (thiazide diuretics, oestrogens, beta blockers, corticosteroids, protease inhibitors for HIV);
> - genetics.

(3) Formation of small, dense LDLs – a highly atherogenic form of the LDL fraction, which is associated with a significant increase in coronary-heart-disease risk.
(4) Predisposition to thrombosis by interaction with coagulation factors.

There is increasing recognition that subtle abnormalities of postprandial TAG metabolism may be equally as important as fasting TAG levels in predicting cardiovascular risk. Prolonged exposure to TAGs after a meal results from overproduction of TAG-rich lipoproteins by the intestine and the liver, or from a decrease in their clearance. Even in patients without overt fasting hypertriglyceridaemia, an abnormal postprandial response to a fat challenge predicts an increased incidence of coronary heart disease.

The causes of elevated TAG levels are summarised in Box 18.2.

Elevated TAG levels may be lowered by a combination of lifestyle changes and drug treatment. Weight reduction, physical exercise, and smoking cessation favourably modify multiple risk factors, including TAGs. Lipid-modifying drugs have been discussed.

18.6 Other dietary factors and coronary heart disease

Antioxidants

Oxidative stress is thought to play an important role in the development of atherosclerosis. Endogenous oxidising agents and free radicals within the vessel wall have multiple adverse actions, including increasing the atherogenicity of LDL, impairing endothelial

Box 18.3 Dietary antioxidants

Vitamins

- vitamin E;
- vitamin C;
- beta-carotene.

Trace elements

- zinc;
- copper;
- manganese;
- selenium.

Others

- *flavanoids* (fruit, berries, tea, wine);
- isoflavones (soybean);
- phenolic compounds (olive oil).

function, and promoting inflammation, smooth-muscle cell proliferation, plaque rupture, and thrombosis. The diet, however, contains many antioxidant compounds, which, once ingested and transported to the vessel wall, may offset these harmful effects. Common antioxidants present in the diet are listed in Box 18.3.

Observational, case-control, and cohort studies show that high antioxidant intake is associated with reduced risk of coronary heart disease. The most convincing evidence is for a protective effect of vitamin E, which, as it is lipid-soluble, is readily able to reduce the oxidation of LDL.

Despite the convincing evidence of a protective effect of antioxidants in epidemiological studies, the results of randomised controlled trials of antioxidant supplements have been disappointing. Several large primary- and secondary-prevention studies have assessed the potential of antioxidants, including vitamin E, vitamin C, and beta-carotene, alone and in combination, to reduce the rates of coronary events. Despite long follow-up periods, antioxidant supplementation failed to effectively reduce the risk of coronary-heart-disease events or mortality in these studies.

The reasons for the lack of success are unknown, but questions have been raised about the methodology of these studies and the types, combinations, and doses of antioxidant supplements used. It has also been suggested that because atherosclerosis develops slowly and the vessel wall is exposed to oxidant stress for many years, antioxidant treatment may need to be started at a very young age to be effective.

There is insufficient evidence at present to recommend the use of antioxidant supplements in the prevention of coronary heart disease. However, consumption of a diet rich in fruit and vegetables (and hence natural antioxidants) is supported by epidemiological data and should be encouraged.

Fibre

Prospective observational studies show an inverse association between the intake of fibre from fruits, vegetables, and cereals and the risk of coronary heart disease. The mechanism appears to be a modest cholesterol-lowering effect of soluble fibres such as pectin, psyllium, and guar gum, attributed to their ability to bind bile acids within the gut. High-fibre diets may also reduce insulin levels and improve insulin-sensitivity and blood-clotting parameters.

There is a lack of clinical trials supporting the benefits of fibre in coronary-heart-disease prevention. Nonetheless, the consumption of fibre is certainly safe and may help to replace high-fat, high-cholesterol foods in the diet.

Soy protein

Data from early animal studies suggest that diets rich in proteins of vegetable origin, such as soy, are less atherogenic than those rich in proteins of animal origin. Replacement of animal protein with soy protein in humans leads to a modest reduction in LDL cholesterol and TAGs, particularly in subjects with high baseline cholesterol levels. Proposed mechanisms for the cholesterol-lowering properties of soy include enhanced bile-acid excretion, increased LDL-receptor activity, potential oestrogen-like effects of soy-based isoflavones, and modulation of other hormones affecting cholesterol metabolism. The role of soy protein in the prevention of coronary heart disease has not been assessed in a randomised trial.

Alcohol

Epidemiological studies show an inverse association between morbidity and mortality from coronary heart disease and the moderate consumption of alcohol. Potential mechanisms mediating the cardioprotective effects of alcohol include an increase in HDL cholesterol and inhibition of platelet aggregation. In addition, red wine contains antioxidant polyphenols, such as catechin, quercetin, and resveratrol. It has been suggested that red wine may offer greater protection that the consumption of other types of alcohol, but the data are conflicting. Moreover, cardioprotective actions of alcohol require the consumption of modest amounts several days per week. This pattern is typical of the consumption of wine with meals in Mediterranean countries.

Higher levels of alcohol consumption and binge drinking are associated with increased mortality. In terms of coronary-heart-disease prevention, it is reasonable to recommend moderate drinking to those who already consume alcohol. The evidence does not, however, justify the recommendation of alcohol intake to a nondrinker for its cardioprotective effect.

Plant sterols and stanols

Plant sterols and stanols are incorporated into foods as 'functional foods' which lower plasma cholesterol levels. They are members of the phytosterol family of compounds, which occur naturally in a variety of plants and vegetable oils such as soy, corn, and wheat. Stanols are saturated sterols with no double bonds in their molecular structure. They are present in nature only in trace amounts and are manufactured by the hydrogenation of plant sterols.

The chemical structure of plant sterols and stanols is very similar to that of cholesterol, allowing them to inhibit cholesterol absorption in the intestine and thereby lower plasma cholesterol levels. Plant sterols and stanols themselves are poorly absorbed.

Recently, spreads enriched with plant sterol/stanol esters have become commercially available. When consumed on a regular basis, these lead to significant reductions in plasma total cholesterol and LDL levels of around 10%. The absorption of fat-soluble vitamins is not affected by plant sterol/stanol intake, though some studies reveal a reduction in carotenoid levels. This may be offset by increasing the intake of fruit and vegetables.

Plant sterol/stanol-enriched spreads may be useful adjuncts to a diet low in saturated fat in terms of lowering plasma cholesterol levels. When used in conjunction with statins, the cholesterol-lowering effects are additive.

More recently, data have emerged which suggest that plant sterols may have a beneficial effect on endothelial function.

Tea

Tea has been suggested to have cardioprotective properties due to its high content of flavonoids and other antioxidants. Epidemiological studies suggest a lower risk of coronary heart disease in subjects with a high intake of flavonoids from tea and other sources, though the evidence is conflicting. A recent meta-analysis suggested that the beneficial effect towards reducing cardiovascular disease is seen with increased consmption of green tea, rather than black tea. There is, however, insufficient evidence to suggest excessive consumption of green tea as a strategy to reduce the risk of developing cardiovascular disease.

Garlic

Garlic contains a variety of active compounds that may protect against atherosclerosis by a number of mechanisms, including inhibition of cholesterol synthesis, suppression of LDL oxidation, and inhibition of platelet aggregation and thrombus formation. Pooled data from clinical studies reveal that garlic or garlic extracts are able to lower plasma cholesterol and reduce blood pressure by a modest degree. There is, however, currently insufficient evidence from robust clinical trials to support an important role for garlic in coronary-heart-disease prevention.

Nuts

Despite their high overall fat content, there is now good evidence to suggest that nut consumption is linked with a reduction in cardiovascular disease. In the Physicians' Health Study, consumption of nuts was linked with a reduction in risk of sudden cardiac death. In addition, as part of a diet in which around one-third of total calorie intake is derived from fat, nut consumption appears to be associated with lower total cholesterol and lower LDL.

Dark chocolate

High-cocoa-content dark chocolate contains high levels of chemicals with antioxidant properties and there is relatively good evidence to suggest that the poly-phenol content of dark chocolate is able to improve lipid profile by raising HDL cholesterol and lowering LDL cholesterol. Compounds found within cocoa are also known to be beneficial in hypertension.

Fish, n-3 fatty acids, and sudden death

Interest in a potentially cardioprotective role of die-tary fish dates back to the 1950s, with recognition of the fact that Inuit Eskimos had very low rates of coro-nary heart disease despite consuming a diet high in fat. It subsequently became clear that long-chain n-3 fatty acids, present in fish and fish oils, possess important cardioprotective effects, and their con-sumption in large amounts by the Inuits may explain the 'Eskimo Paradox'. More recently, several large epidemiological studies have demonstrated an inverse relationship between the intake of long-chain n-3 polyunsaturated fatty acids and mortality from coronary heart disease.

Before continuing, it is important to note that while the evidence which supports the use of marine-derived n-3 fatty acids (eicosapentoic acid and doco-sahexanoic acid) in improving cardiovascular outcomes is relatively robust, there is less evidence that alpha linolenic acid (the n-3 fatty acid found in soybean, flax seed, walnuts, and canola oils) has the same effect.

n-3 fatty acids protect from coronary heart dis-ease through a number of mechanisms that inhibit atherosclerosis, prevent vessel occlusion, and reduce the predisposition to malignant cardiac arrhyth-mias, a common cause of sudden death. Replacing dietary saturated fats with long-chain n-3 polyun-saturated fatty acids reduces TAG levels and tends to increase HDL levels. The protective effects of these changes in the lipid profile have been previously dis-cussed. Moreover, increasing dietary n-3 fatty acid content shifts the balance of eicosanoid production, favouring the synthesis of vasodilatory and anti-aggregatory metabolites in the vessel wall. These effects promote endothelium-dependent vasodila-tation, lower blood pressure, and reduce platelet aggregation. In addition, n-3 fatty acids reduce the production of pro-atherosclerotic growth factors by mononuclear cells.

Interestingly, epidemiological studies suggest that n-3 fatty acids may offer particular protection from sudden cardiac death. In animal studies, n-3 fatty acids reduce the predisposition to ventricular fibril-lation, a fatal cardiac arrhythmia that is a common cause of sudden death in humans. It is thought that incorporation of n-3 fatty acids into the cell mem-brane of heart muscle cells provides resistance to arrythmias, perhaps by modulating the electrical conductance of membrane ion channels.

Support for a clinically important cardioprotective action of n-3 fatty acids derives from two recent ran-domised controlled secondary-prevention trials. The Diet and Reinfarction Trial (DART) gave 2033 male survivors of myocardial infarction advice on each of three dietary changes. These were:

(1) A reduction in total fat intake, with an increased ratio of polyunsaturated to saturated fats.
(2) An increase in fish intake (as fatty fish or fish oil capsules).
(3) An increase in cereal fibre intake.

No reduction in coronary events was seen in the groups who reduced their total fat intake or con-sumed more fibre. In contrast, consumption of fatty fish or fish oil supplementation led to a significant 29% reduction in all-cause mortality, with a 29% reduction in coronary-heart-disease mortality.

The Gruppo Italiano per le Studio della Sopravvivenza nell'Infarto Miocardico (GISSI) trial randomised 11 324 patients surviving a recent myo-cardial infarction to a Mediterranean-style diet sup-plemented with n-3 fatty acids (1 g daily), vitamin E (300 mg daily), both, or none, for 3.5 years. Treatment with n-3 fatty acids reduced the risk of death, nonfa-tal myocardial infarction, and stroke by 15%, whereas vitamin E had no effect. Secondary analyses revealed that the mortality benefit was largely attributable to a 45% reduction in sudden death.

It is important to note that since publication of the DART and GISSI trials there have been significant modifications to the treatment which patients receive following myocardial infarction. The OMEGA trial, published in 2010, which perhaps more accurately reflects current clinical practice, did not show a ben-efit from adding pharmacological n-3 fatty acid sup-plementation to conventional treatment in patients following acute myocardial infarction.

More recent studies suggest that pharmacological doses of fish oil may have a beneficial effect in the prevention of cardiac rhythm disorders, and more research into this potential therapeutic avenue is ongoing.

Taken together, the data certainly suggest that increasing consumption of *n*-3 fatty acids, particularly those derived from fatty fish, is likely to have a benefit on reducing the risk of cardiovascular mortality, particularly sudden cardiac death. More research is needed to ascertain whether pharmacological *n*-3 fatty acids have a therapeutic role to play in the treatment of cardiovascular disorders. Whether the consumption of a Mediterranean-style diet, as in the GISSI study, has additional protective effects is discussed in the next section.

The Mediterranean diet

Traditionally, the total energy content of diets low in saturated fat has been maintained by replacing saturated fats with complex carbohydrates. In recent years, however, it has become increasingly clear that the type of fat in the diet, as well as the total amount, is important in determining cardiovascular risk. Mediterranean-type diets, in which saturated fats are replaced with unsaturated fats, are not low in total fat, but there is substantial evidence that such diets offer significant protection from coronary heart disease.

Interest in the potential benefits of a Mediterranean-type diet was triggered by the Seven Countries Study, published in the 1960s, in which low rates of coronary heart disease and long life expectancy were noted in Mediterranean countries. This prompted the hypothesis that protection from coronary events in such countries may be granted by the type of diet consumed in those countries at that time. The traditional Mediterranean diet, typical of Greece and southern Italy in the early 1960s, contained an abundance of plant food (fruit, vegetables, breads, cereals, potatoes, beans, nuts, and seeds) and low to moderate amounts of fish, poultry, meat, dairy products, and eggs. Olive oil was the main source of dietary fat and alcohol was consumed in moderate amounts. Such a diet was rich in fibre and antioxidants and had a high proportion of monounsaturated fats, principally oleic acid from olive oil.

It is well established that replacement of saturated fats by monounsaturates, rather than carbohydrates, lowers LDL cholesterol without an adverse effect on HDL or TAG levels. In addition, monounsaturated

fatty acids possess a number of other favourable properties. Olive oil consumption enriches LDL particles with oleic acid. Oleic acid-enriched LDL is more resistant to oxidation and is therefore less atherogenic. Dietary monounsaturates also improve endothelial function, reduce the expression of adhesion molecules, decrease the tendency to thrombosis, and, in some studies, lower blood pressure to a small degree.

It is likely, however, that constituents other than monounsaturated fatty acids contribute to the protective effects of a Mediterranean diet. Antioxidants are supplied in abundance, largely by fruit and vegetables, but also as constituents of olive oil and wine. Insulin sensitivity and glycaemic control may be improved by the ingestion of complex carbohydrates and fibre. As discussed earlier, moderate alcohol consumption has been shown in epidemiological studies to potentially protect against coronary heart disease.

Support for the recommendation of a Mediterranean-style diet to prevent coronary heart disease in clinical practice comes from the Lyon Heart Study, a large randomised secondary-prevention trial designed to test whether such a diet, compared with a prudent Western diet, might reduce the recurrence of coronary events after a first myocardial infarction. After 46 months of follow-up in a total of 605 participants, there was an impressive 65% reduction in coronary-heart-disease mortality, and a 56% reduction in all-cause mortality in the group consuming a Mediterranean-style diet. The composition of the experimental diet is summarised in Table 18.4. Participants were recommended to eat more bread, root vegetables, green vegetables, fish, and fruit, and

Table 18.4 The Lyon Heart Study Diet. de Lorgeril *et al.* (1999) © Wolters Kluwer Health.

	Absolute value	% of total calories
Total calories	1947	
Total fat		30.4
Saturated fat		8.0
Polyunsaturated fat		4.6
18:1,*n*-9 (oleic acid)		12.9
18:2,*n*-6 (linoleic acid)		3.6
18:3,*n*-3 (linolenic acid)		0.84
Alcohol		5.8
Protein		16.2
Fibre	18.6 g	
Cholesterol	203 mg/day	

to reduce their intake of red meat, replacing it with poultry. A special margarine was supplied to replace butter and cream, and exclusive use of olive oil and rapeseed oil was recommended for salad and cooking. The margarine had a similar fatty acid composition to olive oil, but was supplemented with linoleic acid and, to a larger extent, alpha-linolenic acid.

The experimental diet was very similar, therefore, to the traditional Mediterranean diet consumed in Crete in the 1960s, with the exception of a greater amount of n-3 polyunsaturated fatty acids. This is important, as alpha-linolenic acid possesses many beneficial properties, which may have contributed to the favourable outcome of this trial. To date, no trials have assessed whether Mediterranean-type diets are effective in the primary prevention of coronary heart disease, although these are ongoing. Nonetheless, there is reasonable evidence from epidemiological studies and the Lyon Heart Study to support the use of such diets in coronary prevention.

Weight-reduction diets

There is now little doubt that obesity (particularly central obesity) is linked with an increase in insulin resistance, the metabolic syndrome, and the subsequent development of type 2 diabetes mellitus. There is also good evidence to associate the development of insulin resistance and diabetes with a significantly increased risk of developing cardiovascular disease. Weight management and weight loss, when appropriate, has therefore a central role to play in the prevention of cardiovascular disease.

In obesity reduction of weight, by any means (particularly dietary intervention coupled with exercise), is associated with reduction in blood pressure and improved insulin sensitivity and has favourable effects on lipid profile. Robust evidence based on long-term randomised controlled trials to support one 'diet' over another in terms of reduction in cardiovascular morbidity and mortality is not available. In spite of this, what evidence there is would seem to suggest that calorie restriction (where appropriate) by means of a diet rich in fruit and vegetables, low in saturated and *trans*-fats, and containing complex rather than refined carbohydrates, in combination with appropriate levels of protein and polyunsaturated and monounsaturated fats, is advisable.

For further information, see Chapters 4 and 6.

18.7 Diet and hypertension

Idiopathic (essential) hypertension significantly increases the risk of coronary heart disease and stroke, and promotes left-ventricular hypertrophy, heart failure, renal failure, aortic dissection, and peripheral vascular disease. In many cases, hypertension is associated with the presence of other risk factors such as obesity, insulin resistance, and lipid abnormalities, which together constitute the 'insulin-resistance (or metabolic) syndrome'.

There is a continuous, graded, near-linear relationship between blood pressure and the incidence of coronary events and stroke. Clinical guidelines attempt to target treatment to those at significantly increased risk by defining thresholds of blood pressure above which blood-pressure lowering is recommended. Many hypertensive subjects require drug treatment to achieve satisfactory reductions in blood pressure, and antihypertensive drugs have been shown to substantially lower the risk of stroke and, to a lesser extent, coronary heart disease in clinical trials.

Smaller but important decreases in blood pressure may also be achieved by lifestyle changes, such as weight loss, physical exercise, and dietary modification. The aetiology of hypertension is multifactorial, depending on an interaction between genetic and environmental factors. A substantial body of evidence suggests that a variety of nutritional factors are implicated in blood-pressure regulation. Lifestyle changes such as dietary modification are useful adjuncts to antihypertensive drug therapy in individuals with hypertension and, if adopted on a large scale, may reduce the incidence of coronary heart disease and stroke in the population.

Nutritional factors involved in blood-pressure regulation

A number of nutritional factors are implicated in the pathophysiology of hypertension. Those most studied include the minerals sodium, potassium, calcium, and magnesium, and other factors such as fatty acids, vitamins, and antioxidants.

Sodium intake is weakly associated with blood pressure in population studies. The effect of reducing sodium intake varies between individuals and is most pronounced in the elderly or those of Afro-Caribbean origin, who often have low renin levels. Pooled data from clinical trials show that dietary sodium restriction leads to small but significant reductions in blood pressure. In a recent randomised trial, the Dietary Approaches to Stop Hypertension (DASH) study, the addition of sodium restriction to a diet designed to lower blood pressure led to a further hypotensive effect. Achieving a large reduction in sodium intake can be difficult as salt is a 'hidden' ingredient in many manufactured foodstuffs and a very low-sodium diet can be unpalatable. Moderate reductions, however, are more readily achieved.

Sodium acts in concert with other minerals in influencing blood-pressure regulation, and potassium, magnesium, and calcium are all inversely (but weakly) correlated with hypertension in population studies. However, trials of potassium, magnesium, and calcium supplements in hypertension have yielded inconsistent results.

As discussed, polyunsaturated fatty acids of the n-3 and n-6 groups are essential precursors in the synthesis of eicosanoids, a family of vasoactive molecules with vasoconstrictor and vasodilator properties. Increased consumption of fish oils rich in n-3 fatty acids has been shown to decrease blood pressure in some, though not all, studies – probably by promoting the synthesis of vasodilator eicosanoids.

Vascular production of oxidants and free radicals is increased in hypertension and impairs endothelium-dependent vasodilatation. A number of antioxidants, including vitamin C and vitamin E, have been shown to reduce blood pressure in hypertensive subjects. Vitamin C, in particular, leads to improvements in endothelial function. As discussed previously, however, antioxidants have proved disappointing in reducing coronary heart disease in clinical trials.

The role of other vitamins in blood-pressure regulation is less clear. Vitamin D may play a role through is effect on calcium homeostasis. Vitamin B_6 is implicated in the central control of the sympathetic nervous system and its deficiency leads to hypertension in animal studies. Human data, however, are currently lacking.

Reduction of blood pressure by diet

Given the close relationship between obesity and hypertension, weight loss is a fundamental part of blood-pressure reduction in obese and overweight individuals, and it has been shown to lower blood pressure and the requirement for antihypertensive drugs in clinical trials. A reduction in alcohol consumption may decrease blood pressure in those who drink to excess.

The ability of a specific combination of dietary changes to lower blood pressure was assessed in the recent Dietary Approaches to Stop Hypertension (DASH) study. In this trial, 459 participants (with a baseline diastolic blood pressure of 80–95 mmHg and systolic blood pressure of 120–160 mmHg) were provided with a diet high in fruit and vegetables, a specially designed 'DASH diet', or a control diet for 8 weeks. The DASH diet was rich in potassium, magnesium, fibre, calcium, and protein, and was low in saturated fat and cholesterol. In those randomised to the DASH diet, systolic blood pressure fell by 5.5 mmHg and diastolic blood pressure by 3 mmHg after 8 weeks. Smaller, though significant, reductions in blood pressure were seen in the group consuming a diet high in fruit and vegetables. In an extension of the DASH study, the DASH-sodium study showed that addition of sodium restriction to the DASH diet led to further falls in blood pressure. The composition of the DASH diet is shown in Box 18.4.

Several meta-analyses have analysed the effect of reducing sodium on blood pressure. All of them appear to show that reducing sodium does lead to a reduction in both systolic and diastolic blood pressure, an effect which is more pronounced in people

---

Box 18.4 The DASH diet

High in:

- fruit;
- vegetables;
- low-fat diary products;
- fish;
- poultry;
- whole grains;
- nuts.

Low in:

- red meats;
- fats;
- sugar-sweetened foods;
- sugar-sweetened beverages.

with pre-existing hypertension. The overall effect was relatively modest, however: a reduction of between 1.5 and 5 mmHg in systolic blood pressure in those with pre-existing hypertension. It is thus perhaps not surprising that a recent review of evidence published by the Cochrane Collaboration was unable to identify a reduction in cardiovascular morbidity or mortality associated with a reduction in dietary salt intake in either normotensive or hypertensive populations (Taylor *et al.*, 2011b).

Although convincing outcome data do not currently exist, there is little doubt that reducing salt intake has a modest effect on reducing blood pressure. Advocating a moderated salt intake would therefore be generally recommended, particularly in a hypertensive population.

18.8 Diet and stroke

Stroke is the most common life-threatening neurological disorder and is a major cause of death and disability in developed countries. Most strokes are due to cerebral infarction, with the remainder caused by primary intracerebral haemorrhage or subarachnoid haemorrhage. Cerebral infarction arises from occlusion of a cerebral artery either by thrombosis of an atherosclerotic cerebral vessel or by embolism of thrombus from a proximal site. As atherosclerosis underlies a significant proportion of strokes, it is not surprising that nutritional factors may be implicated. The evidence for an association between the intake of dietary fat, plasma lipids, and the incidence of stroke is, however, weaker than that for coronary heart disease. Epidemiological studies fail to show a consistent relationship between saturated fat intake or plasma cholesterol levels and the incidence of stroke. Pooled data from large trials of diet and statins in the primary and secondary prevention of coronary heart disease, however, show a significant ~30% reduction in the incidence of stroke. It is unclear whether the benefit stems from cholesterol reduction or other properties of statins such as anti-inflammatory or antioxidant effects.

Stroke incidence is negatively correlated with the intake of antioxidant vitamins in epidemiological studies. Randomised trials of antioxidant supplements, however, have consistently failed to demonstrate an effect on the risk of stroke.

Mineral intake is important in the control of blood pressure, and the relationship between sodium intake and hypertension, itself a major risk factor for stroke, has been discussed. There is some evidence that increased potassium and magnesium intake may reduce stroke risk independently of blood-pressure changes. Data linking fish consumption with risk of stroke are conflicting. Alcohol consumption increases the risk of haemorrhagic stroke in a dose-dependent fashion but studies of alcohol intake and ischaemic stroke are inconsistent.

In general terms, therefore, observational studies suggest that certain dietary factors play a role in the predisposition to stroke. In contrast to coronary heart disease, however, there is a lack of large interventional studies to support the general recommendation of dietary modification as a means of stroke prevention.

18.9 Diet and peripheral vascular disease

Peripheral vascular disease (atherosclerotic disease) often coexists with coronary heart disease and shares the same risk factors. Very few studies have assessed the contribution of dietary factors to the pathogenesis or treatment of peripheral vascular disease in isolation from other manifestations of atherosclerotic disease. Nonetheless, it is reasonable to assume that dietary modifications that reduce the incidence of coronary heart disease, hypertension, and diabetes will decrease the burden of peripheral vascular disease in the population.

18.10 Diet and chronic heart failure

Chronic heart failure is a clinical syndrome in which cardiac output is insufficient to meet the body's needs, leading to fatigue, breathlessness, and fluid retention. Most cases of heart failure are characterised by impaired myocardial contractile function accompanied by increased activity of the sympathetic nervous and renin–angiotensin–aldosterone systems. Myocardial dysfunction often occurs as a consequence of coronary heart disease, hypertension, or diabetes. Genetic factors and viral infections are important causes of heart failure in a not insignificant proportion of patients.

Diet is important in the pathophysiology and treatment of heart failure for four main reasons:

(1) Dietary factors are implicated in the aetiology of many cases of chronic heart failure as they predispose to coronary heart disease, hypertension, and diabetes.
(2) Sodium retention contributes to fluid retention and oedema in many individuals. Restriction of dietary sodium intake, therefore, may be required.
(3) A variety of micronutrients are involved in the regulation of myocardial function, and supplementation may improve symptoms in some individuals. This will be discussed later in this chapter. Heart failure as a consequence of overt nutrient deficiency is rare in developed countries but does occur (e.g. thiamine deficiency).
(4) Patients with chronic heart failure may lose weight and muscle bulk in a process called 'cardiac cachexia'. Dietary modification may help to avoid this process.

Nutrition and cardiac cachexia

Cardiac cachexia denotes an undernourished state, which affects up to a third of patients with severe chronic heart failure and is associated with a poor prognosis. Several mechanisms are thought to contribute to the loss of lean body mass in these individuals.

Energy requirements often increase in chronic heart failure due to an increased resting metabolic rate and a shift toward catabolism. Energy intake, however, usually falls due to a combination of anorexia and reduced nutrient absorption. Appetite is decreased by a number of mechanisms, including central-nervous-system effects, side effects of drugs, and dyspepsia and early satiety caused by hepatic and splanchnic venous congestion. Oedema of the gut wall may reduce the ability to absorb digested foods, vitamins, and other micronutrients. Skeletal muscle bulk is lost by a decrease in physical activity and by the effects of poor cardiac output on nutrient and oxygen supply to the tissues. Malnutrition may affect the myocardium directly and further impair cardiac performance. Finally, increased circulating levels of catecholamines and proinflammatory cytokines, such as tumour necrosis factor alpha (TNFα), promote a catabolic state.

There are no specific recommendations for nutritional support in chronic heart failure as opposed to other chronic conditions characterised by under-nutrition. A high-energy, limited-sodium diet is recommended and meals should be small and frequent. Clinical trials of high-energy diets in chronic heart failure are small in number and reveal increases in weight with variable effects on function.

18.11 Micronutrients and cardiovascular disease

Micronutrients are implicated in the predisposition to atherosclerosis and in maintaining the contractile function of the heart. Support for an important role of vitamins and minerals in the pathogenesis of coronary heart disease, hypertension, peripheral vascular disease, stroke, and chronic heart failure is provided by observational and case–control studies. Further evidence derives from experimental studies in animals and humans, which emphasise the importance of micronutrients in the biochemical and pathological processes underlying cardiovascular disease. It is also increasingly recognised that subclinical deficiency in certain micronutrients is common in the general population. Randomised clinical-intervention trials, however, fail to show a reliable ability of many micronutrient supplements to reduce the incidence of disease. Nonetheless, adequate levels of 'beneficial' micronutrients must be regarded as an essential component of a balanced diet. Achieving high levels of 'beneficial' micronutrients through diets rich in fruit and vegetables, as with the Mediterranean-style diet, may contribute to the reduced incidence of coronary heart disease in recent trials.

Vitamins

Vitamin A

Carotenoids such as beta-carotene are antioxidants and may reduce the oxidation of LDL. However, an association between dietary intake of beta-carotene and the risk of coronary heart disease is not supported by prospective observational studies. Moreover, beta-carotene supplements fail to reduce coronary-heart-disease events in primary-prevention studies.

Vitamin B$_1$

Vitamin B$_1$ (thiamine) is essential for carbohydrate metabolism. Severe thiamine deficiency leads to heart failure in the condition known as beriberi. Diuretic therapy may reduce thiamine levels and inhibit thiamine uptake in the heart. It is unclear whether subclinical thiamine deficiency contributes to myocardial dysfunction in chronic heart failure. Limited evidence suggests that thiamine supplements may increase cardiac performance and symptoms in patients with moderate to severe heart failure.

Vitamin B$_6$, B$_{12}$, and folate

Vitamin B$_6$, B$_{12}$, and folate are required for the metabolism of homocysteine, an amino acid whose levels are strongly correlated with the risk of coronary heart disease, peripheral vascular disease, and stroke. There is an association between elevated plasmahomocysteine levels and atherosclerosis, and several laboratory studies have shown that homocystine can cause atherosclerosis by promoting LDL oxidation, damaging the endothelium, and adversely affecting platelet function and coagulation.

Homocysteine levels are regulated by its conversion to cysteine, in a reaction requiring vitamin B$_6$, or by its remethylation to form methionine, in a reaction requiring vitamin B$_{12}$ and folate. Dietary levels of vitamin B$_6$, B$_{12}$, and folate are inversely associated with the risk of coronary heart disease. Folate supplementation, either alone or in conjunction with B vitamins, leads to significant reduction in homocysteine levels. Initial interest in the potential therapeutic effect of modulation of homocystine levels by vitamin supplementation arose following studies which showed an improvement in vascular health in patients with homocystinuria who were treated with vitanin B and folate supplemetation. Homcystinuria is a genetic effect associated with extreme elevation of plasma homocystine levels and is certainly associated with the development of premature vascular disease.

Several large-scale trials have investigated the effect of using vitamin B and folate supplementation in both patients with known coronary disease and those at high risk of coronary disease. Although there was significant reduction in homcystine levels following vitamin B and folate supplementation, there was no accompanying demonstrable reduction in mortality or cardiovascular morbidity.

At present, there is no good evidence to recommend supplemenation of vitamin B or folate for the prevention of cardiovascular disease, except to those with homocystinuria.

Vitamin C

Vitamin C intake is inversely correlated with the risk of stroke and coronary heart disease in some, but not all, observational studies. Vitamin C promotes endothelial nitric oxide production and improves endothelium-dependent vasodilatation in animals and humans, probably through antioxidant effects. Supplementation has not been shown to reduce the incidence of coronary heart disease in randomised controlled trials.

Vitamin D

Vitamin D is closely implicated in calcium homeostasis and may have effects on the regulation of blood pressure. Data from observational studies suggest that low levels of vitamin D are associated with increased total mortality, are an independent risk factor for the development of cardiovascular disease, and are strongly associated with an adverse prognosis in patients with heart failure. It is currently unclear if supplementation of vitamin D will help to improve outcomes in any of these patient populations, but trials are ongoing.

Vitamin E

Vitamin E is a powerful lipid-soluble antioxidant that may protect against atherosclerosis by reducing the oxidation of LDL cholesterol and decreasing platelet aggregation. Consumption of vitamin E is inversely associated with the risk of coronary heart disease in epidemiological studies. Large-scale randomised controlled trials of vitamin E supplementation, however, have failed to show a beneficial effect.

Minerals

Sodium

Increased sodium intake leads to extracellular volume expansion and stimulation of the sympathetic nervous system. Its role in blood-pressure regulation has been discussed.

Potassium

Potassium acts along with other minerals to regulate cellular ion balance and vascular tone. Dietary potassium consumption is inversely related to the incidence of hypertension and stroke. The role of supplementation as a preventative measure is controversial. Potassium deficiency or excess may predispose to cardiac-rhythm disturbances.

Calcium

The degree of hardness of drinking water is inversely related to coronary heart disease incidence in epidemiological studies. Since water's hardness is partly determined by its calcium content, it has been suggested that calcium has protective effects. There is some evidence that higher calcium intake is associated with lower blood pressure and lower plasma TAG in observational studies, and dietary calcium reduces platelet aggregation in animal studies, perhaps by interfering with the absorption of saturated fats. Low levels of calcium predispose to cardiac-rhythm disturbances and may cause a cardiomyopathy, particularly in children. In spite of this, a recent review of evidence obtained from more than 12 000 patients suggests that calcium supplementation without concominant vitamin D supplementation is actually associated with increased cardiovascular mortality, with a 30% increased risk of myocardial infarction seen in those taking calcium supplemetation.

Copper

Copper is a constituent of cellular enzymes, including copper–zinc superoxide dismutase and cytochrome c oxidase. Copper deficiency is rare in humans but marginal levels potentially contribute to heart failure and atherosclerosis and elevate plasma cholesterol. Copper restriction in animals leads to myocyte damage and cardiomyopathy.

Magnesium

Epidemiological studies show an inverse association between magnesium intake and the risk of coronary heart disease and stroke. Magnesium may also be important in blood-pressure regulation by modulating vascular tone. Low magnesium levels are common in heart failure, may be promoted by diuretic use, and are associated with a worse prognosis. Magnesium deficiency can itself lead to heart failure in patients with anorexia nervosa. Low magnesium levels may contribute to cardiac-rhythm disturbances and intravenous magnesium is useful in the treatment of ventricular arrhythmias.

Manganese

Manganese is a constituent of the antioxidant enzyme manganese superoxide dismutase. Genetic deletion of this enzyme in mice leads to cardiomyopathy. Reduced levels of manganese superoxide dismutase may also be implicated in the cardiomyopathy induced by the anticancer drug adriamycin.

Zinc

Zinc is a critical component of cell membranes and antioxidant enzymes and blocks apoptotic (programmed) cell death. It maintains endothelial cell integrity and protects against inflammation. Low serum zinc levels are found in heart failure and may reflect diuretic use. Its antioxidant properties may be beneficial in atherosclerosis and heart failure.

Selenium

Selenium is a component of the antioxidant enzyme glutathione peroxidase. Selenium deficiency predisposes to peripartum cardiomyopathy and is the cause of Keshan disease, an endemic cardiomyopathy in China. Selenium deficiency may also cause a cardiomyopathy in patients on long-term parenteral nutrition. Its antioxidant properties are thought to protect against atherosclerosis and low selenium levels have been linked to coronary heart disease and peripheral vascular disease. There is, however, insufficient evidence at present to recommend selenium supplementation in the general population.

Lead

Chronic exposure to low levels of lead has been suggested to cause hypertension in animals and humans. The mechanism is thought to involve increased production of reactive oxidant species.

Arsenic

Arsenic is a toxic mineral that can promote atherosclerosis. Contamination by arsenic of drinking-water wells in Bangladesh and Taiwan causes hypertension and 'blackfoot disease', a form of peripheral vascular disease, in the affected population.

Others

Coenzyme Q$_{10}$

Coenzyme Q$_{10}$ (ubiquinone) is a vitamin-like fat-soluble quinone found in mitochondria, where it acts as an electron carrier in oxidative phosphorylation. It also has antioxidant and membrane-stabilising properties. It is thought that coenzyme Q_{10} depletion may contribute to heart failure, in which low myocardial levels are associated with increased mortality. Statins reduce the production of coenzyme Q_{10}, raising a theoretical concern over their use in patients with chronic heart failure. Limited studies of coenzyme Q_{10} supplements in heart failure have produced inconsistent results.

Carnitine

Carnitine is an organic amine that is involved in fatty acid oxidation. It is administered to treat carnitine deficiency, but its ability to increase energy production and remove toxic metabolites suggests a putative role in the treatment of heart failure, coronary artery disease, and peripheral vascular disease. This has not been adequately assessed in trials.

L-arginine

The amino acid L-arginine is the precursor of nitric oxide, an endothelium-derived free radical with potent vasodilatory and anti-atherosclerotic properties. Although intracellular L-arginine levels are not usually limiting, treatment with exogenous L-arginine has been shown to increase nitric oxide production and improve vasodilatation in animals and humans. A potential role in the prevention and treatment of coronary heart disease has not been tested in large randomised trials.

18.12 Concluding remarks

Our understanding of the role of dietary factors in diseases of the heart and blood vessels continues to improve, with important practical implications. Key dietary factors in the prevention of coronary heart disease are summarised in Box 18.5. Recognition of the association between dietary saturated fat, commerically produced *trans*-fatty acids, and plasma cholesterol levels and coronary-heart-disease risk has led to the adoption of cholesterol-lowering measures as the cornerstone of preventive strategies. Large randomised controlled trials have vindicated this approach, but more work is needed to ensure that all those who might benefit receive appropriate advice and treatment. New functional foods, such as

> **Box 18.5 Key dietary factors in the prevention of coronary heart disease**
>
> - maintenance of an ideal body weight (BMI 20–25 kg/m²);
> - reduction in the consumption of saturated fats and *trans*-fatty acids;
> - use of unsaturated fats, including olive oil and rapeseed oil, for cooking;
> - consumption of fruit and vegetables several times per day;
> - consumption of moderate amounts of complex carbohydrates;
> - consumption of dietary fibre, particularly soluble fibre;
> - increased intake of fatty fish;
> - reduction in salt intake;
> - moderation of alcohol intake.

plant-sterol/stanol spreads, provide a useful adjunct to other dietary measures in the reduction of plasma cholesterol. Interest is also turning to other modifiable risk factors, such as HDL and TAG, as targets for intervention. Recognition that other types of dietary fat, such as *n*-3 polyunsaturated fatty acids, exert cardioprotective effects has led to recent important nutritional studies. Trials of a diet high in fatty fish, for example, have been found to lead to impressive reductions in coronary-heart-disease risk.

The importance of complex interactions between nutrients in the diet is increasingly apparent. While antioxidant supplements have proved disappointing, the adoption of a balanced diet rich in antioxidants is well supported by the evidence. The Mediterranean-style diet may approach the ideal standard of the 'cardioprotective' diet.

Acknowledgements

This chapter has been revised and updated by Kate Gatenby, Stephen Wheatcroft, and Mark Kearney, based on the original chapter by Stephen Wheatcroft, Brian Noronha, and Mark Kearney.

References and further reading

Albert CM, Cook NR, Gaziano JM, Zharris E, MacFadyen J, Danielson E, *et al.* Effect of folic acid and B vitamins on risk of cardiovascular events and total mortality among women at high risk for cardiovascular disease: a randomized trial. JAMA 2008; 299(17): 2027–2036.

Bolland MJ, Avenell A, Baron JA, Grey A, MacLennan GS, Gamble, Reid IR. Effect of calcium supplements on risk of myocardial infarction and cardiovascular events. BMJ 2010; 341: c3691.

Conlin PR. Dietary modification and changes in blood pressure. Curr Opin Nephrol Hypertens 2001; 10: 359–363.

de Lorgeril M, Salen P, Martin JL, Monjaud I, Delaye J, Mamelle N. Mediterranean diet, traditional risk factors, and the rate of cardiovascular complications after myocardial infarction: final report of the Lyon Diet Heart Study. Circulation 1999; 99(6): 779–785.

Fairfield KM, Fletcher RH. Vitamins for chronic disease prevention in adults: scientific review. JAMA 2002; 287: 3116–3126.

Hooper L, Summerbell CD, Higgins JPT, Thompson RL, Clements G, Capps N, et al. Reduced or modified dietary fat for preventing cardiovascular disease. Cochrane database of Systematic Reviews. 2001; (3): CD002137 (updated 2011; (7): CD002137).

Jakobsen MU, O'Reilly EJ, Heitmann BL, Pereira MA, Bälter K, Fraser GE, et al. Major types of dietary fat and risk of coronary heart disease: a pooled analysis of 11 cohort studies. Am J Clin Nutr 2009; 89(5): 1425–1432.

Kato H, Tillotson J, Nichamen NZ, Rhaods GG, Hamilton HB. Epidemiologic studies of coronary heart disease and stroke in Japanese men living in Japan, Hawaii and California: serum lipids and diet. Am J Epidemiol 1973; 97: 372–385.

Keys A. Seven Countries: A Multivariate Analysis of Death and Coronary Heart Disease. London: Harvard University Press, 1980.

Kromhout D, Giltay EJ, Geleijnse JM. *n*-3 fatty acids and cardiovascular events after myocardial infarction. New England Journal of Medicine 2010; 363: 2015–2026.

Kromhout D, Menotti A, Kesteloot H, Sans S. Prevention of coronary heart disease by diet and lifestyle: evidence from prospective cross-cultural, cohort, and intervention studies. Circulation 2002; 105: 893–898.

Martin MJ, Browner WS, Wentworth D, Hulley SB, Kuller LH. Serum cholesterol, blood pressure and mortality: implications from a cohort of 361 662 men. Lancet 1986; ii: 933–936.

Renaud S, Lanzmann-Petithory D. Coronary heart disease: dietary links and pathogenesis. Public Health Nutr 2001; 4: 459–474.

Schaefer EJ. Lipoproteins, nutrition, and heart disease. Am J Clin Nutr 2002; 75: 191–212.

Taylor F, Ward K, Moore THM, Burke K, Davey Smith G, Casas JP, Ebrahim S. Statins for the primary prevention of cardiovascular disease. Cochrane Database of Systematic Reviews. 2011a; (1): CD004816.

Taylor RS, Ashton KE, Moxham T, Hooper L, Ebrahim S. Reduced dietary salt for the prevention of cardiovascular disease. Cochrane Database of Systematic Reviews. 2011b; (7): CD009217.

Witte KK, Clark AL, Cleland JG. Chronic heart failure and micronutrients. J Am Coll Cardiol 2001; 37: 1765–1774.

Worth RM, Kato H, Rhoads GG, Kagan A, Syme SL. Epidemiologic studies of coronary heart disease and stroke in Japese men living in Japan, Hawaii and California: mortality. Am J Epidemiol 1975; 102(6): 481–490.

19

Nutritional Aspects of Disease Affecting the Skeleton

Christine Rodda

Monash University, Australia

Key messages

- Bone health is the result of complex interactions between genetic determinants of peak bone mass, lifestyle factors (including nutrition and exercise), the hormonal milieu, and vitamin D status.
- Adequate sun exposure is the most important determinant of vitamin D status.
- Vitamin D deficiency due to poor sun exposure in at-risk individuals, leading to rickets in infants and children and osteomalacia in adults, is entirely preventable.
- Age-specific issues need to be considered with regard to nutritional requirements in order to ensure normal bone growth during infancy, childhood, and adolescence, for the maintenance of

- bone mass throughout adulthood and minimisation of bone loss during senescence.
- Osteopaenia and osteoporosis are frequent complications of chronic systemic disease and may be exacerbated by dietary mineral ion and protein under-nutrition and vitamin D deficiency.
- Bone metabolism is integrally linked with other organ systems in the body and involves osteocyte function, which is modulated by weight-bearing and shear forces on bone. These cells are also integrally involved with phosphate metabolism. Recently, osteocalcin, produced by osteoblasts, has been shown to be a vital link between metabolic processes and bone health, including modulation of insulin sensitivity.

19.1 Introduction

The skeleton is a complex structure, comprising mineral ions, predominantly calcium and phosphorus, which precipitate to form the crystalline structure of hydroxyapatite, which itself precipitates on the helical collagen framework of bone-matrix proteins to form the rigid, strong structure characteristic of normal bone. This chapter will review the basic concepts of calcium homeostasis and bone metabolism, with particular emphasis on relevant dietary aspects in health and disease, from conception to senescence.

Linear bone growth during infancy, childhood, and adolescence ceases once bone growth plates fuse; however, ongoing bone turnover, with resorption of old bone and formation of new bone, continues throughout life. Normal mineral-ion homeostasis involves multiple organ systems, namely the parathyroid

glands, skin, gastrointestinal system, liver, and kidney. Perturbations of any of these organ systems may affect mineral-ion homeostasis and bone metabolism. Consequently, nutritional deficiencies and various chronic diseases may have profound effects on skeletal health. The complex interactions between mineral-ion nutrition, protein/calorie nutrition, and vitamin D status will be discussed in this chapter, together with aspects of diagnostic imaging techniques and laboratory testing relevant to assessment of the skeleton.

19.2 Overview of bone metabolism and mineral-ion homeostasis

Bone metabolism

Throughout life, bone, like skin and the lining of the gut, is continually turned over, in processes referred

Clinical Nutrition, Second Edition. Edited by Marinos Elia, Olle Ljungqvist, Rebecca J Stratton and Susan A Lanham-New.
© 2013 The Nutrition Society. Published 2013 by Blackwell Publishing Ltd.

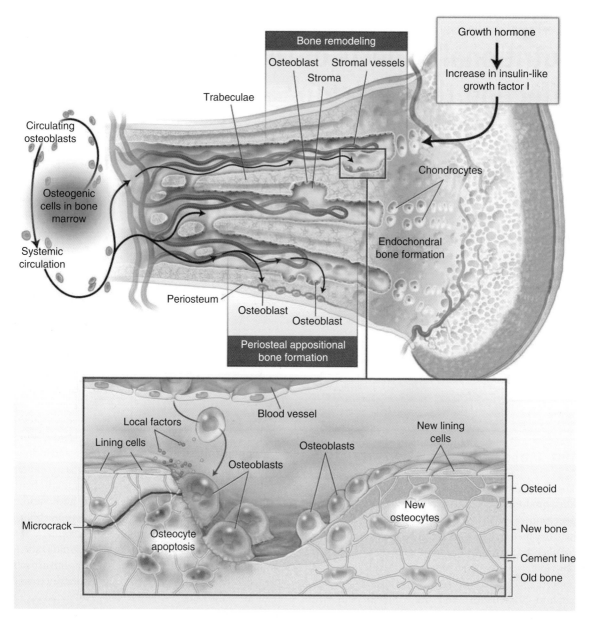

Figure 19.1 Cellular interactions involved in endochondrial bone formation. Canalis E *et al*. Mechanisms of Anabolic Therapies for Osteoporosis, New England Journal of Medicine 2007; 357: 905–916. Copyright © Massachusetts Medical Society.

to as 'modelling' in growing children and 'remodelling' in adults. Bone-resorbing cells (osteoclasts) resorb bone; their action is coupled with that of bone-forming cells (osteoblasts), which lay down new bone (Figure 19.1); osteoblast/osteoclast coupling is mediated via a complex paracrine hormonal

interplay between these two cell types, and involves hormones such as receptor activator of nuclear factor kappa-B ligand (RANKL), fibronectin, and osteoprogerin. Osteocytes, derived from the osteoblastic lineage, are the most numerous type of bone cell. They intercommunicate via cellular processes, to act as

'strain gauges', sensitive to weight-bearing and shear-
ing forces applied to bone, and have a critical role in
stimulating new bone formation. Weight-bearing
exercise is an important determinant of bone
strength; conversely, immobilisation due to prolonged bed rest, or in more recent years, 'weightless-
ness' in prolonged space travel, has been shown to
result in bone loss. Osteocytes also produce fibroblast
growth factor 23 (FGF23) and phosphate-regulating
neutral endopeptidase (encoded on the X chromosome) (PHEX), which act on the kidney and are
major regulators of phosphate homeostasis.

During normal growth in childhood, bone formation exceeds net bone resorption, and bone mass
steadily increases through to adolescence, during
which approximately 40% of bone mass accrual
occurs. By the beginning of the third decade of life,
peak bone mass has been attained and bone mass
reaches a steady state, and in otherwise healthy young
adults bone resorption occurs in balance with bone
formation until menopause in women and late middle age in men, when bone resorption starts to exceed
net bone formation, leading to osteoporosis over the
ensuing decades.

The major determinants of peak bone mass are
listed in Box 19.1.

The nutritional and hormonal (autocrine, paracrine, and endocrine) influences on bone formation
and resorption are complex. Hormonal influences
include parathyroid hormone (PTH), 1,25-dihydroxy
vitamin D_3 (1,25$(OH)_2D_3$), IGF-1 and 2, BMPs, transforming growth factor beta (TGFβ), FGF, osteocalcin, sex hormones, and various cytokines and
lymphokines. Other factors, including (i) nutritional
factors such as obesity, malabsorption syndromes,
and anorexia nervosa, (ii) chronic systemic diseases
such as cystic fibrosis and chronic renal failure, and
(iii) pregnancy and lactation, also affect bone metab-

olism. In recent years the hormone osteocalcin, produced by osteoblasts, has been identified as an
important link between regulators of nutrition, such
as insulin, and bone metabolism.

Mineral-ion homeostasis

Mineral-ion homeostasis is important for both normal
metabolism and structural skeletal rigidity. The major
ions concerned are calcium and phosphorus. Bone
osteoid comprises bone-matrix proteins, predominantly collagen, which are laid down in a complex
helical structure and provide tensile strength to bone.
The mineral ions calcium and phosphorus precipitate within this helical structure as hydroxyapatite
crystals $(Ca_{10}(PO_4)_6(OH)_2)$ to form a strong, rigid
structure characteristic of mature bone.

In growing infants and children, this process predominantly occurs at the metaphyseal growth plates,
within the long bones. Once these growth plates have
fused and linear growth has ceased, bone formation
and resorption occur in a coupled fashion throughout
the healthy adult skeleton. During senescence, new
bone formation diminishes with ongoing bone resorption, leading to osteoporosis. Unmineralised osteoid,
which occurs in rickets in children and osteomalacia
in adults, results in soft, pliable bones. Defective mineralisation will result as a consequence of either calcium
or phosphate depletion, or a combination of both.

Calcium

The adult skeleton contains 1–1.5 kg calcium
(20–25 mg/kg fat-free tissue) and represents 99% of
total body calcium. Less than 1% of calcium circulates in a soluble form, and it is this fraction that plays
a vital role in neuromuscular and cardiovascular
function, in coagulation, and as an intracellular second messenger for cell-surface hormone action, in
addition to its roles in gene transcription and cellular
growth and metabolism. In the presence of dietary
calcium insufficiency, circulating blood calcium is
maintained at normal concentrations, primarily
through the actions of PTH, which maintains circulating calcium at the expense of bone mineralisation
(Figures 19.2 and 19.3).

Dairy foods are the richest, most bioavailable natural
food sources of calcium. The recommended daily
intakes (RDIs) for calcium are listed in Table 19.1 and
dietary sources in Table 19.2. Infant RDI is almost

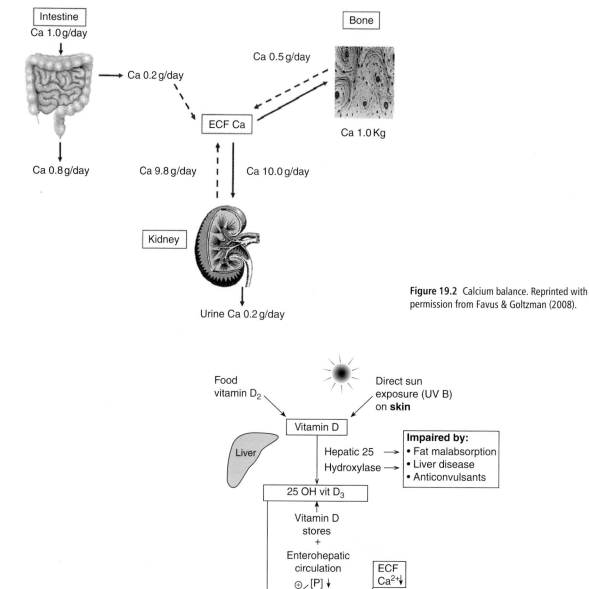

Figure 19.2 Calcium balance. Reprinted with permission from Favus & Goltzman (2008).

Figure 19.3 Vitamin D/calcium metabolism: PTH, parathyroid hormone, produced by the parathyroid glands as shown; [Ca], serum calcium; [P], serum phosphate; UCa, urinary calcium; UP, urinary phosphate.

Table 19.1 Estimated average requirement (EAR) and recommended dietary intake (RDI) for calcium. Adapted from Australian National Health and Medical Research Council (2006).

	EAR	RDI
Children and adolescents		
All		
1–3 years	360 mg/day	500 mg/day
4–8 years	520 mg/day	700 mg/day
Boys		
9–11 years	800 mg/day	1000 mg/day
12–13 years	1050 mg/day	1300 mg/day
14–18 years	1050 mg/day	1300 mg/day
Girls		
9–11 years	800 mg/day	1000 mg/day
12–13 years	1050 mg/day	1300 mg/day
14–18 years	1050 mg/day	1300 mg/day
Adults		
Men		
19–30 years	840 mg/day	1000 mg/day
31–50 years	840 mg/day	1000 mg/day
51–70 years	840 mg/day	1000 mg/day
>70 years	1100 mg/day	1300 mg/day
Women		
19–30 years	840 mg/day	1000 mg/day
31–50 years	840 mg/day	1000 mg/day
51–70 years	1100 mg/day	1300 mg/day
>70 years	1100 mg/day	1300 mg/day
Pregnancy		
14–18 years	1050 mg/day	1300 mg/day
19–30 years	840 mg/day	1000 mg/day
31–50 years	840 mg/day	1000 mg/day
Lactation		
14–18 years	1050 mg/day	1300 mg/day
19–30 years	840 mg/day	1000 mg/day
31–50 years	840 mg/day	1000 mg/day

always met, as breast milk or formula feeds are the sole dietary intake of infants under 3 months of age, and should continue to form the bulk of their diet until 9–12 months of age. Calcium intake beyond this age may be inadequate due to cultural food practices, food faddism, or exclusion diets due to cow's-milk allergy or lactase deficiency. Fortification of fruit juices, bread, and cereal with calcium may provide alternative dietary sources of calcium for those on such exclusion diets. In the event that the RDI for calcium cannot be met, there are a number of commercially available preparations of calcium supplements.

The effectiveness of calcium absorption from commercial preparations is to some degree depend-ent on the type of calcium salt, timing in relation to meals, and number of doses. Calcium citrate-malate (CCM) preparations have been found to be absorbed better than calcium carbonate salts, but CCM is not universally available and is unobtainable in some countries. However, overall the benefits of one calcium salt over another are not substantial.

The efficiency of calcium absorption is affected by pH and other components of food, such as oxalates and phytates, and calcium supplements are best taken in multiple doses rather than as a single daily dose, to maximise absorption efficiency. However, as the number of daily doses of supplements increases, subject compliance is also likely to decrease.

Reduced gastric acid secretion secondary to atrophic gastritis, which is commonly seen in elderly populations, may also contribute to dietary calcium deficiency in the elderly, and it is important that calcium carbonate supplementation is actually taken with meals to optimise calcium bioavailability under these circumstances.

Calcium retention may be suboptimal due to either decreased calcium absorption, as in vitamin D deficiency, or excessive urinary excretion due to high-protein or high-salt diets. High-oxalate (e.g. spinach) and high-phytate (e.g. chapatis) diets also reduce calcium absorption. Carbonated drinks with high phosphoric acid content may impair calcium absorption, and may also be preferred to milk drinks. Aluminium in antacids taken in excess may increase urinary calcium excretion. Dietary factors that impair calcium retention are listed in Box 19.2.

Phosphorus

The human body contains about 0.8–1.0 kg of phosphorus (11–14 mg/kg fat-free mass), and, like calcium, less than 1% of this circulates in a soluble form. Unlike calcium, however, only 85% of total body phosphorus is in the skeleton, because it also has a major role in soft-tissue growth, with 15% present in muscle and other body tissues. In addition, phosphorus has wide-ranging influences on metabolism, and is an important component of basic molecules such as phospholipids, phosphoproteins, and nucleic acids. Phosphate is also integral to normal muscle function, and has an important role in the synthesis and storage of chemical energy as high-energy phosphate bonds such as adenosine triphosphate (ATP).

Table 19.2 Dietary sources of calcium. Prepared by members of the Department of Dietetics, Monash Medical Centre, Clayton, Victoria, Australia.

Food type	mg calcium	Food type	mg calcium
Beverages (per 250 ml)		*Dairy products*	
Skim milk	380	Powdered full-cream milk 2 tbs	95
Full-cream milk	300	Powdered skim milk 2 tbs	130
Fat-reduced milk	375–440	Cheddar cheese 30 g	260
Calcium-enriched soy milk	300–370	Swiss cheese 30 g	290
Soy milk (no added calcium)	30	Edam cheese 30 g	280
Orange juice (no added calcium)	30	Mozzarella 30 g	225
		Parmesan 2 tsp	60
Meat, eggs, and fish		Camembert 30 g	100
Red or white meat av. serve	15	Processed cheese 1 slice	150
Egg (1)	27	Cottage cheese 1 cup	115
Fish (no bones) 150 g	50	Yoghurt, plain 200 g	290
Salmon (canned) 100 g	185	Yoghurt, low fat 200 g	360
Sardines (canned) 100 g	350	Ice-cream 150 ml	70
Tuna (canned) 100 g	10	Cream 2 tbs	35
Oysters (12)	230	Butter 1 tbs	3
Scallops (6)	120		
Prawns (6 medium)	225	*Grain and cereals*	
		Rolled oats ½ cup, raw	25
Beans and nuts		Cornflakes 30 g	2
Baked beans ½ cup	50	Rice (brown) 1 cup, cooked	15
Soya beans 1 cup, cooked	130	Bread (wholemeal) 2 slices	16
Tofu 100 g	130	Bread (white) 2 slices	10
Almonds 50 g	120		
Cashews 50 g	20	*Vegetables*	
Peanuts 50 g	30	Asparagus 6 spears	25
Walnuts 50 g	45	Beans (green) av. serve	30
Sesame seeds 20 g	230	Broccoli av. serve	75
Sunflower seeds 24 g	24	Brussel sprouts av. serve	25
Coconut milk 200 ml	60	Cabbage av. serve	45
		Carrots 1 medium	50
Vegetables		Cauliflower av. serve	15
Apple 1 medium	9	Corn 1 cob	5
Banana 1 medium	10	Mushrooms ½ cup	17
Blackberries ½ punnet	80	Olives each	4
Fig 1 medium	35	Onions 1 small	15
Grapes (sultana) 150 g	30	Peas ½ cup	30
Lemon 1 medium	110	Potato 1 medium	12
Melon 1 cup	40	Pumpkin av. piece	40
Orange 1 medium	55	Silverbeet av. serve	75
Paw paw (medium slice)	30	Spinach av. serve	360
Rhubarb ½ cup (cooked)	105	Tomato 1 medium	20
Strawberries ½ punnet	35	Zucchini ½ cup	20
Pear 1 medium	10		
Raisins 50 g	30	*Miscellaneous*	
		Molasses 1 tbs	120
		Milk chocolate	145
		Dark chocolate	20

Phosphate is an almost ubiquitous component of food, so dietary deficiency is uncommon unless total dietary intake is severely restricted, as may occur in anorexia nervosa or other causes of severe malnutrition, including untreated insulin-dependent diabetes mellitus, or when demand outstrips supply, as may occur in sick, extremely low-birth-weight infants. When it does occur, phosphate depletion has major consequences, affecting neuromuscular, cardiovascular, renal, haematological, and bone metabolism.

Vitamin D metabolism

Renal 1,25 $(OH)_2$ vitamin D_3 production is dependent on multiple organ systems, namely the skin, liver, kidney, gut, and bone. In populations where there are no vitamin D-supplemented foodstuffs, approximately 90% of vitamin D is obtained from vitamin D_3 synthesised in the epidermis from 7-dehydrocholesterol (7-DHC), in a reaction catalysed by ultraviolet B (UVB) light with a wavelength of 288 nm. For this reaction to take place, there must be direct exposure to sunlight or other sources of UVB, as this wavelength of UV radiation is not transmitted through glass or clothing. The efficiency of vitamin D synthesis in the skin tends to decrease with ageing, and is a contributory risk factor for vitamin D deficiency in the elderly. The remaining 10% of vitamin D is derived from dietary sources such as cod liver oil, eggs, and oily fish. Skin production of vitamin D is dependent on: (i) skin pigmentation, (ii) latitude, (iii) clothing practices, and (iv) time spent outdoors in direct sunlight. Skin pigmentation influences the efficiency of vitamin D_3 production from sunlight exposure, and vitamin D production in the skin is inversely proportional to melanin production, as melanin competes with 7-DHC for UVB protons. Consequently, black-skinned individuals need approximately six times more sunlight exposure than fair-skinned individuals to maintain equivalent vitamin D status. The amount of UVB exposure from sunlight is also inversely proportional to latitude, so that UVB exposure is greater in equatorial regions than in regions at higher latitudes. Furthermore, UVB exposure is greater during summer than winter

at higher latitudes, so that the greatest risk for vitamin D deficiency in such regions is in late winter and early spring. The incidence of Vitamin D deficiency is rising in urbanised areas, since as mentioned UVB is not transmitted through glass or clothing, and time spent doing indoor sedentary activities is increasing. These lifestyle changes have also contributed to the rising epidemic of obesity, another risk factor for vitamin D deficiency, likely to be mediated through increased vitamin D catabolism within fat. In the skin, vitamin D_3 is bound to vitamin D-binding protein and is transported in the bloodstream to the liver, where it is rapidly hydroxylated.

Both dietary vitamins D_2/D_3 and skin-synthesised vitamin D_3 are hydroxylated in the liver to form 25-hydroxy vitamin D_3 (25OH D_3), which is the storage form of vitamin D. This hydroxylation step is largely unregulated and vitamin D stores can remain replete for many months without further sun exposure. Vitamin D_3 and its metabolites are fat-soluble vitamins and undergo enterohepatic circulation by cosecretion of 25OH D_3 and bile salts into the duodenum, with subsequent reabsorption of 25OH D_3 within the gut. This reabsorption process may be inhibited by binding of 25OH D_3 to dietary phytates and fibre, or in fat malabsorption syndromes such as coeliac disease or cystic fibrosis. Further hydroxylation of 25OH D_3 to form 1,25$(OH)_2D_3$ occurs in the kidney through the regulation of 1 alpha hydroxylase by PTH, IGF-1, and FGF23, with feedback inhibition of PTH secretion by 1,25$(OH)_2D_3$ (Figure 19.3). The 1,25-hydroxylated form of vitamin D (1,25$(OH)_3D_3$, calcitriol) is the active metabolite of vitamin D, acts via the vitamin D receptor present in multiple tissues of the body, and should more appropriately be regarded as a hormone rather than a vitamin, as its production is under the tight control of PTH and there is a negative feedback loop whereby calcitriol inhibits PTH secretion in turn (Figure 19.3). Other hormones such as FGF23 and IGF-1 also regulate 1 alpha hydroxylase activity. In recent years, the wide tissue distribution of extrarenal 1 alpha hydroxylase and the role of 1,25 $(OH)_2$ vitamin D in immunomodulation, autoimmunity, and tissue growth are being increasingly recognised, although PTH and FGF23 do not regulate extrarenal vitamin D metabolism. Both renal and extra-renal 1,25$(OH)_2D_3$ are inactivated by the enzyme 24 hydroxylase (*CYP24R1*) to form the inactive metabolite, 1,24,25$(OH)_2D_3$.

Table 19.3 Age-related recommended daily intake (RDI) for vitamin D. AI, adequate intake; EAR, estimated average requirement; RDA, Recommended Dietary Allowance; UL, tolerable upper intake level. Holick *et al*. (2011), copyright 2011, The Endocrine Society.

Life stage group	IOM recommendations				Committee recommendations for patients at risk for vitamin D deficiency	
	AI	EAR	RDA	UL	Daily requirement	UL
Infants						
0–6 months	400 IU (10 μg)			1000 IU (25 μg)	400–1000 IU	2000 IU
6–12 months	400 IU (10 μg)			1500 IU (38 μg)	400–1000 IU	2000 IU
Children						
1–3 years		400 IU (10 μg)	600 IU (15 μg)	2500 IU (63 μg)	600–1000 IU	4000 IU
4–8 years		400 IU (10 μg)	600 IU (15 μg)	3000 IU (75 μg)	600–1000 IU	4000 IU
Males						
9–13 years		400 IU (10 μg)	600 IU (15 μg)	4000 IU (100 μg)	600–1000 IU	4000 IU
14–18 years		400 IU (10 μg)	600 IU (15 μg)	4000 IU (100 μg)	600–1000 IU	4000 IU
19–30 years		400 IU (10 μg)	600 IU (15 μg)	4000 IU (100 μg)	1500–2000 IU	10 000 IU
31–50 years		400 IU (10 μg)	600 IU (15 μg)	4000 IU (100 μg)	1500–2000 IU	10 000 IU
51–70 years		400 IU (10 μg)	600 IU (15 μg)	4000 IU (100 μg)	1500–2000 IU	10 000 IU
>70 years		400 IU (10 μg)	800 IU (20 μg)	4000 IU (100 μg)	1500–2000 IU	10 000 IU
Females						
9–13 years		400 IU (10 μg)	600 IU (15 μg)	4000 IU (100 μg)	600–1000 IU	4000 IU
14–18 years		400 IU (10 μg)	600 IU (15 μg)	4000 IU (100 μg)	600–1000 IU	4000 IU
19–30 years		400 IU (10 μg)	600 IU (15 μg)	4000 IU (100 μg)	1500–2000 IU	10 000 IU
31–50 years		400 IU (10 μg)	600 IU (15 μg)	4000 IU (100 μg)	1500–2000 IU	10 000 IU
51–70 years		400 IU (10 μg)	600 IU (15 μg)	4000 IU (100 μg)	1500–2000 IU	10 000 IU
>70 years		400 IU (10 μg)	800 IU (20 μg)	4000 IU (100 μg)	1500–2000 IU	10 000 IU
Pregnancy						
14–18 years		400 IU (10 μg)	600 IU (15 μg)	4000 IU (100 μg)	600–1000 IU	4000 IU
19–30 years		400 IU (10 μg)	600 IU (15 μg)	4000 IU (100 μg)	1500–2000 IU	10 000 IU
31–50 years		400 IU (10 μg)	600 IU (15 μg)	4000 IU (100 μg)	1500–2000 IU	10 000 IU
Lactation[a]						
14–18 years		400 IU (10 μg)	600 IU (15 μg)	4000 IU (100 μg)	600–1000 IU	4000 IU
19–30 years		400 IU (10 μg)	600 IU (15 μg)	4000 IU (100 μg)	1500–2000 IU	10 000 IU
31–50 years		400 IU (10 μg)	600 IU (15 μg)	4000 IU (100 μg)	1500–2000 IU	10 000 IU

[a]Mother's requirement, 4000–6000 IU/day (mother's intake for infant's requirement if intake is not receiving 400 IU/day.

Furthermore, this enzyme also protects the body from vitamin D toxicity, by inactivating 25 OH vitamin D_3 to 24,25(OH)$_2$D$_3$.

Gut absorption of both calcium and phosphate is increased by the action of 1,25(OH)$_2$D$_3$ on the gut, both directly and via upregulation of the calcium-binding protein calbindin-D. Although both calcium and phosphate are absorbed throughout the length of the small intestine, the majority of phosphate is absorbed from the jejunum and ileum, and the majority of calcium from the duodenum. To maintain normal mineral-ion homeostasis, particularly in growing children, the RDIs of both vitamin D (Table 19.3) and calcium (Table 19.1)

must be met. However, the RDI for vitamin D remains controversial given the wide variation in direct sun exposure around the world, and variable skin-pigmentation, latitude, and lifestyle factors. In Australia, for example, there are no national RDIs for vitamin D, as it is assumed that Australians have adequate sunlight exposure for their vitamin D requirements. The RDIs for vitamin D cited in this chapter are based on the recently published US Guidelines (Table 19.3). Dietary sources of vitamin D are listed in Table 19.4.

The skeletal effects of 1,25(OH)$_2$D$_3$ are complex and beyond the scope of this chapter. However, in broad terms, 1,25(OH)$_2$D$_3$ affects both bone

Table 19.4 Dietary sources of vitamin D. Holick MF. Vitamin D Deficiency. N Engl J Med 2007; 357: 266–281. Copyright © Massachusetts Medical Society.

Source	Vitamin D content
Natural sources	

Vitamin D_2
(Ergocalciferol)

Vitamin D_3
(Cholecalciferol)

Source	Vitamin D content
Cod liver oil	~400–1,000 IU/teaspoon vitamin D_3
Salmon, fresh wild caught	~600–1,000 IU/3.5 or vitamin D_3
Salmon, fresh farmed	~100–250 IU/3.5 oz vitamin D_3, vitamin D_2
Salmon, canned	~300–600 IU/3.5 or vitamin D_3
Sardines, canned	~300 IU/3.5 oz vitamin D_3
Mackerel, canned	~250 IU/3.5 oz vitamin D_3
Tuna, canned	236 IU/3.5 oz vitamin D_3
Shiitake mushrooms, fresh	~100 IU/3.5 oz vitamin D_2
Shiitake mushrooms, sun-dried	~1,600 IU/3.5 oz vitamin D_2
Egg yolk	~20 IU/yolk vitamin D_3 or D_2
Sunlight/UVB radiation	~20,000 IU equivalent to exposure to 1 minimal erythemal dose (MED) in a bathing suit. Thus, exposure of arms and legs to 0.5 MED is equivalent to ingesting ~3,000 IU vitamin D_3.
Fortified foods	
Fortified milk	100 IU/8 oz, usually vitamin D_3
Fortified orange juice	100 IU/8 oz vitamin D_3
Infant formulas	100 IU/8 oz vitamin D_3
Fortified yogurts	100 IU/8 oz, usually vitamin D_3
Fortified butter	56 IU/3.5 oz, usually vitamin D_3
Fortified margarine	429 IU/3.5 oz, usually vitamin D_3
Fortified cheeses	100 IU/3 oz, usually vitamin D_3
Fortified breakfast cereals	~100 IU/serving, usually vitamin D_3
Pharmaceutical sources in the Untied States	
Vitamin D_2 (ergocalciferol)	50,000 IU/capsule
Drisdol (vitamin D_2) liquid	8,000 IU/cc
Supplemental sources	
Multivitamin	400, 500, 1000 IU vitamin D_3 or vitamin D_2
Vitamin D_3	400, 800, 1000, 2,000, 5,000, 10,000, and 50,000 IU

IU = 25 ng. [Reproduced with permission from M. F. Holick: *N Engl J Med* 357:266–281, 2007 (3). © Massachusetts Medical Society.]

formation and resorption in the ongoing modelling/remodelling process of bone. At a cellular level, osteoblasts express $1,25(OH)_2D_3$ receptors and may modulate the synthesis of a number of osteoblast-derived products, such as alkaline phosphatase (ALP) and osteocalcin, in addition to the stimulation of proliferation of osteoblasts themselves. During pregnancy, the placenta is also an extrarenal source of 1 alpha hydroxylase and $1,25(OH)_2D_3$. In disease states such as sarcoidosis, tuberculosis, and neonatal subcutaneous fat necrosis, hypercalcaemia may develop as a result of excessive and largely unregulated extrarenal 1 alpha hydroxylase-induced $1,25(OH)_2D_3$ production within these tissues.

19.3 Age-appropriate biochemical reference ranges

Specific reference ranges will not be presented, but it is important to be aware of age-appropriate reference ranges which affect the following biochemical parameters.

Alkaline phosphatase

ALP is mostly bone-derived in infants and children, and consequently is normally up to 3–4 times the upper limit of the normal adult reference range in these age groups, with peak levels corresponding to periods of rapid linear growth, as occur in infancy and the pubertal growth spurt. The isoenzyme bone-specific ALP (BSAP) may now be readily measured using commercially available assays.

Phosphate

Phosphate tends to directly correlate with growth rate and is highest in premature infants and during the first few months of life, and continues to be higher than adult reference ranges throughout growth.

Insulin-like growth factor 1

IGF-1 also tends to directly correlate with growth rate and is highest during the pubertal growth spurt, and continues to be higher than adult reference ranges throughout growth, from the age of 2 years. IGF-1 is also an important marker of overall nutritional status and will be abnormally low in under-nutrition and malnutrition, particularly in children and adolescents.

Osteocalcin

Osteocalcin is one of the most abundant proteins of the bone extracellular matrix, is secreted by osteoblasts, and is a measure of bone formation. Carboxylated osteocalcin (Gla-osteocalcin) binds tightly to hydroxyapatite within bone, while its undercarboxylated form (Glu-osteocalcin) enters the circulation. Recent evidence suggests that this form of osteocalcin has an important role in the regulation of insulin secretion (Figure 19.4). Osteocalcin is also age- and pubertal stage-dependent.

Others

PTH, magnesium, and calcium concentrations do not appear to be age-dependent.

19.4 Pharmaceutical agents commonly used in bone disease

Treatment of vitamin D-deficient rickets and osteomalacia

Vitamin D preparations used for vitamin D deficiency include ergocalciferol (D_2) and cholecalciferol (D_3), and either preparation is effective in restoring vitamin D stores in vitamin D deficiency. The active form of vitamin D, $1,25(OH)_2D_3$

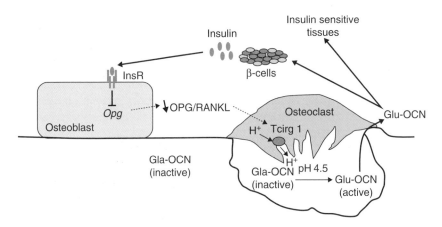

Figure 19.4 A feed-forward regulation loop links insulin, bone resorption, and osteocalcin. Reprinted from Clemens & Karsenty (2011), copyright © American Society for Bone and Mineral Research.

(calcitriol), should not be used to treat vitamin D deficiency as it 'bypasses' the regulating step of 1 alpha hydroxylation in the kidney and may lead to hypercalcaemia.

Treatment of hypoparathyroidism and genetic forms of metabolic bone disease

Calictriol is required for treatment of (i) hypoparathyroidism, (ii) renal osteodystrophy, (iii) X-linked hypophosphataemic rickets, and (iv) congenital disorders of vitamin D metabolism. An alternative, less-expensive pharmacological agent used in some countries is 1 alpha hydroxyvitamin D_3, which undergoes rapid hepatic conversion to $1,25(OH)_2D_3$.

Treatment of osteoporosis

(1) Bisphosphonates are a class of therapeutic agent that chemically resemble naturally occurring pyrophosphate and inhibit bone resorption. Bisphosphonates are commonly used in the treatment and prevention of senile osteoporosis and post-transplant, glucocorticoid (GC)-induced, and other osteoporotic conditions, where bone resorption is considered to be a major mechanism of osteoporosis. It is important to ensure that dietary calcium intake and vitamin D status are adequate to prevent hypocalcaemia, particularly immediately following intravenous administration of bisphosphonates.

(2) Calcitriol may be used an adjunct to the treatment and prevention of GC-induced bone disease.

(3) Dinosamab is a relatively recently developed fully human monoclonal antibody which acts by binding to and inhibiting RANKL, to inhibit bone resorption.

(4) Other recently developed osteoporosis treatments include parathyroid hormone and teriparatide (both anabolic agents), strontium ranelate, and selective oestrogen-receptor modulators (SERMs).

19.5 Diagnostic imaging assessment of the skeleton

Diagnostic imaging techniques are important in the evaluation of skeletal disease. In growing children, 'bone age' is determined by analysing a plain X-ray of the wrist, to assess the pattern of mineralisation in the carpal (wrist) bones, and epiphyses. Bone age is delayed by constitutional delay in growth, malnutrition, endocrine deficiencies such as hypothyroidism and growth-hormone deficiency, pubertal delay, chronic systemic disease, GC treatment, and untreated rickets. Bone age is accelerated by obesity, hyperthyroidism, and precocious puberty. Although skeletal radiography remains the most useful diagnostic imaging technique in the assessment of bone age and rachitic metabolic bone disease, it is insufficiently sensitive for the assessment of bone density. Consequently, a number of diagnostic imaging techniques have been developed, including single- and dual-photon absorptiometry, which have now been superseded by dual-energy X-ray absorptiometry (DEXA), which is currently the most widely used modality in clinical practice, and quantitative computed tomography (QCT), a more precise technique which measures actual volumetric bone density, but is currently used mainly as a clinical research tool. Ultrasound techniques have also been developed to assess bone density.

DEXA bone density

DEXA analyses photon absorption at two different energies to calculate the amount of bone mineral as bone-mineral content and bone-mineral density (BMD). It is able to measure both total body BMD and BMD at regional (clinically relevant) sites such as the lumbar spine, femoral neck and head, and Ward's triangle. DEXA also has the advantage of low radiation exposure, equivalent to approximately one-tenth that for a chest X-ray. BMD measured by DEXA is an areal bone density and actually assesses bone 'density' in cross-sectional area, and hence is expressed as g/cm^2 and is size dependent. Total body and regional (e.g. vertebral) cross-sectional area increases with increasing height and bone size, so for the same true volumetric bone density (g/cm^3), a short individual will be expected to have a lower areal bone density than a tall individual.

Adult BMD is expressed in terms of 'T' scores, which are standard deviation scores (SDSs) compared with a sex-matched healthy young adult reference range. According to World Health Organization (WHO) criteria, a T score of −1.5 to −2.49 SDS is defined as osteopaenia, and osteoporosis is defined as a T score of less than or equal to −2.5 SDS.

In growing children, the T score is clearly meaningless. Consequently, the BMD is compared with age- and sex-matched healthy children, and is expressed as a 'Z' score. However, even this approach has its limitations, because areal BMD increases with increasing bone size, and areal BMD thus increases during growth in childhood and adolescence. The Z score may appear to be within the osteopaenic or osteoporotic range because a child is smaller than his or her age-matched peers due to constitutional delay in growth and puberty, for example, when bone density would be expected to 'catch up' following the onset of puberty.

By assuming a cylindrical shape for the vertebra (for example), a true volumetric bone density may be calculated using DEXA technology. It has been shown that true volumetric bone density in normal, healthy growing children and adolescents remains relatively constant during growth.

QCT

QCT measures true volumetric bone density and can assess bone quality in more detail than is possible with DEXA, as cortical bone volume and trabecular bone volume can be assessed separately. The disadvantages of this method include scant reference data at the present time for children and adolescents, increased radiation exposure compared with DEXA, and the limitation to specific skeletal sites, as only the lumbar spine can be measured in a whole-body QCT, while other specific sites (e.g. involving upper or lower limb) may be assessed using peripheral QCT (pQCT).

Bone ultrasound

Bone ultrasound is another diagnostic imaging technique under development for the assessment of bone density. Paediatric and adolescent reference data remain limited, however. Once again, total body bone density cannot be assessed using this technique.

In summary, at the present time, DEXA using specific paediatric software remains the most widely available and best-validated method by which to assess BMD in children and adolescents, and in fact these features of DEXA apply across all age groups. Provided that the underlying assumptions of areal BMD are understood, DEXA currently remains the preferred method of initial clinical assessment of BMD.

19.6 Rickets/osteomalacia (vitamin D deficiency)

There is still no internationally agreed definition of rickets, particularly with regard to a 'cut-off' value for serum 25OH D_3 concentrations. In older infants and children, radiological changes (as outlined later) invariably occur with unequivocally low 25OH D_3 values, and the presence of rachitic radiological changes confirms a diagnosis of rickets in this age group, irrespective of other biochemical features present. The definition of osteomalacia, which occurs in adults, is arguably more uncertain, as adults no longer have 'growth plates', so that the characteristic metaphyseal changes seen in children do not occur.

In order to prevent vitamin D deficiency, milk products have been routinely fortified in the USA since 1957. Although milk was fortified previously, from the mid 1920s to the 1950s, with provitamin D_2 (ergosterol), and irradiated, this practice was stopped due to the development of hypercalcaemia in some individuals as a result of grossly excessive vitamin D exposure. Quality control for fortification of milk with vitamin D remains an issue, as hypercalcaemia has also occurred in recent years. Most European countries also now routinely provide vitamin D supplementation to exclusively breast-fed infants and fortify milk products with vitamin D, although in 'sunny countries' such as Australia there are no systematic public health measures to provide vitamin D supplementation. Yet in Australia sun avoidance is increasing due to the risk of developing melanoma and other skin cancers from excessive UVB exposure, and 'broad-spectrum' sunscreens which block both UVA and UVB from sunlight have been developed; with excessive use, these may also reduce skin exposure to UVB sufficiently to cause vitamin D deficiency.

Risk factors

General risk factors for vitamin D deficiency include those with:

- limited direct sunlight exposure
- highly pigmented skin
- malabsorption syndromes

Individuals at risk of vitamin D deficiency due to specific social and cultural settings include:

- those who are institutionalised and 'housebound', especially the frail elderly and chronically disabled;
- Islamic women who observe clothing practices such as hijab, in which they are almost entirely covered for reasons of modesty;
- highly pigmented individuals who are socially isolated, particularly apartment dwellers, who spend minimal time exposed to direct sunlight;
- exclusively breast-fed infants of vitamin D-deficient mothers (breast milk contains only 12–60 IU/l; see Table 19.4).

In the absence of vitamin D-fortified foods or vitamin D supplements, individuals living in polluted cities at high latitudes are at increased risk of vitamin D deficiency. Child-bearing women, infants, and young children are at greatest risk, and if environmental factors remain unchanged, individualised ongoing vitamin D supplementation is recommended (see Table 19.3). For lightly pigmented individuals, just 10–20 minutes' direct sun exposure of the face and forearms every day or so over summer should prevent the development of vitamin D deficiency.

Rickets in infants and young children

The association of rickets with sunlight deprivation was not recognised until the early twentieth century, although some physicians had recognised the antirachitic properties of cod liver oil before this. At the beginning of the twentieth century, 85% of children living in northern-hemisphere urban industrialised cities had rickets. In industrially developed countries today, rickets most commonly occurs in exclusively breast-fed infants born in cities at high latitudes to mothers who are also at risk of vitamin D deficiency due to poor sunlight exposure, unfortified food sources (such as milk), social isolation, increased skin pigmentation, or cultural clothing practices, independently or in combination.

In utero, the foetus receives 25OH D_3 through transplacental transfer from the maternal circulation. Hence neonatal 25OH D_3 levels reflect maternal stores. Premature infants and infants of vitamin D-deficient mothers are at high risk of vitamin D deficiency if vitamin D supplementation is not instituted routinely in the neonatal period. Breast milk is a relatively poor source of viatmin D, containing only 12–60 IU/l, even when mothers are vitamin D replete.

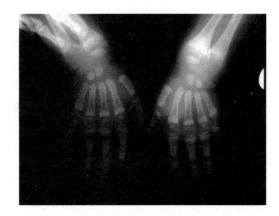

Figure 19.5 Upper-limb X-rays of an 18-month-old boy with vitamin D-deficiency rickets. Note the expanded metaphyses, particularly of the radius and ulnar at the wrist.

Clinical features

Hypocalcaemic seizures are a common presenting feature of rickets in infants aged less than 9 months, but are seen less frequently in older infants and toddlers. Older infants and toddlers tend to present with gross motor delay, leg bowing, or occasionally fragility fractures. However, the diagnosis may be made incidentally on biochemical testing or on chest X-ray performed for other reasons, such as investigation for failure to thrive or fever of unknown origin. The clinical characteristics of rickets include slowing of linear growth, rachitic rosary, wrist and ankle swelling, craniotabes (softening of the skull bones), a widely patent anterior fontanelle, frontal bossing, and reluctance to weight-bear/delayed walking. Rachitic bones are characteristically soft and pliable, as a result of growth of unmineralised bone osteoid (Figure 19.5). Consequently, wrist and ankle swelling and leg bowing become more marked as infants start weight-bearing through crawling, cruising, and walking. Rachitic rosary corresponds to the flaring of the costochondral junctions seen radiologically, and may be palpated anteriorly along the 'nipple line'; it is sometimes also visible on the anterior chest wall in infants and children in the setting of failure to thrive.

It is also important to be aware that other dietary deficiencies may coexist in prolonged, essentially exclusively breast-fed infants and toddlers through the second and into the third year of life, including iron-deficiency anaemia. If the mother is a vegan, consuming no dairy products, vitamin B_{12} deficiency may also be present. Older infants and children may also have abnormal dentition, due to enamel hypoplasia.

Radiological features

Rachitic X-ray changes include flaring of the costochondral junctions and frayed, cupped long-bone metaphyses, with generalised osteopaenia. The typical radiological appearance of rickets is shown in Figure 19.5. These radiological changes represent ongoing osteoid being laid down in bone, which is then poorly mineralised. Radiologically, gross metaphyseal changes are frequently not seen in infants under 3 months of age; however, generalised osteopaenia remains characteristic, and occasionally 'periosteal reactions' are also seen in the long-bone X-rays, giving rise to the radiological differential diagnosis of osteomyelitis or scurvy, which may be excluded on clinical grounds.

Biochemical features

Characteristic biochemical features include:

- raised ALP (BSAP), due to increased bone turnover;
- raised PTH, in response to hypocalcaemia;
- low or undetectable $25OH\ D_3$.

Other biochemical changes, such as serum $1,25OH$ D_3, calcium, and phosphate levels, are variable and dependent on the course of the disease. $1,25(OH)_2D_3$ may often be within the upper end of the reference range or frankly elevated. Both serum calcium and serum phosphate may be low or within the normal range, hence measurement of these parameters is unhelpful in diagnosis. Serum phosphate is characteristically decreased in long-standing rickets, due to the phosphaturic action of PTH.

Prevention

Pregnant and lactating mothers have an increased vitamin D requirement, two to four times the RDI for adults at other times. Identification of pregnant mothers at risk for vitamin D deficiency and providision of vitamin D supplementation during pregnancy will protect both the mother and the foetus from vitamin D deficiency. Postnatal administration of vitamin D to vitamin D-deficient lactating mothers needs to be approximately six times the adult RDI to correct the infants' vitamin D deficiency, indicating that it is preferable to give vitamin D replacement to the mother and infant separately. Vitamin D supple-

mentation of 400 IU daily to exclusively breast-fed at-risk infants, or vitamin D-supplemented infant formula feeds, totally prevent the development of vitamin D-deficiency rickets in otherwise normal infants.

Osteomalacia in adults

Vitamin D-deficiency osteomalacia in adults is an entirely preventable cause of osteoporotic fracture; however, it is often asymptomatic, or else individuals may present with vague symptoms of musculoskeletal aches and pains, depression, and lethargy. Occasionally adults may become significantly hypocalcaemic and present with carpopedal spasm or fitting. Characteristic biochemical changes and poorly mineralised osteoid on bone biopsy provide confirmation of vitamin D-deficiency osteomalacia in adults.

Vitamin D deficiency in the institutionalised and frail elderly

Institutionalised individuals with severe chronic physical and/or intellectual disability associated with epilepsy, such as severe cerebral palsy, are at risk of developing vitamin D-deficiency rickets or osteomalacia due to both limited direct sunlight exposure and anticonvulsant medication, which reduces vitamin D stores by increasing hepatic vitamin D inactivation through induction of the *CYP24R1* (24 hydroxylase) gene. The institutionalised elderly are also at risk of vitamin D deficiency through reduced direct sun exposure, compounded by ageing effects on the skin. This reduces the efficiency of vitamin D production in the skin, and on the gut, which results in reduced calcium absorption. Vitamin D deficiency is an important preventable cause of muscle hypotonia in the elderly. Screening for vitamin D deficiency in this group is recommended, in order to prevent hypotonia and an increased risk of falls and fracture in this vulnerable group.

Vitamin D deficiency in fat malabsorption

The 25-hydroxylated form of vitamin D is a fat-soluble vitamin and is 'recycled' within the enterohepatic circulation (Figure 19.3). Diseases which cause fat malabsorption, such as coeliac disease, and conditions associated with pancreatic exocrine insufficiency, such as cystic fibrosis (see Chapter 24) and chronic liver disease, are added risk factors for vitamin D deficiency across all age groups.

Other causes of rickets/osteomalacia

Chronic renal disease

Chronic renal disease generally, and in dialysis and immediately post-transplant patients in particular, is frequently associated with the following disorders:

- Protein-energy malnutrition and loss of lean muscle mass occurs in 18–75% of dialysis patients, depending on dietary protocols used. Protein restriction in chronic renal failure has been recommended in the past to reduce the degree of uraemia and to minimise further renal damage from excessive hyperfiltration. In more recent years, earlier institution of dialysis and renal transplant, especially in children, has improved protein-energy nutritional status in patients with chronic renal failure.
- Calcium deficiency is exacerbated by impaired $1,25(OH)_2D_3$ production, which results in hyperparathyroidism.
- Rickets/osteomalacia occurs in chronic renal disease via basically two mechanisms, either alone or in combination. These mechanisms are characterised by secondary hyperparathyroidism and adynamic renal bone disease.
- Secondary hyperparathyroidism develops due to associated impaired renal $1,25(OH)_2D_3$ production, which results in hypocalcaemia, which in turn causes secondary hyperparathyroidism. Hyperparathyroidism in this context is an appropriate response to $1,25(OH)_2D_3$ and dietary calcium deficiency, and may be reversed by ensuring sufficient dietary calcium intake and administration of calcitriol. Prolonged, poorly controlled secondary hyperparathyroidism may then progress to tertiary, or unregulated, hyperparathyroidism, which may require surgical intervention and total parathroidectomy, if other medical interventions are ineffective.
- Adynamic renal bone disease resembles senile osteoporosis, as it is characterised by decreased bone turnover, associated with low ALP and other bone-formation markers, and bone resorption

exceeds bone formation. The underlying causes of adynamic renal osteodystrophy are not well understood, but may include: aluminium toxicity in dialysis patients; poor protein/calorie nutrition and/or inappropriate mineral-ion nutrition; hormonal factors such as decreased IGF-1 bioactivity, either due to low IGF-1 associated with poor nutritional status or due to decreased bioavailabilty as a result of increased circulating IGF-binding proteins due to reduced glomerular filtration rate (GFR); and reduced weight-bearing activity due to lethargy associated with chronic illness.

Severe dietary calcium deficiency in young children

Rachitic features may also be observed after weaning when children have minimal access to dairy and other calcium-rich foods. Rachitic changes may also develop as a consequence of a combination of vitamin D and calcium deficiency, highlighting the need to take a very careful dietary history of calcium intake when assessing rachitic infants. Vitamin D replacement alone, without increasing dietary calcium, will result in persistent rachitic changes, radiologically and biochemically, with persisting raised ALP and PTH, in the presence of adequate vitamin D stores ($25OH D_3$ levels).

Genetic disorders

Genetic disorders causing renal phosphate wasting, such as X-linked and autosomal dominant hypophosphataemic rickets, usually present with leg bowing in toddlers and older children, with characteristic rachitic radiological changes, but differ biochemically, as hypocalcaemia and secondary hyperparathyroidism do not occur in untreated individuals with this condition. Affected individuals are treated with phosphate supplements and $1,25(OH)_2 D_3$ (calcitriol).

Genetic abnormalities of vitamin D metabolism are rare, but do need to be considered when children with rickets are clearly vitamin D sufficient. These include the autosomal recessive conditions of 1 alpha hydroxylase deficiency, which may be treated with calcitriol, and vitamin D-resistant rickets, due to genetic mutations within the vitamin D receptor, which may respond to high-dose calcitriol, although severely affected individuals may require parenteral calcium administration as the only means of treatment.

19.7 Mineral-ion homeostasis in preterm infants

A proportion of infants born prematurely will develop metabolic bone disease, but it is difficult to provide accurate figures for the true incidence as there are no widely accepted diagnostic criteria. Bone disease in preterm infants is principally due to substrate (calcium and phosphate) deficiency. Additional factors such as the administration of steroids and diuretics, and the effects of immobilisation or inactivity, also merit consideration for their independent effects on skeletal development.

Bone disease in preterm infants is characterised in the short term by a sequence of events which begins with biochemical evidence of disturbed mineral metabolism, continues with reduced bone mineralisation (as assessed by quantitative absorptiometric techniques), and results in abnormal bone remodelling and reduced linear growth velocity. In extreme forms, fractures of ribs and the distal ends of long bones and craniotabes have been reported. In the longer term, height may be reduced, and bone-mineral accretion in later childhood may also be affected.

Biochemical changes typically observed as part of metabolic bone disease in preterm infants

Whole-blood ionised calcium falls within 18–24 hours of delivery. This is a physiological rather than pathological event, reflecting continued calcium accretion into bone in the face of reduced exogenous calcium input, and a postnatal surge in calcitonin production of unknown aetiology. An increase in calcitonin will stimulate calcium uptake into bone, resulting in a reduction in calcium in the blood, until milk feeds are established. Hypophosphataemia characteristically develops at between 7 and 14 days of age, with plasma phosphate falling below 1.0 mmol/l, and is accompanied by hypophosphaturia, with tubular reabsorption of phosphorus typically >90%, indicating renal phosphate-conserving mechanisms in the infant.

Plasma ALP activity typically rises over the first 3 weeks of postnatal life to levels two- to three-fold greater than the maximum of the adult normal range. ALP increases further (from age 5 to 6 weeks) in infants who receive diets low in mineral substrate compared with those who receive diets with increased mineral content. In the short term, plasma ALP activity greater than five times the maximum of the adult normal range is associated with progressive slowing of linear growth velocity.

In phosphate-depleted infants, both hypercalcaemia (corrected plasma calcium >2.7 mmol/l) and hypercalciuria are frequently observed, possibly in response to elevation of $1,25(OH)_2D_3$. Where routine vitamin D supplementation of milk and cereals is practised, cord blood levels of 25OH D_3 are typically >50 nmol/l, indicating vitamin D sufficiency. Maternal supplementation with vitamin D results in higher cord blood levels of 25OH D_3, but not $1,25(OH)_2D_3$. Where maternal vitamin D intake during pregnancy has been poor, or where there is pre-existing maternal vitamin D deficiency, neonatal vitamin D stores may be low, and supplemental vitamin D of more than the normal 400 IU/day may be required.

A number of studies have identified low/borderline plasma 25OH D_3 and elevated $1,25(OH)_2D_3$ levels in the plasma of preterm infants fed unsupplemented human milk, suggesting an increased requirement for vitamin D during rapid bone turnover in phosphate-depleted infants. Many studies indicate that vitamin D supplementation does improve calcium absorption and retention, although the magnitude of this improvement is variable, possibly reflecting mineral as well as vitamin D status. There are no data indicating improved long-term outcome for infants receiving higher doses of vitamin D. There is no good evidence suggesting frank vitamin D deficiency in the majority of routinely vitamin D-supplemented preterm infants.

Radiological changes seen in preterm infants with metabolic bone disease of prematurity

Radiological abnormalities are occasionally seen at birth in very growth-retarded infants, presumably secondary to inadequate transplacental substrate supply. The majority of infants developing radiological abnormalities (rachitic changes, fractures) either weigh <1000 g at birth or receive diets grossly deficient in mineral substrate. Such diets include intravenous solutions formulated with inorganic mineral salts and expressed breast milk that is not supplemented with phosphate.

A useful scoring system based on single-view radiographs of the wrist or ankle at postnatal ages 5 and 10 weeks was described over 25 years ago by Koo, and it has been found that the majority of infants weighing less than 1000 g have evidence of abnormal remodelling using this system. In older reports, before the routine use of vitamin D supplementation of premature infants, epiphyseal cupping, splaying and fraying, and craniotabes were observed in up to 50% of the population of infants of less than 33 weeks' gestation. Fractures of the ribs and long bones were also widely reported.

Debate continues over the natural history of bone-mineral accretion in preterm infants after discharge from hospital. Some suggest a period of rapid 'catch-up', usually by 8–16 weeks post-term age, such that appendicular bone-mineral content estimated for preterm infants is similar to that of term infants. Increasing the mineral content of the post-discharge diet is associated with improved bone-mineral accretion rates. Many infants show a continuing deficit in radial bone-mineral content up to age 1 year. Beyond this time, there appears to be a gradual catch-up, and then continued increased mineral accretion (when compared with children born at term) from the age of 2 years.

Substrate delivery

Ideally, an intake of 2 mmol/kg per day of phosphate and 3 mmol/kg per day of calcium should be achieved in premature infants. Breast milk contains on average 0.5 mmol/100 ml of phosphate and 1 mmol/100 ml of calcium. Volumes of any milk greater than 240 ml/kg/day are rarely given in hospital. Without phosphate supplementation, a phosphate intake close to that needed to sustain normal bone-mineral accretion can only be achieved in an infant that has linear growth arrest.

In general, studies show that almost all the phosphate is absorbed whatever kind of milk is given, but that only 30–50% of the calcium is absorbed. The issue is much more critical for phosphate than for calcium, however, since 99% of calcium is in the bones, but only 60–70% of the phosphate. Phosphate is needed for many essential processes in the body, and in the face of phosphate insufficiency, bone resorption will occur to provide the balance required.

In summary, sick preterm infants, weighing <1000 g, on fluid restriction, diuretics, and steroids are at greatest risk of mineral-ion deficiency and osteopaenia of prematurity, and require careful attention, particularly in their recovery phase, to ensure that they receive appropriate mineral-ion supplementation in order to allow for normal bone mineralisation and linear growth.

19.8 Corticosteroid-induced bone disease

GCs are widely used pharmacologically for diverse diseases such as asthma, malignancy, and a variety of chronic inflammatory conditions. High-dose GCs are also increasingly being used as part of the immunosuppressive therapy required post-organ transplant. Unarguably GCs are very effective therapeutic agents; however, in high dose (equivalent to greater than prednisolone 2 mg/kg/day) they have a variety of actions on calcium homeostasis and bone itself which together contribute to reduced dietary calcium retention and the development of steroid-induced osteoporosis.

Actions mediated by PTH

The classical view of the effect of GCs was that they induced renal calcium efflux and inhibited calcium uptake from the intestine, leading to a fall in serum calcium and the development of secondary hyperparathyroidism. Increased peripheral sensitivity to actions of PTH has also been reported. The consequences of continuously elevated PTH levels are an increase in bone resorption and reduction in bone formation. This pattern of effects has been widely reported immediately after initiating GC therapy, but the increase in bone resorption does not usually continue. There is a relative increase in bone resorption versus formation, which suggests reduced osteoblastic activity or reduced osteoblastogenesis.

PTH has specific effects on the growth plate, acting through the PTH/PTH-related protein (PTHrP) receptor to inhibit chondrocyte differentiation. This may contribute to the slowing in growth observed clinically and in *in vivo* model systems. There are also thought to be direct effects of steroids on cartilage cells. Fewer cells exit the resting zone to progress through differentiation in animal-model systems of direct steroid infusion into the growth plate area. These underlying mechanisms are consistent with clinical observations of slowing linear growth and bone-age delay in children and adolescents on high-dose steroids, with observed catch-up in both bone age and linear growth following cessation of GCs.

Additional effects of GC excess on systems that modulate bone remodelling

Sex hormones, and oestrogen in particular, have a major role in maintaining normal bone health. Growth hormone (GH) and IGF-1 are also considered to have an important role in bone growth. GC excess causes a reduction of secretion of these hormones via several pathways:

- *Pituitary*: GCs inhibit secretion of GH, luteinising hormone/follicle-stimulating hormone, and adrenocorticotropic hormone. Although serum GH and IGF-1 levels are normal, IGF-1 bioactivity is reduced, possibly due to increased IGF-binding protein 1.
- *Gonadal function*: GCs inhibit synthesis of oestrogen by the ovary and testosterone by the testes.
- *Adrenal*: decrease in secretion (due to suppression of ACTH) of adrenal androgens, dehydroepiandrosterone (DHEA), and androstenedione.
- *Cellular transport*: GCs decrease transport of calcium and phosphate, particularly from the gut.

Direct effects on bone cells

There is debate about the effects of steroids directly on bone cells. While *in vivo* GCs are inhibitory, *in vitro* GCs can either stimulate or inhibit bone formation, depending on the model system, the conditions pertaining, and the amount of steroid in the system. It is important to distinguish between the developmental and regulatory effects of GCs on bone formation. GCs may enhance the differentiation of osteoblastic cells, thus providing more cells to contribute to new bone formation (see later), but in the complete organ they will also inhibit the functions of the differentiated cells and may induce apoptosis.

In the normal bone-remodelling cycle, bone resorption (which lasts about 2 weeks in any individual site) is followed by bone formation (which lasts about 2.5 months). In children, the amount of bone replaced in each 'packet' is 3% more than that removed, thus maintaining an increase in bone mass as part of skeletal linear growth.

In GC-induced bone disease in animals and humans, bone resorption is initially increased (for about a week after starting therapy) but then continues at the normal rate. However, the amount of new bone which is formed to 'fill in' the defects created by resorption is reduced, reflecting both an apparent reduction in osteoblastogenesis and an increased apoptosis of osteoblasts. Increased osteoblast and osteocyte apoptosis have been widely reported in sections of bone from GC-treated humans and animals. In the light of the recent data on the speed of onset/offset of fracture risk associated with steroid therapy, it has been suggested that preservation of the integrity of the osteocyte network is a critical factor in preventing fractures in GC-treated patients.

Prevention and treatment of steroid-induced osteoporosis

Because dietary calcium absorption and retention is approximately 20% less efficient with high-dose GC therapy, dietary calcium intake should increase accordingly. However, previous studies have failed to show a clear benefit from the use of calcium and vitamin D in the prevention of fractures in GC-treated adult patients. There is some evidence for beneficial effects with calcitriol and calcium in combination. Bisphosphonates are a class of drug which inhibit bone resorption, and have been found to be useful in the treatment of GC-induced osteoporosis in adults. In organ-transplant patients in particular, bisphosphonates have been given before transplant in an attempt to prevent the major increase in bone resorption post-transplant. There are no data available for children to indicate either the preferred mode of treatment of established osteoporosis caused by GCs, or prophylaxis in this vulnerable group.

19.9 Post-transplant bone disease

Organ transplants are carried out with increasing frequency and success, due to the development of potent immunosuppressive agents, which include GCs, cyclosporine A, azothioprin, tacrolimus, and newer agents such as rapamycin and mycophenolate mofetil. Post-transplant bone loss is multifactorial, and, as with chronic systemic disease (briefly discussed later), prolonged immobilisation, poor protein/calorie nutrition, hypogonadism, and underlying disease all contribute. Of the immunosuppressive agents listed, GCs and cyclosporine A have a major impact on post-transplant bone loss. The mechanisms of GCs are described in Section 19.8. Cyclosporine A causes rapid and severe bone loss by increasing osteoclastic bone resorption markedly in excess of bone formation. A degree of bone loss due to pre-existing disease commonly occurs pre-transplant, and in the initial stages post-transplant bone loss occurs rapidly and severely. It may then continue in the long term at slower rates, depending on disease state and the doses of long-term immunosuppressive agents required. Thus, prevention and treatment of post-transplant osteoporotic fractures is becoming a major challenge.

The severity of post-transplant bone loss varies according to the organ transplanted. For example, after renal transplant the rate of bone loss at the spine varies from 6 to 18% per year, with the highest rates occurring within the first 6 months after transplantation (compared with the average rate of bone loss during ageing of 1% per year), with fracture rates of 10–20% during the first year post-transplant. However, fractures, particularly in small bones, occur in nearly 50% of diabetic patients within the first 1–2 years after renal transplant with or without a pancreatic transplant, implying specific issues in this particular patient group, which may be related to a combination of pre-existing complications, glycaemic control, and nutritional issues. Fracture incidences of ~37% have been reported in lung-transplant recipients and ~65% in patients who have received liver transplants for primary biliary cirrhosis. Bone-marrow transplantation with adequate sex-hormone replacement does not tend to be associated with such severe bone loss and osteoporosis. Although it remains important to optimise calcium intake and absorption and adequate protein/calorie nutrition in this setting, overall the main contributors to post-transplant bone loss would seem to be the use of specific immunosuppressive agents that cause rapid and severe bone loss, and the major improvements in post-transplant bone loss is likely to be through the development of immunosuppressive protocols which use bone-sparing immunosuppressive agents.

19.10 Osteoporosis associated with chronic disease

Reduced sunlight exposure/vitamin D deficiency, immobility, use of GCs and immunosuppressive agents such as cyclosporine A, protein/calorie and mineral-ion under-nutrition/malnutrition, and hypogonadotropic hypogonadism associated with chronic systemic illness all contribute to the development of osteoporosis. Specific issues related to chronic diseases include:

- Cystic fibrosis, where fat malabsorption with vitamin D deficiency, protein-energy malnutrition, use of GCs, and post-lung transplantation are particularly relevant (see Chapter 24).
- Connective tissue diseases such as systemic lupus erythaematosis and rheumatoid arthritis, and cancer treatments, where the use of immunosuppressive agents including GCs may be specific issues in rheumatological and malignant conditions.
- Oxidative stress with increasing age may be a common molecular mechanism contributing to the development of senile osteoporosis, which often co-exists with other age-related pathologies such as atherosclerosis, insulin resistance, and hyperlipidaemia, all of which become more prevalent with advancing age. Furthermore, oxidative stress associated with poorly controlled type 1 insulin-dependent diabetes mellitus may be a common link between peripheral vascular disease, hyperlipidaemia, and osteoporosis observed in chronically poorly controlled type 1 diabetes mellitus. Consequently, dietary antioxidants may play a role in slowing the rate of progression of these diseases of ageing.
- Thalassaemia, in which untreated hypogonadism and extramedullary erythropoiesis and/or iron overload related renal phosphate wasting, may contribute to bone loss.

However, in chronic disease generally, the risk of development of osteoporosis in both children and adults may be reduced by ensuring vitamin D adequacy, optimising mineral-ion and protein/calorie nutrition, and encouraging appropriate weight-bearing exercise, together with consideration of the use of bisphosphonates.

19.11 Anorexia nervosa

Anorexia nervosa affects approximately 1% of adolescent girls in industrially developed countries, and is associated with considerable morbidity and mortality in up to 15% of affected individuals (see also Chapter 7). Recovery only occurs in up to 50–70% of affected individuals. Major skeletal effects include failure to accrue bone mass during the immediate postpubertal years and bone loss leading to osteoporosis, and are most marked in persistent, early-onset (premenarcheal) anorexia nervosa. Osteoporosis in anorexia nervosa is likely to be due to a combination of overall malnutrition, with both the direct effects of protein-energy malnutrition and the consequences of associated hormonal changes such as low serum IGF-1 levels and hypogonadotropic hypogonadism. Furthermore, these effects are not counterbalanced by the increased weight-bearing activity characteristically associated with this condition.

Clinical features

As a result of decreased food intake and increased energy expenditure, with or without self-induced vomiting and purgative abuse, ongoing weight loss of more than 15% below the minimum expected for age and height occurs. Due to food faddism, dietary intake may be inadequate in both quality and quantity. With specific reference to bone health, avoidance of high-fat dairy products may result in significantly reduced calcium-rich dairy food intake, and decreased overall protein/calorie intake may result in hypophosphataemia and insufficient protein for optimal bone growth. Other biochemical abnormalities which have a detrimental effect on bone formation include hypercortisolaemia, low serum IGF-1 levels, and hypogonadotrophic hypogonadism.

Treatment of anorexia nervosa-associated bone disease

Weight loss due to underlying malignancy or other chronic illness must be excluded at the outset, and having established the diagnosis of anorexia nervosa, treatment should result in improved dietary intake, using behavioural techniques and psychotropic drugs either alone or in combination, with institution of nasogastric feeding and strict bed rest if the individual's clinical status becomes life-threatening. Restoration of bone health depends on achievement of near normalisation of weight for height, and once this is achieved menses may also be expected to resume. Recovery from anorexia nervosa is defined as attainment of normal body weight within 15% of that expected for age and height, and resumption of regular menses for three consecutive cycles.

Clinical studies have shown that bone mass improves with recovery from anorexia nervosa, and normalisation IGF-1 with improved nutritional status is a likely important mediator of this observed improvement in bone mass. However, calcium replacement alone or in combination with oestrogen hormone-replacement therapy, in the absence of weight gain indicating overall improvement in protein/calorie nutrition, is ineffective in maintaining or restoring normal bone mass, implying that a combination of restoration of normal gonadal function and adequate calcium and protein/calorie nutrition is required to support normal bone growth and turnover.

19.12 Senile osteoporosis

Osteoporosis, characterised by thin and brittle bones, represents a significant public health issue in the elderly, and is defined by the WHO as bone density less than −2.5 SDS at two or more clinically relevant sites. Osteoporotic bone architecture is characterised by an irreversible destruction of trabecular bone structure and thinning of cortical bone. Osteoporotic fractures are characterised by 'fragility' fractures, which occur after trivial trauma or spontaneously, typically at the following sites:

- wrist (characteristically following a fall on an outstretched hand);
- femoral neck (occurring either spontaneously or following a fall, associated with severe morbidity, and commonly leading to death in the elderly)
- vertebra (usually occurring spontaneously).

Multiple vertebral fractures result in kyphosis, the 'dowager's hump'. Vertebral fractures are associated with chronic pain and stiffness, and may be associated with nerve-compression syndromes. With an increasingly ageing population in industrially developed countries, 25–35% of women and increasing numbers of elderly men will experience osteoporotic fractures, which result in significant morbidity and mortality, and add billions of dollars to healthcare costs worldwide. Male osteoporosis is becoming more common, as male cardiovascular mortality has decreased and a greater proportion of men are living beyond their eighth decade. More recently, it has been proposed that oxidative stress with increasing age may be the final common molecular pathway leading to senile osteoporosis, atherosclerosis, insulin resistance, and hyperlipidaemia, all features of both advancing age and poorly controlled diabetes mellitus. Oxidative stress with increasing age may be a common molecular mechanism contributing to the development of not only involutional osteoporosis, but several other pathologies, such as atherosclerosis, insulin resistance, and hyperlipidaemia, all of which become more prevalent with advancing age.

Pathophysiology

Osteoporosis occurring beyond the sixth decade is likely to be due to a combination of factors, including the menopause in women, unrecognised vitamin D deficiency, and numerous lifestyle factors, the most important of which are insufficient weight-bearing exercise and long-standing dietary calcium deficiency occurring over decades. Factors in the elderly leading to reduced calcium bioavailability are shown in Box 19.3. As a consequence of reduced calcium absorption and vitamin D deficiency, PTH levels tend to rise in the elderly, exacerbating osteoporosis.

Box 19.3 Factors in the elderly leading to reduced calcium bioavailability

- Reduced sunlight exposure in institutionalised or 'housebound' elderly.
- Ageing skin, reducing skin production of vitamin D.
- Decreased gastrointestinal absorption due to impaired $1,25(OH)_2D_3$ action on the gastrointestinal tract.
- Increasing incidence of atrophic gastritis with age, resulting in reduced gastrointestinal absorption of calcium.
- Thiazide and loop diuretics, increasing urinary calcium excretion.

Preventative strategies

Established osteoporosis is characterised by irreversible bone loss. Consequently, in recent years there has been a major emphasis on osteoporosis prevention through modification of lifestyle factors, such as optimising dietary calcium intake, ensuring vitamin D adequacy, taking regular weight-bearing exercise, and avoiding excessive alcohol consumption and smoking, together with oestrogen hormone-replacement therapy in younger post-menopausal women and testosterone replacement in hypogonadal men. Walking is the most appropriate weight-bearing exercise in the elderly. Although swimming may be soothing for arthritic joints and beneficial for cardiovascular health, it is non-weight-bearing and consequently in itself is not helpful in maintaining or improving bone strength.

Screening at-risk adults with the widespread availability in recent years of the DEXA assessment of bone density has enabled identification of individuals with osteopaenia and/or ongoing bone loss, so that intervention strategies, particularly with administration of bisphosphonates, may be instituted before the development of established osteoporosis and presentation with osteoporotic fractures, at which stage all current interventions for osteoporosis are much less effective. Other environmental factors, including fluoride deficiency, also contribute to enamel hypoplasia in teeth and osteoporosis, prompting water fluoridation in deficient areas. However, fluoride therapy at pharmacological doses has not been shown to decrease the rates of osteoporotic fracture in the elderly.

19.13 Concluding remarks

The interaction between nutrition and metabolic bone disease from infancy to senescence has been discussed in broad, general terms, with particular emphasis on the complex interactions between drugs, lifestyle factors, hormonal factors, and chronic systemic disease. There are a number of organ systems directly involved with mineral-ion homeostasis, namely the parathyroid glands, skin, liver, gastrointestinal system, and kidneys, and it may be perturbed by dietary mineral-ion deficiency, either directly or via vitamin D deficiency, by a number of other factors affecting the above organ systems and by the hormonal milieu of various systemic diseases.

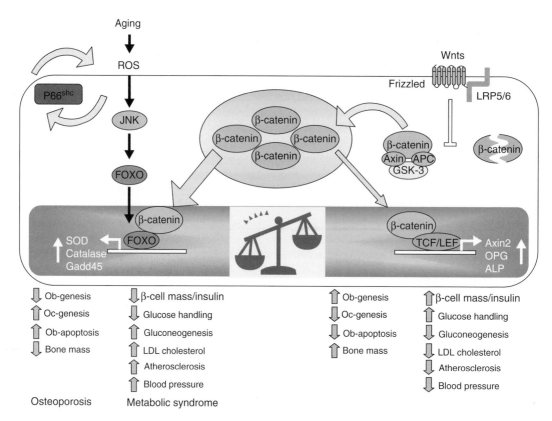

Figure 19.6 The increase of reactive oxygen species (ROS) with age antagonises the skeletal and metabolic effects of Wnt/β-catenin by diverting β-catenin from T-cell factor (TCF)- to forkhead box O (FOXO)-mediated transcription. Manolagas & Almeida (2007), copyright 2007, The Endocrine Society.

Advancing molecular techniques have provided further insights into the underlying mechanisms of age-related bone loss, and it has been proposed that oxidative stress with increasing age may be the final common molecular pathway leading to senile osteoporosis, atherosclerosis, insulin resistance, and hyperlipidaemia, all features of both advancing age and poorly controlled diabetes mellitus (Figure 19.6), and measures to reduce oxidative stress may also ameliorate the progression of senile/involutional osteoporosis.

Osteoporosis, the end point of a number of chronic systemic diseases, is usually the result of the interplay between a number of factors, and therapeutic interventions likewise need to be multifactorial, not only ensuring adequacy of dietary mineral-ion intake and vitamin D status, but also instituting modifications to lifestyle factors, such as optimising weight-bearing exercise, avoiding excessive alcohol, caffeine, and smoking, and instituting appropriate sex-hormone

replacement, with consideration of the use of bisphosphonate or other osteoporosis treatment modalities as appropriate. The clinical implications of appropriate prevention of vitamin D deficiency and treatment of rickets/osteomalacia and osteoporosis cannot be overemphasised, due to the significant associated long-term morbidity, with particular emphasis on osteoporosis and increased mortality, particularly in the elderly.

With an increasingly ageing population, there is a pressing need for nutritional preventative strategies to optimise dietary calcium and protein intake throughout life, in both healthy individuals and the chronically ill, as one of the many interventions required for the prevention and treatment of osteoporosis, an ever-increasing burden on health providers. Despite the widening use of antiresorptive agents such as bisphosphonates in the prevention and treatment of osteoporotic fractures, the challenge remains to develop safe and effective stimulators of bone formation. In recent years, there have been promising results to show the benefit of the use of PTH in the treatment of established osteoporosis in the elderly. However, the wider application of PTH in osteoporosis in growing children is currently precluded as there are data from animal experiments to show that the use of PTH may increase the incidence of osteosarcoma.

References and further reading

Australian National Health and Medical Research Council. Nutrient Reference Values for Australia and New Zealand: Including Recommended Dietary Intakes. Australia: Commonwealth of Australia, 2006.

Bikle D. Nonclassic actions of vitamin D. J Clin Endo Metab 2009; 94: 26–34.

Bishop N. Rickets today – children still need milk and sunshine. N Engl J Med 1999; 341: 602–604.

Canalis E, Giustina A, Bilezikian JP. Mechanisms of anabolic therapies for osteoporosis. JP New England Journal of Medicine 2007; 357: 905–916.

Chan GM, Mileur L, Hansen JW. Calcium and phosphorus requirements in bone mineralization of preterm infants. J Pediatr 1988; 113: 225–229.

Clemens TL, Karsenty G. The osteoblast: an insulin target cell controlling glucose homeostasis. J Bone Miner Res 2011; 26: 677–680.

Dawson-Hughes B. Calcium supplementation and bone loss: a review of controlled clinical trials. Am J Clin Nutr 1991; 54: 274S–280S.

Elder G. Pathophysiology and recent advances in the management of renal osteodystrophy (review). J Bone Miner Res 2002; 17: 2094–2105.

Epstein S, Inzerillo AM, Caminis J, Zaidi M. Disorders associated with rapid and severe bone loss (review). J Bone Miner Res 2003; 18: 2083–2094.

Favus M, Goltzman D. Regulation of calcium and magnesium. In: Primer on the Metabolic Bone Diseases and Disorders of Mineral Metabolism, 7th edn (Rosen CJ, Compston JE, Lian JB, eds). Washington, DC: American Society of Bone and Mineral Research, 2008, Chapter 21, pp. 104–108.

Grindulis H, Scott PH, Belton NR, Wharton BA. Combined deficiency of iron and vitamin D in Asian toddlers. Arch Dis Child 1986; 61: 843–848.

Holick MF. Vitamin D deficiency. N Engl J Med 2007; 357: 266–281.

Holick MF, Binkley NC, Bischoff-Ferrari HA, Gordon CM, Hanley DA, Heaney RP, et al. Evaluation, treatment, and prevention of vitamin d deficiency: an Endocrine Society clinical practice guideline. J Clin Endo Metab 2011; 96: 1911–1930.

Klaus G, Watson A, Edefonti A, Fischbach M, Rönnholm K, Schaefer F, et al. Prevention and treatment of renal osteodystrophy in children on chronic renal failure: European guidelines. Pediatric Nephrology 2006; 21(2): 151–159.

Manolagas SC, Almeida M. Gone with the Wnts: catenin, T-cell factor, forkhead box O, and oxidative stress in age-dependent diseases of bone, lipid, and glucose metabolism. Molecular Endocrinology 2007; 21: 2605–2014.

Martin TJ, Ng KW, Nicholson GC. Cell biology of bone (review). Baillière's Clin Endocrinol Metab 1988; 2: 1–29.

NIH Consensus Statement. Optimum Calcium Intake 12(4). Washington, DC: NIH, 1994.

Peacock M. Calcium absorption efficiency and calcium requirements in children and adolescents. Am J Clin Nutr 1991; 54: 261S–265S.

Pittard WB III, Geddes KM, Sutherland SE, Miller MC, Hollis BW. Longitudinal changes in the bone mineral content of term and premature infants. Am J Dis Child 1990; 144: 36–40.

Rizzoli R, Bonjour JP. Dietary protein and bone health (editorial). J Bone Miner Res 2004; 19: 527–531.

Rosen CJ. Vitamin D insufficiency. New Engl J Med 2011; 364: 248–254.

Salle BL, Glorieux FH, Delvin EE. Perinatal vitamin D metabolism (review). Biol Neonate 1988; 54: 181–187.

Salle BL, Glorieux FH, Lapillone A. Vitamin D status in breastfed term babies. Acta Paediatr 1998; 87: 726–727.

Sambrook PN, Kotowicz M, Nash P, Styles CB, Naganathan V, Henderson-Briffa KN, et al. Prevention and treatment of glucocorticoid-induced osteoporosis: a comparison of calcitriol, vitamin D plus calcium, and alendronate plus calcium. J Bone Miner Res 2003; 18: 919–924.

Schwartz RS. Genetic disorders of renal phosphate transport. New Engl J Medicine 2010; 362: 2399–2409.

Seeman E, Szmuckler G, Formica C, Tsalamandris C, Mestrovic R. Osteoporosis in anorexia nervosa: the influence of peak bone density, bone loss, oral contraceptive use, and exercise. J Bone Miner Res 1992; 7: 1467–1474.

Teegarden D, Lyle RM, McCabe GP, McCabe LD, Proulx WR, Michon K, et al. Dietary calcium, protein, and phosphorus are related to bone mineral density and content in young women. Am J Clin Nutr 1998; 68: 749–754.

Thomas MK, Lloyd-Jones DM, Thadhani RI, Shaw AC, Deraska DJ, Kitch BT, et al. Hypovitaminosis D in medical inpatients. N Engl J Med 1998; 338: 777–783.

20
Nutrition in Surgery and Trauma

Olle Ljungqvist[1] and Ken Fearon[2]

[1]Örebro University Hospital and Karolinska Institutet, Sweden
[2]University of Edinburgh, UK

Key messages

- The response to stress involves a cascade of neuroendocrine and proinflammatory events, which interact and influence each other.
- Together, these responses can have profound catabolic effects on body metabolism, especially following major surgery or trauma.
- A series of measures needs to be taken in the surgical/traumatised patient in order to ensure an adequate provision of and tolerance for nutritional support.

- In critical illness, blood glucose levels should be controlled (if necessary with insulin) to avoid hyperglycaemia.
- No single action will be sufficient to counteract the stress of injury, but a multimodal enhanced-recovery programme should be undertaken in order to turn the patient from catabolism towards an anabolic phase and hence recovery.

20.1 Introduction

Surgery and trauma constitute a major part of modern medicine. In the Western world, every year about 5% of the population has an operation, and some 40% of patients in hospitals undergo an operation as part of their treatment. Accidental major trauma is substantially less frequent, but these patients often require intensive care for prolonged periods of time.

While elective surgery represents an elective type of treatment in which deliberate actions are undertaken to remove or reconstruct organs, and hence can be well planned, trauma represents quite a different situation. Trauma involves a variety of different injuries and affects different parts of the body in different combinations: uncontrolled injuries have occurred, the patient is in a variable state of resuscitation, and the trauma team has to adapt to the situation as best possible. The objective of treatment is to preserve as many organs and bodily functions as possible with a minimum of further trauma.

Although the injuries can be very different, the response to injury is quite similar in surgery and in accidental trauma. The difference between the two lies in the ability to prepare the patient for the injury and to control homeostasis and the stress response in the elective surgical patient, which is not possible in the traumatised patient. The fact that elective surgery care programmes can be proactive, and the surgery performed under well-controlled and planned perioperative conditions, opens the possibility of enhancing recovery after elective surgery. The situation is different in trauma, where many of the proactive initiatives cannot be undertaken, for obvious reasons. Nevertheless, the global strategy for metabolic control and nutritional support is similar in both situations.

Clinical Nutrition, Second Edition. Edited by Marinos Elia, Olle Ljungqvist, Rebecca J Stratton and Susan A Lanham-New.
© 2013 The Nutrition Society. Published 2013 by Blackwell Publishing Ltd.

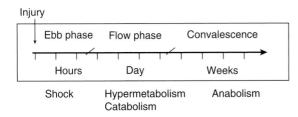

Figure 20.1 Phases of the physiological response to injury. After Cuthbertson (1982).

20.2 The stress response to trauma and its effects on metabolism

It is now about 70 years since Sir David Cuthbertson introduced the terms 'ebb' and 'flow' to describe the metabolic response to long-bone fracture (Figure 20.1). His was the first attempt to introduce some chronological order into the response to trauma and to include 'shock' as an integral part of the response, rather than as a complication. It is important to recognise that the main features of the metabolic response are initiated at the time of the injury and that this is probably the time at which modulation will be most effective. The mediators of such change include the classical neuroendocrine hormones, along with proinflammatory mediators.

The complexity of the interaction between the different components involved in traumatically induced stress is illustrated in Figure 20.2. The injury caused by the operation initiates an inflammatory response, causing the release of cytokines and acute-phase proteins and the activation of stress hormones. The release of these mediators causes a change of metabolism into a catabolic state. However, even in situations in which the inflammatory and endocrine responses are minimised, stress metabolism can occur. This indicates that other mechanisms are likely to be involved in causing the change in metabolism following surgery. Figure 20.2 also shows that fasting before elective surgery adds to the stress, by enhancing the endocrine stress response. In patients in whom stress-induced catabolism is pronounced or prolonged, the risk of complications increases. The development of complications will further aggravate the inflammatory and endocrine stress responses, which may become a vicious circle.

It is perhaps no longer useful to think of the 'ebb' phase as a period of depressed metabolism, but rather

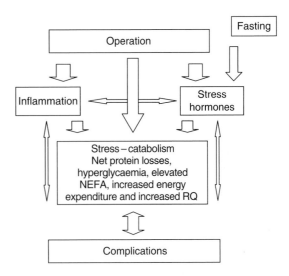

Figure 20.2 Schematic overview of the sequence of events that occurs in response to surgical trauma. NEFA, non-esterified fatty acids; RQ, respiratory quotient.

as the early stage after trauma during which tissue energy production is not limited by oxygen delivery. It is a neuroendocrine response and depends on the magnitude of blood loss and somatic afferent nervous stimuli arising from damaged tissues. These stimuli inhibit homeostatic reflexes subserving both the thermoregulatory and cardiovascular systems. After very serious injuries with failure of oxygen delivery, the 'ebb' phase of altered control mechanisms may be short-lived, as the patient enters into the potentially irreversible spiral of cell and tissue death known as 'necrobiosis'. The 'flow' phase is characterised by an increase in body temperature, metabolic rate, and urinary nitrogen excretion, associated with net protein breakdown, a reduction in muscle mass, and disturbances in energy substrate disposal.

Hypermetabolism

While it has been accepted since Cuthbertson's pioneering studies that hypermetabolism occurs in the 'flow' phase and that the increase is directly related to the severity of injury, there has been a considerable change in our understanding of the magnitude of that increase. In the early 1970s it was believed that the untreated, critically ill, septic, or trauma patient was expending in the region of 5000 kcal/day, creating major problems for those trying to introduce nutrition to the care of such patients. The introduction of clinically useful indirect calorimeters demonstrated that measured energy expenditures were most commonly less than half such predicted values. There was an understandable reluctance to accept these measured values until it was appreciated that a number of the features of critical illness and its treatment would reduce metabolic rate and therefore counterbalance those factors that tended to increase energy expenditure. Severely injured patients or those having undergone major surgery demanding intensive care will be resting in bed and hence the increase in basal metabolic rate (BMR) will be compensated for by the reduction in physical activity. Such patients may often be in bed for long periods, paralysed, ventilated, nursed in a warm environment, and receiving inadequate feeding, and will lose active muscle mass. It is, however, important to ensure that the metabolic rate is not limited by an inadequate supply of oxygen. Thus the majority of trauma patients have energy expenditures only 15–25% above their predicted healthy resting values. The exceptions may be those with excessive burns, although the introduction of early wound excision and grafting in place of treatment with exposure and delay of grafting has reduced the problem of massively elevated energy demands.

There are several factors leading to hypermetabolism and, therefore, an increase in energy expenditure in critical illness. First, there is an upward resetting of thermoregulation, which mediates an increase in energy production through enhanced activity of the sympathetic nervous system. A positive relationship has been demonstrated between urinary catecholamine excretion and metabolic rate in burn injury. Although plasma catecholamine concentrations are increased during the 'flow'-phase response to burns and severe head injury, they are apparently normal after severe musculoskeletal injuries and sepsis. However, such plasma levels may provide only limited information about the state of sympathetic activation following trauma or sepsis as catecholamine turnover is known to double in sepsis.

An increase in sympathetic activity may stimulate metabolic rate by enhancing substrate cycling between non-esterified fatty acids and triacylglycerol, glucose, and glycolytic products. Similarly, protein–amino acid recycling may equally contribute to the increased BMR. The wound, be it an abscess, burn, or fracture, acts as an extra organ and also contributes to this glucose cycling. Lactate produced by anaerobic glycolysis in the wound is transported to the liver, where it is converted to glucose in the Cori cycle, an energy-consuming process. The wound will also contribute to hypermetabolism in a number of other ways. For example, wounds have a hyperaemic circulation, which is not under neural control, and may require an increase in cardiac output and energy expenditure. Activated inflammatory cells in the wound (and elsewhere) have a high oxygen consumption and release a number of cytokines (e.g. interleukin 1 beta (IL-1β) and tumour necrosis factor alpha (TNFα), which have been implicated in the centrally mediated upward resetting of metabolic activity.

It was believed that the increase in protein turnover associated with the 'flow' phase contributed at least 20% of the increase in the metabolic rate, but this is now believed to be an overestimate, except perhaps in children. Nevertheless, intravenous feeding with amino acids elevates body temperature and can be used as a way of maintaining body temperature during major surgery. There may also be an iatrogenic component to hypermetabolism, especially for those being fed parenterally.

The administration of calories (especially carbohydrates) has been shown to increase sympathetic activity and metabolic rate. This response may be enhanced in sepsis (although this has not been a universal finding). In some patients, glucose-based total parenteral nutrition (TPN) has been associated with an increase in respiratory minute ventilation greater than that expected from the increased metabolic load. This respiratory distress can be ameliorated by replacing some of the glucose with fat emulsion, thereby suggesting that increased CO_2 production (most pronounced when the respiratory quotient (RQ) rises above 1.0) may be an important factor. Amino acid solutions can also increase ventilatory 'drive'. This may be due to their low pH, but can also be secondary to a decrease in the serotoninergic suppression of ventilatory drive following inhibition of tryptophan uptake into the brain by increased levels of branched-chain amino acids in the plasma.

Thus the 'flow' phase of the response to trauma/sepsis is characterised by a moderate degree of hypermetabolism. A number of factors mediate the increase, but the most important seems to be a complex interaction between the wound and the central control of metabolic rate, in which the cytokines may have a pivotal role. The proinflammatory response, in combination with counter-regulatory hormones, may also mediate the changes in peripheral metabolic control, including insulin resistance.

Protein metabolism

Cuthbertson noted an increase in urinary nitrogen excretion after long-bone fracture, which he attributed to increased protein breakdown. A recent study showed that following either severe trauma or sepsis, patients admitted to intensive care sustained, on average, a loss of 17% of body water, 16% of total body protein, and 19% of total body potassium over 21 days. These losses were greater than can be accounted for by bed rest alone and occurred even when the patient was in a positive energy balance. The major site of protein loss was skeletal muscle but nitrogen loss also occurred in respiratory muscles and in the gut, although cardiac muscle appeared to be mostly spared.

Muscle wasting represents an imbalance between protein synthesis and degradation. After minor/moderate surgery there is a decrease in synthesis, mirroring the response to short-term starvation. With a more severe insult, protein synthesis in different tissues can be increased (for example, acute-phase protein synthesis in the liver) or decreased (muscle protein synthesis), while protein degradation in skeletal muscle is increased. Inflammatory conditions are associated with an increase in the hepatic synthesis and plasma concentration of a number of so-called positive acute-phase proteins. The positive acute-phase proteins include fibrinogen, C-reactive protein, alpha-1-acid glycoprotein, haptoglobulin, alpha-1-antitrypsin, alpha-2-macroglobulin, and ceruloplasmin. In the human hepatocyte, the main proinflammatory cytokine regulating this response is interleukin-6 (IL-6). On the other hand, the plasma concentration of a number of liver export proteins (e.g. albumin) falls acutely (negative acute-phase reactants) after injury.

Rather than reflecting a reduced synthesis rate, the fall in the plasma concentration of negative acute-phase proteins is thought to be due mainly to increased transcapillary escape, secondary to an increase in microvascular permeability. Thus, although the plasma concentration of the negative acute-phase reactants falls, the net metabolic demands on the liver increase due to continued synthesis of negative reactants, combined with increased synthesis of positive reactants.

The increased protein degradation that occurs in skeletal muscle following injury may be due to increased activity of three different systems: the lysosomal system, the Ca^{2+}-dependent calpain pathway, and the ubiquitin–proteasome pathway. Recent research has suggested that the ubiquitin–proteasome pathway is the major pathway but that it works in concert with the calpain system. The metabolic significance of increased activity of the ubiquitin–proteasome pathway comes from the fact that the process whereby proteins are tagged with ubiquitin for degradation in the proteasome requires adenosine triphosphate (ATP) and therefore, once activated, this pathway not only contributes to the negative nitrogen balance but also the negative energy balance of the patient.

Insulin resistance

Insulin is the best-known anabolic hormone. It is normally released promptly in response to feeding and ensures the storage of nutrients. Although insulin levels peak within less than an hour after feeding, the effects on metabolism remain for another few hours. Insulin promotes oxidation and storage of carbohydrates and fat, and it has a protein-sparing effect.

Insulin resistance is commonly associated with diabetes mellitus. However, in many situations of stress, such as accidental trauma, sepsis, burns, and elective surgery, a state of transient insulin resistance develops in otherwise healthy individuals. From a theoretical point of view, many of the metabolic changes found following trauma can be explained by a reduction in the effectiveness of insulin in exerting its normal actions. In most clinical situations of stress, the resistance to insulin can be overcome by insulin treatment. This was shown to be of importance in postoperative patients in need of ventilatory support in the intensive-care unit (ICU). When glucose levels were maintained at normal levels, morbidity was markedly reduced and mortality almost halved. Interestingly, the effects of insulin were a reduction in a series of complications usually associated with chronic diabetes, such as sepsis and infections, renal function, and polyneuropathy. It is well known that these complications occur in the ICU, and they are clearly associated with poor metabolic control. While the first studies using intensive insulin treatment had very good results when aiming at normoglycaemia, large-scale follow-up studies in general ICU patients and in postoperative patients revealed risks of adverse outcomes due to hypoglycaemia. Therefore, the target glucose level for this treatment in the ICU has been modified from strict normoglycaemia (4.5–6.0 mmol/l) to a moderate hyperglycaemia of 7–8 mmol/l in order to avoid the risks associated with hypoglycaemia.

Insulin resistance in elective surgery has also been studied in detail. The degree of insulin resistance that develops is related to the magnitude of the operation. Following routine upper-abdominal surgery, insulin resistance prevails for about 2–3 weeks. Surgical technique is also a factor affecting the magnitude of insulin resistance, in that laparoscopic techniques result in less pronounced insulin resistance than open surgery. Many of the changes in glucose metabolism following surgery are similar to those found in type 2 diabetic subjects (Table 20.1). Thus, postoperative hyperglycaemia develops as a result of both an increase in glucose production and a decrease in glucose uptake in peripheral tissues. This reduction is associated with a decreased responsiveness of specific glucose-transporting proteins, GLUT4, that are normally activated by insulin to facilitate glucose uptake in insulin-sensitive tissues. This was recently shown to be due to reduced activity of PI 3 kinase, a key intracellular signal to activate GLUT4. Further, inside the cell there is a reduced capacity to store glucose, while glucose oxidation is maintained or even enhanced. In addition, in muscle, protein breakdown is enhanced, and this has also been shown to be related to changes in the signalling pathways, namely by reducing the activity of protein tyrosine kinase, regulating protein metabolism inside the muscle cells.

The relationship between these changes and fat metabolism is less well understood. However, insulin seems to play an important part in all aspects of post-trauma metabolism. Thus, urea excretion is normalised when glucose is given along with insulin, whereas glucose alone has no effect. In addition, when insulin is given in sufficient amounts to maintain normal glucose levels during TPN following elective colorectal surgery, nitrogen balance is normalised, as are fatty acid levels and substrate

Table 20.1 Changes in glucose metabolism following elective surgery. These changes are compared to the changes seen in type 2 diabetes mellitus. Data derived from studies using insulin stimulation under controlled circumstances while maintaining euglycaemia (hyperinsulinaemic euglycaemic clamp) or by measurement of specific glucose-transporting proteins (GLUT4) on the cell surface before and during insulin stimulation.

Metabolic event	Normal response to insulin	Type 2 diabetes	Postoperative
Whole-body insulin sensitivity	↑	↓	↓
Endogenous glucose production	↓	↑	↑
Glucose uptake	↑	↓	↓
Glucose transport into skeletal Muscle (GLUT4 activation)	↑	→	→
Nonoxidative glucose disposal	↑	↓	↓

oxidation. Furthermore, when insulin resistance is prevented, it allows complete enteral feeding without the development of hyperglycaemia and is associated with a neutral nitrogen balance after major colorectal surgery.

Some very recent studies have shown that insulin resistance is directly related to the risk of postoperative complications. Hence, in a study of almost 300 patients undergoing elective cardiac surgery, the degree of insulin resistance when the patients were leaving the operating table was proportional to the risk for major complications, in particular postoperative infections. Another large observational study showed that poor glucose control following elective colorectal surgery was also related to more complications, again mostly infectious. Hence evidence is mounting to indicate that metabolic control, and retaining of anabolic capacity by retaining insulin action, is a key component to avoiding complications after surgical trauma.

20.3 Nutritional support in perioperative care

The majority of elective surgical patients have a normal nutritional status and normal metabolism prior to surgery and usually the surgery is of minor or moderate extent. These patients can eat and should be given normal hospital food as soon as possible after the operation.

A much smaller group of surgical patients are malnourished. These patients have a higher risk of mortality, complications, prolonged hospital stay, and delayed rehabilitation and convalescence. Although some early studies of perioperative nutritional support were conflicting, over the last 20 years a succession of studies have begun to define those groups of patients who benefit, particularly those with prior severe malnutrition. Because of the risks associated with malnutrition and surgery, all patients about to undergo surgery should be screened and assessed for nutritional status. In severely malnourished patients the overall surgical strategy should be reviewed carefully (e.g. restage cancer patients for occult metastases or irresectability) or the nature of surgery/intervention should be curtailed (e.g. use endoscopic stenting as a bridge to surgery or perform a stoma rather than an anastomosis). Those with severe malnutrition should also be considered for artificial perioperative nutritional support.

The low-risk patient undergoing elective surgery

An overview of how to care for the low-risk patient's nutrition in the perioperative period is given in Table 20.2.

Preoperative management

These patients have a normal nutritional status. They can and should eat normal food up until the evening before surgery. Patients undergoing intestinal resections have traditionally been prepared by bowel cleansing the day before surgery. The idea behind bowel cleansing is that if the large bowel is free from faecal matter, the risk of postoperative infection may be reduced. This routine, and its underlying hypothesis, has recently been questioned. Several recent trials have shown no benefit from the use of mechanical bowel preparation in colonic resection, but rather the disadvantage of possibly increasing postoperative anastomotic leak rates. Most patients should therefore not be prescribed bowel cleansing, but rather a small enema. However, for patients who are prescribed preoperative bowel cleansing, low residue oral nutrition supplements can be recommended during or after the cleansing to ensure that the preoperative fasting period is as short as possible. This type of nutrition is nearly fully absorbed and therefore does not compromise bowel cleansing. Treatment with a preoperative carbohydrate-rich drink 2 hours before the anaesthesia on the morning of the operation will minimise thirst, hunger, and preoperative anxiety. In addition, postoperative insulin resistance will be reduced (see the section on glucose control).

Postoperative management

The therapeutic goal for the postoperative patient is rapid recovery to normal function and well-being, the minimisation of complications, and early discharge home. This aim reflects not just good clinical practice but good economics. Minimising the development of catabolism and returning the patient from the catabolic state to one of anabolism is an important part of this process, in which nutrition has a major role. Pre- and perioperative manoeuvres to minimise stress are important, and postoperative

Table 20.2 Nutrition in the uncomplicated patient undergoing small- to medium-size surgery.

Period	Nutrition	Comments
Preoperative		
Day before surgery	Normal food until midnight before surgery	For most patients, to ensure energy and protein intake
	If bowel cleansing 400 ml sip feeds	
Morning of surgery	Preoperative carbohydrates	To minimise discomfort and reduce insulin resistance
Postoperative		
Day of surgery, when fully awake	Free fluids and light meal (tea and biscuits)	
	Sip feeds 200–400 ml	
Day of surgery, evening	Try regular food	If unable to eat solid food, give 200–400 ml sip feeds
Day after surgery	Regular food	If needed, supplement with sip feeds

early oral intake and mobilisation are useful weapons in this process. Sip feeds should be given to patients who do not meet their nutritional goals with hospital food. In a few cases, artificial feeding by the enteral or even the parenteral route may also have a role.

There is no scientific backing for withholding food from patients after surgery. Most patients undergoing surgery can commence oral feeding within hours after the operation. Oral supplements are a very useful prescription for patients who do not tolerate or only partially cover their energy needs with hospital food. Enteral feeding has also been shown to reduce postoperative complications and reduce length of stay in a recent meta-analysis. However, for various reasons, oral feeding is often delayed. The factors that most often cause a delay in the return of normal food intake are old traditions and beliefs that intake of food will cause an increased rate of anastomotic leakage. In addition, there is the belief that bowel movements must occur before it is safe to allow patients to drink and eat. Many of the factors delaying a return to normal gastrointestinal function and normal feeding are caused by routines that are still in practice. These factors can be overcome by changing the traditional routines that have been shown to be unnecessary or even harmful, as outlined earlier.

The malnourished or complicated surgical patient

The overall goals for the compromised patient or the patient undergoing major surgery are the same as for the uncomplicated patient; that is, to promote more rapid recovery. The basis for treatment is the same, and the general guidelines given for the low-risk surgical patient should form the basis for the higher-risk patient. However, in addition to these principles, high-risk or malnourished patients often present a greater level of complexity, which may demand other measures be taken to ensure adequate nutritional and metabolic support.

Preoperative

Several studies have demonstrated that a week or two of preoperative feeding, enterally or parenterally, improves the outcome from surgery in patients with severe malnutrition. On the other hand, artificial nutritional support in those with normal nutritional status or only mild malnutrition is associated with either no benefit or even an increase in complications. Such an increase for preoperative TPN was demonstrated in studies performed over a decade ago, although the higher infection rates may have been due to an overloading of carbohydrate and subsequent hyperglycaemia. In addition, the TPN solutions used lacked glutamine, which may also have adversely influenced the results.

Postoperative feeding of patients who cannot eat postoperatively

The situation is different for patients who are unable to take normal food than that for the uncomplicated patient. The routine use of postoperative parenteral nutrition has not proved useful in previously well-nourished patients or in those in whom normal eating is possible within 7 days after operation. There is some evidence of benefit from parenteral nutrition under the following conditions:

- As a continuation of preoperative nutritional support in previously malnourished patients.
- In patients with postoperative complications that impair gastrointestinal function and prevent normal oral feeding for 5–10 days postoperatively.
- In previously severely malnourished patients undergoing emergency surgery.
- In previously well-nourished patients who have suffered major trauma or critical illness and who are unable to tolerate enteral feeding.

The weight of evidence suggests that enteral feeding by the nasogastric, nasoenteral, and jejunal routes, or a combination of some enteral and supplementary parenteral feeding, is the preferred method, although, in the presence of prolonged gastrointestinal failure, parenteral feeding may be life-saving. Some trials indicate that early and adequate oral supplementation in the first week after surgery may improve outcome, particularly in the malnourished patient. A flowchart for the management of postoperative nutrition in surgical patients is shown in Figure 20.3.

Glucose control in nutritional support of the critically ill

There is growing and strong evidence that glucose levels should be maintained at near-normal levels

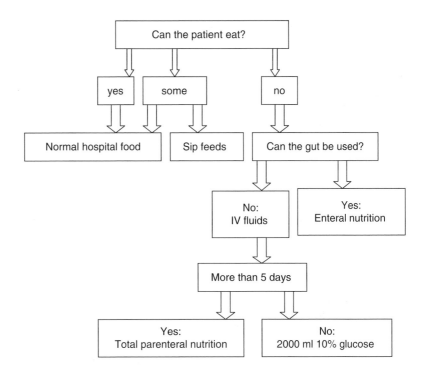

Figure 20.3 Schematic overview of suggested routes to ensure energy and protein intake following surgery.

while feeding the severely stressed surgical patient. Hyperglycaemic diabetic patients undergoing surgery have long been known to run a substantially higher risk of complications (mainly infectious) than nondiabetic patients, or those in whom glucose control has been optimised. It has been shown that this also holds true for patients without diabetes. It was first demonstrated in a study from Belgium that postoperative patients (mainly thoracic surgery) in need of ventilatory support in an ICU setting benefit from intensive insulin treatment to normalise glucose levels (aiming at 4.5–6 mmol/l). Normalising glucose levels using insulin resulted in marked reductions in septic episodes, renal failure, time on ventilator, polyneuropathy, and mortality. The results show that insulin action seems to be key to successful immediate postoperative feeding, but also to avoiding complications that will cause further catabolism. Later studies, however, revealed the danger of adverse hypoglycaemia as a result of too much insulin, and hence the current general recommendations suggests targeting blood glucose at between 7 and 8 mmol/l to reduce the risk of hypoglycaemia.

The use of insulin to maintain glucose control is likely to be a better approach than semi-starvation through carbohydrate restriction. Whether the beneficial effects of insulin are confined to the maintenance of near normoglycaemia or include the previously demonstrated reduction in net protein catabolism and cell-membrane function remains to be determined.

Growth hormone has been tested in a series of clinical trials as a method of inducing anabolism in critically ill patients. It is of interest that the increased mortality experienced with the use of growth hormone in critical-care patients has been ascribed to growth hormone-induced insulin resistance.

Adverse effects of traditional perioperative care in elective surgery patients

Traditional perioperative surgical practice has focused on prolonged fasting both before surgery, to reduce the risks of aspiration, and after surgery, in the face of 'natural' postoperative ileus. In addition, little effort has been made to reduce the classical neuroendocrine stress response, which has been accepted as an inevitable consequence of surgical intervention. Finally, patients have been given excess intravenous fluids based on the principle developed

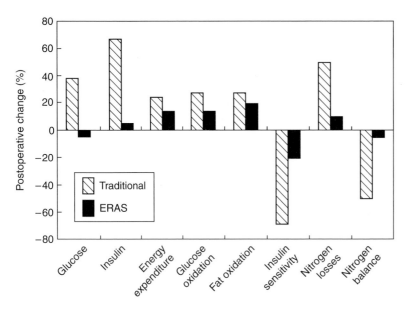

Figure 20.4 The relative changes in different parts of the metabolic response to surgery using traditional perioperative methods compared to perioperative care according to enhanced recovery after surgery (ERAS) programmes. The ERAS concept is described in more detail in the text. Reprinted with permission from Soop M. Effects of perioperative nutrition on insulin action in postoperative metabolism (PhD thesis). Stockholm, Sweden: Karolinska Institutet, 2003.

in trauma resuscitation that 'wet is best'. Recent evidence has shown that ad lib administration of intravenous saline results in oedema of the gut, with delayed gastric emptying, delayed return to normal nutrition, and prolonged hospital stay. The adverse influences of prolonged fasting, unmodulated stress, and saline overload are thought to contribute to net catabolism, postoperative fatigue, and prolonged recovery time from conventional surgery. Several other measures traditionally used in the perioperative period have been shown to be outdated. These include the use of opioids for pain control, bed rest, the use of nasogastric tubes, and prolonged use of catheters and drains.

Enhanced recovery after surgery: modern techniques to minimise stress and support nutrition in elective surgery

When endocrine hormones were discovered and became measurable in the last century, early reports showed that even medium-size open surgery (such as uncomplicated open cholecystectomy) evoked marked release of all the classical stress hormones (catecholamines, cortisol, glucagon, and growth hormone). This in turn was associated with insulin resistance leading to hyperglycaemia, elevated free fatty acid levels, and protein loss caused by increased protein breakdown and reduced protein synthesis.

Since then, modern anaesthesia, minimally invasive surgery, and other perioperative developments have allowed the same operation to be performed with no or minimal stress response. The difference between the classical responses to surgery some 10 years ago and what can be achieved using modern techniques is shown in Figure 20.4.

It is important to understand that postoperative metabolic changes still play an important role in the development of secondary complications and in recovery in general. It is therefore not surprising that nutritional regimens play an important role in the postoperative phase. Recovery from surgery requires a reversal of trauma-induced catabolism and a move towards anabolism. There are several ways by which the catabolic responses can be minimised and anabolism supported. Nutrition – the supply of macro- and micronutrients – represents an essential part of perioperative treatment.

When applied properly, enhanced recovery after surgery (ERAS) protocols have been shown to reduce recovery time and need for hospital stay by 2–3 days following colonic resections, and at the same time reduce complications by up to 50%. Recent studies have shown that the better the compliance to best practice – that is, ERAS treatment elements – the better the outcome. The ERAS programme represents a major change for traditional care, as will be outlined in this section.

Nutrition in enhanced recovery after surgery programmes

ERAS protocols, or 'fast-track' surgery programmes, involve an integrated series of steps aimed at minimising the stress of a surgical operation and informing and involving the patient in their recovery. The various events and treatments in the perioperative period have been scrutinised for supportive evidence in the literature and old routines with no scientific backing have been exchanged for routines shown to have positive effects on recovery. These programmes have been shown to minimise reduced physiological function and to enhance the return to normal function. A key aspect is the support of normal gastrointestinal function and an early return to normal fluid and food intake. Many of the programmes have targeted patients undergoing gastrointestinal (primarily colon) surgery, and have shown clearly that the time of recovery after this type of surgery is prolonged by the use of old traditions and outdated routines.

Preoperative carbohydrate treatment instead of overnight fasting

It has been assumed that the traditional preoperative overnight fast is useful and not harmful. However, over the last decade many national anaesthesia societies have changed preoperative fasting guidelines and now recommend free intake of clear fluids until 2–3 hours before anaesthesia for elective procedures. This change has been proven safe and was introduced to reduce the discomfort of thirst. This routine also helps to avoid preoperative dehydration.

It has been shown recently that the metabolic changes that occur during an overnight fast influence the response to stress. In studies in which a patient's metabolic status has been changed from the overnight-fasted state to the carbohydrate-fed state by intake of an iso-osmolar carbohydrate-rich drink, marked effects on postoperative insulin resistance have been observed. This treatment not only reduces thirst but also improves hunger and preoperative anxiety. For patients who are excluded from using modern fasting guidelines, intravenous glucose with or without insulin has been shown to have the same benefits. Provided the glucose load is sufficient (5 mg/kg/minute, often by use of 20 or 30% glucose solutions), the metabolic change from that of overnight fasting to a fed state can be achieved along with

glycogen loading. This regimen has been shown to reduce cardiac complications after cardiac surgery and protein losses, and to improve muscle function, patient well-being, and recovery.

Continuous epidural analgesia

A central part of the multimodal approach to recovery after open surgery is the preoperative placement and activation of a continuous epidural based primarily on the infusion of local anaesthetic with or without opiates. For open abdominal surgery, the epidural should be placed in the lower thoracic region. This places a block over the abdominal wall and the adrenals, hence attenuating the release of catecholamines. By activating the epidural before the operation, it can be determined that the block covers the region of the proposed incision and that it will function well as the basis for postoperative pain relief.

An effective and functional epidural has several effects. Blocking the adrenals and minimising catecholamine release can reduce postoperative insulin resistance. Effective pain relief also has positive effects on insulin sensitivity. Finally, systemic opioids can be avoided. Opioids have a negative effect on both gastric emptying and gastrointestinal motility in general.

Balancing fluids to support postoperative gastrointestinal function

Overloading the patient with fluids and sodium chloride perioperatively causes oedema and delays the return of normal gastrointestinal function. Balancing postoperative maintenance fluids at 2000 ml and NaCl at 77 mmol/day has been shown to substantially enhance gastric motility and speed up recovery. Stopping intravenous fluids on the first postoperative day is one of the key factors in the ERAS approach to recovery.

Minimally invasive surgical techniques

With the widespread use of laparoscopic techniques in surgery, it has become evident that minimally invasive techniques play an important role in the recovery of the patient after surgery. Laparoscopic surgery allows the same procedure to be performed with substantially less pain, discomfort, and metabolic derangement. Specifically, the proinflammatory cytokine response is attenuated, while the neuroen-docrine stress response is dampened to a lesser degree. For many procedures, laparoscopic surgery has become the method of choice. This is particularly true for upper gastrointestinal procedures, but is becoming increasingly so for lower gastrointestinal procedures.

Interestingly, a recent report showed that patients undergoing laparoscopic cholecystectomy had sub-stantially lower rates of postoperative nausea when given a preoperative dose of corticosteroids well before the onset of the operation. This finding sug-gests that even with a relatively minor operation, beneficial effects can be demonstrated by blocking the inflammatory response prior to the procedure. Hence, even with minimally traumatic and invasive techniques, multimodal postoperative care should be considered.

Drains, tubes, and catheters

There is evidence that postoperative 'drip and suck' regimens are used excessively and unnecessarily in traditional patterns of postoperative care. Nasogastric drainage tubeshave been shown in a large meta-analysis of published studies to be associated with increased complication rates, particularly respiratory infections. They should therefore be used only when absolutely necessary, as in gastric outlet obstruction.

The metabolic effects of a combined treatment programme

It has been shown recently that when preoperative carbohydrate-rich drinks and epidural anaesthesia are combined with feeding of an almost complete enteral diet from the day of surgery onwards, a neu-tral nitrogen balance can be maintained after major colorectal surgery. In addition, near-normal glucose levels (average 5.8 mmol/l) were maintained during ongoing feeding. Postoperative insulin resistance was kept low and comparable with that reported after more minor surgery, such as laparoscopic cholecys-tectomy or inguinal hernia repair. These data show that if the metabolic response is kept at a minimum, feeding is possible, and it results in minimal losses of body proteins – a complete transformation of the classical ebb-and-flow catabolic spiral originally described by Cuthbertson.

20.4 Feeding the severely traumatised patient

The severely traumatised patient represents quite a different situation to that of the elective surgical patient. First and foremost, several organs may have been damaged directly. Key organs in this respect are the thoracic organs, the brain, the liver, and the kid-ney. Such injuries will potentially have a marked impact on the treatment needed to maintain vital organ function and hence subsequent nutritional management. An obvious example is the patient with a head injury demanding ventilatory support, per-haps body-temperature cooling, and sedation. These measures will have clear influences on the route of nutrient administration, as well the amounts given.

Another important aspect differing in these patients is that they will have a full-scale stress response, having been injured in the awake state, with no preparation possible. Hence, these patients will develop a greater degree of metabolic distur-bance and often present with hyperglycaemia as a result of marked insulin resistance in response to haemorrhage and other sequelae from the injury. Fluid resuscitation to maintain cardiovascular function will further influence metabolism and nutritional therapy later in the patient's course. Furthermore, many of these patients need surgery in a critical state and various measures required to maintain vital functions during such procedures will impact on nutritional intake and how well the body tolerates nutrients supplied.

The overall strategy for severely injured trauma patients is to secure vital organ function upon arrival and thereafter during surgery. Once these measures have been stabilised, nutritional support can begin. Pre-emptive planning for postoperative nutrition via the enteral route can be achieved by placement of an enteral feeding tube in the stomach, or more often in the jejunum. This will facilitate enteral feeding in the postoperative/post-traumatic phase. Enteral feeding begun in small amounts even within hours after emer-gency trauma surgery has been shown to be feasible and advantageous. This often needs to be comple-mented by parenteral feeding. Glucose levels should be kept within the slight supranormal range with insulin. However, for patients with multiple injuries, a severe degree of insulin resistance may be expected, and for these patients it is also necessary to monitor acid–base balance. Reports from major burn injury have revealed that in severe insulin resistance, glucose may not be fully oxidised, due to inhibition of intracellular metabolism, and hence there is a risk of excess lactate formation from excessive glucose uptake. In this situation, glucose delivery must be reduced.

Once the patients stabilise and the initial phase is over, the general principle of moving from parenteral to enteral and finally to oral and normal feeding can be employed. During this course, it may be useful to monitor energy demands by using indirect calorimetry, which is available in some ICUs.

Prescription of feed

The major aim of perioperative care is the early introduction of normal food. Regular hospital food should be the first choice for nutrition in most postoperative patients. However, it is essential to monitor and record the adequacy of such an intake.

For patients unable to consume sufficient food to meet their needs, the following guidelines can be applied. The supply of nutrients by the enteral route is limited by gastrointestinal tolerance in the postoperative period. For those patients consuming some but not sufficient regular food, sip feeds can be recommended. For patients able to take only minor portions of normal food or none at all, enteral tube feeding using a standard polymeric feed should be used in most cases, starting at 20–30 ml/hour and increasing as tolerance improves, based on gastric aspirate residuals. Several positive trials of postoperative enteral feeding have used quite low intakes of 18–20 kcal/kg body weight in the first few days, with beneficial results, particularly in terms of infection. Some studies in major trauma and in cancer surgery suggest that immune-enhancing feeds may have some advantage over standard feeds in these conditions.

In a series of recent studies it has been suggested that addition of specific immune-enhancing nutrients such as arginine, *n*-3 fatty acids, and dietary nucleotides may be of benefit for the patient undergoing major surgery. When these formulas have been given perioperatively in major surgery, reductions in infectious complications and reduced length of stay have been reported in a large meta-analysis. From the design of the studies, it is not clear whether the effects were related to the addition of nutrients as such or the addition of any one of the specific components. Hence,

it remains unclear which component carries the potential effects. In contrast to the elective surgical patient, in the critical-care setting there is recent trial evidence suggesting that increased mortality is associated with the use of particular immunonutrition formulations.

With parenteral nutrition, particular attention should be paid to avoiding too little or too much salt and water and to avoiding hyperglycaemia. For many patients, insulin may be needed to maintain normoglycaemia. Otherwise, standard prescriptions can be used to give 25–30 kcal/kg/day, with 30–40% of total calories from fat (see Chapter 9). Intakes of 0.15–0.2 g N/kg/day are usually adequate, with an energy-to-nitrogen ratio of approximately 150 : 1. The usual recommended amounts of minerals and micronutrients should also be supplied. The addition of glutamine or glutamine dipeptides to standard TPN has been associated with improved long-term outcome from critical care. Further studies are awaited.

20.5 Concluding remarks

With adequate precautions against postoperative ileus, most patients undergoing surgery can return to normal oral feeding almost immediately. Several traditional routines need to be changed. Proper anaesthetic techniques for pain control will help to facilitate a return to the use of the oral route for feeding and to avoid postoperative ileus. Preoperative feeding improves the outcome from surgery in patients with severe malnutrition, and preoperative carbohydrates reduce postoperative insulin resistance and protein catabolism in elective surgery. Postoperative enteral nutrition reduces postoperative complications. There is some evidence of benefit from postoperative enteral and/or parenteral nutrition in previously malnourished patients, in those with postoperative complications, and after major trauma or burns. Most importantly, feeding should be part of an integrated protocol of management throughout the patient's clinical course.

Acknowledgements

This chapter has been revised and updated by Olle Ljungqvist and Ken Fearon, based on the original chapter by Olle Ljungqvist, Ken Fearon, and Rod A Little.

References and further reading

Allison SP, Kinney JM. Perioperative nutrition. Curr Opin Clin Nutr Metab Care 2000; 3: 1–3.

Beattie AH, Prach AT, Baxter JP, Pennington CR. A randomised controlled trial evaluating the use of enteral nutritional supplements postoperatively in malnourished surgical patients. Gut 2000; 46: 813–818.

Cuthbertson DP. The metabolic response to injury and other related explorations in the field of protein metabolism: an autobiographical account. Scot Med J 1982; 27: 158–171.

Heyland DK, Montalvo M, MacDonald S, Keefe L, Su XY, Drover JW. Total parenteral nutrition in the surgical patient: a meta-analysis. Can J Surg 2001; 44: 102–111.

Kehlet H. Multimodal approach to control postoperative pathophysiology and rehabilitation. Br J Anaesth 1997; 78: 606–617.

Knight, David JW. Immunonutrition: increased mortality is associated with immunonutrition in sepsis. BMJ 2003; 327: 682–683.

Ljungqvist O. Modulating postoperative insulin resistance by preoperative carbohydrate loading. Best Pract Res Clin Anaesthesiol 2009; 23(4): 401–409.

Ljungqvist O. Insulin resistance and outcomes in surgery. J Clin Endocrinol Metab 2010; 95(9): 4217–4219.

Kanagaraj M, Varadhan KK, Ljungqvist O, Lobo DN. A meta-analysis of the effect of combinations of immune modulating nutrients on outcome in patients undergoing major open gastrointestinal surgery. Ann Surg 2012; 255(6): 1060–1068.

Sato H, Carvalho G, Sato T, Lattermann R, Matsukawa T, Schricker T. The association of preoperative glycemic control, intraoperative insulin sensitivity, and outcomes after cardiac surgery. J Clin Endocrinol Metab 2010; 95(9): 4338–4344.

Smith I, Kranke P, Murat I, Smith A, O'Sullivan G, Soreide E, et al. Perioperative fasting in adults and children: guidelines from the European Society of Anaesthesiology. Eur J Anaesthesiol 2011; 28(8): 556–569.

van den Berghe G, Wouters P, Weekers F, Verwaest C, Bruynickx F, Schetz M, et al. Intensive insulin therapy in the critically ill patients. N Engl J Med 2001; 345(19): 1359–1367.

van den Berghe G. How does blood glucose control with insulin save lives in intensive care? J Clin Invest 2004; 114(9): 1187–1195.

Varadhan KK, Lobo DN. A meta-analysis of randomised controlled trials of intravenous fluid therapy in major elective open abdominal surgery: getting the balance right. Proc Nutr Soc 2010; 69(4): 488–498.

Varadhan KK, Neal KR, Dejong CH, Fearon KC, Ljungqvist O, Lobo DN. The enhanced recovery after surgery (ERAS) pathway for patients undergoing major elective open colorectal surgery: a meta-analysis of randomized controlled trials. Clin Nutr 2010; 29(4): 434–440.

Varadhan KK, Lobo DN, Ljungqvist O. Enhanced recovery after surgery: the future of improving surgical care. Crit Care Clin 2010; 26(3): 527–547.

21
Infectious Diseases

Nicholas I Paton,[1] Miguel A Gassull,[2] and Eduard Cabré[2]

[1]*National University of Singapore, Singapore*
[2]*Hospital Universitari Germans Trias i Pujol, Spain*

Key messages

- Advanced human immunodeficiency virus (HIV) infection and tuberculosis are chronic infections that are commonly associated with wasting.
- Reduced nutrient intake is the main cause of wasting, although metabolic disturbances may promote lean-tissue loss.
- Increasing nutrient intake is the key to treatment, although pharmacological management approaches may also sometimes be helpful.
- Anti-HIV drug treatment is frequently complicated by body fat changes and metabolic disturbances.

- Acute infections such as malaria and acute infectious diarrhoea have important effects on nutritional status, especially in children, and are an important cause of death in developing countries.
- Malnutrition increases the risk of malaria.
- Rehydration therapy, achieved using the World Health Organization (WHO) rehydration mixture or similar solution, is the key to management of acute infectious diarrhoea.

21.1 Introduction

Chronic infections often have profound effects on nutritional status. Two chronic infections are of particular importance in terms of global morbidity and mortality in the early twenty-first century: tuberculosis and human immunodeficiency virus (HIV) infection. The interaction between malnutrition and tuberculosis has long been recognised, although there has been little scientific research in this area. This is in contrast with HIV infection, a relatively new infection, where intense research efforts in the last 25 years have resulted in a body of knowledge about the effects of infection on nutrition and metabolism and the treatment of wasting, which far exceed the existing knowledge accumulated for any other infectious disease. This chapter will therefore focus on HIV infection, and to a lesser extent on tuberculosis, in order to outline the existing knowledge about the nutritional issues

accompanying chronic infections. Many of the principles probably apply to other infectious diseases.

The effects of acute infection on host nutrition and metabolism are similar to those of many other stress conditions, and are largely independent of the causative pathogen. The interaction between nutrition and acute infection is especially important in developing countries, where pre-existing malnutrition may increase the frequency and severity of acute infections, and certain acute infections may precipitate malnutrition. Acute gastroenteritis and malaria will be described in this chapter, as they are extremely common infections in the developing world and are both good examples of the infection–nutrition interaction.

Infectious diseases are extremely heterogeneous in their clinical presentation, although a number of nutritional features (such as anorexia, catabolism, increased basal metabolic rate (BMR), decreased physical activity, and increased requirements for some micronutrients) are common to most of them. In addition to these general manifestations, there are other, more specific features of some infectious diseases that may have nutritional consequences. Examples include the requirement for special forms of nutritional support in patients with severe infections who require intensive care and mechanical ventilation; the oesophageal dilatation and dysmotility of Chagas' disease; and the fluid and electrolyte disturbances of patients with severe gastrointestinal infections, such as cholera.

21.2 Human immunodeficiency virus infection

Transmission and epidemiology

HIV is transmitted by sexual intercourse (homosexual or heterosexual), by transfusion of infected blood or blood products, by needles contaminated with blood (usually in intravenous drug abusers who share needles, rarely in the context of accidental injury to healthcare workers), or vertically (i.e. from mother to baby *in utero*, intrapartum, or by breast milk). Whereas the principal mode of transmission in developed countries is sexual contact between men, the majority of infections worldwide are acquired by heterosexual transmission and vertical transmission.

The acquired immune deficiency syndrome (AIDS) pandemic looks set to be among the most devastating events in human history. There were estimated to be 34 million people living with HIV infection at the end of year 2010, more than 3 million of whom are children. There are approximately 2.7 million new infections and 2 million deaths from AIDS each year, thus placing HIV infection in the same league as the traditional scourges of tuberculosis and malaria as the principal infectious causes of mortality in global terms. The disease has decreased life expectancy by 20 years in some of the worst-affected countries.

Clinical features

The course of HIV infection can be divided into four stages. The seroconversion illness (stage I) occurs in 50–90% of patients at an average of 2–4 weeks following acquisition of infection. There follows an asymptomatic phase (stage II) without overt clinical manifestations, although active replication of virus and destruction of CD4 cells continues. This asymptomatic phase may last indefinitely in a small proportion (less than 5%) of patients, but will progress to symptomatic infection in the majority. The earliest indication of progression to immune failure and symptomatic disease is usually mucocutaneous conditions, such as oral candidiasis (thrush) and oral hairy leucoplakia. Persistent generalised lymphadenopathy is the first definitive condition to signify the end of the asymptomatic phase and its occurrence defines stage III disease.

With further depletion of immune function, patients become at risk of opportunistic infections and malignancies. When one of a defined set of indicator conditions develops (such as *Pneumocystis carinii* pneumonia (PCP), cytomegalovirus (CMV) colitis, or Kaposi's sarcoma), the patient is deemed to have developed AIDS or stage IV disease. Until the recent advent of highly effective combination antiretroviral therapies, AIDS was invariably fatal within a few years. It has recently been recognised that HIV-infected patients are also at increased risk of a variety of diseases in addition to the traditional AIDS-defining conditions, such as cardiovascular disease, renal disease, and bone disease.

Treatment of HIV disease

The therapeutic approach may be divided into prevention of disease progression and treatment of complications that arise. Considerable progress in the development and utilisation of antiretroviral drugs has been made in the last 15–20 years. Nucleoside analogues, which block the action of the HIV reverse transcriptase enzyme and drugs that inhibit the HIV protease enzyme and the processes of viral fusion and integration have been developed and have a powerful effect in the treatment of HIV. Combination of a protease inhibitor (or alternative drug) with two nucleoside analogues is now regarded as the standard of care in developed nations. This highly active antiretroviral therapy (HAART) has been shown to be effective in halting and even reversing the progression of HIV disease. Widespread adoption of HAART in developed nations has markedly decreased the population rates of progression from asymptomatic HIV disease to

AIDS and the rate of death from AIDS-related illnesses. A retrospective cohort study of nearly 8000 patients in France demonstrated drops in hospitalisation days by 35%, new AIDS cases by 35%, and deaths by 46% within 1 year following the introduction of HAART into routine usage.

In cases where severe immune compromise has already occurred, prophylactic antibiotics can be used to prevent opportunistic infections such as PCP and *Mycobacterium avium* infection. Most of these agents can be discontinued after a period on effective antiretroviral therapy. In patients who present for the first time with an episode of acute opportunistic infection, antimicrobial treatment is initially directed towards overcoming the infection.

For patients living in settings where antiretroviral therapy is not universally available, the approach to therapy of HIV disease may be limited to the treatment of specific complications (especially tuberculosis) and prophylaxis of other infections where affordable agents are available.

Wasting in HIV infection

Definition of HIV wasting syndrome

Involuntary weight loss is a common feature of advanced HIV infection, and 'HIV wasting syndrome' is recognised as one of the conditions that can define a patient as having advanced disease or AIDS. The definition of HIV wasting syndrome is given in Box 21.1.

Epidemiology of HIV wasting syndrome

Surveillance studies in the USA conducted in the early 1990s estimated that between 20 and 25% of patients who had AIDS developed wasting syndrome at some time during the course of their disease. In the late 1990s, the widespread use of HAART had a dramatic effect on the incidence of opportunistic infections and has probably halved the incidence of wasting syndrome in developed countries. Factors contributing to the pathogenesis of HIV-associated wasting are listed in Box 21.2.

The figures for large patient populations are encouraging, and demonstrate convincingly that HAART can prevent wasting. However, it is uncertain whether body weight and BCM recover fully following the introduction of HAART in patients who have established wasting at the time of initiation of therapy. Few clinical trials of HAART collected

> ### Box 21.1 Definition of HIV wasting syndrome
>
> Profound involuntary weight loss greater than 10% of baseline body weight plus either chronic diarrhoea (at least two loose stools per day for ≥30 days) or chronic weakness and documented fever (for ≥30 days, intermittent or constant) in the absence of a concurrent illness or condition other than HIV infection that could explain the findings (e.g. cancer, tuberculosis, cryptosporidiosis, or other specific enteritis).

> ### Box 21.2 Summary of the pathogenesis of HIV-associated wasting
>
> - HIV-associated wasting is largely a phenomenon of advanced HIV disease (AIDS).
> - Wasting usually occurs in association with opportunistic infections.
> - Reduced food intake is central to the pathogenesis of wasting.
> - There are numerous causes of reduced food intake in HIV patients.
> - Malabsorption is common, but is likely to act only as an exacerbating factor rather than the sole causative factor in wasting.
> - Numerous metabolic derangements accompany HIV disease, but their role in wasting is unclear.
> - Body-composition studies show preferential lean-tissue and body cell mass (BCM) loss, indicating that metabolic factors may have an influence.
> - Hypogonadism contributes to BCM loss in a subset of patients.

even simple body-weight measurements, let alone body-composition data. Clinical experience suggests that some patients with severe wasting do regain weight, but carefully conducted prospective studies are needed to quantify this.

One further important point is that the majority of people infected with HIV live in the developing world and, in spite of enormous international efforts to expand access to treatment, in many places less than 50% of those who need treatment with combination antiretroviral therapy actually receive it. HIV-related wasting is therefore likely to remain a significant problem in the populations of developing countries. In some African countries, wasting is such a universal feature of HIV disease that the name 'slim disease' has become synonymous with AIDS.

Definition of HIV-associated wasting

The prevalence of wasting syndrome, as defined above, gives only an approximate indication of the true problem of malnutrition in HIV disease. The definition itself is unsatisfactory as it technically excludes wasting associated with recognised opportunistic infections (which are the commonest cause). Malnutrition is considerably more complex than the clinical concept of wasting syndrome. In one study of HIV patients in Germany, 27% of patients had weight loss of >10% but did not meet the other criteria (fever or diarrhoea) for a diagnosis of wasting syndrome. The true incidence of malnutrition in any population of HIV-infected patients will depend on the social, cultural, and medical characteristics of the patients in a practice, but it is probably true to say that a majority of patients will at some stage experience problems with nutrition.

Thus, due to the inadequacy of the term 'HIV wasting syndrome', which, *sensu strictu*, probably excludes the majority of cases of malnutrition, the term 'HIV-associated wasting' will be used throughout this chapter to refer to the occurrence of weight or lean-tissue loss, irrespective of the presence of other clinical symptoms or disease complications. There is no widely accepted definition of HIV-associated wasting, but possible indicators are listed in Box 21.3.

Clinical importance of HIV-associated wasting

There is good evidence that wasting affects survival in HIV-infected patients. One early retrospective study demonstrated that there is progressive depletion of body weight and BCM up to the time of death in AIDS patients, to a body weight of 66% and a BCM of 54% of ideal values. These are very close to values prior to death seen in malnourished people in the siege of Leningrad in 1941–1942, and it is therefore likely that in some patients with HIV the timing of death relates to the magnitude of weight and BCM depletion rather than the specific disease process that causes the wasting. Furthermore, some patients die from malnutrition alone, without other active complications of HIV infection being apparent.

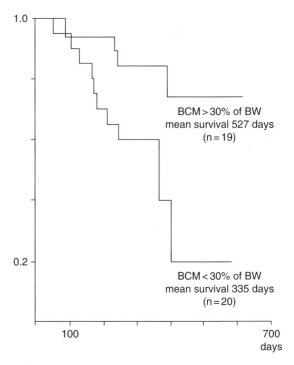

Figure 21.1 Graph of relationship between body cell mass (BCM) and survival. BW, body weight. Adapted from Süttmann *et al.* (1995) © Wolters Kluwer Health.

Other prospective studies have confirmed the relationship between weight loss and survival, and have suggested that even 5% weight loss can have an independent adverse impact on the disease progression. Depletion of BCM appears to have a more direct effect than body weight. A prospective study of BCM measured by bioelectrical impedance in a German cohort has shown that patients with BCM >30% of body weight had significantly longer survival than those with BCM <30% of body weight at baseline (Figure 21.1).

Apart from the effects on survival, loss of lean tissue has been shown to significantly affect physical function in patients with HIV infection. Involuntary weight loss can also cause profound psychological stress and is often mentioned as one of the most disturbing features of the illness. Patients who have chosen not to disclose their illness to family and friends find it increasingly difficult to maintain the deception, and this may result in social isolation.

The interaction between malnutrition and immune function is well recognised, and wasting may increase morbidity by prolonging recovery from opportunistic infections, thereby lengthening hospital stay and further impairing resistance to nonfatal infections such as oral candidiasis. The consequences of HIV-associated wasting are summarised in Box 21.4.

Patterns of weight change in HIV infection

Weight loss tends to occur in association with disease complications, especially intercurrent infection. A prospective study of weight change in a group of AIDS patients followed for periods of 9–49 months with regular body-weight measurement revealed two distinct patterns of weight loss. Episodes of acute rapid weight loss (median 9.1 kg in 1.7 months) were commonly associated with non-gastrointestinal opportunistic infections such as PCP, bacterial chest infections, and septicaemia. Episodes of chronic unremitting progressive weight loss (median 13.2 kg in 9.5 months) occurred, usually in conjunction with diarrhoeal disease such as cryptosporidium infection. Periods of weight stability or weight gain (usually associated with recovery from opportunistic infections) were also observed (see Figure 21.2).

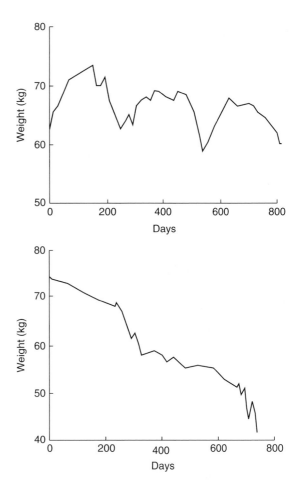

Figure 21.2 Patterns of weight change in HIV infection. Adapted from Am J Clin Nutr 1993; 58(3): 417–424. Copyright © American Society for Nutrition.

Patterns of body-composition change in HIV infection

An influential early cross-sectional study in which BCM was measured using total body potassium demonstrated that BCM was lower in patients with AIDS than in controls. There was a relative increase in extracellular water volume, and body fat mass was also decreased, although to a lesser extent than the BCM loss. This pattern of BCM loss with preservation of fat is indicative of a metabolic basis for the wasting process.

Longitudinal studies using dual-energy X-ray absorptiometry (DXA) revealed subsequently that when HIV patients develop wasting they do indeed lose fat, approximately in the proportions that would be expected if calorie restriction were the

sole aetiology. There also appears to be a sex difference, with HIV-infected women tending to lose a greater proportion of fat than men when they develop wasting. These differences may reflect differences in the baseline fat mass that influence the pattern of weight loss, or perhaps endocrine differences that influence the wasting process. Some of the variability between patients in body-composition change may also relate to the specific opportunistic infections from which the patients suffer. One study comparing different opportunistic infections found that patients with protozoal diarrhoea had decreased body fat, whereas those with systemic *Mycobacterium avium intracellulare* infection had decreased skeletal muscle mass. The

---

Box 21.5 Body composition in HIV-associated wasting

- body weight ↓
- fat mass ↓
- fat-free mass ↓
- BCM ↓↓
- extracellular water ↑

---

effects on body composition in HIV-associated wasting are listed in Box 21.5.

Energy metabolism in HIV infection

A number of studies have measured one or more component of energy balance in patients with HIV infection. These have shown somewhat conflicting results, but make sense if they are interpreted in conjunction with the clinical characteristics of the patient cohort studied.

In asymptomatic HIV infection, energy intake appears to be normal or slightly increased (by about 15%), possibly as a voluntary or involuntary attempt to compensate for occult malabsorption. This is consistent with the observation of weight stability in early disease. In later stages of HIV disease, energy intake is much more variable, depending on the presence or absence of disease complications at the time the measurement is made. Patients undergoing rapid weight loss (usually in association with an intercurrent infection) have markedly decreased energy intake, and those undergoing weight gain (usually following recovery from opportunistic infections) have normal or increased energy intake. Factors causing a reduced food intake are listed in Box 21.6.

Numerous investigators have shown that resting energy expenditure (REE) is elevated in patients with HIV infection. In those free from acute opportunistic infections, mean REE is elevated by an average of 8–12% irrespective of whether the patient has asymptomatic disease, or has experienced prior weight loss and opportunistic infections. Individual patients show greater variability, with some showing reduced REE suggestive of a starvation response. Others measured at the time of secondary infection have been shown to have a mean REE of around 30% above that of controls in some studies. The differing findings may reflect the heterogeneity of advanced HIV disease. One study found that patients with protozoal

---

Box 21.6 Causes of reduced food intake in HIV infection

- nausea and vomiting;
- taste disturbances;
- dysphagia;
- early satiety;
- anorexia;
- depression;
- dementia;
- food access or preparation problems;
- voluntary (to avoid diarrhoea);
- voluntary (dietary manipulation to more 'healthy' diet).

---

diarrhoeal disease had reduced REE, whereas patients with acute PCP and *Mycobacterium avium* infection had raised REE. The differences in REE between infections may also reflect alterations in the amount of BCM, as well as altered cellular metabolism.

Due to the difficulty of measurement, few studies of total energy expenditure (TEE) have been conducted in patients with HIV infection. The definitive study using the doubly labelled water method demonstrated an overall reduction in TEE compared with reference control values for normal men. There was a significant positive relationship between TEE and rate of weight change (i.e. patients with rapid weight loss had the lowest TEE). In the same study, physical-activity level (the ratio of TEE/REE) was significantly reduced in patients with rapid weight loss compared with patients with slow weight loss and stable weight (values of 1.3, 1.6, and 1.9, respectively). Thus, increase in TEE cannot be responsible for HIV-associated wasting.

Protein metabolism in HIV infection

Again there is some variability in the findings of studies of whole-body protein metabolism in HIV infection. For example, a study using the ^{15}N glycine technique demonstrated that asymptomatic patients with AIDS had reduced protein turnover indicative of a starvation-type response. A study using the ^{13}C leucine technique to measure whole-body protein metabolism in both the fasted and the fed state (using parenteral nutrition) demonstrated that patients with symptomatic AIDS had significantly increased protein turnover compared with controls, with both synthesis and degradation being increased. There was a normal anabolic response to feeding in the

HIV-infected patients. The variability of results may reflect the heterogeneity of clinical conditions of the patients that were studied.

Fat and carbohydrate metabolism in HIV infection

Various disturbances of fat metabolism have been described in HIV infection. Fasting triglyceride levels increase with progression of disease, lipoprotein lipase activity is decreased, and the clearance of triglycerides is reduced. *De novo* lipogenesis, the synthesis of fatty acids from other substrates in the liver, is increased. It is unlikely that these changes in triglyceride metabolism have a significant causal role in the wasting process. They are probably an epiphenomenon reflecting increased activity of cytokines in patients with HIV infection.

In contrast to the insulin resistance that usually accompanies infection, it appears that patients with HIV infection (not on HIV treatment) have increased insulin sensitivity and increased rates of insulin clearance. However, insulin resistance is seen frequently in patients receiving antiretroviral drugs.

Endocrine abnormalities and HIV-associated wasting

Hypogonadism has been well documented in HIV infection, occurring in up to 30% of men with AIDS, although this appears to be becoming less common in the era of effective HIV drug therapy. Various aetiologies have been suggested, including primary testicular disease, the effects of drugs, and hypothalamic dysfunction. It has been shown that androgen levels in hypogonadal men with HIV infection are closely correlated with BCM and exercise functional capacity, suggesting that androgen deficiency plays a role in the pathogenesis of HIV wasting.

There is some evidence for disturbance of the growth-hormone axis in HIV infection, although the data are conflicting. One study found that HIV-infected adults had insulin-like growth factor 1 (IGF-1) levels at the lower limits of normal and had a blunted response to exogenously administered growth hormone. Another found that growth-hormone pulse frequency, amplitude, and area under the curve did not differ between HIV-infected patients and controls.

Cytokines and HIV-associated wasting

It is thought that cytokines may mediate some of the metabolic changes induced by infection, including wasting. Tumour necrosis factor alpha (TNFα), a cytokine produced by macrophages and monocytes that is a mediator of the immune response, may be responsible for some of the systemic effects of chronic infection. Several studies have found raised levels of serum TNFα or TNF receptors in HIV patients, although others have not. Interleukin-1 (IL-1), interleukin-6 (IL-6), and interferon-alpha have also been proposed as mediators of wasting. Although these cytokines appear to be linked to disturbances in fat metabolism *in vitro* and *in vivo*, the association between serum levels of these factors and the wasting process *in vivo* remains unproven.

Treatment of HIV-associated wasting
General approach to treatment

The aim of treatment is to increase lean body mass (BCM in particular) and thereby improve quality of life, physical functioning, and survival. The initial step should be to identify and remove any underlying cause of the wasting. Treatment and recovery from opportunistic infection are often accompanied by repletion of body weight. Initiation of treatment of HIV infection with antiretroviral drugs may also result in some weight gain, although this may be offset by lipodystrophy changes.

Given that the predominant cause of wasting is a decrease in energy intake, the first step in the management process must be to increase calorie intake. However, the disturbances in intermediary metabolism which may be present in HIV disease, particularly at the time of opportunistic infections, may have some impact on the efficacy of nutritional interventions. An intervention which just results in the accumulation of fat and water may be deleterious. Assessment of the composition of any weight gain is a critical part of the evaluation of any therapeutic intervention in HIV wasting. A summary of the treatment of wasting is shown in Figure 21.3.

Nutritional therapy
Nutritional counselling

This is likely to be an important first step, although controlled-trial evidence for its efficacy is lacking.

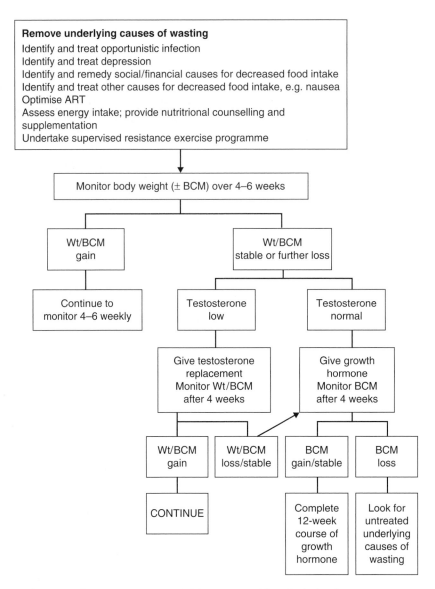

Figure 21.3 Summary of treatment of wasting. ART, antiretroviral therapy; Wt, weight; BCM, body cell mass.

Alternative diets for 'healthy living' are popular in the HIV community but may be lacking in important nutrients. Identification of such diets and provision of appropriate advice may result in worthwhile weight gain.

Oral supplements

Many nutritional supplements are available, although few have been subjected to controlled clinical trials comparing them with counselling alone. It appears that these supplements do achieve a worthwhile increase in energy intake (i.e. are not simply substituting for energy intake from normal diet), and this increase in energy intake may result in bodyweight gain. However, supplements do not appear to improve immunological recovery (i.e. increase CD4 T-cell count) or improve control of HIV viral replication.

Enteral tube feeding

The simplest approach is to use a fine-bore nasogastric tube, but although this is sometimes well tolerated for short periods of time, it can be uncomfortable and unsightly for the patient. Percutaneous endoscopic gastrostomy (PEG) has been demonstrated to be a safe and effective method of providing nutrition in selected situations where conventional nutritional intake is difficult (e.g. patients with swallowing difficulties and those in intensive care). Several uncontrolled studies have shown that PEG feeding appears to be a useful and relatively safe method of providing long-term nutritional support in selected AIDS patients. Most of the descriptive studies have documented substantial gains in weight and BCM, without an excessive rate of complications from the procedure.

Parenteral nutrition

This modality of feeding is usually reserved for situations in which the small intestine is inaccessible or nonfunctional. It is probably not effective for patients with severe ongoing systemic infections (e.g. CMV or *Mycobacterium avium* infection). A prospective controlled multicentre trial of total parenteral nutrition (TPN) versus dietary counselling has been conducted in France. Thirty-one severely malnourished AIDS patients were randomly assigned to receive either TPN or dietary counselling over a period of 2 months. Body weight, fat-free mass, and BCM all increased in the TPN group (by 13, 9, and 15%, respectively) and decreased in the dietary-counselling group (by 6, 5, and 12%, respectively). The TPN group had better long-term survival. This trial demonstrated that TPN can offer significant benefits in selected patients with AIDS, and the demonstration that a nutritional intervention increases survival is a landmark. The drawbacks of this therapy are that it is costly, logistically difficult to administer for long periods, and may have a net adverse effect on quality of life (this has not been addressed in studies).

Progressive-resistance exercise

A supervised programme of progressive-resistance exercise has been shown to increase lean body mass and may have other health benefits, such as increasing high-density lipoprotein (HDL) cholesterol. Encouraging patients to undertake a formal exercise programme (usually conducted in a gym) should therefore be considered as part of the management plan for wasting.

Pharmacological therapy
Megestrol acetate

Megestrol acetate is a synthetic orally active progestational agent which causes an increase in appetite and weight gain. The mechanism of appetite stimulation is unclear. Two large randomised controlled clinical trials have investigated this drug for patients with HIV-associated wasting. Both have shown that high-dose (800 mg/day) megestrol effectively increases energy intake and causes weight gain. However, it appears that the gain is almost entirely composed of fat, and lean tissue may actually decrease. This might result from the fact that megestrol may cause hypogonadism and thus have an anti-anabolic effect in addition to its appetite-stimulating effect. Therefore, megestrol has little to do in the treatment of HIV wasting, although it may have some role in the palliation of anorexia for patients in whom increasing survival is not the primary objective.

Testosterone

Hypogonadal HIV-positive men may benefit from physiological testosterone replacement, which can be given by either intramuscular injection (e.g. testosterone enanthate 300 mg every 3 weeks) or by a cutaneous patch. Supraphysiological doses of testosterone administered for a few months increase lean body mass in eugonadal HIV-positive men, but more safety data are needed before this approach can be advocated for long-term use.

Anabolic steroids

Chemically synthesised testosterone derivatives may have relatively greater anabolic and lesser androgenic activity in comparison with testosterone. However, there are insufficient data from controlled clinical trials to recommend their use and there are concerns over safety (especially in patients with concomitant hepatic disease).

Growth hormone

Growth hormone has been shown to reverse negative nitrogen balance and increase lean body mass in many situations: post-surgical, cancer, burns, and hypocaloric feeding. It has also been shown to reverse the body-composition changes associated with ageing. A definitive multicentre, double-blind, placebo-controlled study of growth hormone for

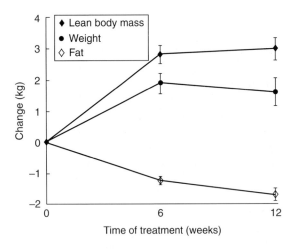

Figure 21.4 Body-composition changes with growth hormone. Reproduced from Schambelan *et al.* (1996) with permission from American College of Physicians.

HIV-associated wasting has been conducted (see Figure 21.4). A total of 178 men with HIV-related wasting were randomised to receive either placebo or subcutaneous growth hormone (0.1 mg/kg per day) for 12 weeks. Patients who received growth hormone had significant increases in body weight (1.6 kg) and lean body mass (3.0 kg), and a significant decrease in fat mass. There were no significant changes in body weight or body composition in the placebo group. Patients treated with growth hormone also showed significantly greater treadmill-work performance than placebo patients. Growth-hormone therapy was well tolerated. On the basis of this and similar studies, growth hormone has been licensed for the treatment of AIDS wasting in the USA and some other countries. However, the treatment is expensive and this factor severely limits its use.

Others

Thalidomide, an inhibitor of the cytokine TNF, has been shown to induce metabolic changes that lead to lean body mass increase, especially in patients with HIV and concomitant tuberculosis. However, the use of thalidomide is limited by side effects, particularly drug rash and peripheral neuropathy in long-term use, and of course its notorious teratogenic effects, which prohibit its use in women of childbearing age.

Dronabinol, the synthetically manufactured active ingredient of marijuana, has been shown to be effective in controlling nausea and vomiting in patients with cancer. A randomised controlled trial has demonstrated improvements in appetite and decreased nausea in patients with HIV-related wasting, although there was no significant effect on body weight.

HIV-associated lipodystrophy syndrome

Less than 2 years after widespread adoption of HAART into clinical practice, anecdotal reports began to emerge of unusual changes in body appearance. The most noticeable feature initially was an increase in the size of the dorsocervical fat pad, termed 'buffalo hump'. Subsequent reports identified patients who had marked fat gain in the abdominal area. Studies using computed tomography (CT) and magnetic resonance imaging (MRI) scans demonstrated that the increased abdominal girth was caused by excessive intra-abdominal fat rather than the subcutaneous fat that is usually seen with ageing or obesity (subcutaneous fat over the abdomen appeared to be decreased in these patients; see Figure 21.5). Some patients experience a disfiguring loss of fat pads in the cheeks and loss of subcutaneous fat from the arms and legs, resulting in abnormally prominent veins and muscles.

Many patients also have elevated levels of triglycerides, cholesterol, insulin, and C-peptide, suggesting a pattern of insulin resistance, and some have raised lactate levels. The term 'lipodystrophy syndrome' was coined to describe patients with changes in fat (increase or decrease) in one or more area of the body, together with deranged metabolic parameters. The presentation is very heterogeneous, with some patients having fat changes without metabolic disturbances and vice versa. It is unclear at this stage whether this is a single syndrome or multiple superimposed conditions. Metabolic and body-shape disturbances in antiretroviraltreated HIV patients are listed in Box 21.7.

The aetiology of the lipodystrophy syndrome has not been definitively ascertained, but is likely to be multifactorial. Initially it was thought that protease inhibitors were the likely culprits, but it is now clear that nucleoside reverse-transcriptase inhibitors (RTIs) may also be implicated (possibly reflecting

(a)   (b)

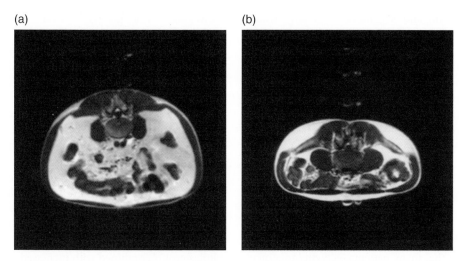

Figure 21.5 Abdominal magnetic resonance images of an HIV-infected man (a) with visceral adiposity syndrome and of a non-HIV-infected man (b) similar in race, weight, and total adiposity to the patient in image (a). Am J Clin Nutr 1999; 69(6): 1162–1169. Copyright © American Society for Nutrition.

Box 21.7 Some of the metabolic and body-shape disturbances in antiretroviral-treated HIV patients ('lipodystrophy syndrome')

- facial lipoatrophy;
- arm and leg lipoatrophy/prominent veins;
- buttock lipoatrophy;
- buffalo hump;
- central fat accumulation;
- generalised fat accumulation or atrophy;
- raised cholesterol;
- raised triglycerides;
- insulin resistance/diabetes;
- asymptomatic hyperlactataemia/lactic acidosis.

mitochondrial toxicity caused by these drugs). Furthermore, large epidemiological studies have shown that several factors other than drugs (e.g. age, race) are important additional determinants of lipodystrophy. Stavudine, one of the nucleoside RTIs, has been identified as the main causative factor for lipoatrophy in the face, arms, and legs, and this has led to its gradual withdrawal from clinical use in situations where there are affordable alternatives.

Treatment for body fat changes

The development of effective treatments for these problems is hampered by the clinical heterogeneity and the lack of a clear understanding of the pathogenesis of the condition. Stopping or switching HIV drugs does not usually result in significant reversal of body-shape changes, although it may benefit the hyperlipidaemia and insulin resistance. Peripheral fat loss is the most difficult to manage. There are anecdotal reports of improvements using collagen implants into the cheeks to improve appearance. There is no treatment available for fat loss in the arms or legs at present.

Central fat gain is perhaps more amenable to therapy. Diet and aerobic exercise should be the first step, and resistance training may also have some beneficial effects. A low dose of growth hormone has been shown to decrease visceral abdominal fat and truncal obesity in HIV-infected patients with fat accumulation, and a similar effect has been seen with tesamorelin, a growth hormone-releasing factor. However, the effects of these pharmacological interventions appear to be transient and the changes reverse when the treatment is stopped. Also, they may worsen insulin resistance, and their place in clinical management is therefore unclear.

Lactic acidosis

This is a side effect of nucleoside-analogue RTIs, in particular the drug stavudine. It is defined by elevated venous lactate levels (>2.0 mmol/l) and low arterial pH (<7.3). The main clinical features are nausea, abdominal pain, and shortness of breath. Milder cases may present more subtly, with fatigue and weight loss. Underlying liver disease may be a risk factor for the development of drug-induced lactic acidosis. The condition may sometimes be fatal.

Management is uncertain, although some interventions have been used with success in the treatment of other mitochondrial diseases. These include riboflavin and thiamine, antioxidants such as vitamin C, and L-carnitine, although controlled trials of these agents in the treatment of lactic acidosis in the setting of HIV infection are lacking.

Insulin resistance and diabetes

It is apparent that many patients receiving treatment for HIV infection have insulin resistance, although frank diabetes is relatively rare. It is not known whether the insulin resistance will ultimately progress to diabetes, although this is certainly possible. Fasting glucose levels are most often normal, and an oral glucose tolerance test, or better the measurement of fasting insulin levels, is needed to make a diagnosis of insulin resistance. The importance of insulin resistance is that it can increase the risk of atherosclerosis (even without raised glucose levels) and is associated with hypertriglyceridaemia that is also atherogenic. It is unclear whether the insulin resistance is related to body fat abnormalities or whether it is mainly related to the use of protease inhibitors that cause both phenomena.

When considering treatment of insulin resistance, other risk factors for atherogenesis should be looked for (e.g. smoking, high blood pressure, etc.) and modified wherever possible. As with the treatment of type 2 diabetes mellitus, diet and exercise form an essential first component of therapy. The diet should comrpise 50–60% carbohydrate, 30% fat (maximum 10% saturated fat), and 10–20% protein. Insulin-sensitising agents such as metformin may be useful.

Hyperlipidaemia

Severe increases in total cholesterol, low-density lipoprotein (LDL) cholesterol, and triglycerides can occur in patients receiving HIV drugs. These appear to be mainly, although not exclusively, related to therapy with protease inhibitors. The consequences of elevated cholesterol and triglycerides are likely to be as great – if not greater – for HIV-infected people as they are in the HIV-negative patient.

Treatment should mainly be targeted at LDL cholesterol and can follow standard guidelines that are applicable to the HIV-negative population, although attention to triglycerides and reduced HDL is also warranted. Diet and exercise are the most important initial interventions, along with cessation of smoking and treatment/reversal of any other risk factors. The diet should involve progressive restriction of dietary fat and total cholesterol until acceptable limits are achieved. Drug therapy may be indicated, and low doses of the statins pravastatin or atorvastatin may be useful. Fibrates (e.g. gemfibrozil) may also be useful, especially where increased cholesterol is combined with increased triglycerides, or in the situation of isolated hypertriglyceridaemia. Bile-sequestering resins should not be used due to their effect of increasing serum triglycerides and their potential effect of decreasing HIV-drug absorption.

Micronutrients and HIV

In addition to the marked reductions in intake of macronutrients described earlier, many HIV-infected patients do not consume the Recommended Dietary Allowance (RDA) of several micronutrients, such as B-complex vitamins, vitamin E, and zinc. This situation may be exacerbated by malabsorption, which is common in patients with HIV, especially those in the advanced stages of disease. Fat malabsorption may adversely affect the absorption of fat-soluble vitamins. Furthermore, inadequate intake may be further exacerbated by the possibility that the requirements for micronutrients in HIV-infected patients exceed the RDA in some cases. The prevalence of micronutrient deficiency varies considerably with the patient group, the stage of HIV disease, and the setting, but frequencies of up to 65% for vitamin A deficiency (in pregnant women) and of 20–30% for deficiencies of vitamins E, C, B_6, B_{12}, zinc, and iron have been reported.

A number of studies have linked micronutrient deficiency to accelerated progression of HIV disease. For example, vitamin A deficiency is associated with increased mortality, increased risk of vertical (mother-to-child) transmission of HIV, growth failure in HIV-infected children, and increased HIV in breast milk and the genital tract.

More than 30 clinical trials of micronutrient supplementation have been conducted, but they are generally of small size and the effects may be specific to the population studied. One large-scale study has been conducted, and it had convincing findings. In Tanzania, 1000 pregnant women were randomised to receive a daily multivitamin supplement, a supplement of vitamin A and beta-carotene, both, or neither (all received daily iron and folate). Those who received the multivitamin supplement had a 40% decrease in foetal death and low birth weight, and a significant increase in CD4 counts. The vitamin A and beta-carotene supplement did not appear to have any additional effect. More trials are needed to determine whether these findings of a benefit of multivitamin supplementation can be generalised to other populations.

None of the trials of supplementation with vitamin A or beta-carotene have shown beneficial effects in adults, although there is evidence of benefit in children. Zinc supplementation improved diarrhoea in children but not in adults. Selenium supplementation appeared to reduce diarrhoea in pregnant women in one study and HIV viral replication in two small studies. There is no evidence of a benefit of vitamin D supplementation alone.

Micronutrient interventions are particularly appealing for developing countries, where the prevalence of micronutrient deficiencies is likely to be relatively high and the cost-effectiveness and feasibility of specific interventions are favourable. In these circumstances, provision of a multivitamin supplement seems reasonable. More data are needed before micronutrient supplementation can be recommended to other groups, although micronutrients are widely consumed by HIV patients in developed countries, at varying and sometimes excessive doses.

Breast-feeding and HIV

HIV can be transmitted from infected mother to uninfected child through breast-feeding, and this route represents one of the major contributors to the HIV epidemic in children. The timing of transmission through breast milk (early versus late) is hard to define, for practical reasons. Several factors may influence the risk of transmission, including the viral load in the breast milk, the presence of mastitis, nipple disease, and variation in feeding practices (such as alternating between bottle- and breast-feeding, which seems to increase the risk above that of breast-feeding exclusively).

It is therefore recommended that HIV-infected mothers do not breast-feed their children. Avoidance of breast-feeding has been shown to reduce the transmission of HIV by around 50%. However, complete avoidance of breast-feeding and substitution of formula may not be possible in some developing countries due to financial or practical constraints. Also, there is a concern that reliance on formula-feeding may increase mortality from other causes, which might offset the advantage of reduced mortality from HIV. However, a randomised clinical trial of formula- versus breast-feeding in infants of HIV-infected mothers in Kenya showed that the incidences of diarrhoea, pneumonia, and overall mortality were similar in the two groups. Furthermore, the rate of survival free of HIV infection at 2 years was much higher in the formula-fed group, and this would be expected to yield longer-term survival benefits in favour of formula-feeding. Thus, it appears that formula-feeding can be a safe alternative to breast-feeding for HIV-infected mothers in a developing-country setting, provided that there is appropriate education and access to clean water.

If breast-feeding is essential, two approaches may help to reduce the risk of HIV transmission to the baby: first, the baby should be breast-fed exclusively, receiving only breast milk for the first few months of life (as opposed to breast-feeding supplemented by the feeding of other liquids or solids); and second, the baby should be given antiretroviral therapy while being breast-fed.

21.3 Tuberculosis

Epidemiology and importance

It is estimated that approximately one-third of the world's population is infected with *Mycobacterium tuberculosis*, the bacterium that causes clinical tuberculosis. Usually the infection is contained by the immune system, so that only a small proportion of the infected population (approximately 15 million) has clinical disease at any one time. However, the disease results in the deaths of approximately 2 million people per year, which places it amongst the most important infectious diseases in global terms. Most of these deaths occur in the developing world, and in many countries the disease has a large social and economic impact. The incidence of tuberculosis started to increase in the late 1980s and early 1990s, partly due to the advent of HIV infection (which increases tuberculosis risk) and partly due to complacency in tuberculosis control programmes. After a concerted international effort, per capita incidence rates are now stable or falling again in most areas of the world. However, rates of drug resistance are climbing and multi-drug-resistant tuberculosis (MDR-TB) now represents an important emerging disease, affecting around 500 000 people annually and causing over 100 000 deaths per year. Extensively drug-resistant tuberculosis (XDR-TB) – resistant to the major first- and second-line drugs – is now being reported from many countries.

Causative agent and transmission

The tuberculosis bacterium is transmitted mainly by the inhalation of aerosols from individuals suffering from pulmonary disease. The risk factors for infection are proximity to and duration of contact with an infected individual, so the family members and other household contacts of infected individuals are at highest risk. Although vaccination with bacille Calmette–Guérin (BCG) is widely used, the degree of protection offered is variable and certainly not 100%.

Clinical presentation, treatment, and course

Initial infection with tuberculosis is usually asymptomatic. However, a small proportion of infected people develop clinical symptoms such as cough, chest pain, and shortness of breath. Systemic symptoms such as fever, night sweats, and weight loss may also occur. Primary infection may progress to severe lung disease or disseminate throughout the body.

Most cases of tuberculosis are caused by reactivation of infection acquired many years earlier. The trigger for reactivation may be immunosuppression due to disease (e.g. malignancy, diabetes, or HIV infection) or drugs (e.g. in transplant patients). The usual site of disease is the lung. The commonest symptoms of reactivation of pulmonary tuberculosis are cough, fever, night sweats, weight loss, and fatigue.

The disease can be diagnosed by chest X-ray and by staining sputum samples to show the mycobacteria. Tuberculosis can reactivate at many sites other than the lungs (e.g. lymph nodes, bones, abdominal viscera, brain, and heart). In addition to the symptoms specific to the region affected, systemic symptoms such as fever and weight loss may sometimes be prominent.

Bloodborne dissemination of *Mycobacterium tuberculosis* can lead to miliary tuberculosis, especially in those with more severe immunosuppression. Miliary tuberculosis can manifest with symptoms associated with the organs involved (usually several) or as a pyrexia of unknown origin. In chronic cases, cachexia may be prominent and specific clinical signs may be few.

The treatment for tuberculosis is essentially the same irrespective of the site of disease. Combination therapy is essential for cure, and direct observation of therapy may also improve the outcome. The usual treatment involves taking a combination of three or four drugs (including rifampicin and isoniazid) for 2 months, followed by continuation of the rifampicin and isoniazid for a further 4–7 months, depending on the site of infection and the individual patient's state of immunosuppression. Hepatitis is the main complication of standard combination therapy. Isoniazid interferes with niacin metabolism and this may result in a peripheral neuropathy. This can be prevented by pyridoxine. In malnourished patients, isoniazid may precipitate pellagra. Treatment of MDR-TB and XDR-TB is much more challenging, involving the use of multiple drugs for prolonged periods of time (at least 18 months) and having substantial associated toxicity.

Nutritional and metabolic effects of tuberculosis

Wasting has been recognised for centuries as one of the cardinal signs of tuberculosis: the disease was known to Greek physicians as '*phthisis*', meaning 'to waste away', and in the eighteenth and nineteenth centuries tuberculosis was popularly called 'consumption'. Even in the modern era, where prompt diagnosis is possible, patients have often become severely cachectic by the time treatment is initiated. This is especially true in developing countries. A study from Malawi showed that unselected patients presenting for treatment of tuberculosis had their body weights reduced approximately 20% below normal values.

In the last 20 years the wasting associated with tuberculosis has been compounded by the fact that many patients with tuberculosis are co-infected with HIV. It is not surprising, given that both are associated with wasting, that the coincidence of the two diseases in the same patient often leads to very severe malnutrition. Indeed, in a post-mortem study of HIV-infected patients dying with 'slim disease', undiagnosed tuberculosis was found to be present in a large percentage.

Importance of the interaction between malnutrition and tuberculosis

Malnutrition is known to be detrimental to the host immune response to mycobacterial infection, and therefore increases susceptibility to tuberculosis infection. Tuberculosis is a frequent complication of malnutrition, and is a major cause of mortality among malnourished children of developing countries. The reactivation of tuberculosis in the elderly may also partly be the result of malnutrition in this population. Although it is hard to establish, because of many confounding factors, malnutrition is likely to contribute to the increased risk of reactivation of tuberculosis seen in HIV-infected people, alcoholics, and the homeless. Deficiency of vitamin D is known to increase susceptibility to tuberculosis, and there is some evidence that vitamin A and C deficiencies also increase susceptibility to tuberculosis.

As well as increasing the susceptibility to tuberculosis, malnutrition alters its clinical manifestations: malnourished patients have an atypical presentation of tuberculosis. Malnutrition also impairs recovery from tuberculosis. A study that examined the predictors of mortality in a group of patients who had tuberculosis diagnosed during hospitalisation showed that malnutrition was an independent predictor of death.

Furthermore, surgery (resection of affected lung) is increasingly being employed for the treatment of difficult cases of MDR-TB in specialist referral centres. Severe malnutrition is associated with a poor outcome and with increased complications following surgery. Patients with MDR-TB are also often amongst the most severely malnourished, as they have endured a prolonged inflammatory process and long courses of toxic drugs.

Aetiology of malnutrition in tuberculosis

The aetiology of the malnutrition in tuberculosis has not been fully ascertained. A few studies have shown that BMR/REE is slightly increased in tuberculosis, although total daily energy expenditure is unlikely to be greatly raised, because physical-activity energy expenditure is usually reduced in such patients. Anecdotal experience suggests that the key cause of wasting in tuberculosis is decreased energy intake, as a result of anorexia associated with the infection. However, no studies have formally investigated this aspect of the disease.

The cause of the anorexia associated with tuberculosis has not been established, although several potential mediators can be suggested. One of the most likely is TNF, as this cytokine is known to cause cachexia in animal models. Increased production of TNF is known to accompany tuberculosis. Drugs used to treat tuberculosis are frequently associated with gastrointestinal side effects that may further impair food intake.

Body composition in tuberculosis

The nature of body-composition changes in tuberculosis has not been well studied. One study showed a relative increase in extracellular water in patients with tuberculosis. A cross-sectional study of the effects of tuberculosis in patients with underlying HIV infection demonstrated a marked reduction in intracellular water and a relative increase in extracellular water in patients co-infected with tuberculosis compared to those without tuberculosis. The depletion of BCM was severe in patients with tuberculosis. Other markers of nutritional status, such as serum albumin, are also frequently reduced in this disease.

Nutritional therapy for wasting in tuberculosis

There is commonly an improvement in appetite and later a gain in body weight following the initiation of antituberculous therapy. Although clinicians often use weight gain to assess the response to antituberculous chemotherapy, the relationship between weight gain and clinical outcome is uncertain, and in one study microbiological response was not associated with weight gain. Few prospective studies have examined the composition of the weight gain and it may be distorted from normal (e.g. more fat or water gain) by the underlying disease process. One study which used simple anthropometric measurements to investigate the response to therapy found that body weight, arm circumference, and triceps skinfold all improved after 2 months of chemotherapy in 122 patients with sputum-positive tuberculosis in Malawi, suggesting that at least some fat accrual occurs, but more detailed prospective studies are needed.

In view of the frequency of severe malnutrition and its importance in adversely affecting the immune response to tuberculosis, optimising the nutritional status of these patients may confer some benefit on the host and the speed of recovery. Although spontaneous nutritional recovery may occur, it is possible that treating both the infection and malnutrition simultaneously will be more successful. However, there are few good data to support the use of nutritional interventions in patients with tuberculosis. Those studies that have been conducted are generally too small to provide reliable indication of benefits on mortality or cure of tuberculosis, but the evidence suggests that there may be improvements in body weight gain and possibly physical function. The protein requirements are not known. Early work suggested that increasing the protein intake to very high levels might be beneficial. However, increasing nitrogen intake may place additional demands on the respiratory function of tuberculosis patients and hence this approach should be avoided in patients with extensive lung damage and respiratory compromise.

Thus, in general, the evidence would support attempts to achieve an increased energy intake, with normal or slightly increased protein composition. This can be done most easily by means of dietary alteration and by use of energy and protein supplements. It is important to treat any drug-induced nausea and vomiting with antiemetics, and the use of antipyretics for fever is also likely to help appetite. In severely malnourished patients who are unable to consume sufficient calories and protein with these approaches, use of nasogastric feeding or PEG feeding may be warranted.

Micronutrient supplementation

There have been few controlled trials of micronutrient supplementation in TB and hence the evidence for the efficacy of multimicronutrient supplementation is

weak. It appears that there is no benefit on mortality, sputum clearance, or body-weight change. Vitamin D was used to treat patients with cutaneous tuberculosis prior to the advent of modern antituberculous drugs. Cod liver oil and sunlight were popular therapies for tuberculosis in the nineteenth century. Consideration should be given to vitamin D supplementation, especially in those who are vegetarians.

Pharmacological treatments for wasting in tuberculosis

A few studies have been conducted on the use of pharmacological treatments to accelerate weight gain. One small study found benefit in using anabolic steroids for patients with tuberculosis, although this needs to be further investigated before it can be recommended. Several studies have found increased weight gain with the use of thalidomide. However, at present there are no accepted drugs for enhancing weight gain in tuberculosis and treatment is purely nutritional.

21.4 Malaria

Epidemiology and importance

Malaria is the most important protozoal infection in humans, with more than one-third of the world's population exposed to the risk of infection. There are an estimated 150–270 million clinical cases per year, and approximately 780 000 deaths. The greatest burden of disease is in Africa, and African children account for most of the deaths worldwide.

In recent years significant progress has been made in malaria control efforts, thanks to renewed international commitment, the availability of substantially increased resources, and better preventive approaches. An effective vaccine may be on the horizon and, for the first time since the failed control programmes of the 1950s and 1960s, some are beginning to speculate about the possibility of eradication within the next generation.

Clinical presentation and treatment

The main symptom is fever that may become periodic, occurring only every few days, once infection is well-established. Other nonspecific symptoms include headache, vomiting, and diarrhoea. Although malaria is a mild and self-limiting infection in most cases, patients infected with the *Plasmodium falciparum* parasite can develop a range of complications, which may result in death. Common complications include cerebral malaria (manifesting as decreased consciousness, convulsions, or other neurological signs), pulmonary oedema, hypoglycaemia, anaemia, and renal failure. Secondary infections are frequent (e.g. pneumonia or gram-negative septicaemia).

The non-falciparum malarias are treated with chloroquine over a period of 2–3 days, followed by primaquine over a period of 2 weeks to eradicate the liver forms of the parasite. Chloroquine is usually well tolerated. Falciparum malaria is usually treated with artemisinin-based combination therapy, which is well tolerated and effective.

The role of protein–energy malnutrition in malaria

Early studies suggested that protein–energy malnutrition or protein deficiency protected the host against malaria morbidity and mortality. More recent studies, with more rigorous methods, have indicated the opposite to be the case. Cohort studies have shown that malnutrition is associated with increased rates of infection and increased frequency of clinical attacks of malaria. Studies conducted in hospitalised malaria patients in several African countries have shown that malnourished patients are 1.3–3.5 times more likely to die or have permanent neurological sequelae than normally nourished patients. However, although malnutrition does appear to exacerbate malaria, the impact is smaller than that seen with malnutrition on diarrhoea or pneumonia. In addition, there may be age-dependent relationships between malnutrition and malaria that explain some of the inconsistencies in the data. The situation of starvation and famine may present a special case. It has been shown that refeeding humans in situations of famine can reactivate low-grade malaria infections.

Micronutrients and malaria

Multiple nutrients may play a role in protecting against or exacerbating malaria. However, the relationships are complex and the immunological basis is unclear. The effects may be due to effects on the host and/or parasite.

A number of cross-sectional studies have shown an inverse relationship between vitamin A levels and the concentration of malaria parasites in the blood. A definitive study on the effects of vitamin A supplementation on clinical malaria was conducted in Papua New Guinea. It showed that giving vitamin A supplementation reduced the frequency of *P. falciparum* malaria episodes by 30% among preschool children.

Several cross-sectional studies and intervention studies also indicate a relationship between zinc deficiency and malaria. A placebo-controlled trial showed that zinc supplementation reduced the frequency of health centre attendance due to falciparum malaria by 38% and reduced the frequency of malaria accompanied by high levels of parasitaemia by 69%. However, a recent large trial in 612 Tanzanian children did not demonstrate an effect of zinc supplementation, so the benefits or otherwise of zinc supplementation on malaria remain unclear.

Several studies of iron supplementation in malaria-endemic areas have shown that iron supplementation increases the risk of developing or reactivating malarial illness. However, a definitive systematic review of all the evidence has shown that iron does not increase the risk of malaria. The improvements in anaemia following iron supplementation are substantial, suggesting that iron-supplementation programmes in accordance with international dosing guidelines are appropriate for iron-deficient populations residing in malaria-endemic areas. This remains a somewhat controversial area.

The effects of folate are unclear. Riboflavin deficiency appears to protect against malaria, although high-dose riboflavin therapy may be advantageous in patients who have clinical malaria. Thiamine deficiency may predispose to more severe malaria. Vitamin E deficiency tends to protect against clinical malaria. The effects of other antioxidants are unknown.

21.5 Gastrointestinal infections

Definition and aetiopathogenesis

A large number of pathogens, including bacteria, viruses, and protozoa, can infect the small bowel and colon, mostly causing diarrhoeal illness, such as acute gastroenteritis, food poisoning, and traveller's diarrhoea – which are not necessarily clearly distinguishable from each other – and more specific

---

Box 21.8 Organisms causing gastrointestinal infections

Bacteria

- *Vibrio cholerae*;
- *Vibrio parahaemolyticus*;
- *Aeromonas* spp.;
- enterotoxigenic *E. coli* (ETEC);
- enteroinvasive *E. coli* (EIEC);
- enteropathogenic *E. coli* (EPEC);
- enterohaemorrhagic *E. coli* (EHEC);
- enteroaggregative *E. coli* (EAggEC);
- diffusely adhering *E. coli* (DAEC);
- *Shigella* spp.;
- *Salmonella* spp.;
- *Campylobacter* spp.;
- *Yersinia* spp.;
- *Staphylococcus aureus*;
- *Clostridium perfringens*;
- *Bacillus cereus*;
- *Lysteria monocytogenes*;
- *Clostridium difficile*.

Viruses

- rotavirus (mainly group A);
- calicivirus (Norwalk virus, Norwalk-like virus);
- enteric adenovirus;
- astrovirus.

Protozoa

- *Giardia lamblia*;
- *Entamoeba histolytica*;
- *Cryptosporidium*;
- *Isospora*;
- *Cyclospora*;
- *Microsporidium*;
- *Balantidium coli*;
- *Blastocystis hominis*.

---

conditions such as typhoid fever, cholera, and dysentery (Box 21.8).

Bacterial diarrhoea can be classified into toxigenic and invasive types. The prototype organisms for toxigenic diarrhoeas are *Vibrio cholerae* and ETEC. These pathogens do not invade intestinal epithelium, but adhere to the enterocytes, where they produce enterotoxins of the cytotonic type, which lead to watery diarrhoea and dehydration. Invasive diarrhoea is caused by pathogens, such as *Salmonella*, *Shigella*, EIEC, *Campylobacter*, and *Yersinia*. Although some of these organisms can also produce enterotoxins, they cause an intense inflammatory reaction in the intestinal, and mostly colonic, mucosa, leading to prostaglandin-mediated diarrhoea, often with blood and leukocytes in the faeces (dysenteric stools). In some food poisoning (e.g. *Clostridium perfringens*, *Staphylococcus aureus*, *Bacillus cereus*), acute diarrhoea is caused by preformed bacterial toxins found in the contaminated food.

Viruses responsible for gastrointestinal infections can be grouped into four categories: rotavirus, calicivirus (including Norwalk virus), enteric adenovirus, and astrovirus. All of them usually produce watery diarrhoea, often accompanied by vomiting. Protozoan infections include giardiasis, amebiasis, and infections caused by *Cryptosporidium*, *Isospora*, and *Cyclospora*. Clinical consequences of these infections range from asymptomatic cases or mild diarrhoea to severe malabsorption or devastating diarrhoeal illness.

Epidemiology: the magnitude of the problem

Acute infectious diarrhoea is the first or second cause of death in most developing countries, being responsible for 3–4 million deaths annually worldwide, particularly in children. In fact, 20–30% of deaths in infants and children are due to enteric infections. Even in industrialised countries, gastrointestinal infections are a major health problem. In the USA, most children under 5 years of age experience an average of two episodes of diarrhoea per year.

Food poisoning, defined as an illness caused by the ingestion of contaminated food, usually occurs in the form of outbreaks worldwide. Bacteria (or their toxins) cause about 80% of food-poisoning outbreaks for which an aetiology can be identified. However, it has to be kept in mind that only 40% of such outbreaks fulfil the microbiological standards for confirmed aetiology.

Annually, more than 250 million people travel from one country to another, of which at least 15 million go from industrialised to developing countries. Acute diarrhoea often occurs among these individuals (traveller's diarrhoea), with an attack rate ranging from 25 to 50%. About 30% of patients with traveller's diarrhoea are sick enough to be confined in bed, and another 40% must alter their planned activities. The aetiology of traveller's diarrhoea depends on the country, but on average, most cases are due to ETEC, EAEC, *Campylobacter* spp., and *Shigella* spp. Other bacteria, viruses, and protozoa can also be identified as causative agents. However, in about 40% of cases an individual pathogen cannot be found.

Diarrhoea is the most frequent and often most symptomatic gastrointestinal manifestation of AIDS, occurring in 50–90% of these patients. In some cases, diarrhoea is due to the so-called 'Idiopathic AIDS enteropathy', which is thought to be caused by a combination of villus hypoplasia, altered cytokine production, ileal dysfunction, exudative enteropathy, intestinal dysmotility, and bacterial overgrowth. Most often, however, diarrhoea is directly related to different intestinal pathogens, particularly protozoa and viruses (Box 21.9). In general, infectious diarrhoea is more prevalent and more severe in AIDS patients that in healthy immunocompetent individuals. The effects of gastrointestinal infections associated with AIDS often aggravate the wasting syndrome present in these patients.

Specific (antimicrobial) therapy of gastrointestinal infections

Giving a comprehensive, in-depth description of the specific antimicrobial treatment of all gastrointestinal infections is beyond the scope of this chapter. Such treatment is summarised in Table 21.1, and the reader should search for detailed information on this field elsewhere. However, as a general guideline, antimicrobial therapy is mandatory in shigellosis, typhoid fever, and some cases of non-typhoid salmonellosis, cholera, and EIEC. Nontoxigenic strains of E. coli should be treated only in infants. Antimicrobial treatment is also advised in giardiasis and amebiasis. A short empirical course of ciprofloxacin in recommended for traveller's diarrhoea. Other bacterial diarrhoeas should be treated with antibiotics only in the presence of bacteraemia, as well as in immunodeficient (e.g. AIDS) or seriously ill patients. No drug treatment is recommended for ETEC or viral diarrhoea. There is no satisfactory antimicrobial therapy for some prevalent protozoal infections in AIDS (e.g. *Cryptosporidium, Isospora, Cyclospora*, and *Microsporidium*).

Nutritional and metabolic management of gastrointestinal infections

Despite the use of antimicrobial therapy when indicated, the management of patients with acute infectious diarrhoea mostly relies on dietary and,

Box 21.9 Pathogens most often causing diarrhoea in AIDS

Protozoa

- *Cryptosporidium;*[a]
- *Microsporidium;*[a]
- *Isospora;*[a]
- *Cyclospora;*
- *Giardia lamblia.*

Viruses

- CMV;[a]
- herpes simplex;
- rotavirus;
- calicivirus (Norwalk virus);
- enteric adenovirus;
- HIV itself (?).

Bacteria

- *Salmonella* spp.;[a]
- *Shigella* spp.;[a]
- *Campylobacter* spp.;[a]
- *Mycobacterium avium* complex;
- *Mycobacterium tuberculosis.*

Fungi

- *Histoplasma capsulatum;*
- *Coccidioides;*
- *Candida albicans;*
- *Cryptococcus neoformans.*

[a]Most frequent.

particularly, supportive rehydration therapy. Appropriate rehydration and replacement of electrolyte losses may be lifesaving, particularly in children and in developing countries, where superimposed malnutrition and famine are also frequent.

In chronic diarrhoea, stool output is usually not greater than 1500 g/day, whereas in acute diarrhoea between 1 and 20 kg/day may be passed, the highest amounts occurring in cholera. Normal stools contain relatively low concentrations of sodium (less than 10 mmol/kg) but are high in potassium (90 mmol/kg). As daily stool output increases, faecal sodium concentration rises and potassium falls. At 500 g stool/day they are equimolar (55 mmol/kg), and values approach those of plasma at stool outputs higher than 5 kg/day (130 mmol/kg for sodium and 4 mmol/kg for potassium).

Table 21.1 Antimicrobial therapy in infectious diarrhoea. PO, *per os*; IV, intravenous; IM, intramuscular; TMP-SMX, trimethoprim-sulfamethoxazole; EPEC, enteropathogenic *E. coli*; EAggEC, enteroaggregative *E. coli*; DAEC, diffusely adhering *E. coli*; EIEC, enteroinvasive *E. coli*.

	Drug of choice	Alternative drugs
Recommended in symptomatic patients		
Shigella spp.	Ampicillin (PO or IV)	Fluoroquinolones
	TMP-SMX (PO)	Nalidixic acid
Clostridium difficile	Metronidazole (PO)	
	Vancomycin (PO)	Other fluoroquinolones
Traveller's diarrhoea	Ciprofloxacin (PO)	TMP-SMX
EPEC, EAggEC, and DAEC in infants; EIEC	TMP-SMX (PO)	
Typhoid fever	Ciprofloxacin (PO)	Ceftriaxone
		Amoxycillin
		Chloramphenicol
		TMP-SMX
Cholera	Tetracycline (PO)	Doxycycline
		Cipro/Norfloxacin
		Amoxycillin
		TMP-SMX
Salmonella	Ampicillin (PO)	Ciprofloxacin
	TMP-SMX (PO)[a]	
Amebiasis	Metronidazole (PO), followed by	Tetracycline (PO) plus
	iodoquinol (PO) or paromomycin (PO)	dehydroemetine (IM)
Giardiasis	Metronidazole (PO)	Quinacrine
		Furazolidinone
		Paromomycin
Not recommended, except for immunodeficient, septic, or seriously ill patients		
Campylobacter spp.	Erythromycin (PO)	Ciprofloxacin (PO)
Yersinia spp.	Fluoroquinolones (PO)	Aminoglycosides
	TMP-SMX (PO)	Tetracycline
	Chloramphenicol (PO)	
Aeromonas spp.	TMP-SMX (PO)	Tetracycline
	Cephalosporins (PO)	Chloramphenicol
	Fluoroquinolones (PO)	
Vibrio (non-cholera)	Tetracycline (PO)	
EPEC, EAggEC, and DAEC in adults; EHEC	TMP-SMX (PO)	
Not recommended		
ETEC		
Viral diarrhoea		

In ampicillin-resistant strains.

Oral rehydration solutions

The traditional way to provide fluids and electrolytes has been the intravenous route, but in recent years oral rehydration solutions (ORSs) (Table 21.2) have proven to be equally effective and logistically more practical in developing countries. ORSs are based on the reliable physiological principle that glucose (and other organic compounds, such as amino acids) enhances sodium absorption in the small bowel, even in the presence of secretory losses caused by bacterial toxins, and that in addition colonic pathways for water and electrolyte absorption remain largely intact in acute diarrhoea.

Initially used for treating acute infectious diarrhoea in children in developing countries, ORSs have been shown to be useful in managing several types of diarrhoeal disease, in both children and adults, and not only of infectious origin (e.g. early stages of short-bowel syndrome and idiopathic AIDS enteropathy).

For years, the most widely used ORS was the World Health Organization (WHO)/UNICEF mixture, which

Table 21.2 Compositions of some oral rehydration solutions (ORSs).

	Electrolytes		Carbohydrates	
	Sodium (mmol/l)	Potassium (mmol/l)	Glucose (g/l)	Rice syrup (g/l)
WHO/ UNICEF	75	20	13.5	–
Pedialyte	45	20	25	–
Rehydralyte	75	20	25	–
Dioralyte	60	20	16	–
Glucolyte	35	20	36	–
Ricelyte	50	25	–	30
Ceralyte	70	20	–	40

was provided in packets containing glucose (20 g) and three salts – sodium chloride (3.5 g), potassium chloride (1.5 g), and either trisodium citrate (2.9 g) or sodium bicarbonate (2.5 g) – to be diluted in 1 l of water. It has been shown to be lifesaving in mild and moderate diarrhoea, but is suboptimal for cholera because, in spite of improving hydration and reducing mortality, it does not shorten the duration of diarrhoea.

An early modification of the standard solution was the addition of glycine or other amino acids, but this resulted in little improvement. A subsequent modification was to use some type of starch, usually rice, instead of glucose. A meta-analysis including almost 1400 adult and paediatric patients showed that rice-based ORSs reduced stool output in the first 24 hours by 36% in adults and 32% in children with cholera as compared to the WHO/UNICEF mixture. However, in non-cholera diarrhoea, the reduction was only 18%. Other studies have shown no major benefit. Attempts with maltodextrins and cereals have also been disappointing.

Water absorption is more efficient if the gut content is relatively hyposmolar (200–250 mosmol/l) rather than isosmolar (330 mosmol/l). It has been suggested that low-osmolarity ORSs, in which glucose and sodium concentrations are lowered, improve stool output, duration of diarrhoea, and the total amount of ORS and intravenous fluids required, in both cholera and non-cholera diarrhoea, without inducing hyponatraemia. If confirmed, reduced-osmolarity ORSs may replace WHO-based solutions in the future.

Diet

Dietary management of acute infectious diarrhoea has been influenced more by fads and fancies than by scientific knowledge. The traditional approach is absolute dietary abstinence. However, it is better to eat judiciously during an attack of diarrhoea than to drastically restrict oral intake. Soft, easily digestible foods are most acceptable to the patient with acute diarrhoea. In the early stages of the disease, a diet based on foods such as rice, carrots, and boiled meat or fish is advisable. Beverages containing caffeine or methylxanthine (coffee, tea, cola) and alcohol should be avoided, as they increase bowel motility.

In children, it is important to restart oral feeding as soon as the child is able to accept oral intake. Recent studies indicate that most infants with acute diarrhoea could be successfully managed with continued feeding of undiluted non-human milk, and routine dilution of milk or the use of lactose-free products is not necessary.

21.6 Concluding remarks

Although the HIV pandemic continues to have a disastrous impact on society in many of the worst-affected countries, there are grounds for optimism. Various international funding initiatives such as the Global Fund have allowed a dramatic increase in the numbers of patients who can access HIV treatment in resource-poor settings, which in turn has brought about major improvements in survival from this disease. However, with wider access to HIV drugs, the metabolic side effects of these drugs may become a problem at the population level, especially in societies where smoking is also prevalent. Increasing rates of drug resistance in tuberculosis are resulting in a greater proportion of patients who have a chronic debilitating disease requiring longer treatment, and these patients require more attention to be paid to nutritional aspects of their care. Further research work is needed to define appropriate treatment strategies for the management of nutritional and metabolic consequences of these major infections, and progress in this area is likely to be slow.

References and further reading

Atia A, Buchman AL. Treatment of cholera-like diarrhoea with oral rehydration. Ann Trop Med Parasitol 2010; 104: 465–474.

Brown TT, Glesby MJ. Management of the metabolic effects of HIV and HIV drugs. Nat Rev Endocrinol 2012; 8: 11–21.

Engelson ES, Kotler DP, Tan Y, Agin D, Wang J, Pierson RN Jr, Heymsfield SB. Fat distribution in HIV infected patients reporting truncal enlargement quantified by whole-body magnetic resonance imaging. Am J Clin Nutr 1999; 69(6): 1162–1169.

Giannella RA. Infectious enteritis and proctocolitis and bacterial food poisoning. In: Sleisenger & Fordtran's Gastrointestinal and Liver Disease, 8th edn (M Feldman, LS Friedman, LJ Brandt, eds). Philadelphia: Saunders-Elsevier, 2006, pp. 2333–2392.

Huston CD. Intestinal protozoa. In: Sleisenger & Fordtran's Gastrointestinal and Liver Disease, 8th edn (M Feldman, LS Friedman, LJ Brandt, eds). Philadelphia: Saunders-Elsevier, 2006, pp. 2413–2434.

Iriam JH, Visser MME, Rollins NN, Siegfried. Micronutrient supplementation in children and adults with HIV infection. Cochrane Database Syst Rev 2010; 12: CD003650.

Koethe JR, Chi BH, Megazzini KM, Heimburger DC, Stringer JSA. Macronutrient supplementation for malnourished HIV-infected adults: a review of evidence in resource-adequate and resource-constrained settings. Clin Infect Dis 2009; 49: 787–798.

Macallan DC, Noble C, Baldwin C, Foskett M, McManus T, Griffin GE. Prospective analysis of patterns of weight change in stage iv human immunodeficiency virus infection. Am J Clin Nutr 1993; 58(3): 417–424.

Okebe JU, Yahav D, Shibita R, Paul M. oral iron supplments for children in malaria-endemic areas. Cochrane Database Syst Rev 2011; 10: CD006589.

Schambelan M, Mulligan K, Grunfeld C, Daar ES, LaMarca A, Kotler DP, et al. Recombinant human growth hormone in patients with HIV-associated wasting: a randomized, placebo-controlled trial. Ann Intern Med 1996; 125: 873–882.

Sinclair D, Abba K, Grobler L, Sudarsanam TD. Nutritional supplements for people being treated for active tuberculosis. Cochrane Database Syst Rev; 2011: 11: CD006086.

Süttmann U, Ockenga J, Selberg O, Hoogestraat L, Deicher H, Muller MJ. Incidence and prognostic value of malnutrition and wasting in human immunodeficiency virus infected outpatients. 1995; 8(3): 239–246.

22
Nutritional Support in Patients with Cancer

Federico Bozzetti

University of Milan, Italy

Key messages

- Cancer is a condition that can affect nearly every organ system in the body. Its prognosis is enormously variable, from nearly 100% survival to almost 100% mortality depending on the site of the primary cancer.
- The majority of patients with cancer amenable to a curative therapy can maintain nutritional status with a normal diet, with or without the need for oral nutritional supplements. Some patients will require nutritional support in the form of enteral or parenteral nutrition at some stage of their disease in order to meet their nutritional needs.
- Many studies have examined the effects of enteral and parenteral nutrition on the outcome of cancer in different settings, with differing results.

- Modern approaches to the optimisation of nutritional status in cancer include the use of appetite stimulants, the modulation of nutrients, and supplementation with immunonutrients or anabolic/anticatabolic agents.
- The prevalence of weight loss observed in people with cancer varies enormously, from 30 to 90%. There is a relationship between weight loss and poor quality of life, and high morbidity and mortality rates have been demonstrated in both medical and surgical malnourished cancer patients.
- Cancer cachexia is a syndrome that occurs in approximately 70% of cancer patients during the terminal course of the disease and may be evident as a clinical presentation in 10–30% of subjects.

22.1 Introduction

Cancer needs to be considered differently from most other challenges in clinical nutrition. As opposed to diseases affecting the bowel, liver, kidney, or lung, which have been discussed in detail in Chapters 11, 12, 14, and 16, cancer can exert its effect on nearly every organ of the body. In addition, cancer and its clinical management need to take into account many other variable factors, such as age, widely variable survival rates, and differing therapeutic options. Because of this variability, cancer serves to illustrate an important principle in standards of clinical nutrition.

Given this level of variability, it is extremely difficult to conduct studies in which the outcomes are not confounded by a wide variety of factors. For this reason, this chapter will set out to demonstrate the evidence supporting the use of nutritional support in this heterogeneous group of patients.

This chapter is laid out in two main sections. The first concentrates on cancer cachexia, outlining the factors thought to be involved in the development of this condition. The second will deal with nutritional management in cancer, including the effects of nutritional support on nutritional status and clinical outcome, and the different modes of nutritional support given to patients with cancer.

Clinical Nutrition, Second Edition. Edited by Marinos Elia, Olle Ljungqvist, Rebecca J Stratton and Susan A Lanham-New.
© 2013 The Nutrition Society. Published 2013 by Blackwell Publishing Ltd.

22.2 Cancer cachexia

Definition and prevalence

The word 'cachexia' is derived from the Greek words 'kakos' meaning 'bad' and 'hexis' meaning 'state'. Cancer cachexia is a syndrome that occurs during the terminal course of the disease in approximately 70% of cancer patients and may be evident at clinical presentation in 10–30% of subjects. A recent, consensus-based definition of cancer cachexia was published in the Guidelines for Parenteral Nutrition on behalf the European Society for Clinical Nutrition and Metabolism (ESPEN): 'Cancer Cachexia is a complex syndrome characterized by a chronic, progressive, involuntary weight loss which is poorly or only partially responsive to the common nutritional support and it is often associated with anorexia, early satiation and asthenia. It is usually amenable to two main components: a decreased nutrient intake (which may be simply due a crucial involvement of the gastrointestinal tract by the tumour or by cytokines or similar anorexia-inducing mediators) and metabolic alterations due to the activation of systemic proinflammatory processes.'

Resulting metabolic derangements include insulin resistance, increased lipolysis, and normal or increased lipid oxidation with loss of body fat, increased protein turnover with loss of muscle mass, and an increase in production of acute-phase proteins.

These cytokine-induced metabolic alterations appear to prevent cachectic patients from regaining body cell mass during nutritional support, are associated with a reduced life expectancy, and are not relieved by exogenous nutrients alone.

Quite recently, other definitions of cancer cachexia have been proposed: Fearon et al. (2011) define cancer cachexia as 'a multifactorial syndrome characterized by an ongoing loss of skeletal muscle mass (with or without loss of fat mass) that cannot be fully reversed by conventional nutritional support and leads to progressive functional impairment. Its pathophysiology is characterized by a negative protein and energy balance driven by a variable combination of reduced food intake and abnormal metabolism. The agreed diagnostic criterion for cachexia was weight loss greater than 5%, or weight loss greater than 2% in individuals already showing depletion according to current bodyweight and height (body-mass index <20 kg/m(2)) or skeletal muscle mass (sarcopaenia).'

Although both these definitions detail the main clinical and metabolic features of cancer cachexia, they are not yet validated for routine use in clinical practice. Only two definitions are validated in the literature. One defines cancer cachexia as being characterised by three main factors: body weight loss $\geq 10\%$, nutrient intake ≤ 1500 kcal/day, and level of C-reactive protein (CRP) ≥ 10 mg/l. This definition is supported by a strong clinical and pathophysiological rationale, is prognostically validated, and represents the first true attempt to define cachexia according to objective criteria.

Nevertheless it has some limitations. First, it defines cachexia but it does not classify it in different stages of severity. Second, there is an objective difficulty in assessing the energy content of the diet of cancer patients in a nonspecialistic setting and without the help of a dietitian, and, furthermore, this definition requires a blood examination, and consequently the patient must be assessed twice. Finally, this definition was validated in a population of patients with pancreatic cancer only.

More recently, Bozzetti & Mariani (2009) have defined cancer cachexia as 'a complex syndrome characterized by a severe, chronic, unintentional and progressive weight loss, which is poorly responsive to conventional nutritional support, and may be associated with anorexia, asthenia and early satiation.'

Unlike the previous definitions, this pragmatic statement focuses mainly on clinical self-evident features and emphasises some specific aspects (chronic, unintentional, and progressive weight loss, unresponsiveness to conventional nutritional support). Furthermore, it includes anorexia and early satiety or fatigue, not only for their high prevalence in weight-losing cancer patients but also because their pathogenesis is closely related to the same factors (interleukin-6 (IL-6), tumour necrosis factor alpha (TNFα), etc.) responsible for the derangement of metabolism and for the weight loss. Hence their presence might reflect the role of some common specific mechanisms underlying both the clinical appearance and the metabolic picture of cancer cachexia.

Depending on the degree of the weight loss and the presence/absence of one/all of these symptoms, it is possible to stratify patients in four different classes

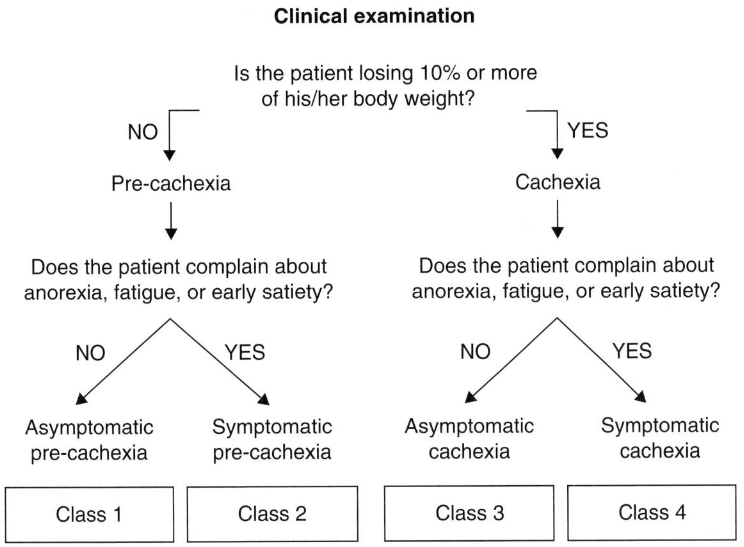

Clinical examination

Figure 22.1 Classification of cancer cachexia proposed by SCRINIO (SCReenIng Nutritional status In Oncology). Modified from Bozzetti & Mariani (2009), copyright © 2009 by SAGE Publications. Reprinted by permission of SAGE Publications.

(Figure 22.1). These classes (from 1 to 4) represent stages of progressive severity of the cachexia. Moving from 'asymptomatic precachexia' (class 1) to 'symptomatic cachexia' (class 4), there are statistically significant trends ($P < 0.0001$) in the percentage of gastrointestinal versus non-gastrointestinal tumours, severity of cancer stage, percentage of weight loss, number of symptoms per patient, Eastern Cooperative Oncology Group (ECOG) performance status, and nutritional risk score.

Other characteristics of cancer cachexia include anaemia, depletion, and alterations in body compartments, disturbances in water and electrolyte metabolism, and the progressive impairment of vital functions. Specific investigations into the composition of the body compartments of cancer patients have shown an increase in the ratio of total body water to total body potassium compared with normal subjects. A recent study in cachectic patients, which determined total body water and total body potassium isotopically, concluded that total body water can be accurately predicted, whereas measured values of total body potassium were significantly lower than predicted. Total body water, therefore, significantly overestimated the metabolically active tissue in weight-losing cancer patients.

Unlike patients with simple anorexia nervosa, in whom weight loss accounts for a more or less propor-

tional decrease in the size of all organs, patients with malignant cachexia have preferential sparing of the liver, kidney, and spleen, as well as significant involvement of other parenchyma. Lieffers *et al.* (2009) recently reported that increases in mass and in the proportion of high-metabolic-rate tissues (liver, spleen, and tumour) represent a cumulative incremental resting energy expenditure (REE) of approximately 17 700 kcal during the last 3 months of life and may contribute substantially to cachexia-associated weight loss.

Patients with malignant tumours have the highest prevalence of malnutrition of any segment of the hospitalised population. The prevalence and severity of cachexia are not always directly related to calorie intake, histological variety, or type of tumour spread; nor are they related to tumour size, since weight loss may be present even when the tumour represents less than 0.01% of the total body weight. In some cancer patients, weight loss may be the most frequent presenting symptom, affecting up to 66% of patients during the course of their disease. The overall prevalence of weight loss may be as high as 86% in the last 1–2 weeks of life.

A weight loss greater than 10% of the pre-illness body weight may occur in up to 45% of hospitalised adult cancer patients. In a recent prospective investigation aiming to define the nutritional status of cancer outpatients, Mariani *et al.* (2012) reported the degree and prevalence of malnutrition in 1500 patients (Table 22.1).

Table 22.1 Prevalence and severity of weight loss in different primary cancers. GI, gastrointestinal. Reprinted from Mariani *et al.* (2012), © Springer.

	Primary % weight loss (median)	% of patients with ≥10% weight loss
Upper GI	6.6	35
Oesophagus	15.1	66
Stomach	11.7	57
Pancreas	14	64
Small bowel	4.4	21
Colon rectum	4.8	28
Lung	6.4	35
Upper respiratory	5.4	25
Others	8.1	45

Pathophysiology

Our understanding of the aetiopathogenesis of cancer cachexia is limited and based more on knowledge of abnormalities in nutritional behaviour and metabolic patterns than on the identification of specific mediators. Three theories have been suggested:

(1) metabolic competition;
(2) under-nutrition;
(3) alterations of metabolic pathways.

Metabolic-competition theory

The metabolic-competition theory suggests that neoplastic cells compete with host tissues for amino acids, functioning thereby as a sort of 'nitrogen trap'. This may be true in experimental tumours, where neoplastic tissue accounts for a very high percentage of the carcass weight, but it is unlikely to be an important mechanism in human tumours, where the common experience is the opposite. There are cases of both cachectic patients with tumours of only a few grams and patients with a rather good general status with huge abdominal masses. Therefore, such a theory can only explain a very small fraction of cases of nutritional deterioration in cancer patients.

Under-nutrition

The second theory supports the role of under-nutrition as the main cause underlying the development of cancer cachexia. The reason for the reduced intake of nutrients in patients with lesions of the upper digestive tract is clear. A study carried out by the Istituto Nazionale Tumori, Milan, showed that the prevalence of subjective anorexia ranged from 33 to 40% of patients (depending on the type and site of the tumour), and that most of the nutritionally related variables were significantly worse in anorectic patients than in nonanorectic patients. Studies in the 1970s and 1980s found that anorexia is seen as a presenting symptom of malignancy in around 14–50% of newly diagnosed cancer patients, since abnormalities of food intake and feeding patterns occur. More recent studies report a prevalence of anorexia of about 60–64%, and up to 85% in patients with advanced disease.

However, regardless of the tumour's location, anorexia is the most common cause of reduced intake and usually consists of a loss of appetite and/or a feeling of early satiety. Anorexia often precedes the development of malnutrition and may be a presenting symptom of malignancy in 25% of patients. However, Bosaeus (2008) has reported that weight loss cannot be accounted for by the diminished dietary intake, since energy intake in absolute amounts is not different and intake per kilogram body weight is higher in weight-losing patients than in weight-stable patients, although long-term dietary intake may be difficult to assess precisely.

The presence of anorexia adversely affects quality of life: in systematic analyses of symptoms of advanced cancer, anorexia, together with pain and fatigue, is consistently among the 10 most prevalent and one of the top five most distressing symptoms reported by patients.

The mechanisms involved in the onset of anorexia are poorly understood. Older studies supported the role of intermediate metabolites (lactate, ketones, low-molecular-weight peptides, oligonucleotides) coupled with a state of relative hypoinsulinaemia.

Parabiotic experiments, in which a nonmetastasising tumour is implanted in an animal whose circulation is connected surgically to that of another non-tumour-bearing animal, demonstrate that anorexia, metabolic changes, weight loss, and cachexia occur in the non-tumour-bearing animals as well, despite the lack of evidence of metastatic tumour at necroscopy. Since the two surgically connected animals only share 1.5% of their total circulation, this suggests the presence of a tumour factor such as a cytokine.

Increased serotoninergic activity within the central nervous system (CNS) has been proposed as a possible cause of anorexia. Such activity is secondary to the enhanced availability of tryptophan to the brain, since a close relationship between elevated plasma-free tryptophan and anorexia was observed in cancer patients with a reduced food intake. The uptake into the brain of tryptophan is competitive with that of branched-chain amino acids (BCAAs), and administration of BCAAs by increasing the plasma levels of these competitors at the level of the blood–brain barrier may lead to a decrease in the occurrence of anorexia.

Cytokines may have a pivotal role in long-term inhibition of feeding, through mimicking the hypothalamic effect of excessive negative-feedback signalling from leptin. This can be achieved by persistent stimulation of anorexigenic neuropeptides such as adrenocorticotropic hormone (ACTH)-releasing factors, as well as by inhibition of the neuropeptide Y orexigenic network, which consists of opioid peptides and galanin, in addition to the newly identified melanin-concentrating hormone orexin and agouti-related peptide.

Leptin, the hormone produced by fat that suppresses appetite and increases energy expenditure to maintain weight stability, has been found in appropriately low levels in weight-losing cancer patients during initial studies.

Reduced intake has also been related to the presence of dysgeusia – a distortion or absence of the sense of taste. The decreased ability to perceive sweet flavours has been linked to anorexia, whereas a decrease in the threshold for bitter flavours has been linked to an aversion to meats rich in bitter substrates (amino acids, purines, polypeptides). Altered smell perception is also related to aversion to food.

In underfed patients there are secondary changes in the gastrointestinal tract, such as a decrease in secretions and atrophy of the mucosa and musculature, which may be responsible for the feeling of fullness and delayed emptying, the defective digestion, and the poor absorption of nutrients. Delayed gastric emptying and gastroparesis are also common in patients with advanced cancer. A comprehensive review on cancer anorexia was published by Laviano *et al.* (2003).

Alterations of metabolic pathways

The third theory underlying the pathogenesis of cancer cachexia relates to metabolic abnormalities. These span overall energy balance, the individual macro- and micronutrients, and the acute-phase response.

Energy balance

It is generally accepted that resting energy expenditure (REE) in patients with cancer is more variable than in normal subjects and is frequently increased by 50–300 kcal/day. The metabolic basis of this increase is poorly understood. One possibility concerns the mass and metabolic rate of malignant tissue. The mass of human tumours rarely exceeds 4% of body weight, so if it is assumed that the associated metabolic rate (per kilogram of tissue) of this tissue is similar to that of the rest of the body, a large increase in REE will not be expected. However, information about the energy expenditure of human malignant tissue *in vivo* is lacking. It is possible that a metabolically active tissue might contribute disproportionally to REE. By analogy, four organs (brain, kidney, heart, and liver), which account for about 5% of body weight, are responsible for about half of the REE in a healthy adult. Another possibility concerns the energy costs of metabolic processes induced by the tumour, such as increased gluconeogenesis, increased glucose–lactate recycling, and protein synthesis, all of which require adenosine triphosphate (ATP). This increased requirement will be associated with increased heat production.

A further explanation for the alteration in energy expenditure is based on the observation that cancer patients tend to oxidise a higher quantity of non-esterified fatty acids (NEFAs) than control subjects, even in the presence of other energy substrates. This indirectly implies a channelling of carbohydrate intermediates towards lipogenesis before oxidation, which represents a costly metabolism in terms of the consumption of ATP. It has also been reported that protein turnover can account for up to 50% of REE, with the liver usually accounting for 20–25% of overall oxygen consumption. Investigations in humans have shown that while the synthesis of muscle protein is diminished in cancer patients, the hepatic synthesis of secretory proteins, acute-phase reactants, fibrinogen, glycoproteins, and immunoglobulins can be increased.

The activity of the sympathetic nervous system may also contribute to basal hypermetabolism. It is difficult to explain the large variability in REE by a single metabolic process and it is likely that a combination of metabolic processes is involved, and that the combination varies with the type of cancer and stage of disease.

Total energy expenditure (TEE), which includes REE plus the physical-activity energy expenditure,

Year	No. of patients	Type of tumour	% hypermetabolic patients (REE ≥ 110% PEE)
1869–1924	34	Leukaemia	97
1914	33	Gastric carcinoma	45
1924	71	Leukaemia	86
1950	41	Leukaemia/lymphoma	100
	23	Carcinoma	91
1951	5	Leukaemia/lymphoma	5
1956	12	Solid tumours	67
1965	4	Solid tumours	75
1978	10	Miscellaneous	80
1980	65	Miscellaneous	58
1980	42	Gastroenteric tumours	↓ in males
1982	16	Miscellaneous	0
1982	200	Miscellaneous	63
1982	43	Gastroenteric tumours	↓
1983	173	Gastroenteric tumours	54
1983	73	Colorectal carcinoma	30
1983	5	Carcinoma of the lung	100[a]
1984	31	Lung cancer	100
1984	31	Carcinoma of the lung	100
1986a	24	Colorectal carcinoma	0
1986b	98	Miscellaneous	0
1988	7	Sarcoma	100[a]
1988	83	Colon and lung carcinoma	0[a]
1988	58	Colon and lung carcinoma	0[a]
1992	–	Hepatocarcinoma	–

Table 22.2 Studies on resting energy expenditure (REE) in cancer patients. PEE, predicted energy expenditure. Bozzetti F. Nutrition support in patients with Cancer. In: Artificial Nutrition Support in Clinical Practice (J Payne-James, G Grimble, D Silk, eds) 2001, Greenwich Medical Media, now published by Cambridge University Press, reproduced with permission.

[a] Referred to a control group.

may not be increased in cancer patients, as shown by tracer studies in free-living patients with cancer and other techniques in other malignancies. In fact, TEE may appear decreased in advanced cancer patients when compared to predicted values for healthy individuals, mainly because of a reduction in the physical activity. Recent data with the use of a wearable device, the SenseWear Armband (SensorMedics Italia Srl), would indicate that the TEEs of weight-stable leukaemic patients and of weight-losing bedridden patients with gastrointestinal tumours are about 24 and 28 kcal/kg/day, respectively.

In conclusion, the decrease in physical activity, which is very common in advanced malignant diseases, offsets or more than offsets any increase in REE. This implies that the loss of energy stores which may eventually lead to cancer cachexia is more likely to be due to a decrease in energy intake than an increase in energy expenditure.

Data on the prevalence and severity of hypermetabolism are shown in Tables 22.2 and 22.3.

Carbohydrate metabolism

Carbohydrate metabolism can be considered as whole-body and skeletal-muscle glucose metabolism, hepatic glucose metabolism, and tumour glucose metabolism. In this context, the main alterations in carbohydrate metabolism include decreased oral glucose tolerance, which occurs in 37–60% of tumour-bearing patients. By using the intravenous glucose tolerance test, it has been demonstrated that head and neck cancer patients have reduced first-phase insulin response, similar to that seen in type 2 diabetes, and a reduced glucose disposal. This result seems to be directly correlated, at the multiple-regression analysis, not only with acute insulin response but with triiodothyronine concentration. The reduced glucose disposal indicates that there is insulin resistance, with reduction in the normal ability of the insulin-sensitive tissues (e.g. muscle, gut) to take up glucose.

Investigations using the euglycaemic hyperinsulinaemic clamp technique have generally shown that there is a significant reduction in glucose utilisation

Table 22.3 Resting energy expenditure (REE) and type of tumour. Bozzetti F. Nutrition support in patients with Cancer. In: Artificial Nutrition Support in Clinical Practice (J Payne-James, G Grimble, D Silk, eds) 2001, Greenwich Medical Media, now published by Cambridge University Press, reproduced with permission.

Site/type	No. of patients	% patients with increase in REE	Median increase of REE (%)
Lung	5	100	–
	31	100	31
	22	0	–
	38	0	–
Leukaemia	133	74	35
Lymphoma	18	–	22
Sarcoma	9	–	14–18
Localised	4	–	33–41
Metastatic	7	100	35
Gastric carcinoma	28	40	10
	7	–	20
Colorectal carcinoma	73	22	20
	24	0	–
	16	–	28
	38	0	–
	45	0	–
Gastroenteric carcinoma	42	–	↑ in males
Localised	24	–	4
Metastatic	19	–	8

when the insulin concentration is in the physiological range, and that this effect is not overcome with administration of supraphysiological insulin concentrations. Fasting serum insulin is normal or low. On the whole, these studies imply that glucose may not be utilised in the whole body of cancer patients as well as lipids or amino acids. Since glucose oxidation appears to only be mildly reduced, the major defect in glucose utilisation probably resides in non-oxidative glucose disposal or in the synthesis of glycogen.

Hepatic glucose metabolism can also be altered during cancer cachexia. Approximately 75% of studies report an increase in the rate of hepatic glucose production in cancer patients. Gluconeogenesis from several precursors (lactate, alanine, glycerol) has been reported to be increased, as have total glucose production, turnover, and recycling. Cancer patients also have an increased glucose flux, which could consume up to 40% of the carbohydrates ingested and may contribute to the weight loss. The outpouring of lactic acid by some tumours leads to an increase in the conversion of lactate to glucose by the liver. This process – the Cori cycle – is energy-consuming, because the conversion of 2 moles of lactate to glucose requires 6 moles of ATP, whereas only 2 moles of ATP are recovered in the reconversion of glucose to lactate, and it has been estimated to account for 300 kcal of energy loss per day.

Although the Cori cycle normally accounts for 20% of glucose turnover, this rises to 50% in cachectic cancer patients and accounts for disposal of 60% of the lactate produced. Both glucose production rates were found to be higher in malnourished cancer patients than in non-cancer patients with comparable weight loss. The increase in glucose recycling, equivalent to 40% of the daily glucose intake of the cancer patient, has been estimated to lead to a potential loss of 0.9 kg of body fat per month.

The tumour itself can contribute to changes in carbohydrate metabolism. There is some evidence that a disproportionate requirement for glucose by the tumour accounts for the increase in glucose turnover and consumption. Perfusion experiments determined that glucose uptake by tumour tissue in patients with soft-tissue sarcomas was approximately 160 mg/minute (230 g glucose/day) when uptake remained constant for 24 hours. Glucose uptake is proportional to tumour size and corresponds to approximately 1.4 g/day/gram of tumour, a value which would account for the increase in glucose metabolism (170 g/24 hours) observed in sarcoma-bearing patients.

Most solid tumours, either because of isoenzyme alterations or because of their poor vascularisation and hence hypoxic nature, rely almost exclusively on the anaerobic metabolism of glucose as their main energy source, with most being converted to lactate. Glucose uptake and lactate release by human colon carcinoma have been found to exceed the peripheral tissue exchange rate by 30-fold and 43-fold, respectively. This extra requirement for glucose by the tumour is accompanied by a marked decrease in glucose utilisation by host tissue, particularly the brain, which resembles the situation found in starvation.

In conclusion, tumours have been demonstrated to affect the rate of glucose utilisation in a number of tissues. Given that there are only 1200 kcal stored in the body as liver and muscle glycogen, blood glucose levels would be expected to fall. This does not occur, because of the parallel increase in the hepatic glucose production. This production of endogenous glucose cannot be suppressed by the administration of exogenous glucose, which would be effective in healthy volunteers. In fact, studies in hepatic cell cultures from tumour-bearing subjects have demonstrated a dose-related increase in glucose synthesis from physiological concentrations of lactate and alanine (and a further increase in the presence of an excess of precursor), which probably takes place through a mechanism of induction of the gluconeogenic enzymes.

Hypoglycaemia has been reported in patients with carcinoma of the stomach, cecum, or bile ducts, with pseudomyxoma, and with paraganglioma, sometimes occurring before the presence of a tumour is suspected. Hypoglycaemia was originally thought to be a result of high glucose consumption by the tumour, but recently it has been suggested that it arises through the ability of some tumours, other than insulinoma, to produce insulin or insulin-like substances. Since insulin levels have been shown to be low in cases of tumour-associated hypoglycaemia, the production by a tumour of an insulin growth factor has been suggested as the cause of enhanced peripheral glucose uptake. The most likely candidate for the pathogenesis of extrapancreatic tumour hypoglycaemia is the production of a high-molecular-mass (15–25 kDa) insulin-like growth factor type 2 (IGF-2) by the tumour. Thus, patients with cancer have an increased glucose production and turnover, which may be enhanced by the production of IGF-2. Such changes contribute to an increased energy expenditure by the host.

The main abnormalities of carbohydrate metabolism are summarised in Box 22.1.

Box 22.1 Metabolic abnormalities in the cancer patient

Carbohydrate

- decreased glucose tolerance;
- insulin resistance in insulin-sensitive tissues (muscle, gut, etc.);
- defect in non-oxidative glucose disposal or in glycogen synthesis;
- increase in gluconeogenesis from lactate, alanine, and glycerol;
- increase in total glucose production, turnover, and recycling.

Lipid

- depletion of fat stores and lipid content in muscle;
- increased lipolysis and fat oxidation;
- increased fatty acid and glycerol turnover.

Protein

- unchanged or decreased muscle protein synthesis;
- unchanged or increased protein breakdown;
- increased hepatic synthesis of acute-phase proteins;
- specific alterations of plasma amino acid profile.

Lipid metabolism

Under normal conditions of feeding and fasting, two adipose-tissue enzymes, hormone-sensitive lipase and lipoprotein lipase, control the uptake and breakdown of fat from adipose tissue. During early starvation, decreased insulin levels and increased glucagon and adrenaline result in cyclic adenosine monophosphate (cAMP) activation of a protein kinase, which phosphorylates and activates the hormone-sensitive lipase. This enzyme hydrolyses the lipid droplet of the adipocyte into NEFAs to be released into the circulation. Conversely, the activated lipoprotein lipase hydrolyses the core of the circulating triacylglycerol-rich lipoproteins into NEFAs and monoacylglycerol. These NEFAs are the major source of substrate for adipocyte triacylglycerol (TAG) synthesis, since adipocytes synthesise very small amounts of fatty acids *de novo*. This mechanism seems to be disrupted in anorexic weight-losing cancer patients. In patients with cancer cachexia there is an overall depletion of fat stores and lipid content in muscle samples. The rates of depletion are equal, as suggested by the relative increase in fractions (phospholipid and free cholesterol) of polyunsaturated fatty acid (PUFA). The increased serum concentration of NEFAs, when present, could explain the decreased post-receptor insulin resistance. Fasting plasma glycerol concentrations have been shown to be higher in weight-losing cancer patients than in weight-stable cancer patients, thus providing evidence for an increase in lipolysis. The main abnormalities of lipid metabolism are summarised in Box 22.1.

Some patients, especially if undernourished, exhibit a clear state of hyperlipidaemia and have a decrease in plasma lipoprotein lipase. The elevated plasma lipid level may be immunosuppressive, and thereby affect ultimate survival. Several clinical studies have observed an increased mobilisation of fatty acids before weight loss occurs, suggesting the production of lipid-mobilising factors (LMFs) either by the tumour or by host tissue. This could contribute to tumour growth. Patients with ovarian or endometrial tumours were found to have lower concentrations of linoleic acid in subcutaneous adipose tissue than cancer-free subjects, suggesting mobilisation to supply lipid to the tumour. Linoleic acid has been found to act as a stimulator of tumour growth both *in vitro* and *in vivo*. Whole-body lipid metabolism was found to be increased in cancer patients with weight loss. The increase of lipolysis may be due to an increase in the hormone-sensitive lipase.

Cancer patients with weight loss have an increased glycerol and fatty acid turnover compared with normal subjects and cancer patients without weight loss. There is also an increased oxidation of fat, which is proportional to the stage of disease and to the severity of the malnutrition, and an increased rate of removal of infused lipids from the blood, suggesting that host tissues may increase their utilisation of fatty acids as an energy source even in the presence of high plasma glucose concentration. It is interesting that the administration of glucose fails to inhibit fat mobilisation and oxidation, as usually occurs in normal patients.

Protein metabolism

Abnormalities of protein metabolism in cancer patients (shown in Box 22.1) include nitrogen depletion (lean body mass and visceral protein) in the host, changes in hepatic and muscular protein turnover, an increase of gluconeogenesis from amino acids, and abnormal patterns of plasma amino acids. Investigations into protein kinetics have shown conflicting results. Whole-body protein turnover has been reported as being not significantly different from control, or even increased. Discrepancy in absolute values among different studies may reflect

heterogeneity in the investigative methods, whereas differences between cancer patients and controls may be related to the type of cancer population and choice of controls. The exceptionally high protein turnover rate found in some patients with hepatocellular carcinoma has been demonstrated to be a consequence of elevated endogenous protein breakdown and oxidation of amino acids.

Some authors have reported specific alterations of plasma amino acid profile. A recent extensive collective review by Lai *et al.* (2005) has summarised the alterations in the levels of the single amino acid and, interestingly, has reported that in patients with cancer of the head and neck or of the gastrointestinal tract (i.e. the patient population which most often requires nutritional support), the plasma level of all of the essential amino acids (except threonine) is always decreased.

Compared with normal colon tissue, human colon tumours were observed to have a specific requirement for serine and for BCAAs.

There is some discrepancy in the results of the literature in the area of protein metabolism in muscle.

The more consistent finding is that there is a decrease in protein synthesis, but normal and increased rates have also been reported. The negative net balance is explained by a normal breakdown concurrent to a decreased synthesis, or by an increase in breakdown.

Recent research supports the concept that muscle wasting is associated with an increased gene expression and the activity of the calcium/calpain and ubiquitin/proteasome proteolytic pathways in addition to the classic proteolytic mechanisms due to the lysosome cathepsins B, H, D, and L. Calcium/calpain-regulated release of microfilaments from the sarcomere is an early and perhaps rate-limiting component of the catabolic response in muscle. Released microfilaments are ubiquinated in the N-end rule pathway, regulated by the ubiquitin-conjugating enzyme $E2_{14k}$ and the ubiquitin ligase $E_{3\alpha}$, and degraded by the 26S proteasome. Several proinflammatory cytokines, including TNF, IL-1 and IL-6, and glucocorticoids, stimulate production of ubiquitin mRNA. In muscle loss, pale fibres are affected more than red fibres, and predominantly myofibrillar proteins are involved, as shown by measurements of 3-methylhistidine.

As regards hepatic protein metabolism, studies with radiolabelled leucine have shown that while in normal subjects 53% of hepatic protein synthesis derives from muscle, it accounts for only 8% in malnourished cancer patients. Synthesis of structural liver proteins is normal, and that of the acute phase is increased.

There is a correlation between hypoalbuminaemia and tumour bulk. Studies with labelled precursors have reported a reduction in albumin synthesis, which is partially corrected by increased protein intake, and an increase in the catabolised fraction. However, recent investigations have shown that synthesis of negative acute-phase reactants such as albumin is maintained despite reduced circulating concentrations, whereas synthesis of positive acute-phase reactants (e.g. fibrinogen) is significantly increased. There is also an increase in transcapillary escape, with a decrease in the intravascular and extravascular ratio.

In rare cases, hypoalbuminaemia is also caused by its sequestration in pathological compartments or by loss to the outside (nephrotic syndromes, protein-losing enteropathy, aminoaciduria in acute leukaemias). Such findings could explain the frequent occurrence of hypoalbuminaemia even when degradation is normal and synthesis is increased, as reported in recent investigations. Chronic administration of TNF in tumour-bearing animals results in a reduction of whole-body protein synthesis and net loss of skeletal protein, but in an increase in liver protein synthesis.

The tumour itself can interfere with protein metabolism. The metabolic-competition theory suggests that the tumour acts as a 'one-way nitrogen trap', and that this may have an influence on body economy when the mass accounts for 20% of the body weight of the host. However, it has been found that experimental tumours containing less than 6% of total body nitrogen have a protein metabolism equal to 35% of all protein synthesis. In humans it has been demonstrated that when the tumour is localised and resectable (i.e. in colorectal cancer), there is no substantial impact on the overall protein kinetics, while measurement of the difference in arteriovenous concentrations of amino acids in tumour-bearing limbs versus normal extremities has shown that less than half of the output of amino acids is released in the circulation by the tumour-bearing limb.

Some studies have demonstrated that the amino acid appearance rate is related to tumour bulk. Measurements in tumour tissue of protein metabolism have established that the tissue has a very high fractional protein synthesis rate of 50–90% per day. This is very similar to the liver and contrasts with a rate of 1–3% for skeletal muscle. In a recent study it was found that those cancer patients who had an elevated plasma amino acid appearance rate survived and those with a normal rate died. Although this issue is controversial, it would appear that an adequate acute-phase response to tumour may reflect a more effective fight against cancer.

Acute-phase response

The development of cancer cachexia may elicit an acute-phase response to malignancy, which is a basic defensive and phylogenetically primitive response of the body against injury. This includes reductions in serum iron and zinc levels, alterations in amino acid distribution and metabolism, and increases in acute-phase globulin synthesis and gluconeogenesis, negative nitrogen balance, and sometimes fever. This process is due to cytokines secreted by macrophages at the tissue site of the tumour, which inhibit albumin synthesis and stimulate the synthesis of acute-phase proteins.

These include:

- *CRP*, which promotes phagocytosis, modulates the cellular immune response, and inhibits the migration of white blood cells into the tissues.
- *Alpha-1-antichymotrypsin*, which minimises tissue damage due to phagocytosis and reduces intravascular coagulation.
- *Alpha-1-macroglobulin*, which forms complexes with proteases and removes them from circulation, maintains antibody production, and promotes granulopoiesis and synthesis of other acute-phase proteins.

An acute-phase protein response is seen in a significant proportion of patients bearing tumours that are frequently associated with weight loss (e.g. pancreas, lung, oesophagus) and is more frequent in the advanced stages of disease. The presence of such a response in patients with pancreatic or renal cancer is associated with a shortened survival, perhaps due to the exaggerated muscle breakdown required to supply amino acids for the acute-phase-response protein synthesis.

Vitamin and mineral deficiencies

Deficiencies in vitamins may be present in some undernourished cancer patients. The most significant include reductions in plasma levels of folate, vitamin A, and vitamin C. Between 19 and 52% of hospitalised patients have been noted to have reduced serum folate levels and 18–35% of patients who die of cancer and subsequent infections have severe liver deficiency of vitamin A at autopsy. Recently it has been found that many cancer patients have low levels of 25(OH)D (<50 nmol/l); such low levels are associated with a high incidence of cancer and are a marker of poor prognosis.

Mineral deficiencies can occur in some cancer patients as part of the cytokine-mediated inflammatory response (in addition to being a consequence of common causes such as poor oral intake, increased dietary requirements, and excessive urinary and stool losses). Zinc concentrations in the blood can drop as an early response to cytokines, which may be elevated in cancer patients. In cancer patients who are hospitalised, a low serum zinc (<0.7 mg/l) is not uncommon and usually normalises after a 3-week administration of 50 mg zinc/day. Serum copper is normal or elevated in cancer patients, with a pattern similar to that of serum zinc. Serum iron levels usually fall as result of cytokine-mediated response.

Hormonal milieu

Many patients develop insulin-resistance syndrome as a result of cancer and exhibit a small but significant elevation in serum insulin concentration. As a consequence, as in the case of diabetes, they have reduced glucose utilisation, loss of first-phase insulin response, and sometimes increased fasting hepatic glucose production. As already mentioned, the weight-losing cancer patients frequently have an increase in fatty acid oxidation and plasma fatty acid appearance rate. The rate of TAG hydrolysis is much higher than that of fat oxidation, so that albumin-bound fatty acids are partially utilised for energy, but many are utilised for re-esterification or substrate cycling back to TAGs.

Multiple studies have failed to demonstrate elevation in the counter-regulation of hormones, with the exception of a mild elevation in urinary free cortisol secretion. Catecholamines and glucagon are usually normal, but growth hormone (GH) was found to be increased at 24-hour analysis and by random sampling in malnourished cancer patients. Levels of GH are further increased by the infusion of arginine and

insulin. Hypogonadism has been reported in male cancer patients and free triiodothyronine and triiodothyronine concentrations can both be low.

As a normal response, to save energy in the injured subject, the body's ability to convert the stored form of a thyroid hormone (thyroxin or T_4) into the active form of thyroid hormone (triiodothyronine or T_3) becomes impaired and T_4 is converted to an inactive form known as reverse-T_3 hormone (rT_3). This process can occur in aggressive cancers, when the patient's response is similar to that of an injury response. There is no evidence of increased thyroid hormone levels during refeeding.

Mediators

Cytokines

The cytokines which were identified as mediators of cancer cachexia include TNF, IL-1, -2, -4, and -6, and interferon α, β and γ. These cytokines are produced by immunocytes as an endogenous immune response to the tumour and regulate many of the nutritional and metabolic disturbances that occur in the host with cancer, leading to:

- decreased appetite;
- stimulation of the basal metabolic rate (BMR);
- stimulation of glucose uptake;
- stimulation of the mobilisation of fat and protein stores;
- reduction in adipocyte lipoprotein lipase activity;
- enhanced muscle amino acid release;
- stimulation of hepatic amino acid transport activity.

Elevated concentrations of tissue and circulating cytokines have been found in cancer patients and enhanced hepatic cytokine gene expression has been found in tumour-bearing animals.

Recent studies have reported that in patients with different solid tumours, TNF polimorphism was associated with anorexia (lung cancer), IL-1β gene polimorphism was associated with cachexia (gastric cancer), IL-1β genetic polymorphisms were shown to have a possible modulatory role in the cancer anorexia/weight-loss syndrome in patients with metastatic gastric and oesophageal cancer, and pro-inflammatory cytokine haplotypes (IL-6 CC, IL-10 GG, TNFα) were associated with adverse prognosis in pancreatic carcinoma.

Table 22.4 Cytokine-mediated effects on protein, carbohydrate, and lipid metabolism. TNF, tumour necrosis factor; IL, interleukin; LPL, lipoprotein lipase; IFN, interferon.

Cytokine	Protein	Carbohydrate	Lipid
TNF	Increased muscle proteolysis	Increased glycogenolysis	Decreased lipogenesis
	Increased protein oxidation	Decreased glycogen synthesis	
	Increased hepatic protein synthesis	Increased gluconeogenesis	
		Increased glucose clearance	
		Increased lactate production	
IL-1	Increased hepatic protein synthesis	Increased gluconeogenesis	Increased lipolysis
		Increased glucose clearance	Decreased LPL synthesis
			Increased fatty acid synthesis
IL-6	Increased hepatic protein synthesis		Increased lipolysis
			Increased fatty acid synthesis
IFNγ			Decreased lipogenesis
			Increased lipolysis
			Decreased LPL activity

A comprehensive review on this topic can be found in Seruga *et al.* (2008).

The clinical effects of the administration of some cytokines to experimental animals are reported in Table 22.4 and are covered in the next section.

Both animal and human studies show that administration of TNFα causes an initial drop in body weight followed by a decreasing response with repeated administration. Acute administration of TNFα causes effects similar to those seen in cancer cachexia, including an increase in metabolic rate (by 30%), plasma TAGs, glycerol turnover (by more than 80%), and NEFA turnover (by more than 60%), as well as in temperature, heart rate, and epinephrine and ACTH levels. Similar effects were seen on protein metabolism, where whole-body protein turnover, total amino acid efflux, and acute-phase protein response were increased. It is noteworthy that in human studies where TNF was given to cancer patients intermittently, it did not cause weight loss, perhaps because it was not possible to consistently elevate TNF levels. In the studies, these responses were blunted by ibuprofen despite the absence of changes in the plasma levels of TNFα. However, in chronic administration the alterations were resolved, despite continuous administration of TNFα.

Moreover, in no phase I clinical investigation of TNFα was cachexia a major side effect; instead, fluid retention through damage to the vascular endothelium and increased capillary permeability were reported. Only hypertriacylglycerolaemia persisted despite the development of tachyphylaxis, but this seems to be unrelated to cachexia, since, for instance, hypertriacylglycerolaemic AIDS patients maintain their weight for prolonged periods of time.

Experimental studies suggest that the increase in serum TAGs due to TNFα administration is mainly due to hepatic synthesis and secretion of very low-density lipoproteins (VLDLs) rather than adipose tissue. Depletion of skeletal muscle would be due to the induction of oxidative stress and nitric oxide synthase, and consequent decreased myosin creatine phosphokinase expression and binding activity. It is possible that naturally occurring TNFα inhibitors in the circulation may hide TNFα production by the host's monocytes. In fact, these inhibitors were found to be circulating freely in healthy volunteers and to be increased in individuals with ovarian cancer. The inability to detect TNFα in cachectic patients has led to the suggestion that it acts as a paracrine/autocrine mediator rather than as the circulating messenger in cachexia.

Production of TNF by isolated peripheral blood mononuclear cells has been shown to be elevated in weight-losing pancreatic cancer patients with an acute-phase protein response, suggesting that local rather than systemic production may be the more relevant.

Some investigators did not find elevated TNFα levels in weight-losing or weight-stable cancer patients and this may be due to the presence of circulating inhibitors or to their action as paracrine/autocrine inhibitors. Nevertheless, there was a two-fold increase in the relative levels of messenger ribonucleic acid (mRNA) for hormone-sensitive lipase in the adipose tissue of cancer patients compared with controls. These findings suggest that TNFα may not contribute to the development of cachexia in cancer, but indicate a stimulation of lipolysis in adipose tissue. Anti-TNFα antibodies have had minimal effects in tumour-bearing animals, even if in a human squamous cell carcinoma of the maxilla, grown as a xenograft in nude mice, anti-TNFα antibodies partially reversed, but did not completely normalise, body weight.

IL-1 has been shown to have many effects similar to those of TNFα, including suppression of lipoprotein lipase and enhancement of intracellular lipolysis. Elevated IL-1 plasma levels are seldom found in cancer patients, but antibodies against an IL-1 receptor mitigate cachectic symptoms in tumour-bearing mice to a similar degree to anti-TNFα antibodies.

Unlike TNFα and IL-1, increased levels of IL-6 are measured in the serum of cancer patients. IL-6 is the main cytokine involved in the induction of acute-phase proteins and fibrinogen synthesis, and elevated levels have been reported in 39% of patients with lung or colon cancer and an ongoing acute-phase protein response. However, since all of the patients had lost weight, it is difficult to determine whether IL-6 was elevated in cachectic patients alone. Antibodies to IL-6 administered to patients with AIDS-related lymphoma produced weight gain in those losing weight and stabilised the levels of the acute-phase-reactant CRP. The increase in circulating IL-6 is closely related to tumour burden and is thought to originate from tumour cells as well as from various tissues of the cancer-bearing host (e.g. liver, kidney, small intestine, etc.) and to be induced by the IL-1 production of tumour-infiltrating macrophages. Again, local production of IL-6 by peripheral blood mononuclear cells is important, and its production seems to be elevated in patients with pancreatic cancer and an acute-phase protein response.

Interferon gamma (IFNγ) is known to have effects on fat metabolism similar to those of TNFα, namely the inhibition of lipoprotein lipase and of protein synthesis, and polyclonal antibodies anti-IFNγ partly mitigate cancer-induced anorexia and weight loss. Increased serum IFNγ levels have been found in 53% of patients with multiple myeloma. However, no association was observed between the level of IFNγ and the clinical parameters of the disease. These findings suggest that IFNγ alone may not be responsible for the induction of wasting. In the long term, a vicious cycle is activated that results in anorexia and widespread abnormalities in carbohydrate, protein, and lipid metabolism (Figure 22.2).

The acute response to TNFα in healthy volunteers appears to be a rise in CRP, a decrease in serum zinc level, and a doubling of the forearm amino acid efflux, primarily attributable to increases in the glucogenic amino acids alanine and glutamine. This accelerated nitrogen release may be due to starvation effects. These results have been replicated in animals and with IL-1. It is unclear, however, which distal mediators in the cytokine cascade are the key players. The mechanisms underlying host cachexia have been suggested to be due to cytokines, elaborated by activated immunocytes in response to the tumour and having secondary effects which exhibit an acute-phase reaction, rerouting nutrients from the periphery to the liver.

Studies evaluating the effects of cytokine administration on the circulating glucose concentration indicate that the plasma glucose level rises or falls depending on the dose of cytokine administered, the timing of the measurement, and the specific cytokine given. There are experimental data which indicate that TNFα administration can induce a marked increase in whole-body glucose utilisation even though glucose uptake does not increase equally in all organs or tissues. It is likely that the loss of fat stores in patients with cancer is due in part to the ability of TNFα and IL-1 to mobilise fat stores. In the experimental setting, TNFα is able to reduce the adipocyte lipoprotein lipase activity and heparin-releasable lipoprotein lipase activity and to increase the serum TAG levels, which also depend on a stimulation of the hepatic lipid secretion. IL-6 is also able to reduce adipose-tissue lipoprotein lipase activity and heparin-releasable lipoprotein lipase activity.

Catabolic factors

In addition to cytokines, some studies have reported circulating human factors that act directly on skeletal muscle and adipose tissues in a hormone-like manner. The most important are the LMFs, and to a lesser extent the protein-mobilising factors (PMFs). LMFs include the toxohormone-L isolated from the ascitic fluid of patients with hepatoma and that isolated from culture media of the human A375 melanoma

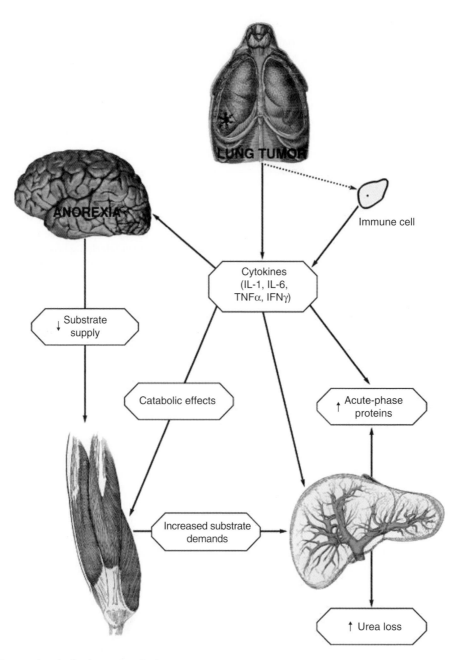

Figure 22.2 Suggested mechanism for cancer cachexia.

cell line. LMFs act directly on adipose tissue, with release of free fatty acid and glycerol, in a manner similar to that of lipolytic hormones. The mechanism involved could be the continuous stimulation of LMFs on the cAMP, which results in the activation of protein kinase, which in turn phosphorylates an inactive form of TAG lipase, otherwise known as hormone-sensitive lipase.

There is strong evidence that LMFs produced by tumours are related to the process of cachexia: LMF is absent or released in reduced amounts from tumours that do not induce cachexia, and is also absent from normal serum, even under conditions of starvation. The level of LMF in the sera of cancer patients has been found to be proportional to the extent of weight loss, and is reduced in patients responding to chemotherapy.

Following some preliminary *in vitro* investigations showing inhibition of the tumour LMFs by the PUFA eicosapentaenoic acid (EPA), cachectic patients suffering from pancreatic cancer were treated with fish oil capsules containing 18% EPA and 12% docosahexaenoic acid (DHA). This supplementation reversed the weight loss of 2.9 kg/month and led to a weight gain of 0.3 kg/month, which was associated with a temporary reduction of acute-phase proteins and stabilisation of the REE.

There is some evidence that PMFs play a role in human cancer cachexia. Some investigators found the presence of u- and m-calpains, a group of cytosolic, calcium-dependent proteases capable of inducing proteolysis when incubated with rat diaphragm, in the serum of cachectic patients, and subsequently succeeded in isolating the 24 kDa proteoglycan from the urine of cachectic patients, regardless of the tumour type. This factor was able to accelerate the breakdown of skeletal muscle *in vitro* and *in vivo* and to produce weight loss *in vivo* by a process that did not involve anorexia.

Iatrogenic malnutrition
Hypophagia

Anorexia and hypophagia may involve a psychological component that is related to the communication of the diagnosis or of therapeutic decisions such as the need for hospitalisation or disabling therapies. In paediatric patients in particular, conditioning mechanisms can lead to anorexia or food aversion. Nutritional changes resulting from iatrogenic lesions of the alimentary tract are also important. Table 22.5 lists the nutritional changes related to the radical resection of organs of the digestive tract. Malnutrition is only rarely related to reduced caloric and protein intake resulting from certain procedures (interference in chewing and swallowing due to glossectomy, dysphagia, total gastrectomy), although the long survival which is now possible thanks to advances in the oncological therapies exposes a higher number of cancer patients to the risk of under-nutrition. Malnutrition may also be due to malabsorption.

Table 22.5 Nutritional consequences of radical resection of alimentary-tract organs.

Organ	Nutritional consequences
Tongue or pharynx	Need for enteral feeding (due to dysphagia)
Thoracic oesophagus	Gastric stasis (due to vagotomy) Malabsorption of fats (due to vagotomy)
Stomach	Dumping syndrome; anaemia; malabsorption of fats, iron, calcium, and vitamins
Duodenum	Biliary–pancreatic deficiency
Jejunum (up to 120 cm)	Reduced absorption of glucose, fats, protein, folic acid, vitamin B_{12}, etc.
Ileum (60 cm) or ileocecal valve	Malabsorption of vitamin B_{12}, biliary salts, and fats
Small intestine (75%)	Malabsorption of fats, glucose, protein, folic acid, vitamin B_{12}, etc.; diarrhoea
Jejunum and ileum	Complete malabsorption
Colon (subtotal or total resection)	Water and electrolyte loss
Pancreas	Malabsorption and diabetes
Liver	Transient hypoalbuminaemia

Nutritional complications associated with radiotherapy are frequent (Table 22.6). It has been demonstrated that approximately 90% of patients submitted to intensive treatment in the head and neck region, the abdomen, or the pelvis lose weight unless nutritional support is provided. More than 10% of patients lose over 10% of their usual weight when radiotherapy is continued for a period of 6–8 weeks. The pathophysiology of malnutrition from radiotherapy is twofold: direct hypophagia in patients receiving radiotherapy to regions of the head and neck and chest, and hypophagia associated with malabsorption in patients receiving radiotherapy to the abdomen.

The minimum tolerated dose for other regions (i.e. the dose that may cause severe complications within 5 years of completion of radiotherapy using the standard high-energy therapeutic modality fractioned into 10 Gy a week, with five sessions a week) varies from 35 to 50 Gy, depending on the organs and tissue in question (Table 22.7). Head and neck irradiation interferes with nutrition because it causes a rapid exponential loss in the sense of taste. After 3–4 weeks, patients begin to suffer from an affected taste sensation due to lesion of the microvilli of the gustatory

Region irradiated	Early effects	Late effects
Head and neck	Odynophagia	Ulceration
	Xerostomia (dry mouth)	Xerostomia
	Mucositis	Dental caries
	Anorexia	Osteoradionecrosis
	Dysosmia	Trismus
	Hypogeusia (reduced ability to taste)	Hypogeusia
Thorax	Dysphagia	Fibrosis
		Stenosis
		Fistula
Abdomen and pelvis	AnorexiaNausea	Ulceration
	Vomiting	Malabsorption
	Diarrhoea	Diarrhoea
	Acute enteritis	Chronic enteritis
	Acute colitis	Chronic colitis

Table 22.6 Nutritional complications associated with radiotherapy.

Table 22.7 Radiation tolerance of the parts of the gastrointestinal tract. TD 5/5 = total dose of radiation which will give rise to a 5% increase in significant complications in 5 years; TD 50/5 = total dose of radiation which will give rise to a 50% incidence of significant complications in 5 years.

Organ	TD 5/5 (rads)	TD 50/5 (rads)
Stomach	4500	5000
Small intestine	4500	6000
Colon	4500	6500
Rectum	5500	8000

cells or their surfaces. This condition returns to normal 2–4 months after the end of treatment.

Another change caused by head and neck irradiation is the decrease in salivation that occurs in the first 3–4 days of therapy, causing nausea and dysphagia and facilitating the onset of caries. Erythema, mucositis, and oropharyngeal ulceration with odynophagia may develop during the second or third week.

Radiotherapy to the chest may lead to dysphagia when the field of irradiation includes the oesophagus; it occurs with fractioned doses of approximately 30 Gy over 3 weeks and may persist for several weeks after completion of therapy. Radiotherapy to the abdomen and pelvis may cause two different types of nutritional disturbance: those related to decreased food intake due to anorexia, nausea, and vomiting, and those due to chronic X-ray enteropathy.

Negative side effects from chemotherapy occur in several forms (Table 22.8): anorexia due to changes in the sense of taste, with perception of a metallic tinge; dysphagia due to ulceration of the mucosa of the lip, tongue, oropharyngeal cavity, and oesophagus; decrease in food intake due to nausea and vomiting; and constipation or adynamic ileus.

The combination of chemo- and radiotherapy produces cytotoxicity as a result of their simple additive effect and of synergism (the final response is greater than the sum of the effects of the single modalities as a result of the use of sensitising drugs).

Examples of common negative effects of combinations of therapy used in cancer treatment are summarised in Box 22.2.

Box 22.2 Common examples of the negative effects of combinations of therapy used in cancer treatment

- Antitumour antibiotics (adriamycin, actinomycin D, bleomycin) are generally more toxic when administered to patients undergoing radiotherapy.
- The incidence and severity of oesophagitis from irradiation increase with the use of actinomycin D, vinblastine, hydroxyurea, procarbazine, and the combination of cyclophosphamide, vincristine, and actinomycin D.
- Adriamycin and daunomycin are sensitising agents which, when combined with radiotherapy, may cause oesophageal stenosis.
- Fluorouracil, actinomycin D, and adriamycin may enhance damage from irradiation in other regions of the digestive tract.
- Actinomycin D and adriamycin are responsible for the so-called 'recall reaction', in which there is a reactivation of the latent effects of irradiation during medical therapy. In this case, severe irritation of the gastrointestinal mucosa may recur periodically.

Table 22.8 Negative side effects of chemotherapy.

Drug	Severity and duration
Chemotherapeutic drugs commonly associated with severe nausea and vomiting	
Nitrogen mustard (mustine hydrochloride; mechlorethamine hydrochloride USP)	Occurs in virtually all patients May be severe, but usually subsides within 24 hours
Chloroethyl nitrosoureas	Variable, but may be severe
Streptozotocin (streptozocin)	Occurs in nearly all patients Tolerance improves with each successive dose given on a 5-day schedule
Cis-platinum (cisplatin)	May be very severe Tolerance improves with intravenous hydration and continuous 5-day infusion Nausea may persist for several days
Imidazole carboxamide (DTIC; dacarbazine)	Occurs in virtually all patients Tolerance improves with each successive dose given on a 5-day schedule
Chemotherapeutic drugs commonly associated with mucositis	
Methotrexate	May be quite severe with prolonged infusions or if renal function is compromised Severity is enhanced by irradiation May be prevented by administration of adequate citrovorum rescue factor (folinic acid, leucovorin)
5-fluorouracil (fluorouracil USP)	Severity increase with higher doses, frequency of cycles, and arterial infusions
Actinomycin D (dactinomycin USP)	Very common; may prevent oral alimentation Severity enhanced by irradiation
Adriamycin (doxorubicin)	May be severe and ulcerative Increased in the presence of liver disease Severity enhanced by irradiation
Bleomycin	May be severe and ulcerating
Vinblastine	Frequently ulcerative

Malabsorption

The malabsorption that occurs in cancer patients can be iatrogenic in origin, or directly related to disease. Recently, in fact, it has been reported that patients with advanced breast cancer exhibit a markedly reduced capacity for active and facilitated absorption of some substrates. However, it should be noted that intestinal enzyme deficiency and significant biochemical changes in the intestinal mucosa (with consequent malabsorption of protein) appear very early under conditions of fasting and hypoalbuminaemia, even in the absence of morphological changes. For this reason, it is difficult to determine whether there is an actual 'neoplastic enteropathy', or if malabsorption is attributable to simple malnutrition and to what degree.

As far as postoperative malabsorption is concerned (Table 22.5), pancreatectomy may cause digestive enzyme deficiency, with loss through the stool of fats and proteins as well as a considerable quantity of vitamins and minerals. Radiotherapy to the small and large intestine may cause immediate and late damage, since the epithelium of the small intestine is second only to bone marrow in radiosensitivity. Damage from irradiation, which appears in 70–80% of patients who receive abdominopelvic radiotherapy, is clinically expressed as malabsorption of glucose, fat, electrolytes, and, in part, proteins (due to peptidase deficiency). Morphological lesions consistent with flattening of the villi and a reduction in mitosis have been demonstrated in asymptomatic patients after a dose of 20 Gy over 3 weeks or 33 Gy over 4 weeks. Spontaneous recovery usually occurs within 2 weeks of completion of radiotherapy. One-third of patients who have had acute enteritis subsequently develop late enteritis.

More recently, the adoption of special measures to dislodge small bowel from the pelvis (Trendelenburg

Table 22.9 Drug-induced nutrient deficiencies.

Drug	Nutrient(s) affected
Aminoglycoside	Magnesium, zinc
Ammonium chloride	Vitamin C
Antacid	Phosphorus, phosphates
Aspirin	Vitamin C
Cholestyramine	Triglycerides, fat-soluble vitamins
Coumadin	Vitamin K
Diphenylhydantoin	Niacin
Diuretics	Sodium, potassium, magnesium, zinc
Doxorubicin and vidarabine	Carnitine
Estrogen and progesterone compounds	Folic acid, vitamin B_6
Hydralazine	Vitamin B_6
Isoniazid	Vitamin B_6, niacin
Laxatives	Sodium, potassium, magnesium
Penicillamine	Vitamin B_6
Phenobarbital and phenytoin	Vitamin C, vitamin D
Phenothiazines	Vitamin B_2
Platinum	Magnesium, zinc
Steroids	Vitamin A, potassium
Tetracycline	Vitamin C
Tricyclic antidepressants	Vitamin B_2

Box 22.3 Incidences in which malabsorption is directly related to the tumour

- The pancreas is involved and there is obstruction of the biliary–pancreatic ducts.
- There are lesions in the small intestine from leukaemic foci or lymphoma, or solid tumours that can directly infiltrate the wall, obstruct lymphatic flow, or affect the mucosa and villi.
- There are protein-losing syndromes present in patients with lymphoma or gastric carcinoma.
- The digestive tract is the target organ of strong pharmacological substances secreted by certain tumours (e.g. apudomas), such as trophic hormones, steroids, hormonal polypeptides with low molecular weight, quinines, and prostaglandins.
- There are alterations in the villi and their function in patients with tumours whose origin is extra-gastrointestinal.

---

position, use of belly board, maintenance of a full bladder during radiotherapy) has decreased the frequency of severe radiation enteropathy.

Treatment with growth-inhibiting compounds may also cause malabsorption. Folic-acid antagonists may cause changes in the intestinal mucosa which are similar to those of sprue, with a reduction in epithelial cell mitosis and absorption of xylose and other nutrients. The administration of fluorouracil leads to a dipeptidase deficiency, and a single intravenous administration of methotrexate (2–5 mg/kg) is followed by inhibition cell mitosis of the jejunal mucosa, as well as other cellular changes. A number of drugs may interfere with normal utilisation or elimination of nutrients and precipitate the onset of (sub)clinical deficiency (Table 22.9). Malabsorption that is directly related to the tumour may be present in a series of circumstances, as summarised in Box 22.3.

22.3 Nutritional support in cancer

Rationale for the use of nutritional support

Malnutrition and outcome

Not only can malnutrition and a depletion of muscle mass be caused by multidrug chemotherapy, but malnutrition can adversely affect outcome. Longitudinal studies have demonstrated that the prognosis for cancer patients with weight loss is worse than that for weight-stable patients. Even though the stage of the tumour and the degree of responsiveness to the oncological therapy are major prognostic factors for survival, there are many reports in the literature showing that weight loss is a significant and often independent predictor of decreased survival in both postoperative and in nonsurgical cancer patients. With reference to nonsurgical cancer patients, the prognostic role of the weight loss has been reported by many authors. Under-nutrition was found to be predictive of early mortality after palliative self-expanding metal stent insertion in patients with inoperable or recurrent oesophageal cancer.

With reference to body compartments, it appears that depletion of body proteins or a bioelectrical impedance phase angle (a measure which characterises the distribution of water between the extracellular and the intracellular spaces and reflects the lean body mass) lower than the 5° percentile of the standard reference are also associated with a poorer survival. However, the depletion of fat tissue also matters. Accelerated loss of adipose tissue begins at 7 months and reaches an average loss of 29% of total adipose tissue 2 months before death. Loss of adipose tissue and loss of phospholipid fatty acids occur in tandem and are predictive of survival.

From the clinical perspective, there are several composite scores of malnutrition correlating with prognosis. In patients with cancer of the oesophagus and of the stomach, the Prognostic Nutritional Index was a factor independently associated with long-term survival. The Glasgow Prognostic Score, an index ranging from 0 to 2 depending on the low level of serum albumin (<3.5 mg/dl) or high level of CRP (>10 mg/dl), has been shown to be able to predict on multivariate analysis the survival of patients with inoperable gastrooesophageal cancer. The prognostic role of this score has been confirmed in a variety of solid tumours. Finally, from 4 to 23% of terminal cancer patients ultimately die because of cachexia.

Malnutrition and quality of life

Twenty and thirty per cent of quality of life performance is accounted for by nutrient intake and nutritional status, respectively, and malnourished cancer patients have higher rates of hospital readmissions, longer hospital stay, increased symptom distress, and reduced quality of life. A significant association with weight loss is seen for the main dimensions of quality of life – physical, functional, cognitive, social, fatigue, nausea, pain, loss of appetite, constipation, and diarrhoea – in 907 cancer patients. Malnutrition is a disease-independent risk factor for reduced muscle strength and functional status in cancer patients.

Malnutrition and chemotherapy

Total body nitrogen has been found to be the most powerful predictor of neutropaenia after chemotherapy in breast-cancer patients. There is emerging evidence that malnourished cancer patients are at higher risk for chemotherapy toxicity. Weight loss and hypoalbuminaemia are associated with an increased toxicity from chemotherapy. Total body nitrogen has been found to be the most powerful predictor of neutropaenia after chemotherapy in breast-cancer patients. Assuming that fat-free mass represents the volume of distribution of many cytotoxic chemotherapy drugs, individual variation in fat-free mass may account for up to three-times variation in the effective volume of distribution for chemotherapy administered per unit body surface area of cancer patients. Sarcopaenia is a significant predictor of toxicity and time to progression in metastatic breast cancer patients treated with capecitabine. Similarly, a body mass index (BMI) < 25 kg/m^2 with diminished muscle mass is a significant predictor of toxicity in metastatic renal-cell carcinoma patients treated with sorafenib. In addition, malnourished

cancer patients have a poor response to chemotherapy (rate and duration).

Effects of nutritional support on the nutritional status

The effects of parenteral and enteral nutrition on nutritional status have been reviewed elsewhere and are summarised in Tables 22.10 and 22.11. The beneficial effects of parenteral nutrition are more evident when compared in controlled studies with a standard oral diet (Table 22.12). It is noteworthy that there is a nutritional benefit even when a vigorous nutritional support is administered to patients undergoing an oncological therapy (Table 22.13). Special interest has been focused on the effects of parenteral and enteral nutrition on body cell mass, the component of body compartment which contains the oxygen-exchanging, potassium-rich, glucose-oxidising, work-performing tissue, and on the protein component of the body, which represents the 'functional compartment' *par excellence*.

Table 22.10 Effects of total parenteral nutrition (TPN) on the nutritional status of cancer patients. Adapted from Bozzetti (1989), copyright © 1989 by SAGE Publications. Reprinted by permission of SAGE Publications.

Variable	Response
Body weight	Always increases
Body fat	Usually increases
Muscle mass	
Anthropometry	No change or increase
Urinary creatinine or 3-CH$_3$-histidine	No change or decrease
Lean body mass	
Nitrogen balance	Always positive
Total-body nitrogen	No change or increase
Whole-body potassium	Increase or no change
Serum protein	
Total protein albumin	No change
Transferrin	Usually no change
Prealbumin	Usually no change
Retinol-binding protein	No change or increase
Cholinesterase and ceruloplasmin	Usually increase or no change
Immune humoral response	No change
IgA; C$_3$, C$_4$	No change
IgG, IgM, IgA	No change or sometimes increase
Nonspecific cellular response	
Neutrophils, total lymphocytes, B,T lymphocytes, helper T, suppressor T, chemotaxis	No change
Phagocytosis, killing index, natural killer	No change or increase

Table 22.11 Effects of enteral nutrition on the nutritional status of cancer patients. TIBC, total iron-binding capacity; CHE, cholinesterase; TBPA, thyroxin-binding prealbumin. Adapted from Bozzetti (1989), copyright © 1989 by SAGE Publications. Reprinted by permission of SAGE Publications.

Variable	Response
Body weight	Usually increase, sometimes no change
Body fat	Increase or no change
Muscle mass	
Anthropometry	No change; sometimes increase
Urinary creatinine or 3-CH$_3$-histidine	No change
3-CH$_3$-histidine efflux from the leg	Decrease
Tyrosine, AA and BCAA efflux from the leg	No change
Lean body mass	
Nitrogen balance	Usually positive or equilibrium
Total-body nitrogen	No change
Whole-body potassium	Increase or no change
Serum protein	
Total protein albumin	No change or increase
TIBC, CHE, TBPA	Usually no change; sometimes increase or decrease
Ceruloplasmin	No change or increase
Immune humoral response	No change
IgG, IgA, IgM, CH$_{50}$	No change
C$_3$-C$_4$, C$_3$PA	Increase
Nonspecific cellular response	Increase or no change

Table 22.12 Nutritional effects of total parenteral nutrition (TPN) versus a standard oral diet. CHE, cholinesterase; RBP, retinol-binding protein; TBPA, thyroxin-binding prealbumin. Adapted from Bozzetti (1989), copyright © 1989 by SAGE Publications. Reprinted by permission of SAGE Publications.

Variable	TPN	Oral diet
Weight	↓ or =	= or ↓
N balance	positive	negative
Total-body K	=	=
Urinary 3-methylhistidine	↓	=
Total protein	= or ↑	= or ↓
Albumin	= or ↓	= or ↓
Transferrin	↑ or =	= or ↓ ↑
CHE, RBP	↑	↓
TBPA	=	=
Ceruloplasmin, fibrinogen, IgA	=	=
IgG, IgM, C$_3$A	↑	=

Studies evaluating whole-body potassium (WBK) have generally had more positive results than those evaluating total-body nitrogen (TBN). There are probably several explanations for the discrepancy between the response of WBK and that of TBN, aside

Table 22.13 Effects of total parenteral and enteral nutrition in cancer patients receiving chemotherapy or radiotherapy. TPN, total parenteral nutrition; EN, enteral nutrition. Adapted from Bozzetti (1989), copyright © 1989 by SAGE Publications. Reprinted by permission of SAGE Publications.

Variable	Type of nutrition	Response
Body weight	TPN	Increase or no change
	EN	Increase or no change
Body fat	TPN	Increase
Muscular mass	TPN	Increase
Lean body mass		
Nitrogen balance	TPN	Positive
Total body nitrogen	TPN	No change
Serum protein		
Total protein	TPN	No change
Albumin	TPN	No change
Transferrin	TPN	No change
Retinol-binding protein	TPN	No change
Immune humoral response		
IgA, IgM	TPN	Increase

from the intrinsic error of the two techniques, since neutron activation measures all protein nitrogen (cellular protein + extracellular collagen) equally without differentiating the site or the metabolic activity of the nitrogen measured. In fact, the intracellular potassium concentration is also influenced by the state of cellular hydration, by glycogen stores, and by the level of insulin and catecholamines; and its depletion may be independent of the loss of body protein. In addition, the K/N ratio changes in different tissues of the body (3 mol of K/kg of N in muscle, to about 1.3 mol/kg in the rest of the lean body mass, to 1 mol/kg in adipose tissue).

The low nitrogen accretion with parenteral or enteral nutrition should come as no surprise. Studies on body composition during weight recovery suggest that the initial percentage of body fat is the most important determinant variable in energy partitioning: the higher it is, the lower the proportion of energy mobilised as protein will be, and hence the greater the propensity the body has to mobilise fat during semi-starvation and to deposit it subsequently during refeeding. Consequently, different results may simply reflect different types of tissue depletion and renewal in response to the nutritional support administered.

A number of studies have examined specific protein kinetic responses to parenteral nutrition in malnourished cancer patients. Whole-body protein turnover

Table 22.14 Response to total parenteral and enteral nutrition in cancer versus non-cancer patients. TPN, total parenteral nutrition; EN, enteral nutrition. Adapted from Bozzetti (1989), copyright © 1989 by SAGE Publications. Reprinted by permission of SAGE Publications.

Variable	TPN		EN	
	Cancer	Non-cancer	Cancer	Non-cancer
Weight	↑	↑↑	↑	↑ or ↑↑
Arm circumference				
Triceps skinfold	↑	↑	= or ↑	↑
Arm muscle area	↑	↑↑	↑	↑
Creatinine height Index	↑	↑↑	↑	↑
N balance	+	+	+	+
Total-body K	–	–	↑	↑
Albumin	↑	↑↑	↑	↑
Prealbumin	=	=	=	=
Retinol-binding Protein	=	=	–	–
Balance of:				
Na	+	+	–	+
K	+	+	–	+
Cl	+	+	–	+
Mg	+	+	–	+
P	+	+	+	+
Ca	=	=	+	+

has been shown to increase with parenteral nutrition, but whole-body protein synthesis has been reported both to increase and to decrease. Whole-body protein catabolism has been reported to decrease in cancer patients on parenteral nutrition. Few studies have investigated the two components of protein kinetics, namely the muscle compartment and the extra-muscle compartment, and these have reported an increase in whole-body protein synthesis and in the fractional synthetic rate of protein in muscle, with no change in whole-body protein catabolism. In severely malnourished patients with gastric cancer, whole-body protein synthesis and catabolism do not significantly change from 'before' to 'during' parenteral nutrition, even when the net balance moves from negative to positive. In contrast, the skeletal-muscle protein synthesis, as well as the protein-synthesis rate, significantly increase, converting the net balance to a positive value.

The effect of enteral nutrition on protein metabolism is worthy of note in that in patients with advanced ovarian cancer, oral intake of amino acids (40 g in 3 hours) is capable of acutely stimulating muscle protein synthesis despite an ongoing chemotherapy and an enhanced inflammatory burden. Similarly, oral administration of a whey-based leucine-enriched supplement is able to significantly increase the protein muscle synthesis. Generally it has been shown that parenteral nutrition does not increase the serum level of proteins, albumin transferrin, cholinesterase, or ceruloplasmin.

As regards parenteral nutrition and immunological response, some studies have reported an increase of lymphocyte blastogenesis and production of the helper T lymphocyte lymphokine IL-2 after 7 days of a parenteral-nutrition regimen, but also a significant impairment of basal natural-killer and IL-2-activated natural-killer activity. In contrast, it was recently found that a 10-day course of parenteral nutrition was able to restore to normal a depressed basal or IL- or IFN-stimulated natural-killer activity in cachectic cancer patients.

Taken as a whole, the data show that parenteral and enteral nutrition are usually able to decrease a further deterioration of the nutritional state and may sometimes improve some metabolic indices. These results are probably dependent on the length of the nutritional support, the biological aggressiveness of the tumour, and the efficacy of the available oncological therapy. It must be emphasised that even while the nutritional benefit often seems to be limited to maintaining a 'status quo,' it does so in patients who would be condemned to a progressive chronic 'autocannibalism' without nutritional support. However, the nutritional response of cancer patients is always more sluggish and limited than that of undernourished non-cancer patients (Table 22.14).

A 10-day course of parenteral nutrition, including 29 kcal nonprotein/kg/day + 1.6 g amino acid/kg/day, significantly decreases protein breakdown (by 50 and 59%) and protein synthesis (by 21 and 33%) in cancer and noncancer patients, respectively, while increasing protein turnover (by 15%) in cancer patients only. The utilisation efficiency of infused amino acid for synthesis of body protein is 39% in both cancer and noncancer patients. Table 22.15 reports data comparing parenteral and enteral nutrition, and Table 22.16 summarises the effects of parenteral and enteral nutrition on protein turnover. It is noteworthy that both techniques are able to improve some nutritional indices, such as body weight, fat mass, nitrogen balance, and WBK. Thyroxin-binding prealbumin and retinol-binding protein levels increase only with parenteral nutrition, while some immune-response indices (complement factors and lymphocyte number) improve only with enteral nutrition. TBN shows a small gain only with parenteral nutrition.

The results of three randomised studies comparing parenteral and enteral nutrition were partially conflicting, but only parenteral nutrition showed some significant advantages with regard to weight gain, nitrogen balance, maintenance of serum albumin levels, and some mineral balances (potassium, magnesium, phosphate, sodium, and chloride). However, differences were marginal, and the slight advantage of parenteral nutrition does not support its being used indiscriminately in malnourished cancer patients with a working gastrointestinal tract. In considering the use of parenteral nutrition, some related complications should be considered.

Table 22.15 Effects of total parenteral and enteral nutrition on nutritional variables. TPN, total parenteral nutrition; EN, enteral nutrition; TIBC, total iron-binding capacity; CHE, cholinesterase; TBPA, thyroxin-binding prealbumin; RBP, retinol-binding protein. Adapted from Bozzetti (1989), copyright © 1989 by SAGE Publications. Reprinted by permission of SAGE Publications.

	Response	
Variable	TPN	EN
Weight	↑	↑
Body fat	↑	↑
Muscle mass[a]	=	=
Lean body mass		
N balance	+	+
Total-body K	↑	↑ (=)
Total-body N	= ↑	=?
Serum proteins		
Total protein	=	=
Albumin	=	= ↓
TIBC, CHE	=	= ↑
Ceruloplasmin	=	=
TBPA	↑ or =	= or ↑
RBP	↑	–
Protein flux	↑ or =	=
Synthesis, catabolism	=	=
Immune humoral response		
IgG, IgA, IgM	=	=
C_3, C_4	=	↑
C_3PA	–	↑
CH_{50}	–	=
Immune cellular response		
Neutrophils	=	–
Lymphocytes (total/subpopulations)	=	↑ or =
Chemotaxis/phagocytosis	=	–

[a]3-methylhistidine, amino acid efflux, anthropometry, creatinine-height index.

Effects of nutritional support on clinical outcome

Effects of nutritional support in cancer patients undergoing surgery
Parenteral nutrition

Most of the randomised controlled trials on perioperative total parenteral nutrition (TPN) have been performed in non-malnourished patients, and in many of them were started in the postoperative period. These trials have shown that TPN in these settings is useless or deleterious. Now we are aware that a possible adverse effect of postoperative TPN may be the potentiation of a hyperglycaemic status due to the abrupt load of glucose in conditions where there is already a condition of glucose intolerance and an insulin resistance. On the other hand, at least two randomised controlled trials in cancer patients with a weight loss ≥10% have shown that pre- and postoperative TPN was able to reduce complications, and in one study mortality too, when compared with isotonic fluids administration. It is noteworthy that no apparent correlation was found between reduction of postoperative complications and preoperative improvement of the standard nutritional markers of nutritional risk.

A prospective randomised study involving cirrhotic patients who were submitted to wide hepatic resections for hepatocarcinoma reported that perioperative BCAA-enriched parenteral nutrition can

Table 22.16 Effects of total parenteral and enteral nutrition on daily protein turnover in cancer patients. UGI, upper gastrointestinal; BEE, basal energy expenditure; C/N, kcal/nitrogen; GI, gastrointestinal. Adapted from Bozzetti (1989), copyright © 1989 by SAGE Publications. Reprinted by permission of SAGE Publications.

Tumour	Regimen per day		Synthesis (g/kg)		Catabolism (g/kg)	
	kcal/kg	AA/kg	Pre	Post	Pre	Post
Oesophagus[a]	38	1.68	2.2	2.7	2.8	2.4
Oesophagus[a]	44	0.87	2.4	2.3	2.9	2.3
UGI	BEE × 1.2	C/N = 200	2.0	1.8	2.3	1.1
GI	29	1.6	2.1	1.3	2.6	1.3
GI	25	1.4	–	0.68[b]	–	0.37

[a] Statistically significant.
[b] μmol leucine/kg/minute.

reduce postoperative complications. However, these conclusions have to be accepted with some reservation because the control group may have been treated with an excessive load of fluid and sodium and there is now evidence that an excessive perioperative load of fluid may be deleterious.

Enteral nutrition

The ESPEN Guidelines on Enteral and Parenteral Nutrition 2006 and 2009 state that preoperative fasting from midnight is unnecessary in most patients, and that patients undergoing elective surgery who do not have specific risk of aspiration may drink clear fluids and eat solids until 2 and 6 hours before anaesthesia, respectively. In fact, preoperative intake of a carbohydrate drink the night before (800 ml) and immediately before (400 ml) surgery does not increase the risk of aspiration, and in colorectal patients reduces postoperative insulin resistance, preserves skeletal mass and muscle strength, and improves preoperative well-being.

Since an inadequate oral intake for more than 14 days is associated with higher mortality, enteral nutrition (tube feeding or oral nutritional supplementation (ONS)) is indicated even in patients without obvious malnutrition, if it is anticipated that the patient will be unable to eat for more than 7 days perioperatively. It is also indicated in patients who cannot maintain oral intake above 60% of their requirements for more than 10 days. Enteral nutrition is the preferred route if there is no intestinal obstruction or ileus, severe shock, or intestinal ischaemia.

Randomised controlled trials on preoperative standard enteral nutrition versus routine care are few and show no clinical benefit, or a benefit in minor complications if administered with ONS in the postoperative period. However, many randomised controlled trials have demonstrated that preoperative intake of ONSs (3 × 250 ml) enriched with arginine, n-3 fatty acids, and nucleotides for 5–7 days are able to reduce postoperative morbidity and length of stay after major abdominal cancer surgery, regardless of the nutritional status, when compared with standard enteral nutrition.

No benefit was observed in two randomised controlled trials where postoperative tube standard feeding was compared with routine care, but when fish oil-enriched feeds were used a reduction in gastrointestinal complications was reported in comparison with patients receiving standard control feeds.

Enteral tube feeding versus parenteral nutrition

There is no difference in mortality between postoperative administration of enteral nutrition versus parenteral nutrition regardless of the nutritional status of the patients, but a significant reduction in length of hospital stay is observed with enteral nutrition in both well-nourished and malnourished patients, in complications of any type.

These data are in agreement with a large re-analysis of the databases of randomised controlled trials on perioperative nutrition in gastrointestinal cancer patients, coordinated from Milan and published in the years 1999–2002. This study has shown that regardless of the weight of loss (which is a major independent risk factor for complications), there is a hierarchy of efficiency of the nutritional support, which is better with enteral (especially if enriched with immune substrates) and worse with parenteral nutrition (especially with isotonic formulas) (Figure 22.3).

A detailed update of this topic is found in Bozzetti (2011).

Effects on outcome in oncological patients

To date, 19 randomised controlled trials in adults have explored the effects of parenteral nutrition as an

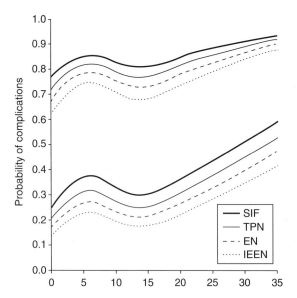

Figure 22.3 Postoperative complication rate by percentage of weight loss, depending on the nutritional regimen. Lower curves represent the class of patients with the lowest risk of complications according to the multivariable analysis. Upper curves apply to the class of patients with the highest surgical risk. It appears that in all patients the risk of postoperative complications is related to the percentage of weight loss and in all classes there is a hierarchy of benefit of nutritional support, ranging from administration of isotonic fluids to immune-enriched enteral nutrition. SIF, standard isotonic fluids; TPN, total parenteral nutrition; EN, enteral nutrition; IEEN, immune-enriched enteral nutrition. Reprinted from Clin Nutr, vol 26. Bozzetti F et al. Postoperative complications in gastrointestinal cancer patients: the joint role of the nutritional status and the nutritional support, p698–709. Copyright 2007, with permission from Elsevier.

adjunct to chemotherapy on survival, remission, and complications. An important meta-analysis from the American Gastroenterological Association is summarised in Table 22.17. However, the results of these meta-analyses have been severely criticised, not only for the quality of the studies and the nutritional regimens in use 30 or more years ago, but mainly because patients were not all malnourished. As a matter of fact, these studies investigated the effects of supraphysiological doses of calories and protein, and nowadays we are aware of the risk of this approach.

Randomised controlled trials on parenteral nutrition versus nonparenteral nutrition (with/without oncological therapy) in malnourished/aphagic cancer patients simply do not exist, mainly for ethical reasons, because it is not acceptable to maintain a control group of malnourished/aphagic patients without nutritional support. Among oesophageal cancer patients, those receiving parenteral nutrition tolerate a higher total dose of chemotherapy and have similar surgical outcomes to those who are able to maintain oral diets. However, if supplementation includes omega-3-enriched supplements, enteral support is followed by a lesser bone-marrow toxicity than parenteral nutrition.

The ESPEN Guidelines (2006, 2009) state that intensive dietary counselling combined with nutritional supplements is able to increase nutrient intake and to prevent therapy-related weight loss and interruption of radiotherapy of gastrointestinal and head and neck areas. If an obstructing upper gastrointestinal tumour or iatrogenic local mucositis interferes with swallowing, enteral nutrition should be delivered by tube.

Evidence-based data from randomised controlled trials are few: whereas the effects on response to treatment of oral nutritional supplements given to patients receiving radiotherapy for head and neck tumour are nil, intensive, individualised, long-term nutritional counselling combined with nutritional supplementation proved to be efficient in preventing further deterioration of the nutritional status and global quality of life. More recently, such an approach was able to improve response to therapy and survival in head and neck and gastrointestinal cancer patients receiving radio- and chemotherapy.

Routine enteral nutrition during autologous or allogeneic haematopoetic stem-cell transplantation is not recommended, since there is no benefit in immunocompromised and thrombocytopenic patients, and there may even be an increased risk of haemorrhage and infection. In these patients, enteral and parenteral nutrition have the same effects on nutritional status and the occurrence of infective complications, but it should be borne in mind that enteral nutrition is rarely exclusive and is not well tolerated.

The addition of glutamine did not show any consistent benefit in four randomised controlled trials in patients undergoing haematopoietic stem-cell transplantation, but in a single study EPA (1.8 g/day) proved efficient in improving complications and survival.

n-3 enriched enteral nutrition

EPA can be administered in capsules as mixed marine triglycerides (fish oil) or as semi-purified ethyl ester. The benefit in clinical practice is much lower than that found in preclinical or phase II studies. There have been four meta-analyses on the clinical effects

Table 22.17 Meta-analysis of randomised clinical trials of patients given total parenteral nutrition (TPN) during chemotherapy. Reprinted from Gastroenterology, vol 121. Koretz R, Lipman T, Klein S. AGA technical review on parenteral nutrition, p970–1001. Copyright 2001, with permission from Elsevier.

Outcome	Absolute risk difference %	Confidence intervals %	Number of studies (patients) included
Mortality	0	−5, +5	19 (1050)
Total complication rate	+40	+14, +66	8 (333)
Infectious complcation rate	+16	+8, +23	8 (823)
Tumour response	−7	−12, −1	15 (910)
Bone-marrow toxicity	+22	−10, +54	3 (134)
Gastrointestinal toxicity	+1	−9, +11	6 (310)

of n-3 supplements and three of them concluded that there were insufficient data to establish whether oral EPA was better than placebo.

The discrepancies between these meta-analyses are probably due to the poor compliance with ingestion of the n-3 preparations (due to the unpleasant taste or having too many capsules to take), the too-short duration of the treatment, the selection of symptomatic gastrointestinal cancer patients, and the failure to combine n-3FA with an adequate nutritional support.

With no firm data to rely on, major international nutrition societies comment cautiously on the use of n-3 fatty acids. The recent ASPEN Guidelines state that n-3 fatty acid supplementation may help to stabilise weight in cancer patients on oral diets experiencing progressive unintentional weight loss (type 2 evidence), whereas the ESPEN Guidelines only say that evidence is contradictory/controversial.

Home parenteral nutrition and enteral nutrition

Many authors define this type of nutritional support as 'palliative' nutrition, but this has been debated for three reasons. (i) Advanced cancer patients very rarely suffer from a symptom of famine or thirst which requires palliation by artificial nutrition. On the contrary, these patients are anorectic, and in the very late stages of their disease just a little fluid and mouth care is sufficient to relieve symptoms of thirst and dry mouth. (ii) Although the World Health Organization (WHO) definition of palliative care includes an amelioration of quality of life as its main goal of the treatment, there is more evidence that parenteral or enteral nutrition can delay death from starvation in some selected aphagic patients than that they can improve their quality of life, and sometimes a wrong indication for nutritional support may indeed exacerbate the quality of life of a patient. (iii) Finally, a correct therapeutic programme in any phase of the disease should always consider, among its priorities,

Table 22.18 Proportion of patients with cancer reported on registers of home parenteral feeding in various countries.

Country	Proportion of cancer patients on HPN
Italy	57%
Japan	55%
USA	46%
The Netherlands	60%
Spain	39%
Belgium	23%
Denmark	8%
UK	5%

the maintenance/improvement of quality of life of the patient, regardless of the stage of disease.

The use of nutritional support (especially home parenteral nutrition (HPN)) in incurable cancer patients is extremely controversial and cancer patients account for quite different percentages in different European countries (Table 22.18). Patients with benign intestinal failure survive many years with the use of HPN, whereas many cancer patients die in a few months despite its use. This has led some institutions and countries to not use HPN for incurable cancer patients on the basis of a low benefit-to-cost ratio.

The main criterion for classifying a patient with incurable cancer (i.e. oncologically but not biologically terminal) relies on the clinical presumption by the oncologist who knows the natural history of the disease that the patient is going to die 'with' the cancer, not 'for' the cancer.

The candidature of a cancer patient for an HPN programme faces formidable problems, which have been critically reviewed in the recent literature. These are:

(1) Estimation of the life expectancy due to the malignancy. Only if the patient is expected to succumb to starvation (which requires approximately 2 months) before dying from tumour

progression can there be a gain in survival through HPN. This point is crucial, and it is well known how inaccurate (and usually over-optimistic) such predictions are.

(2) Awareness of the prognosis by the patient and their relatives. This is required in order for them to give informed consent to the programme. However, especially in southern Europe, the patient's desire/right not to know the truth is often respected. On the other hand, members of the patient's family often ask for artificial nutrition because they believe their relative will not die as long as they are nourished artificially. These problems are often amplified when, during the course of the disease, it is necessary to withdraw parenteral nutrition because it appears futile.

Both of these issues should be discussed and shared by the oncologist, the patient, and the caregiver/relative prior to the start of parenteral nutrition.

Survival data from different series are reported in Table 22.19. In a large ongoing multicentre prospective study on incurable cachectic cancer patients (Figure 22.4), the mean survival was 3 months.

Studies have shown that cancer patients receiving palliative care are interested not only in the quantity of their remaining life, but also the quality. In a recent survey of patients with advanced lung cancer, only 22% chose palliative chemotherapy in preference to supportive care alone if it offered an additional 3-month survival, in contrast to 68% if it substantially reduced adverse symptoms without prolonging life. It is however noteworthy that considerable disparity exists between concurrent ratings of quality of life made by patients and their physicians.

Data on quality of life are sparse. The existing literature is summarised in two excellent reviews by Baxter *et al.* (2006) and Winkler (2005). According to data from the North American Register, 31% of patients appeared to be completely rehabilitated at 1 year, but in recent reports 13–18% in the American and European registries were completely rehabilitated, and another 27% were partially socially rehabilitated.

Sixty-nine advanced, malnourished, and almost aphagic/(sub)obstructed cancer patients enrolled in a programme of HPN were prospectively studied regarding nutritional status, length of survival, and quality of life through the Rotterdam Symptom Checklist questionnaire (Bozzetti *et al*, 2002). These variables were collected at the start of HPN and then at 30-day intervals. Median survival was 4 months (range 1–14), with about one-third of patients surviving more than 7 months, and nutritional indices maintained stable until death. Quality-of-life parameters remained stable until 2–3 months before death. The conclusion was that HPN may benefit a limited percentage of patients, who may survive longer than the time allowed by a condition of starvation and depletion. Provided that these patients survived longer than 3 months, there was some evidence that quality of life remained stable and acceptable for some months.

With reference to HEN, there are retrospective data from large national American and European

Table 22.19 Home parenteral nutrition: retrospective selected series.

Author	Number of patients	Survival (mean values)
Weiss *et al.* 1982	9	67% ≥6 months (15-578 days)
Hurley *et al.* 1990	9	13.6 months
August *et al.** 1991	17	53 days (5-208)
King *et al.*** 1993	61	60 days (82-780), 23% ≥30 days
Mercadante 1995	13	3-121 days (23% ≥30 days)
Cozzaglio *et al.* 1997	75	121 days (30-456)
Pasanisi *et al.* 2001	76	74 days (6-301), 85% ≥30 days
Duersken *et al.* 2004	9	26-433 (2 >1 year)
Hoda *et al.* 2005	52	152 days (30-4620), 31% ≥1 year
Brard *et al.* 2006	28	72 days
Santarpia *et al.* 2006	152	45 days (6-1269), 11% ≥90 days

*33% fistulas, 22% radiation enteropathy
**18% small bowel syndrome/radiation enteropathy

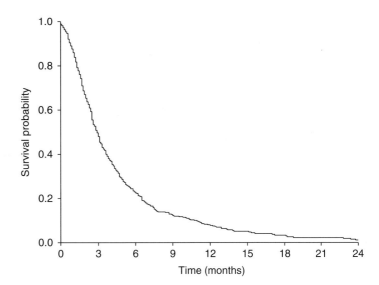

Figure 22.4 Survival of 427 incurable cancer patients on home parenteral nutrition (HPN) (unpublished data from F Bozzetti).

registers showing that three-quarters of patients were able to achieve a full rehabilitation or a subjective improvement. An *ad hoc* study showed a slight improvement in quality of life and symptoms but a decline in body image in one-third of patients.

Nowadays, patients with an incurable malignancy are candidates for HPN if starvation/obstruction are the major problems, the tumour is slow-growing, there is no evolutionary or conspicuous involvement of vital organs, there are no pleural/peritoneal effusions which might abruptly worsen with fluid administration, and other symptoms are absent or easily controlled.

Furthermore, it has to be agreed that if/when these criteria are lacking during the course of the disease, HPN will be progressively tapered and converted to isotonic fluids.

Supplemental parenteral nutrition

This term refers to a partial parenteral nutritional support given to patients who are not fully aphagic and maintain some capability to nourish orally by themselves. Consequently, in this patient population it is possible to perform randomised controlled trials. A supplemental parenteral nutrition was studied in 309 weight-losing patients with solid tumours (primarily gastrointestinal lesions) and an expected survival of at least 6 months using a multimodal palliation which included cyclooxygenase (COX) inhibitors (usually indomethacin, 50 mg twice daily), erythropoietin (15 000–40 000 units per week), and insulin (0.11

units/kg/day) (Fouladiun *et al*, 2005). On an intention-to-treat basis, patients randomised to receive supplemental nocturnal HPN (20–25 kcal/kg/day, 0.10–0.15 g nitrogen/kg/day) had an improvement in energy balance ($p < 0.03$), and the as-treated analysis demonstrated a prolonged survival ($p < 0.01$), improved energy balance ($p < 0.001$), increased body fat ($p < 0.05$), and a greater maximum exercise capacity ($p < 0.04$).

Supplemental nightly parenteral nutrition for about 4 months was able to improve the phase angle and to get at least a temporary benefit or stabilisation of the nutritional status in the majority of the patients investigated.

Much less convincing is the prospective clinical trial of 152 patients with 9.4% weight loss or BMI < 20 who had advanced, mainly gastrointestinal, cancer, and who intermittently received oncological therapy and an intensified oral enteral nutrition (Shang *et al*, 2006). These patients were randomised to receive or not a supplemental parenteral nutrition (680 kcal/day and 26 g protein/day). Median follow-up was at 11.1 months, and at various time intervals a benefit in many nutritional variables, in quality of life, and in survival was shown in patients on home supplemental parenteral nutrition. Since benefit was confined to parenteral-nutrition patients despite both groups receiving the same amount of calories (~2200 kcal/ day), it was speculated that absorption of enteral nutrients was abnormal. What appears definitely unusual in this study is that the control group, despite chemotherapy, radiotherapy, or both, maintained an oral enteral intake of 33 kcal/kg/day during the late phases of progression of the disease, a finding which we never observe in this patient population. The most probable interpretation is that nutrition 'prescribed' by vein was effectively administered, whereas there is no such certainty concerning the prescription of the same amount of nutrients by mouth.

In an uncontrolled study on severely malnourished and very advanced patients who were aphagic (36% of them) or hypophagic (<500 kcal/day; 64% of the series) and often receiving palliative chemotherapy, the median survival was 2 months or less. Finally, quite recently a report on the palliative home care of 68 patients in the Stockholm region noted that parenteral nutrition was more common than tube feeding due to the frequency of gastrointestinal symptoms, such as early satiety, nausea, and vomiting, which make the use of tube feeding difficult. These findings are in keeping with previous prospective investigations into the preferences of cancer patients for type of nutritional support: intravenous versus tube feeding.

In conclusion, an early long-term intravenous nutritional support in less-advanced cancer patients with mild hypophagia and mild malnutrition could protect integrated metabolism and metabolic function in these subjects. This would also support the concept that nutrition is a limiting factor which influences survival when the disease is advanced but the final outcome is not impending. The current availability of commercial all-in-one admixtures (<1 l) able to cover more than half the energy requirements of the average advanced cancer patient enormously simplifies the nutritional approach to weight-losing hypophagic cancer patients.

Nutritional regimen

It has to be pointed out that the recommendations about a specific nutritional regimen are especially valid in three conditions: when patients are frankly cachectic, when parenteral nutrition or enteral nutrition are exclusive (i.e. the contribution of spontaneous oral feeding is negligible), and when nutritional support is expected to last for at least some weeks. In other conditions (perioperative state, supplemental enteral or parenteral nutrition, nutritional support during oncological treatments, etc.) there is less evidence that patients need 'specialised' nutritional support.

Energy

It is well known that an increased REE is relatively frequent in many patients with malignancy and may account for the progressive development of a cumulative energy balance and finally the onset of cachexia. However, if we consider the TEE, which includes the REE plus the physical-activity energy expenditure, this value may appear decreased in advanced cancer patients when compared to predicted values for healthy individuals, mainly because of a reduction in the physical activity.

Recent data with the use of a wearable device, the SenseWear Armband (SensorMedics Italia Srl), would indicate that the TEEs of weight-stable leukaemic patients and of weight-losing bedridden patients with gastrointestinal tumours are about 24 and 28 kcal/kg/day, respectively. For practical purposes, and if not measured individually, total daily energy expenditure in advanced cancer patients may be assumed to be rather similar to that in healthy subjects, ranging between 25 and 30 kcal/kg/day.

Choice of nutrients

Fat: the majority of studies concerning the metabolic utilisation of substrates have been performed during/after an intravenous administration of nutrients, in order to avoid any interference from an unpredictable variation in the intestinal absorption which might occur following enteral administration.

In 1971, Waterhouse & Kemperman showed that fat is efficiently mobilised and utilised as a fuel source in cancer patients. The rationale for the use of lipid emulsions stems from several sophisticated metabolic studies:

(1) Many authors have reported a very efficient mobilisation and oxidation of endogenous fat in the postabsorptive state, ranging from 0.7 to 1.9 g/kg/day (i.e. about 6.3–17.0 kcal/kg body weight/day, or approximately 60–78% of the resting metabolic expenditure) in both weight-stable and weight-losing cancer patients.

(2) Subsequent investigations focused on the effects of different fat emulsions, long-chain triglycerides (LCTs), and medium-chain triglycerides (MCTs). After the administration of LCT or mixed LCT/MCT emulsions, the clearance of lipid was reported to be 1.4 versus 2.3 versus 3.5 or 1.2 versus 1.6 versus 2.1 g/kg/day, respectively,

in healthy subjects versus weight-stable versus weight-losing cancer patients, respectively.

(3) The oxidation rate after intravenous administration of LCT and mixed LCT/MCT emulsions in weight-losing cancer patients was reported to be 1.3–1.6 or 0.62 g/kgBW, respectively.

As regards the effects of fat infusion on the protein metabolism of cancer patients, data from the literature are scanty: the administration of Intralipid, a soybean-based emulsion, at about 29 kcal/kg body weight/day, was able to significantly decrease net protein catabolism in patients with lower gastrointestinal tumours but not in those with upper gastrointestinal ones.

There is, however, some concern about the potential toxicity of long-term parenteral administration of lipids. Previous studies showed that the adverse effects reported with LCT emulsions occured when the lipid infusion rate was greater than 2.6 g/day (i.e. about 20–24 kcal/kg/day), but now many authors suggest not exceeding a dose of 1 g/kg body weight/day if parenteral nutrition is administered for some weeks.

Whereas there is a general agreement that glucose should not account for the overall energy load, the type of fat emulsion to be used is a matter of investigation due to the concern that the excess of *n*-6 PUFA, present in the classic soybean- and safflower-based lipid emulsions might be immunosuppressive and proinflammatory.

This has led to the development of alternative lipid emulsions. Lipid emulsions based on mixtures of LCT and MCT were formulated in order to reduce the *n*-6 PUFA content. The *n*-6/*n*-3 PUFA ratio is similar in soybean and mixed LCT/MCT emulsions, but the content of essential fatty acids (linoleic and alpha-linolenic acid) of LCT/MCT emulsions is half that of soybean-based formulations.

Another approach is the use of olive oil-based emulsions, which contain about 20% *n*-6 PUFA (enough to supply the essential fatty acids requirements) and 65% oleic acid and are rich in alpha-tocopherol.

In this way there is a potentiation of the anti-inflammatory action of the admixture through a downregulation of PGE2 production, activation of peroxisomal proliferators-activated receptors, and suppression of the activation of genes involved in the inflammatory process.

Since chemotherapy and radiation therapy are associated with increased formation of reactive oxygen species and depletion of critical plasma and tissue antioxidant, a potential benefit of olive oil emulsion could be the protective effect of alpha-tocopherol on lipid peroxidation.

More recently, *n*-3-enriched fatty emulsions have become available on the market. There is as yet no specific experience with such emulsions in cancer patients.

Glucose: there are additional advantages to replacing glucose with lipid in the parenteral nutrition regimen.

First, it appears wise to try to limit the infectious risk associated with hyperglycaemia, which, albeit mainly reported in nononcological settings, may be expected in cancer patients with a poor utilisation of both endogenous and exogenous glucose. Furthermore, in a clinical setting it was shown that in patients undergoing allogeneic bone-marrow transplantation for haematologic malignancies there were reduced rates of lethal acute graft-versus-host diseases when receiving high-LCT parenteral nutrition regimens.

Finally, glucose administration tends to cause a deleterious positive water balance, as discussed in the water requirement section.

Protein: the optimal nitrogen supply for cancer patients cannot be determined at present.

Recommendations (based on expert opinion) range between a minimum protein supply of 1 g/kg/day and a target supply of 1.2–2.0 g/kg/day.

As regards the quality of proteins, a prospective, randomised, crossover trial involving patients with advanced intra-abdominal adenocarcinoma concluded that BCAA-enriched TPN resulted in an improved protein accretion and albumin synthesis when compared with standard amino acid solutions. This approach was not subsequently further expanded.

The role of supplementation with glutamine is still controversial, despite some biological rationale, and a recent narrative review has shown that of 24 studies evaluating the effects of oral glutamine on chemotherapy toxicity, only 8 reported a clinical benefit, and of 12 studies with parenteral glutamine supplementation, only 6 reported a reduced clinical toxicity.

Water: a restriction in water administration is advised for several reasons. Cachexia is often associated with the expansion of the extracellular fluid volume. If patients have peritoneal carcinomatosis, an overzealous administration of water, glucose, and sodium can sharply precipitate an impending ascitis. Glucose reduces renal sodium excretion and, for the same reasons, the loss of extracellular fluid. This effect is mediated by insulin, a potent antinatriuretic and antidiuretic hormone (ADH), through an increased sympathetic activity.

In cancer patients, excessive production of ADH may occur due to either the tumour, the presence of nausea (which frequently occurs in advanced stages of disease), or the administration of morphine. Furthermore, cachexia is associated with loss of intracellular water and solutes, which affects the hypothalamic osmoreceptor cells, stimulating ADH release at levels which maintain serum osmolality sodium at subnormal levels.

As a consequence, the clearance of free water is decreased. Free-water clearance is also decreased because the urea load presented to the kidney is reduced secondary to protein under-nutrition, whereas the synthesis of endogenous water is maintained by the oxidation of carbohydrates and fats, and insensible water loss drops due to reduced physical activity.

According to the ESPEN Guidelines (2006, 2009) the total volume of fluid and sodium should not exceed 30 ml and 1 mmol per kilogram per day, respectively.

Effects of nutritional support on tumour growth

It has been widely reported that the intravenous administration of TPN and especially of amino acids to tumour-bearing animals can lead to an increase in absolute tumour volume and weight, mitotic activity, and number of metastases, even if the tumour weight/carcass weight ratio sometimes remained unchanged. This effect has been explained by the fact that some components of the nutritional regimen are able to bring about a uniform reduction of the cell-proliferation cycle or a recruitment of dormant cells from the G0 phase into the active phase of cell replication.

It has to be pointed out that in these experimental studies, refeeding after a period of nutritional deprivation resulted in a measurable increase in tumour volume after only 24 hours, and an increase in the S-phase tumour cell population could be observed by flow cytometry only 2 hours after the start of TPN,

with gradual normalisation of tumour growth kinetics within 24–48 hours of initiating TPN. This short-term effect of TPN on tumour growth kinetics represents a biological response at the cellular level which appears to be independent of the nutritional status of the host. Results from animal studies cannot, however, be extrapolated directly to the clinical field, since animal tumours usually become very large, accounting for up to 20% of the carcass weight. Such a condition never occurs in man, since human tumour mass rarely exceeds 1–2% of the host's weight. Furthermore, these experimental tumours have doubling times of a few days and can kill the animal host in a few weeks from the time of their onset, conditions which are rarely found in human solid tumours. Therefore, the administration of TPN to these animals even for just 1 week means feeding them for a substantial part of the natural history of their tumour, which would correspond to a TPN regimen of several months or years in human cancer patients. The literature on the modulation of tumour cell proliferation in humans by parenteral or enteral nutrition is sparse. Apart from anecdotal reports, the clinical research has followed three main directives: (i) to investigate the relationship between nutritional status and tumour growth; (ii) to evaluate some markers of tumour growth before and after TPN or enteral nutrition; and (iii) to study the metabolic activity of cancer cells in fasting conditions and after administration of different substrates.

(1) In an investigation (Bozzetti et al, 1995) of the relationship between some indicators of nutritional status (weight loss, serum albumin and cholinesterase, number of lymphocytes) and the labelling index in 136 patients with lymphoma, there was no evidence that a good nutritional state could result in faster tumour growth. Instead, the opposite statistical association was found: in depleted patients, tumours grew faster, as though more-aggressive tumours could negatively affect the nutritional status.

(2) A review of the literature by Bozzetti & Mori (2009) identified 12 suitable papers representing a total of 140 patients receiving nutritional support versus 84 controls. The studies were classified as randomised clinical trials (five), comparative nonrandomised clinical trials (three), and trials with patients who were controls for themselves

(four). The indicators of tumour growth used in the studies included the DNA index, ornithine decarboxylase activity, flow-cytometric DNA distribution, and the labelling index with tritiated thymidine or bromodeoxyuridine. It was found that an increased tumour growth was never observed in control patients without nutritional support but was reported in 7 out of 12 studies in patients receiving nutritional support.

(3) Finally, in an investigation into the uptake of [18]2-fluoro-2-deoxy-D-glucose (FDG) by healthy liver and by tumour in fasting conditions and after glucose-based (4 mg/kg/min) or lipid-based (2 mg/kg/min) parenteral nutrition, using positron emission tomography (PET), showed that the FDG uptake by the metastases was 3.0–3.6 times higher than that by healthy liver in fasting conditions, and was not significantly affected by the subsequent administration of glucose or lipid. It is possible that the metabolic activity of the tumour is so high that it cannot be manipulated by the administration of nutrients unless we totally deprive the organism of glucose intake and concurrently block the gluconeogenesis.

The current combined approach

A modern approach to the nutritional support of cancer patients includes adequate administration of nutrients through the enteral route, if possible, and intravenously if not. Provided the enteral route is available and working, appetite should be stimulated pharmacologically if anorexia is present. This may not be sufficient to reverse a catabolic state, and it has been demonstrated that the synthesis rate of export proteins (fibrinogen) is elevated in the fasted state and further rises during enteral nutrition, thus perpetuating and accelerating loss of lean tissue and deterioration of the nitrogen economy. The use of anabolic or anticatabolic agents in combination with nutritional support should thus be warranted.

Appetite stimulants
Megestrol acetate

Megestrol acetate is available in 20 and 40 mg tablets and as a suspension at 40 mg/ml. It is usually reported that about 70% of patients receiving a dose of 800 mg/day (as tablets) or 600 mg (as oral suspension) show an improvement in appetite within 1–2 weeks. The prophagic effect of prostagens as medroxyprogesterone acetate (MPA) and megestrol acetate seems to be mediated by the downregulation of the synthesis and release of serotonin and of proinflammatory cytokines, leading to an increase in hypothalamic concentrations of neuropeptide Y. Although this percentage at first glance suggests that megestrol is highly effective, it should be considered that 44% of placebo-exposed patients also have an improvement in appetite, which reduces the actual percentage of patients who truly benefit from this progestational agent. Moreover, in several randomised controlled trials there is a drop-out rate of about 40% of patients, and according to an intention-to-treat rule this further reduces to 20% the number of patients who respond to this drug. The increase in appetite translates to a gain of weight and patients receiving progestational agents are more than twice as likely to gain weight as those receiving placebo. Unfortunately, the administration of megestrol acetate does not impact on either survival or quality of life, perhaps because it causes weight gain which primarily augments body fat and some fluid, and not lean tissue. Megestrol, in fact, produces antigonadotrophic effects and can stimulate adipocyte differentiation. The administration of megestrol acetate may be associated with adverse events such as thrombophlebitis, oedema, impotence, hyperglycaemia, and menstrual bleeding on withdrawal, as well as Addisonian crisis if abrupt discontinuation is concurrent with a stress. There is a positive correlation between dosage (at least up to 800 mg/day) and outcome, and from a clinical point of view the suggestion is to start with lower doses (160–400 mg/day) and reserve higher doses for resistant patients.

Corticosteroids

Corticosteroids inhibit the synthesis or release of prostaglandins and proinflammatory cytokines such as IL-1 and TNFα. They are able to stimulate the appetite for a short time, have an antiemetic activity, and can reduce asthaenia. Although several randomised placebo-controlled trials have demonstrated that corticosteroids (dexamethasone 0.75–1.5 mg *per os* four times daily; prednisolone 5 mg *per os* three times daily; methylprednisolone 16 mg *per os* twice daily or 125 mg IV once daily) induce a usually temporary (limited to a few weeks) effect on symptoms such as appetite, food intake, sensation of well-being, and performance status, none has shown a benefit on body weight. The administration of these drugs may entail long-term complications such as cataract formation, weakness, mild neuropsychiatric symptoms (in up to 50% of patients), delirium, diabetes, osteoporosis, and immunosuppression. Due to the fact that their activity vanishes after a few weeks, steroids are not indicated to treat anorexia in patients with a survival anticipated to be greater than 8 weeks. For bedridden patients, corticosteroids may be a good option, as exacerbation of muscle wasting is not of particular concern. They may also prove useful in patients who need concurrent co-analgesia with anti-inflammatory agents. Type, dosage, and route of administration remain ill-defined and low dosages (less than 1 mg/kg/day of prednisone equivalent) seem recommendable in daily clinical practice.

Cyproheptadine hydrochloride

The proposed weight-gain mechanism of cyproheptadine is serotonin antagonism. A randomised double-blind trial in cancer patients with anorexia or cachexia failed to prevent weight loss compared with the placebo group, but patients receiving cyproheptadine (8 mg three times daily) had less nausea, less energy, and more sedation and dizziness than placebo patients. Cyproeptadine is now only recommended in patients with carcinoid tumour, because it proved useful in improving diarrhoea and promoting a weight gain. Cyproheptadine is available as 4 mg tablets and as a syrup in a concentration of 2 mg/5 ml.

Dronabinol

The literature reporting on the use of cannabinoids in the treatment of cancer cachexia is sparse. Dronabinol has been shown to alter the cytokine production by human immune cells. It would seem that some benefit in appetite and mood is obtained by an administration of 5 mg/day, with about two-thirds of patients reporting that their appetites are stimulated. There is an increased calorie intake and weight gain with 2.5 mg three times daily 1 hour after meals, but neuropsychological effects are not uncommon, including nausea and slurred speech. Combination of dronabinol with megestrol acetate does not offer any advantage over treatment with megestrol acetate alone. A study compared oral dronabinol (2.5 mg twice daily) versus megestrol acetate liquid suspension (800 mg) versus both; megestrol acetate-treated

patients reported greater appetite improvement (75 vs. 49%) and a 10% weight gain over baseline (11 vs 3%). There was no difference in survival.

Branched-chain amino acids

The use of BCAAs was proposed some years ago, following the rationale that increased hypothalamic serotinergic activity could play a role in the development of anorexia. BCAA might slow down the entry of tryptophan – the precursor to serotonin – into the brain by competing for the same transport system across the blood–brain barrier. Encouraging results have been reported in a pilot study in which anorectic patients received oral supplementation of BCAA for a few days.

A randomised investigation of the benefit of a supplementation with BCAA (11 g/day) for 1 year in patients undergoing chemoembolisation for hepatocellular carcinoma showed lower morbidity, higher serum albumin, and better quality of life than in the control group.

Ghrelin

Ghrelin is a gut–brain peptide expressed in the stomach that stimulates food intake by activating neurons of the arcuate nucleus of the hypothalamus and increases body weight. Its role in clinical practice is doubtful: not only is cancer anorexia in humans associated with increased plasma concentration of ghrelin, which is likely to be secondary to ghrelin resistance in the hypothalamus, but it promotes the release of GH, which may influence tumour growth. The preliminary experience, however, showed that cancer patients receiving ghrelin infusion increased their energy intake, and this effect remained after treatment.

Anabolic agents
Anabolic androgen steroids

Anabolic androgen steroid (AAS) administration induces increases in the mRNA expression of the skeletal-muscle androgen receptor, increases the intracellular utilisation of amino acids derived from protein degradation, and stimulates net muscle synthesis. Despite initial promising data on body-weight maintenance, no significant difference in body-weight loss was observed between weight-losing lung-cancer patients receiving chemotherapy with versus without nandrolone decanoate (200 mg weekly for 1 month). Oxandrolone (10 mg orally twice a day) was reported to improve weight, lean body mass, performance status, and quality of life. A possible explanation is the higher specificity of the oxandrolone in its androgen-receptor binding, as suggested from animal experiments.

Growth hormones

There is some concern regarding the use of GHs, because of the possible stimulation of tumour growth. However, in experimental investigations tumour progression was not shown. One clinical study reported an increase in whole-body protein synthesis greater than the stimulation of whole-body protein breakdown, with no change in muscle protein turnover. In a study in 10 patients, GH administered for 3 days increased plasma IGF-1 levels and decreased urinary nitrogen losses, but an improvement in nitrogen balance was observed only in patients who were not overtly cachectic.

Nonspecific immune modulators
Nonsteroidal anti-inflammatory drugs and COX-2 inhibitors

Nonsteroidal anti-inflammatory drugs (NSAIDs) act by inhibiting prostaglandin production by the rate-limiting enzymes COX-1 and COX-2. COX-1 is expressed constitutively in most tissues and appears to be responsible for the production of prostaglandins, which mediate normal physiological functions, such as maintenance of the integrity of the gastric mucosa and regulation of the renal blood flow. In contrast, COX-2 is undetectable in most normal tissues and is induced by cytokines, growth factors, oncogenes, and tumour promoters. It contributes to the synthesis of prostaglandins in inflamed and neoplastic tissues. Steroids and NSAIDs (indomethacin 50 mg twice daily) have been shown to promote survival benefit in randomised controlled trials in undernourished patients with metastatic solid tumours. More recently, reduced markers of systemic inflammation (CRP and erythrocyte sedimentation rate (ESR)) and reduced energy expenditure were demonstrated with preservation of total body fat. Adding erythropoietin and TPN, they further obtained improved energy balance, increased body fat, and a greater exercise capacity and prolonged survival in a *post hoc* analysis. The effect of the association of ibuprofen with megestrol versus megestrol alone has been investigated in a randomised con-

trolled trial in gastrointestinal cancer patients with weight loss. The combined treatment was associated (after 3 months of therapy) with an increase in body weight (median +2.3 kg) versus a decrease (median −2.8 kg) in patients receiving megestrol alone. Quality-of-life scores were also improved.

A pilot study explored the efficacy of the association of celecoxib (200 mg twice daily) with medroxyprogesterone acetate (500 mg twice daily) and an oral food supplementation, for 6 weeks, in lung cancer patients. This treatment was associated with stability or a gain in weight, and also with an improvement in early satiety, appetite, nausea, and performance status.

Fish oil

Fish oil is particularly rich in long-chain n-3 PUFA, which includes eicosopentaenoic (EPA; C20:5 n-3) and docosahexaenoic (DHA; C22:6 n-3) acids. These derive from linolenic acid (C18:3 n-3) and undergo biological transformation to eicosanoids, which alter the production of inflammatory mediators, including cytokines. Suppression of cytokine production occurs by inhibiting the COX pathway, and hence prostaglandin and leukotriene synthesis. Fish oil and n-3 fatty acid (EPA in particular) are inhibitors of TNFα and IL-1 (but also of IL-2 and IL-6) by macrophages, lymphocytes, and peripheral blood mononuclear cells, and of the effects of proteolysis-inhibiting factor (PIF). EPA also inhibits T-cell proliferation, competes for the incorporation of arachidonic acid into membrane phospholipids, and inhibits arachidonic acid's conversion into prostanoids. In the experimental setting, EPA is able to preserve lean body mass through a reduction of protein degradation without having an effect on protein synthesis. This is achieved by a downregulation of the increased expression of the ubiquitin–proteasome pathway, and this explains why in order to restore the lean body mass it is necessary to combine an inhibition of protein degradation with high protein supplements in order to stimulate protein synthesis. EPA acts at several stages in the signalling cascade induced by PIF in skeletal muscle: it reduces the release of arachidonic acid in response to PIF and its conversion to 15-HETE; it then blocks the action of 15-HETE; and finally it attenuates binding of NF-κB in the nucleus through stabilisation of the NF-κB cytoplasmic complex. EPA would also block the effects of LMFs. EPA is administered at doses 20–40 times the normal

Western dietary intake. In clinical practice, however, its use has not been validated by randomised controlled trials, and four meta-analyses have reported conflicting results on its potential benefits.

Pentoxyphylline

Pentoxyphylline decreases TNFα mRNA levels but failed to increase appetite or weight in a double-blind, randomised placebo-controlled trial in cancer patients who received 400 mg three times daily.

Thalidomide

Thalidomide downregulates COX-2 and TNFα production in monocytes *in vitro* and in other proinflammatory cytokines, and normalises TNFα levels *in vivo*. Furthermore, it inhibits angiogenesis. The mechanism is an inhibition of NF-kB, and in recent clinical studies thalidomide appeared to reverse losses in weight and lean body mass over the trial period, and to improve appetite. At a dose of 100 mg/night, there is an improvement in anorexia (63%), nausea, and insomnia, and in sense of well-being. Boasberg *et al.* (unpublished data) observed weight stability with 100–200 mg/day. Thalidomide (200 mg orally) has been associated with a nutritional supplementation and obtained weight gain and an augmentation of the lean body mass. Despite these promising results, thalidomide cannot at this moment represent the standard of care, due to the frequent, mainly neurological, side effects which can adversely affect the quality of life of the patient.

Clarithromycin

A single experience showed that after 3 months of clarithromycin therapy in patients with unresectable non-small-lung cancer there was a significant decrease in IL-6 serum levels and a significant increase in body weight.

Others
Inhibitors of proteasome

A study from the Mayo Clinic shows that bortezomib, a proteasome inhibitor had negligible favourable effects on cancer-associated weight loss in patients with metastatic pancreatic cancer.

Adenosine 5′-triphosphate

The rationale for using ATP is twofold: it is a key energy source and it can enhance weight stability.

One study randomly assigned lung-cancer patients to receive continuous infusion of ATP or not, and after 1 month reported a 0.2 kg increase in the ATP-treated group versus a 1 kg loss in the nontreated group. In addition, strength and quality of life were more favourable in the ATP-treated group.

Antioxidant

Recently, starting from the concept that in advanced cancer patients (i) there are increased levels of reactive oxygen species and decreased levels of glutathione peroxidase; (ii) these reactive oxygen species are predictive of clinical outcome and survival; and (iii) they may be positively corrected by antioxidant agents, an integrated treatment has been proposed which combines daily *n*-3-enriched PUFA supplements (Prosure, two cans, i.e. 620 kcal, 32 g protein, and 2.2 g EPA), medroxyprogesterone acetate (500 mg orally), Celecoxib (200 mg orally), a diet with high polyphenol content (300 mg) or supplemented with one tablet of Quercetix, and finally an antioxidant treatment *per os* (alpha-lipoic acid 300 mg, carbocysteine lysine salt 2.7 g, vitamin A 30 000 IU, vitamin C 500 mg, and vitamin E 400 mg). In a phase 2 study they preliminarily reported after 4 months of therapy an increase in body weight, lean body mass, appetite, and quality of life. They also observed a statistically significant correlation between lean-body-mass changes and IL-6 levels.

References and further reading

Arends J, Bodoky G, Bozzetti F, Fearon K, Muscaritoli M, Selga G, *et al*. ESPEN Guidelines on Enteral Nutrition: non-surgical oncology. Clin Nutr 2006; 25(2): 245–259.

August DA, Huhmann MB ; American Society for Parenteral and Enteral Nutrition (ASPEN) Board of Directors. ASPEN clinical guidelines: nutrition support therapy during adult anticancer treatment and in hematopoietic cell transplantation. JPEN 2009; 33(5): 472–507.

Baxter JP, Fayers PM, McKinlay AW. A review of the quality of life of adult patients treated with long-term parenteral nutrition. Clin Nutr 2006; 25: 543–553.

Bosaeus I. Nutritional support in multimodal therapy for cancer cachexia. Support Care Cancer 2008; 16(5): 447–451.

Bozzetti F. Effects of artificial nutrition on the nutritional status of cancer patients. JPEN 1989; 13: 406–420.

Bozzetti F. Nutrition support in patients with cancer. In: Artificial Nutrition Support in Clinical Practice (J Payne-James, G Grimble, D Silk, eds). London: Greenwich Medical Media, 2001.

Bozzetti F. Perioperative nutritional support in adult cancer patients. Proc Nutr Soc 2011; 70(3): 305–310.

Bozzetti F, Arends J, Lundholm K, Micklewright A, Zurcher G, Muscaritoli M. ESPEN Guidelines on Parenteral Nutrition: nonsurgical oncology. Clin Nutr 2009; 28(4): 445–454.

Bozzetti F, Boracchi P, Costa A, Cozzaglio L, Battista A, Giori A, La Monica G, Silvestrini R. Relationship between nutritional status and tumor growth in humans. Tumori 1995; 81(1): 1–6.

Bozzetti F, Cozzaglio L, Biganzoli E, Chiavenna G, De Cicco M, Donati D, Gilli G, Percolla S, Pironi L. Quality of life and length of survival in advanced cancer patients on home parenteral nutrition. Clin Nutr 2002; 21(4): 281–288.

Bozzetti F, Gianotti L, Braga M, Di Carlo V, Mariani L. Postoperative complications in gastrointestinal cancer patients: the joint role of the nutritional status and the nutritional support. Clin Nutr 2007; 26(6): 698–709.

Bozzetti F, Mariani L. Defining and classifying cancer cachexia: a proposal by the SCRINIO Working Group. JPEN 2009; 33(4): 361–367.

Bozzetti F, Mori V. Nutritional support and tumour growth in humans: a narrative review of the literature. Clin Nutr 2009; 28(3): 226–230.

Elia M, Van Bokhorst-de van der Schueren MA, Garvey J, Goedhart A. ESPEN Guidelines on Parenteral Nutrition: surgery. Clin Nutr 2009; 28(4): 378–386.

Fearon K, Strasser F, Anker SD, Bosaeus I, Bruera E, Fainsinger RL, et al. Definition and classification of cancer cachexia: an international consensus. Lancet Oncol 2011; 12(5): 489–495.

Fouladiun M, Körner U, Gunnebo L, Sixt-Ammilon P, Bosaeus I, Lundholm K. Daily physical-rest activities in relation to nutritional state, metabolism, and quality of life in cancer patients with progressive cachexia. Clin Cancer Res 2007; 13(21): 6379–6385.

Jatoi A, Qi Y, Kendall G, Jiang R, McNallan S, Cunningham J, et al. The cancer anorexia/weight loss syndrome: exploring associations with single nucleotide polymorphisms (SNPs) of inflammatory cytokines in patients with non-small cell lung cancer. Support Care Cancer 2010; 18(10): 1299–1304.

Koretz R, Lipman T, Klein S. AGA technical review on parenteral nutrition. Gastroenterology 2001; 121: 970–1001.

Laviano A, Meguid MM, Rossi-Fanelli F. Cancer anorexia: clinical implications, pathogenesis, and therapeutic strategies. Lancet Oncol 2003; 4(11): 686–694.

Lieffers JR, Mourtzakis M, Hall KD, McCargar LJ, Prado CM, Baracos VE. A viscerally driven cachexia syndrome in patients with advanced colorectal cancer: contributions of organ and tumor mass to whole-body energy demands. Am J Clin Nutr 2009; 89(4): 1173–1179.

Lundholm K, Nitenberg G, Stratton RJ. Enteral (oral or tube administration) nutritional support and eicosapentaenoic acid in patients with cancer: a systematic review. Int J Oncol 2006; 28(1): 5–23.

Mariani L, Lo Vullo S, Bozzetti F; on behalf of the SCRINIO Working Group. Weight loss in cancer patients: a plea for a better awareness of the issue. Support Care Cancer 2012; 20(2): 301–309.

Seruga B, Zhang H, Bernstein LJ, Tannock IF. Cytokines and their relationship to the symptoms and outcome of cancer. Nat Rev Cancer 2008; 8(11): 887–899.

Shang E, Weiss C, Post S, Kaehler G. The influence of early supplementation of parenteral nutrition on quality of life and body composition in patients with advanced cancer. JPEN 2006; 30(3): 222–230.

Teunissen SC, Wesker W, Kruitwagen C, de Haes HC, Voest EE, de Graeff A. Symptom prevalence in patients with incurable cancer: a systematic review. J Pain Symptom Manage 2007; 34(1): 94–104.

Waterhouse C, Kemperman JH. Carbohydrate metabolism in subjects with cancer. Cancer Res 1971; 31: 1273–1278.

Weimann A, Braga M, Harsanyi L, Laviano A, Ljungqvist O, Soeters P, et al. ESPEN Guidelines on Enteral Nutrition: surgery including organ transplantation. Clin Nutr 2006; 25(2): 224–244.

Winkler MF. Quality of life in adult home parenteral nutrition patients. JPEN 2005; 29: 162–170.

23
Paediatric Nutrition

Anthony F Williams

St George's, University of London, UK

Key messages

- The challenge of optimal childhood nutrition is to match supply with demands throughout the period of growth and development, so that full genetic potential can be realised.
- Worldwide, about 9 million children die each year before reaching the age of 5. Malnutrition is considered to be a sole or contributory cause in about half of these deaths.
- Breast-feeding improves the health of mother and baby, even in industrialised countries.
- Childhood growth involves not only an increase in body size but changes in body proportions, the relative sizes of organ systems, and chemical composition.
- Nutrition has an important role to play in neurological, gastrointestinal, renal, and metabolic maturation.

- Growth monitoring is a fundamental tool in clinical paediatrics and child health surveillance. This necessitates the choice of an appropriate standard or reference.
- Growth faltering among young children in industrialised countries is most commonly the result of chronic energy deficiency arising from inappropriate care practices, rather than underlying physical disease or food shortage.
- A range of dietary products and delivery devices is now available for specialised enteral and parenteral nutritional support of sick children of all ages and sizes.

23.1 Introduction

'Paediatrics' is the treatment of disease during growth and development. As a clinical discipline it is inextricably linked to 'child health' – the promotion and maintenance of health in children. The child, or 'paediatric patient', varies enormously both in maturity and in size, from the 500 g 23-week-gestation neonate to the fully-grown adult. The challenge of optimal childhood nutrition is to match supply with demands throughout this period of age, so that full genetic potential can be realised. Failure to do so compromises the child's health and chance of survival. It also strongly influences health in adult life.

Why are children nutritionally vulnerable?

Worldwide, about 9 million children die each year before reaching the age of 5. Malnutrition is considered

to be a sole or contributory cause in about half. The particular vulnerability of children can be explained by considering influences which act on nutrient demand and supply.

Demands

Growth imposes metabolic demands during childhood. These are particularly high during infancy (the first year of life) and adolescence. Growth is not merely an increase in size. As children grow, their body proportions alter, reflecting maturation in body composition and changes in the partitioning of nutrients between organ systems. These events are developmentally programmed, so that the effects of supply failure depend to a large extent upon the age of the child. For example, severe energy restriction in early childhood, when the normal pace of growth is rapid and the brain is still developing, may never be recoverable. The end

---

Clinical Nutrition, Second Edition. Edited by Marinos Elia, Olle Ljungqvist, Rebecca J Stratton and Susan A Lanham-New.
© 2013 The Nutrition Society. Published 2013 by Blackwell Publishing Ltd.

result is 'stunting', with associated impairment of cognitive development.

Supply

Failure of nutrient supply in children may be attributable to many causes. In the case of babies born too early, immaturity of the absorptive, metabolic, and excretory systems may constrain supply. In older children, illness (acute and chronic, somatic, or psychological) may both increase demands and deleteriously affect supply by reducing appetite or increasing losses. However, the most important factor is simply the availability of food. This is a key distinction between supply failure in children and adults. Adults can more often find the food they need, whereas young children (those with the highest demands) need others to find it for them. Where children are concerned, food shortage is not confined to resource-poor countries; it occurs even in industrialised nations as a result of parenting, educational deficiencies, and socioeconomic deprivation.

Imbalance of supply and demand

Children are more disadvantaged than adults when supply does not meet demand. The smaller the child, the smaller their nutrient stores, and the shorter the period they will last. Additionally, immaturity of the metabolic and excretory systems, coupled with the relatively high demands of essential organs (such as the brain), constrains the capacity for reductive adaptation. The reasons why children are nutritionally vulnerable are summarised in Box 23.1.

These points will be revisited in more detail at later points in this chapter.

Applications of nutritional science in paediatrics and child health

People practising in paediatrics and child health apply nutritional principles daily. Box 23.2 lists some examples relevant to practice in both industrialised and resource-poor countries. Advances in clinical nutrition have had a major impact on child survival globally; for example, well-controlled trials have shown that vitamin A supplementation in resource-poor countries can reduce mortality amongst preschool children by about 30%. In industrialised countries, improved techniques of nutritional support have greatly improved the survival of sick children,

---

Box 23.1 Vulnerability of children

High demands

Demands are related to:

- rate of growth;
- amount of metabolically active tissue (e.g. brain) per unit of body mass;
- occurrence of disease.

Supply limitations

Supply may be limited by:

- immaturity of the absorptive, metabolic, and excretory systems;
- developmental stage (ability to forage and eat);
- neurological impairment;
- psychological disorder;
- social and educational disadvantage;
- effects of disease on appetite, ability to eat, etc.

Body composition

Nutrient stores are related to:

- absolute body size;
- tissue composition (protein, fat, and water).

Box 23.2 How nutritional science is applied in paediatrics and child health

Promotion of child health

- primary prevention, e.g. breast-feeding, vitamin supplementation;
- secondary prevention, e.g. screening for iron deficiency or phenylketonuria (PKU).

Primary treatment of disease

- e.g. exclusion diets (coeliac disease, allergy), therapeutic diets (inborn errors).

Nutritional support

- e.g. feeding the extremely low-birth-weight (<1000 g) baby, or treating sick infants and children with chronic illnesses.

---

such as those born extremely early and those who develop chronic disease or intestinal failure.

Long-term relevance of paediatric nutrition

Optimising nutrition in early life is increasingly seen to have relevance to long-term health (Scientific

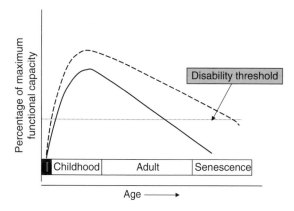

Figure 23.1 Model for promoting lifelong health through optimisation of early nutrition. Maximum functional capacity is achieved as a result of tissue growth and maturation during foetal life (black area) and childhood. Functional capacity then declines during adult life at a rate determined by health, lifestyle, and environmental factors, eventually crossing a 'disability threshold'. The time taken to reach this point is partly determined by the height of the initial peak around adolescence.

Advisory Committee on Nutrition, 2011). Although many of the mechanisms still require clarification, epidemiological data clearly show that patterns of growth in foetal life and infancy are correlated with later risk of cardiovascular disease and the metabolic syndrome. Effects seem most marked amongst individuals whose early growth was severely restricted, but it is important to realise that there is in fact a gradation of risk right across the normal range of body size and shape observed in populations. Thus the potential later health dividends of providing optimal early nutrition could be considerable.

Figure 23.1 shows conceptually how early-life interventions could integrate with later (adult and old-age) interventions to improve health outlook with ageing. If functional capacity is maximised in the early years, the individual has a greater reserve from which decline begins in adult life. Such an approach acts synergistically with interventions in later life aimed at slowing the rate of decline. The effect of both is to prolong the period that elapses before functional capacity crosses a 'disability threshold'. One example of such an effect might be bone health. Bone mass in later years might theoretically be optimised by attainment of peak bone mass during childhood and adolescent growth, coupled with measures (such as optimal nutrition and lifestyle) to slow decline in adult life.

23.2 Growth

Growth and physical and mental development are processes which distinguish children from adults. Physical growth involves an increase in both the size and complexity of body structure, occurring under genetic and endocrine regulation. The pattern of growth has a characteristic tempo which is disturbed if nutrient supply is inadequate or disease impairs nutrient uptake and utilisation. Therefore, growth monitoring is a key clinical tool in paediatrics and child health.

The process of growth has a number of corollaries for nutrient demands. First, depending on the child's age, it is 'expensive'. For example, in early infancy, when growth is most rapid, it may consume half the energy intake. Second, the partitioning of nutrients between organ systems also changes, because their relative size alters substantially with growth, affecting to some extent the balance of nutrient requirements.

Measuring growth: growth references and standards

The pattern of growth can be defined by measuring large numbers of children. Groups of children of differing ages may be measured at the same time (cross-sectional sampling) or a cohort of children may be measured at specified ages as they grow up (longitudinal sampling). The data obtained may be reproduced graphically in the form of growth charts or transformed into the properties of a normal distribution as z-scores (i.e. the number of standard deviations from the mean). The former are most commonly used for day-to-day clinical monitoring of individual children, whereas the latter are most widely used for handling population data. Weight, height (or length), and occipitofrontal circumference (OFC; head circumference) are most frequently measured in clinical practice, though references exist for other measures too, such as skinfold thickness, mid-arm circumference, knee–heel, and foot length. Cross-sectional charts may not adequately depict substantial inter-individual variations in normal growth patterns, particularly during infancy and at adolescence. This observation has clinical implications and is further discussed later.

A key question when designing a growth chart is deciding which children to measure. Two approaches may be followed: one is to measure a group of

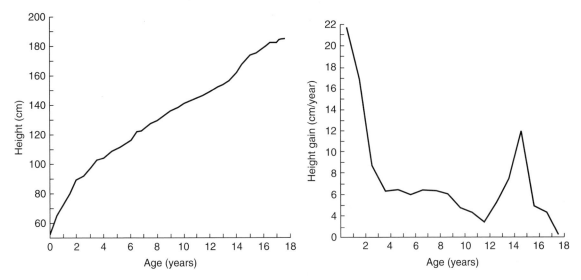

Figure 23.2 Attained-size and growth-velocity plots. Philibert de Montbeillard, an eighteenth-century French aristocrat, made serial measurements of his son's height throughout childhood. These are plotted in two ways: the left-hand plot shows height attained and the right-hand plot the velocity of growth at any particular age. Reprinted with permission from Tanner (1989).

unselected children from a population; the other is to select children identified as healthy and who are known to be optimally nourished. The former approach generates a growth *reference*, whereas the latter generates a growth *standard*. These are conceptually different: a reference describes how a child in the population studied *is* growing, whereas a standard describes how a child *should* grow. The World Health Organization (WHO) chart for children 0–5 years of age is an example of an internationally applicable growth standard. Children were selected from relatively affluent social backgrounds and were all singleton infants born at term to nonsmoking mothers who had been well throughout the pregnancy. The children were then exclusively or predominantly breast-fed for the first 4–6 months of life (mean age at introduction of complementary foods was 5.4 months). Their growth was monitored longitudinally for the first 2 years, and the remainder of the chart is derived from cross-sectional data on a similar sample. Children from six countries were studied (Brazil, the USA, Norway, India, Oman, and Ghana), making this a truly international growth standard.

The growth charts in current use in the UK employ a combination of these approaches. From 2 weeks to 4 years of age the WHO standard is used, and from 4 to 18 years of age the UK 1990 growth reference is used. The latter was compiled from over 25 000 cross-sectional weight and height measurements of white English, Welsh, and Scottish children sampled in seven separate studies conducted 1978–1990. These were normalised to the year 1990. Further explanation of how to use the UK-WHO chart, which was introduced in 2009, may be found elsewhere. The UK growth charts are open-access and may be freely downloaded from the Royal College of Paediatrics and Child Health (RCPCH) Web site (http://www.rcpch.ac.uk/child-health/research-projects/uk-who-growth-charts-early-years/uk-who-growth-charts-early-years). Fact sheets, teaching presentations and plotting exercises can also be found at this site (http://www.rcpch.ac.uk/child-health/research-projects/uk-who-growth-charts-early-years/uk-who-0-4-years-growth-charts-initi).

Distance and velocity charts

Growth data may be displayed in terms of either absolute attainment (i.e. distance traveled) for age or the speed of growth at a particular age (Figure 23.2). Clinical monitoring is most commonly performed using charts of the former type, inter-individual variation being depicted in the form of centile lines. Both the UK-WHO 0–4 (Figure 23.3) and the UK 1990 4–18 growth charts show nine lines. These

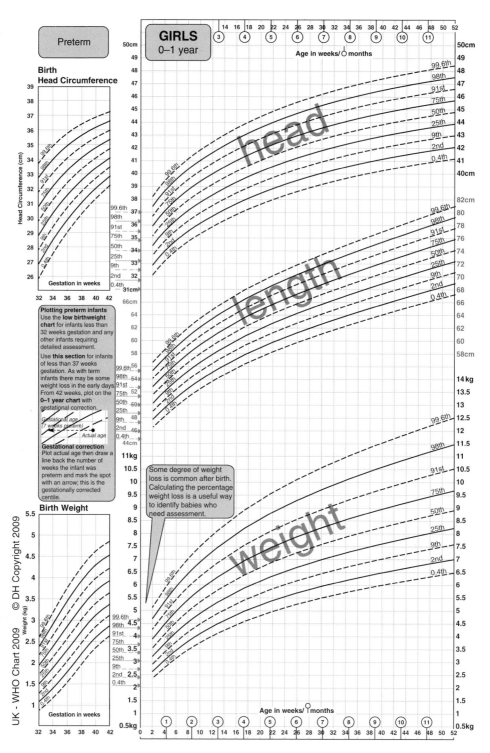

Figure 23.3 The new UK-WHO 0–4 growth chart. Between the ages of 0 and 4 years, the charts show weight, length, and head circumference data from the WHO Multicentre Growth Reference Study. The birth weight and size data on the ordinate are pooled data for all British births between 37 and 42 weeks included in the UK 1990 growth reference. UK WHO Growth Charts, Girls 0–4 years, A4, Department of Health. © Crown Copyright, 2009.

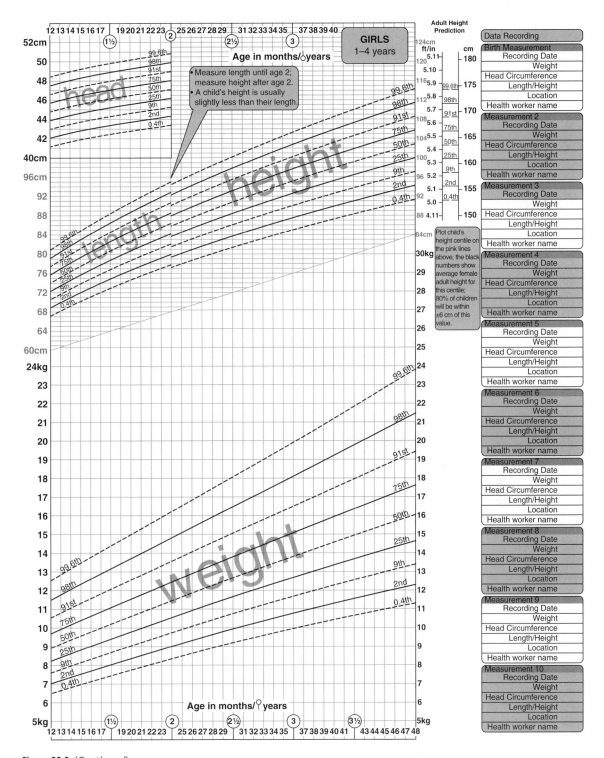

Figure 23.3 *(Continued)*

represent the 0.4th, 2nd, 9th, 25th, 50th, 75th, 91st, 98th, and 99.6th centiles, each band being spaced two-thirds of a standard deviation above or below the next. Thus it is easy to see how many standard deviations a child's height (or weight) is above or below the mean (Figure 23.4).

A key assumption in using growth charts for clinical monitoring is that an individual child's growth trajectory parallels the centile lines on the chart: a phenomenon known as 'channelling' or canalisation. With a few physiological exceptions, deviation from such a course signifies under- or over-nutrition, or the presence of an underlying disease process which modifies nutrient assimilation, demands, or losses.

Growth data depicted in velocity/age format are now less commonly used clinically. They have a specialist use in investigation and monitoring in endocrine/growth clinics, but the need for extremely accurate measurements limits their clinical value, as the error in any difference estimate is double that of the individual measurements used. Nevertheless, for the purpose of considering nutrient demands, a useful insight into the overall pattern of growth can be obtained by examining a velocity chart. In fact, the pattern can be resolved mathematically into three overlapping curves: the infant, child, and pubertal phases (Figure 23.5). This is known as the ICP model of infant growth and reflects changes in the dominant influences of growth with age:

- Infant growth is primarily nutrient/insulin- and insulin-like growth factor (IGF)-led, an extension of the foetal pattern.
- Childhood growth is predominantly growth hormone-led.
- Pubertal growth is primarily driven by the influence of sex steroids on growth hormone secretion.

The increase in velocity at puberty is called the pubertal growth spurt. This occurs at a substantially younger age in girls, first because they enter puberty earlier than boys and second because their growth spurt occurs at an earlier stage of puberty, so that it is subsiding by menarche (Figure 23.6), helping to ensure both that the girl's growth is completed before pregnancy occurs and that foetal nutritional demands are anticipated by the deposition of maternal body stores.

Optimal growth: the place of international standards

Children in resource-poor countries are generally smaller than their counterparts in industrialised ones and it might be argued that local references are more relevant to growth monitoring in such communities. However, studies that have compared the growth of better-off and poor children *within* such countries have shown large differences in rates of growth, the former often matching patterns seen in richer industrialised countries. This argues strongly for application of international growth standards as a measure for improving the nutritional status of children globally.

The US NCHS (National Center for Health Statistics) reference was used as such a standard for many years, though it had many shortcomings. First, important secular changes in the twentieth century have been associated with changes in the growth patterns of children even in rich countries. The NCHS standards drew on growth data over 50 years old, and today's children are taller and heavier. Second, many of the infants included in the NCHS reference were artificially fed, and methods of infant feeding exert major influences on the pattern of growth in infancy. For these reasons, the chart has been replaced by the new WHO international growth standard mentioned earlier. Analysis of the growth data from six countries in the WHO Multicentre Growth Reference Study demonstrated that rates of linear growth to 5 years of age showed extremely low intercentre variation, justifying the use of this chart as an international standard.

Physiological deviations from growth references

Although the phenomenon of 'channelling' underpins the clinical use of growth charts for longitudinal monitoring, individual children can show patterns of growth which deviate from the centile lines for valid physiological reasons. This tendency to cross up or down centile-line channels is particularly marked at two stages of life: infancy and puberty.

Infancy

As charts are compiled from cross-sectional data, there is a tendency for babies at the extremes of the birth-weight range to show regression towards the mean during the early months, crossing centiles up or

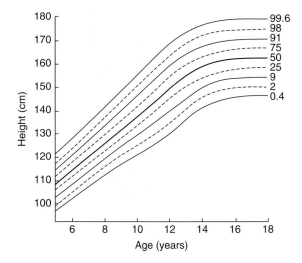

Figure 23.4 A 'nine-centile' growth chart, showing centile bands spaced at intervals of two-thirds of a standard deviation (i.e. z-score 0.66). This presentation is now most commonly used in UK clinical practice. Data shown here are for British girls aged 5–18 included in the UK 1990 growth reference. Reproduced from BMJ, Cole TJ, 308: 641–642, 1994 with permission from BMJ Publishing Group Ltd.

down (Figure 23.7). At a given gestational age, birth size is principally affected by placental function (nutrient supply) and maternal, rather than paternal, size. An infant constrained by intrauterine environment will, if optimally nourished after birth, grow in such a way as to seek out his or her genetic potential by exhibiting catch-up growth. Conversely, an infant over-nourished *in utero*, such as the infant of a diabetic mother, may exhibit catch-down growth. These processes are usually completed by the end of the first year of life, but in extreme cases may continue into the second year. It is sometimes important to distinguish clinically between the catch-down growth of an unusually heavy baby (e.g. the infant of a diabetic mother) and weight faltering. It is therefore essential to know fully the parental measurements and perinatal history when interpreting growth patterns in infancy.

Puberty

The age at onset of puberty varies greatly between individuals. For example, although pubic hair appears at an average age of 11.9 years in girls, the 2nd and 98th centiles for this stage are 5 years apart, at 14.4 and 9.4 years, respectively. Because the 50th-centile line on the growth chart reflects the growth trajectory of a child entering puberty at the average age, one exhibiting late puberty may show an

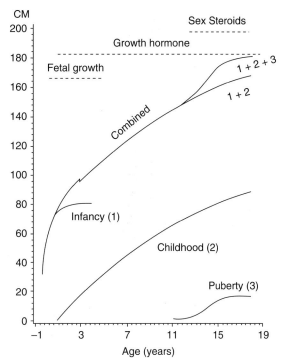

Figure 23.5 The Karlberg 'ICP' model of human growth. The chart shows three lines, which represent the infancy (1), childhood (2), and puberty (3) curves. These summate to form the 'combined growth' curve. Reprinted by permission from Macmillan Publishers Ltd: Eur J Clin Nutr (Karlberg *et al.* (1994), Linear growth retardation in relation to the three phases of growth. Eur J Clin Nutr, vol 48 Supp 1, pages S25–43). Copyright (1994).

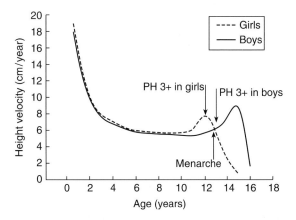

Figure 23.6 Differences in timing of the pubertal growth spurt. Height-velocity curves for boys and girls are overlapped. Comparable stages of puberty (Tanner's pubic hair (PH) rating 3) are indicated by the arrows. The growth spurt is clearly an earlier pubertal event in girls than in boys.

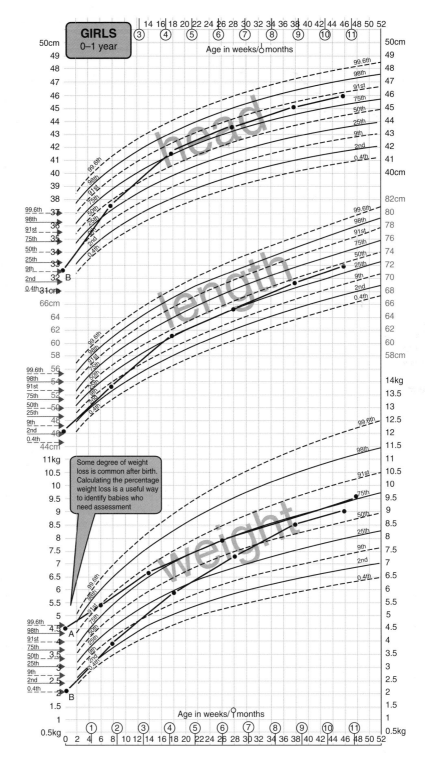

Figure 23.7 'Catch-up' and 'catch-down' in infancy. Growth curves are plotted for two babies on the UK 1990 growth reference chart. Baby A, the infant of a diabetic mother, has a birth weight above the 97th centile. Excessive weight gain *in utero* was the result of maternal, hence foetal, hyperglycaemia and hyperinsulinism. After birth, she 'catches down' towards her genetically determined size. Baby B was born at term with birth weight less than the 0.4th centile and head circumference at the 9th centile. This indicates 'head sparing' and is typical of late intrauterine growth retardation (IUGR). After birth, the baby crosses several centiles upwards, a pattern indicative of 'catch-up' to genetically determined size following release from intrauterine constraint. Chart developed by RCPCH/WHO/Department of Health, Copyright © 2009 Department of Health.

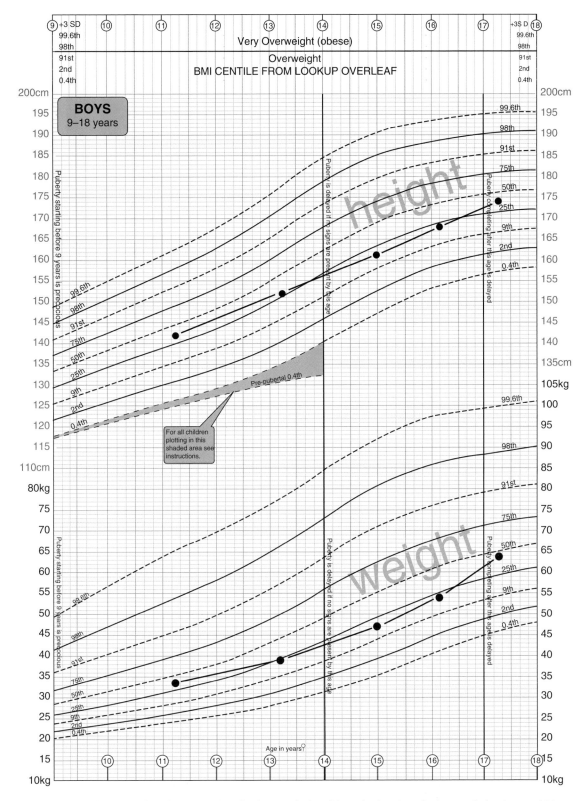

Figure 23.8 Late puberty plotted on the UK-WHO growth reference. This boy did not develop signs of puberty until after the age of 14 years ('delayed puberty'). Because his pubertal growth spurt is relatively late, there is the apparent effect of crossing down one centile space for both weight and height, with recovery after the onset of puberty. This is because the cross-sectional chart best reflects the growth trajectory of boys entering puberty at average age. Chart developed by RCPCH/WHO/Department of Health, Copyright © 2009 Department of Health.

apparent downward crossing of centile lines at this age, with later apparent catch-up as puberty occurs (Figure 23.8). The converse may also obtain in early puberty: a child may show apparent early upward and later downward centile crossing. Earlier growth charts (Tanner–Whitehouse, based on data collected in the 1960s) made some allowance for this by showing as a shaded area the age at which variations attributable to puberty might occur. Interpretation may be further confounded by the observation that taller, heavier children tend to develop puberty earlier than those who are shorter and lighter, whereas those with chronic disease may show later puberty. This adaptation may help them catch up to their genetically determined final height despite long-term disease-associated under-nutrition. In 2012, the new UK-WHO growth chart for children aged 2–18 years was published. This incorporates a new system of pubertal assessment and, like the other growth charts, is openly accessible from the RCPCH Web site (www.rcpch.ac.uk).

Body composition and growth

Childhood growth involves not only an increase in body size but changes in body proportions, the relative sizes of organ systems, and chemical composition. These changes have implications for:

- The nature and amount of body nutrient stores.
- The partitioning of nutrients between organ systems.
- The potential for nutrient restriction to have lifelong effects.

Sexual-dimorphism body composition becomes very apparent after puberty but is present to a limited extent well before.

Nutrient stores

Changes in the amount and distribution of body fat reserves exemplify the implications of growth for nutrient stores. Figure 23.9 shows how the body mass is distributed between fat, protein, and water as a child grows to 10 years. The extracellular fluid compartment is relatively large at birth but quickly decreases in size, a process which largely accounts for the normal weight loss of newborn infants in the first week of life. In the first 6 months, body weight more than doubles and the proportion of fat increases from about 14 to 25%. Thus the average fat mass of a

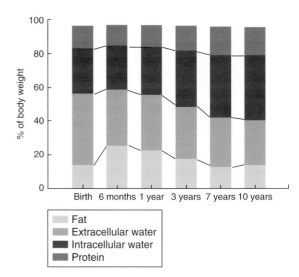

Figure 23.9 Change in the relative sizes of body compartments with age. Drawn using data from Fomon *et al*. (1982). Reproduced with permission by the Am J Clin Nutr (1982; 35: 1169–1175), American Society for Nutrition.

Table 23.1 Percentage of body weight accounted for by various tissues and organs at various stages of human development. This article was published in Widdowson EM. Changes in body composition during growth. In: Chapter 17 in Scientific Foundations of Paediatrics, Davis JA, Dobbing J (eds). Second edition. Copyright Heinemann, 1981.

	24-week foetus	Full-term newborn	Adult
Muscle	25	25	40
Bone	22	18	14
Heart	0.6	0.5	0.4
Lungs	3.3	1.5	1.4
Liver	4	5	2
Kidneys	0.7	1	0.5
Brain	13	12	2.0

6-month-old baby is about fourfold greater than that of a normal newborn – some 2 kg as opposed to 500 g. This need to deposit large amounts of fat (9 kcal/g) partly explains why growth is so energetically demanding at this stage of development, consuming up to 50% of a baby's energy intake.

The connotations for surviving a period of starvation are equally important, and are even more dramatic if the extremely preterm baby is considered. The fat compartment of a 500 g 25-week-gestation baby represents only 2–3% of body weight: about 10–15 g or 90–130 kcal. Provision of nutritional support is therefore a matter of urgency in such a patient.

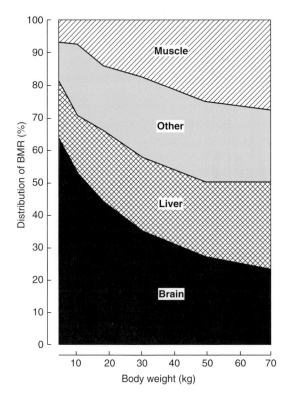

Figure 23.10 Change in energy partitioning with age. Reproduced with permission from Pediatrics, Vol. 47, p169–179, Copyright © 1971 by the AAP.

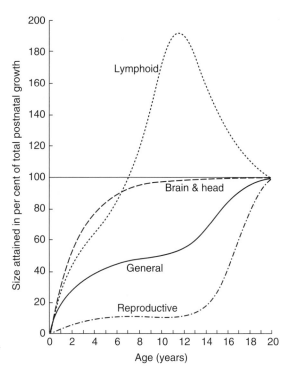

Figure 23.11 Changes in the relative sizes of organ systems with age. The graph shows the ages at which organs attain a given percentage of their size at age 20 (100%). Note that 90% of brain growth is completed in the first 3 years, and that the relative size of the lymphoid organ in childhood significantly exceeds that in the adult. Reprinted with permission from Tanner (1989).

Organ systems and nutrient partitioning

Table 23.1 illustrates the relative contribution of various organ systems to body weight in the infant and adult. A notable difference is the relative size of the brain, which is growing at peak velocity around term and completes much of its growth in the first 2 years of life. These changes have major effects on the contribution brain metabolism makes to resting energy expenditure (REE) (Figure 23.10). As glucose is the principal brain fuel, it also explains why glucose requirements change so greatly with age. In the adult, hepatic gluconeogenesis can be suppressed by an intravenous infusion of 1–2 mg glucose/kg body weight/minute. However, the term newborn needs 3–5 mg/kg body weight/minute and the preterm, growth-retarded newborn (with a relatively much larger brain) some 6–8 mg/kg body weight/minute. If glucose requirements were expressed instead per 100 g of brain weight, a different picture would emerge: requirements are similar across the age spectrum.

This example clearly shows how changes in body composition associated with growth affect nutrient partitioning between organ systems and hence nutrient requirements if expressed on a per-unit-body-weight basis.

Nutrient restriction and critical growth periods

Figure 23.11 shows the stages in childhood at which various organ systems undergo the most rapid growth. It is particularly important to note that brain growth is virtually completed in the early years of childhood. Prolonged and severe nutrient restriction at this age may be associated with lifelong functional deficit.

Chronic early-life under-nutrition results in stunting (linear growth restriction), which is extremely common in resource-poor countries, with as many as one-third to one-half of all children being affected. At 2 years of age, in such settings, a height greater than 2 standard deviations below the mean on WHO charts (z-score -2.0) seems to be associated with a later IQ deficit of around 10 points. The extent to which this reflects deprivation of nutrients, as

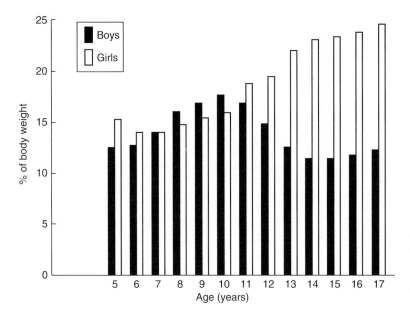

Figure 23.12 Differences between boys and girls in development of the fat compartment. The bars represent fat as a percentage of body weight. Difference between sexes becomes significant only after puberty. Data from Widdowson (1981), copyright Heinemann.

Box 23.3 Growth

- A growth *reference* and a growth *standard* are cocnceptually different.
- A growth chart can be compiled from cross-sectional or longitudinal data.
- Growth references can be represented graphically (centile charts) or statistically (z-scores).
- Cross-sectional charts can conceal normal variation in growth patterns during infancy and at puberty.
- Growth is a sensitive measure of health, nutrient supply, and socioeconomic status. These influences are much stronger than ethnic background.
- The pattern of growth can be resolved into infant, child, and pubertal phases (the Karlberg ICP model). These reflect differing endocrine influences.
- Body composition and the relative sizes of organ systems change as growth proceeds. The timing of a nutritional insult therefore determines the outcome.
- Sex differences in body composition appear at puberty.
- The growth spurt occurs early in female puberty and late in male puberty.

---

opposed to the effects of numerous confounders (e.g. poverty, illness, and low birth weight) is uncertain. Mechanisms exist to spare brain nutrition in the presence of nutrient shortages. For example, the newborn who has suffered intrauterine growth retardation (IUGR) as a result of placental failure has a small body with thin limbs and a large head because blood flow and nutrients are diverted away from the somatic organs to the brain. To a lesser extent, brain sparing, with similar changes in body proportions, is also evident in malnourished young children.

Sexual dimorphism in body composition

Differences in the body compositions of boys and girls are present throughout childhood but become very marked after puberty, as shown in Figure 23.12. In girls, fat represents a much higher proportion of pubertal weight gain than in boys, who deposit more lean body tissue. These differences reflect the dominance of androgenic steroids in boys, but functionally also ensure that girls have more adequate energy reserves to meet the later demands of pregnancy and lactation.

Key points about growth and body composition are summarised in Box 23.3.

23.3 The impact of development on nutrition

'Children are not just small adults' – they are growing and exhibit developmental changes which better equip them to meet metabolic demands. For example, developmental changes in the gastrointestinal system enhance the efficiency of nutrient absorption, while those in the liver and kidney progressively increase the child's ability to adapt to over- or under-supply

of nutrients. Most important of all is the child's neurological maturation, which facilitates transition from total dependence during infancy to the independent adult, capable of seeking out and selecting a food supply. This section examines some of the major nutritional changes that occur as the child develops.

Neurological maturation

Infancy, the first 12 months of life, is a particularly rapid period of developmental change during which the typical term infant will treble in weight and move from total dependence on milk to the acceptance of a mixed diet compatible with the family's culture. This process of nutritional diversification is gradual and the pace of change needs to respect the timing of normal psychomotor and mental developmental changes, often referred to as 'developmental milestones'. Those particularly relevant to the development of eating behaviour are shown in Table 23.2. Note that these are approximations only and there can be substantial normal variation between individual children.

When considering Table 23.2, it may be useful to know that paediatricians generally think about developmental milestones in four groups (or 'fields'):

- gross motor function and maintenance of posture;
- fine motor function (manipulation) and vision;
- speech and hearing;
- psychological and social.

Table 23.2 Developmental 'milestones' of neurological maturation relevant to feeding.

Milestone	Age achieved
Sucking and swallowing	From about 34 weeks of gestation
	Reflex sucking disappears about 4 months
Rooting reflex	Present at term
	Disappears about 4 months
Coordinated acceptance of a spoon	About 6 months
Puts hands to mouth	About 5–6 months
Sits unsupported	About 7 months
Transfers objects from hand to hand	About 8 months
Pincer grip	About 10 months
Full rotary chewing movements	1–2 years
Holds spoon or cup to feed	12–18 months
Feeds self (but messily)	18 months–2 years

Successful feeding requires convergence in all fields. The child must be able to sit comfortably, hold their head erect and be able to turn (gross motor), have coordinated oropharyngeal movements in order to sweep a spoon, swallow (speech), locate food with their hand and transfer it to their mouth (vision and fine motor), and interact with a carer (psychological). As a result, children with cerebral palsy (a disorder of posture and movement caused by a nonprogressive lesion of the developing brain, in which muscles become stiff or 'spastic', making coordinated movements hard to achieve) often have major feeding problems. They need help with body positioning and careful attention must be paid to the texture and consistency of foods offered in order for them to learn to eat.

Thinking about the development of complementary feeding skills in this way emphasises a number of other points:

- The child needs to be 'developmentally ready': there is no point in offering solids before the child is ready to take them. Indeed, to do so may result in force-feeding and negatively affect eating behaviour.
- The introduction of complementary feeding at appropriate times may also help to reinforce the coordinated use of muscle groups. Sucking from the breast or bottle teat requires the tongue to move only in a sagittal plane, whereas forming solids into a bolus requires the gradual attainment of rotary tongue movements necessary for speech. Anecdotally, there is a frequent association between early feeding problems and speech delay, though whether one is a consequence of the other, or both reflect the underlying delay in neurological maturation is not clear.

The impact of neurological development on nutrition is summarised in Box 23.4.

Box 23.4 Impact of neurological development on nutrition

- Children mature neurologically in a well-defined sequence marked by 'milestones'.
- The development of feeding requires integration of milestones in all fields: gross motor, fine motor, speech, and psychosocial.
- Appropriate timing and progression of complementary feeding must recognise this process.

Gastrointestinal maturation

The gut is anatomically mature by about 24 weeks of gestation and there is transit of fluid through the upper intestine from early in the second trimester of pregnancy. Foetal swallowing can be observed on ultrasonography, and obstruction related to congenital anomalies (e.g. oesophageal or duodenal atresia) results in accumulation of excessive amniotic fluid (polyhydramnios). Swallowed water is absorbed in the small intestine and excreted through the foetal kidneys; there is thus turnover of the water compartment of the amniotic fluid. There is no net transit through the large intestine, which accumulates meconium, a sticky dark green material. Meconium is usually excreted within 24 hours of birth (excretion during labour may be an indication of foetal stress resulting from hypoxia and ischaemia). Delayed excretion of meconium is often an indication of lower intestinal obstruction or dysmotility, such as Hirschsprung's disease.

Animal studies have shown that feeding is the important trophic stimulus to further postnatal development of the gut. Milk feeding results in both a hypertrophy (increase in cell size) and a hyperplasia (increase in cell number) of the small intestine, and milk of the animal's own species is more effective than artificial milks in this respect. The newborn's capacity for mucosal absorption increases rapidly after birth in response to enteral feeding, which also stimulates the release of 'gut hormones', including cholecystokinin, motilin, and enteroglucagon, helping to stimulate bile flow, intestinal transit, and the integration of liver metabolism with feeding.

Despite the observation that about half the infant's energy intake is provided by fat, the pancreas is relatively small at birth, and secretion of pancreatic lipase is reduced. This apparent paradox is explained by the existence of other effectors of luminal fat digestion, including the initiation of fat digestion in stomach, through the release of lingual lipase during sucking, and the presence in breast milk of a bile salt-stimulated lipase active at duodenal pH and stimulated by bile salts. Thus breast-milk lipids are more effectively absorbed than those in formula or other milks. When infants are born prematurely, fat digestion is even less well developed than at term, and initiation of enteral feeding is further hampered by poorly coordinated propulsion due to delay in the

propagation of a migrating motor complex. The latter appears at a gestation of about 34 weeks, concomitant with the presence of effectively coordinated sucking and swallowing. It is known, however, that the initiation of feeding can effectively 'call forward' the maturation of motility patterns. Enteral feeding in even very preterm infants (from about 24 to 26 weeks' gestation) is usually therefore commenced in small quantities as soon as possible after delivery, increasing gradually in volume as tolerated.

Another important aspect of gut maturation is the evolution of immune protection during infancy. Diarrhoeal disease is a leading cause of death in infants and young children. Moreover, mechanisms must develop which allow the infant to recognise harmful antigens yet become tolerant to foods. A number of factors are important in this respect:

- The provision of specific passive secretory immunity (secretory immunoglobulin A) through the enteromammary axis of breast-feeding.
- The presence of nonspecific immune factors in breast milk (e.g. lysozyme, lactoferrin, the lactoperoxidase system).
- The promotion of a large-bowel flora dominated by bifidobacteria, rather than coliform organisms. This is partly attributable to the prebiotic effect of nonabsorbable oligosaccharides in breast milk, in which they constitute about 10% of the carbohydrate content.

Although the last has long been cited as important in protecting the gut from infection, the nature of large-bowel flora may also be important in the determination of systemic immune tolerance through regulation of the relative balance of T-helper/suppressor activity (see Chapter 8).

Important factors in gastrointestinal maturation are summarised in Box 23.5.

Renal maturation

At birth, both glomerular filtration rate (GFR) and renal tubular concentrating capacity are reduced. This limits the amount of solute that can be cleared from the blood and increases the demand for free water needed to eliminate dietary excess in a relatively dilute urine. The term 'renal solute load' (RSL) is used to describe the amount of absorbed dietary solute surplus to growth demands that must be eliminated through the kidneys. Stressors such as fever or diarrhoea may further compromise excretory capacity by increasing insensible and stool water losses, reducing water availability for urine. Retention of solute then leads to hyperosmolar dehydration.

Carbohydrate and fat do not contribute to RSL because they are entirely eliminated through non-renal routes (oxidation to CO_2 and water). The principal components of RSL are sodium (Na), potassium (K), chloride (Cl), and absorbed phosphorus (P_a), together with the amount of urea formed by oxidation of protein excess to growth demands. These form the potential renal solute load (PRSL). However, the actual RSL depends not only on the composition of the feed, but on the baby's rate of growth (which influences the rate of solute retention) and non-renal water losses. In the absence of diarrhoea, the latter can be ignored, so that RSL can be calculated as:

$$\text{Estimated RSL} = \text{PRSL} - (0.9 \times$$
$$\text{weight gain in g/day}) \, \text{mosmol/l}$$

PRSL can in turn be expressed by the formula:

$$\text{PRSL} = N/28 + Na + Cl + K + P_a \, \text{mosmol/l}$$

In both formulas, elemental composition is expressed in mmol/l. The factor 0.9 in the first equation is an estimate which allows for the disposal of solute by deposition in growing tissue (0.9 mmol for each gram of weight gained). This observation re-emphasises R.A. McCance's dictum that growth constitutes the infant's 'third kidney', and explains the paradox by which infants tolerate protein intakes that would be proportionally far too high for an adult with similarly low GFR resulting from kidney disease (see Chapter 14). The divisor of 28 in the second equation, applied to the total fraction of nitrogenous solute

(N/mg), assumes that the modal number of nitrogen atoms per molecule of urinary nitrogenous solute is 2; in other words, that it is urea.

A final complication is that the amount of water consumed is partly determined by the energy density of a feed: infants consuming an energy-dense feed will take a lower volume, hence less water. Thus, whereas the calculations above show PRSL in terms of mosmol/l, it is more logical to express it as mosmol/100 kcal. Table 23.3 shows the PRSLs of various feed types calculated in both ways. On both theoretical and epidemiological grounds (risk of hypernatraemic dehydration), it can be shown that feeds with a PRSL < 27 mosmol/100 kcal are safe, whereas those > 38 mosmol/100 kcal are associated with increased risk of developing hyperosmolar dehydration. For regulatory purposes, limits of 30–35 mosmol/100 kcal have been proposed for infant formulas.

The role of renal maturation in nutrition is summarised in Box 23.6.

Metabolic maturation

At birth, the normal newborn must switch rapidly from continuous transplacental nutrient supply to a pattern of intermittent enteral feeding. Initially, during the onset of stage II (postpartum) lactogenesis, the amount of energy delivered by breast milk is small. Typically volumes of only 50–100 ml may be taken on the first day of life, rising to 600–800 ml by the end of the first week. Counter-regulatory mechanisms are well developed, in keeping with the need to meet high obligatory metabolic demands (at this stage, cerebral metabolism accounts for over half of the REE: see Figure 23.10) at this time of low intake. With the cessation of transplacental glucose supply, there is a surge in glucagon secretion, resulting in glycogenolysis. About 1% of the term newborn's body weight is glycogen, which forms an important short-term energy reserve. The glucagon surge also promotes gluconeogenesis, with glycerol (from fat stores), alanine (from muscle), lactate, and pyruvate acting as substrates.

Adrenaline secretion is also important in opposing the action of insulin, which dominates the foetal metabolic milieu. It stimulates lipolysis in fat stores and protein breakdown in muscle (releasing alanine to fuel gluconeogenesis) during the early hours of

Table 23.3 Calculation of potential renal solute load (PRSL) for various milks. Reprinted from J Pediatr, 134, Fomon SJ & Ziegler EE. Renal solute load and potential renal solute load in infancy, 11–14. Copyright (1999), with permission from Elsevier.

| Type of milk feed | Nutrient concentrations | | | | | PRSL | | | |
| | Protein (g/l) | Na (mmol/l) | Cl (mmol/l) | K (mmol/l) | P_a (mmol/l) | Constituents | | Total | |
						Urea (mosmol/l)	Σ elecs (mosmol/l)	mosmol/l	mosmol/100 kcal
Human milk	10	7	11	13	5	57	36	93	14
Milk-based formula	15	8	12	18	11	86	49	135	20
Whole cow's milk	33	21	30	39	30	188	120	308	46

Box 23.6 Renal maturation

- Young infants, especially those born preterm, have both reduced GFR and reduced tubular concentrating capacity.
- The amount of dietary solute in excess of the need for growth is known as the 'renal solute load' (RSL).
- Low GFR, particularly in the very preterm baby, reduces clearance of RSL through the kidneys, contributing to uraemia.
- Impaired tubular concentrating capacity requires that the infant be given sufficient water to eliminate RSL, or else the plasma will become hyperosmolar.
- The PRSL of a feed is normally greater than the RSL because growth consumes solute, effectively acting as a 'third kidney'.

Box 23.7 Metabolic maturation

- Counter-regulatory mechanisms are well developed in the healthy term newborn.
- They are instrumental in effecting the change from continuous transplacental delivery of nutrients to intermittent enteral feeding controlled by appetite.
- High metabolic demands and the immaturity of some metabolic steps mean that a greater number of amino acids is essential or conditionally essential for the young infant.
- The protein quality of breast milk is high.
- High protein quality and the existence of mechanisms promoting nitrogen economy in the baby explain why the nutritional protein content of breast milk at first sight seems low.

---

life. Growth hormone and cortisol also play important roles; indeed, children with growth-hormone or cortisol deficiency may present with significant neonatal hypoglycaemia. This switch from carbohydrate to fat metabolism is evident as:

- A fall in respiratory quotient from 1.0 in the first hour to 0.8–0.85 by about 8–12 hours of age.
- The appearance of significant ketonaemia at 24–48 hours of age ('suckling ketogenesis').

In contrast, some pathways important to the metabolism of protein are less mature in the young infant, particularly if preterm. The ability to synthesise urea following deamination of amino acids is reduced, as is capacity to interconvert certain essential amino acids. The latter particularly increases metabolic requirements for cysteine and taurine (less easily synthesised from methionine) and for tyrosine (synthesised from phenylalanine at older ages).

These apparent metabolic constraints possibly reflect the observation that the young infant is strongly anabolic and in health has little need to dispose of excessive amino acid. Indeed, the young infant's metabolic milieu is characterised more by the need to conserve nitrogen in the interests of protein economy. Thus the intake of nitrogen from breast milk is relatively low, but the infant is able to maintain nitrogen balance by virtue of:

- The high quality of breast-milk protein (conventionally used as the reference for calculating the amino acid scores of alternative proteins – such as cow's milk or soya – used in infant formulas).
- The existence of mechanisms for colonic salvage. Almost a quarter of the nitrogen in breast milk is 'non-protein nitrogen' (much of it urea), and there is good evidence that the infant can incorporate this into body protein. (The observation of a high level of non-protein nitrogen has caused some to observe that it is not appropriate to express the protein content of breast milk by applying the conventional factor of 6.25 to nitrogen measured using the Kjeldahl technique. A factor of 5.18 probably reflects more closely the nutritional protein content.)

The role of metabolic maturation in nutrition is summarised in Box 23.7.

23.4 Infant feeding

Previous sections have shown that infancy is a period of particular nutritional vulnerability: the potential rate of growth is rapid, body stores are small, and functional immaturity constrains adaptation to both over- and under-supply. Feeding during infancy therefore warrants close attention.

Breast-feeding

The establishment of successful breast-feeding is crucial to the general health of mother and baby in all environments (see *Public Health Nutrition* in this series). In summary, the principal health gains associated with breast-feeding are reduced vulnerability to gastrointestinal and respiratory (including ear) infections and suppression of ovulation, leading to a reduction in demands on family resources. Long-term gains also include an advantage in the child's cognitive development, a reduced risk of obesity in later life, and a reduction in the mother's risk of pre-menopausal breast cancer. Although these factors were once considered less relevant to industrialised countries, cohort studies in the UK have clearly shown that babies who are not breast-fed suffer more gastrointestinal and respiratory infections and are more likely to be admitted to hospital. Since exclusive or predominant breast-feeding is associated with the highest standards of health, the growth pattern of infants so fed is regarded as a standard for all infants, regardless of feeding method (see the earlier sections of this chapter).

Key points about breast-feeding are listed in Box 23.8.

Box 23.8 Breast-feeding

- Breast-feeding is associated with better health outcomes for mother and baby, even in industrialised countries.
- Data on the consumption and composition of breast milk constitute a dietary reference for young infants.
- The growth pattern of exclusively or predominantly breast-fed infants is regarded as the ideal (or 'standard' pattern; see Section 23.2).
- The production of breast milk is controlled by infant demand: unrestricted access to the breast and an effective feeding technique are both important to success.
- There are technical problems in measuring precisely both the amount of milk the infant consumes and its composition.

Composition of breast milk

Nutritionally, breast milk alone is viewed as the reference diet for infants younger than 6 months of age. Table 23.4 summarises its composition and compares it with that of a typical infant formula and of unmodified cow's milk. There is pronounced inter-individual variability in the composition of breast milk. This is attributable to a number of factors, including the gestational age of the baby, the postnatal age of the baby, the volume produced, and the time of day. Even within a single mother–baby pair, the fat concentration rises significantly during a feed.

The nitrogen moiety of breast milk is particularly complex, for a number of reasons. First, many of the proteins serve 'non-nutritional' biological functions, such as specific and nonspecific immune protection of the gut and mucosal surfaces. For example, about 10% of the protein is secretory immunoglobulin A (IgA), which is not absorbed. Second, about a quarter of the nitrogenous compounds exist as the so-called 'non-protein nitrogen' fraction, which comprises free amino acids, urea, and other small peptides. There is evidence that much of this can be salvaged in the colon. For these reasons, the true, nutritionally available protein content of breast milk is not easily measurable and cannot be simply expressed as a fraction of the total nitrogen content.

The economic utilisation of the nitrogenous compounds in breast milk to match the demands of growth helps to prevent the accumulation of urea, which would otherwise need to be eliminated through the kidneys. This, together with the low macro-element content, minimises the PRSL of breast milk to the extent that the breast-fed baby need not be offered additional free water to facilitate renal solute clearance. Thus breast milk alone is sufficient as both a food and a drink for the first 6 months of life.

Establishment of breast-feeding

The endocrine control of lactation ensures that breast-milk supply matches demands made by infant sucking. In practical terms, the key requirements for successful establishment of breast-feeding at birth are:

- unrestricted access to the breast when the infant is hungry;
- effective milk removal by the infant.

Table 23.4 Summary of the composition of human milk, infant formula, and cow's milk. IgA, immunoglobulin A. Data for the composition of infant formula are taken from Ministry of Agriculture Fisheries and Food (1995), © Crown Copyright 1995 and subsequent amendments, taking the mid-point of the legally permissible range unless otherwise stated. Data for the composition of cow's milk and human milk are taken from Williams (1991).

	Constituent	Human milk	Infant formula	Cow's milk
Protein nitrogen	Total protein (g/l)	8.9[a]	18	31
	Secretory IgA (g/l)	0.5–1.0	0	trace
	Lactoferrin (g/l)	1	0	trace
	Lysozyme (g/l)	0.05–0.25	0	trace
Non-protein nitrogen	(% of total N)	25	0	5
Carbohydrate	Lactose (g/l)	65	25 (minimum)	45
	Oligosaccharides (g/l)	12	Not exceeding 8 (as 90% oligogalactosyl-lactose and 10% oligofructosyl saccharose)	1
	Other (e.g. glucose polymer) (g/l)		Up to 10 g in total as: lactose, maltose sucrose, glucose syrup, starch, or maltodextrins	
Fat	Total (g/l)	40 (very variable – see text)	35	40
Energy	kcal/l	600–>800	600–750	600–800
Minerals	Na (mmol/l)	7	12	20
	K (mmol/l)	15	20	39
	Ca (mmol/l)	9	10	30
	Mg (mmo/l)	1	3	5
	P (mmol/l)	5	14	30
	Ca:P ratio (by weight)	2:1	0.5:1 to 2:1	1.3:1
	Fe (mmol/l)	0.014	0.125	0.01

[a]See note in the text about the uncertainty surrounding the true (nutritional) protein content of human milk.

Many clinical problems with breast-feeding, such as breast pain, cracked and sore nipples, mastitis, early dehydration, and poor weight gain, result from errors in breast-feeding technique which hamper the second of these requirements. In order for the baby to remove milk from the breast effectively, he or she must be properly positioned (or held correctly by the mother) and attached at the breast (i.e. take sufficient breast tissue into the mouth, not just the nipple). An account of the skills required to assess and correct such problems is beyond the scope of this text, but early referral to a professional skilled in breast-feeding management is essential should such problems develop.

Consumption of breast milk

The volume of breast milk consumed by a breast-feeding baby has been measured in a number of ways. The oldest is 'test-weighing' – measuring the difference in the baby's (or occasionally the mother's) weight before and after a feed. Although improvements in the accuracy of scales have reduced the errors inherent in weighing a moving baby, there remains considerable variation in the volume of milk consumed from day to day. The procedure is also intrusive and may alter the mother and baby's feeding pattern, making measurements of limited value. For these reasons, test-weighing is no longer used for clinical purposes, the most practical measure of breast-feeding adequacy being the baby's growth rate judged using the UK-WHO chart, which was derived by observation of healthy breast-fed babies. For research purposes, measurements of the breast-milk intake of 'free-living' breast-fed babies have been made using isotopic dilution techniques, administering either ^2H_2O or $^2H_2^{18}O$ to the baby or to the mother and baby. These suggest that breast-fed babies consume some 400–800 ml/day of breast milk.

The composition of the milk which the baby consumes is also difficult to measure, because it changes during the feed. A number of solutions to this problem have been tried:

- *Expressing the entire content of the breasts at a feed.* An objection to this is that the baby may not remove all milk from the breast, but choose to leave some behind. Because the fat concentration rises progressively as the breast empties, the expressed sample may overestimate the energy content of milk consumed.

- *Expressing samples before and after a feed.* This technique has been widely used, but the assumption that changes in concentration follow a linear trend during a feed may not be valid.
- *Doubly-labelled water ($^2H_2^{18}O$) technique.* As the ^{18}O exchanges with both the CO_2- and ^2H-labelled water pools, differences in the rate of elimination can be used to calculate both energy expenditure and milk intake, allowing energy intake to be inferred (see Chapter 2 of *Introduction to Human Nutrition* in this series).

Formula feeding

Unmodified animal milks (for example, cow's milk) are unsuitable for young infants for several reasons:

- Protein and mineral content impose too high an RSL.
- Micronutrient content (e.g. iron, folic acid, vitamin D, vitamin A) is inadequate.
- Fat and protein are relatively indigestible.

When a mother chooses not to breast-feed, therefore, the infant should be fed an infant formula. According to UK and European law, this label defines a commercial product which provides the nutritional requirements of infants in good health for the first 4–6 months of life, as set out in legally enforceable compositional requirements. The Infant Formula and Follow-on Formula Regulations 1995 (Ministry of Agriculture Fisheries and Food 1995) (revised in 2007) define the terms 'infant formula' and 'follow-on formula', setting out legally permissible minimum and maximum nutrient concentrations.

Infant formula must be based on a cow's-milk or soy-protein source, the amount and type of protein (whey:casein ratio) being adjusted to the baby's metabolic needs. The carbohydrate moiety of infant formula is usually supplied by lactose and other permissible carbohydrates (Table 23.4) in amounts intended to approximate those of breast milk (about 70 g/l). Vegetable oil blends usually provide the fat: these are substituted for cow's-milk fat because the latter is less digestible, having a higher saturated fatty acid content. The mineral content of infant formulas is also adjusted. Notably, the sodium content is reduced and the ratio of calcium:phosphorus increased. Finally, infant formulas are fully supplemented with trace minerals and vitamins.

The non-breast-fed infant should receive infant formula for at least the first 12 months of life – alone for the first 4–6 months and later as part of a progressively diversified weaning diet (see the next subsection). Infants over 6 months are, however, sometimes given a follow-on formula. The composition of 'follow-on formulas' is also defined in UK and European law, but, unlike infant formulas, they are not required to meet the infant's whole nutritional requirements. Like infant formulas, they are micronutrient-enriched and promoted commercially as having value in preventing iron deficiency. Although there is good evidence that they are superior to whole cow's milk in this respect they have not been shown to be any better than infant formula, which remains a suitable choice at this age for the non-breast-fed infant.

All powdered infant formulas need careful reconstitution:

- All utensils must be sterilised.
- Water must be boiled and of appropriate electrolyte composition. It should be tap water drawn from the mains supply (not through an ion-exchange softener) or bottled water of similar composition. The main concern here is the sodium concentration: EU regulations set a maximum [Na] of 200 mg/l at the tap.
- Level measures in the correct measuring scoop (usually supplied with the tin) must be used.
- Powder should be added to the measured amount of water, not *vice versa*, or the feed may be hazardously overconcentrated.

The amount of formula infants consume averages about 150 ml/kg/day at 2–3 months of age. However, this is merely a guideline and, as with breast-feeding, there is large inter-individual variation. For example, in a well-known study of a group of 3-month-old American infants, consumption varied from 120 to over 220 ml/kg/day.

Key points on infant formula are summarised in Box 23.9.

Complementary feeding

Complementary feeding is the introduction of foods other than breast milk or infant formula into the infant's diet. The term is now generally considered preferable to 'weaning', which misleadingly implied a role in the cessation of breast-feeding. In fact, the

---

Box 23.9 Infant formula

- An infant formula is based on cow's milk or soya protein modi-fied to meet compositional standards such as those set out in UK law and European Commission directives. Infant formula is designed to provide the entire nutritional requirements of healthy, full-term infants for the first 4–6 months of life but lacks the many immune factors found in breast milk.
- Extensive modification of cow's milk reduces PRSL, enhances pro-tein quality, alters macronutrient balance, and adjusts Ca:P ratio.
- Infant formula is enriched with trace minerals and vitamins.
- Powdered infant formulas must be reconstituted carefully, according to the manufacturer's instructions.
- The amount of formula consumed averages about 150 ml/kg/day at 3 months of age, but varies greatly between babies.

---

primary role of complementary feeding is to increase dietary diversity, not to reduce breast-milk intake. Complementary foods themselves are sometimes also referred to in the literature as beikost (USA) or solids (UK).

Although complementary feeding is generally thought of as a mechanism for increasing the nutrient density of the diet, it serves a number of other devel-opmental functions too (see Section 23.3). There has been much controversy over the optimum time at which to introduce foods other than breast milk into the infant's diet. Introducing them too early will undesirably increase RSL, reduce breast milk intake, compromise the maintenance of lactational amenor-rhoea, and expose the infant to dietary antigens such as gluten (see Chapter 8). Leaving complementary feeding too late, on the other hand, may impair growth, because the nutrient density of a liquid diet is relatively low. Moreover, the concentration of some important micronutrients in breast milk (such as iron) is low, and that of some, particularly zinc, declines with the length of lactation.

Historically, a number of different philosophical approaches have been applied to defining the appro-priate age for introducing complementary foods:

- *Factorial calculation of the intake required to support 'optimal growth'.* If the expected rate of growth is known, it is possible to calculate what energy intake is required after making allowance for losses and maintenance expenditure. Although this approach seems intuitively sensible, consider-able problems arise in agreeing what is meant by 'optimal growth' and it is now acknowledged that

older growth references (such as NCHS) did not accurately describe the early growth pattern of breast-fed infants. The use of such charts was one factor which historically led to overestimation of the energy and protein requirements of growing breast-fed infants. Others were underestimation of breast-milk intake and miscalculation of the nutrient content of breast milk. Better estimation of these quantities subsequently led to a postponement of the recommended age for complementary feeding from 'about 3 months' to '4–6 months'. More recently, recommendations have been further revised to 'about 6 months' on the basis of evidence discussed later.

- *Consideration of developmental and biological fac-tors.* An alternative way of considering the prob-lem is to ask by what age infants are developmentally prepared to receive foods other than breast milk. Maturation of neurological, gastrointestinal, renal, and immune function can be taken into account and considered together with available data on the morbidity associated with complementary feeding at particular ages. On this basis, the WHO review concluded that exclusive breast-feeding can be continued with benefit for 'about the first six months' in healthy infants of appropriate birth weight, though alternative strategies may need to be considered for at-risk groups such as those of low birth weight.

- *Controlled studies of interventions.* A limited amount of information is available from small controlled trials, mainly conducted in less-developed-country settings. Commercially prepared complementary foods were introduced at 4 or 6 months and the effects on growth and breast-milk intake studied. Introduction at 4 months did not confer a detecta-ble growth advantage, although it was associated with a reduced breast-milk intake. Clearly such studies are difficult to perform and a particular problem with the controlled work described was differential dropout from the study groups, which could have biased the findings.

Taking all this evidence together, there seems no good reason to suppose that introduction of com-plementary foods earlier than 6 months benefits the majority of breast-fed infants. Traditionally first foods have been pureed and offered from a spoon 2–3 times a day after breast feeds, increasing the

Box 23.10 Growth and complementary feeding

- The timing of complementary feeding should reflect the pace of the individual baby's development.
- Controlled studies suggest that introducing complementary foods at 4 months (as opposed to 6 months) does not lead to faster growth but is associated with compensatory reduction in breast-milk intake.
- Breast- and bottle-fed babies show different patterns of growth in the first year of life, breast-fed babies being lighter at a year of age.
- There is no evidence that these growth differences are due to shortage of breast milk.
- The mechanisms which explain these growth differences and their long-term significance are currently unclear.

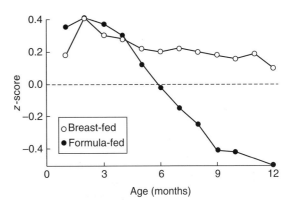

Figure 23.13 Differences in weight gain between breast- and bottle-fed infants. The curves show weight as a variation (in fractions of a z-score) from the 50th centile of NCHS reference. Thus breast-fed babies, on average, quickly rise 0.4 standard deviations above the 50th centile, then fall 0.4 standard deviations below by the end of the first year of life. Adapted from Am J Clin Nutr (1993; 57: 140–145), copyright © American Society for Nutrition and Pediatrics, 96, 495–503, copyright 1995 by the AAP.

amounts as accepted. Salt, sugar, and strong spices must not be added. Once well accepted, solid foods that will dissolve in the mouth (e.g. banana, toast) offer a useful stage in the transition to finely, then coarsely, chopped and ultimately lumpier foods which require chewing or which the infant can hold. Diversification of the diet in infancy has generally been viewed as a gradual process, but the key concern is that it should be conducted at a pace compatible with the infant's development. Thus children who are first offered solids at around 6 months can progress to lumpier foods at a much more rapid pace than those introduced at 4 months. The eventual aim should be that by 1 year of age the infant is having three main meals a day, plus snacks and three or four breast feeds to supply the fluid portion.

Key points on growth and complementary feeding are summarised in Box 23.10.

Effect of feeding on infant growth

Breast- and bottle-fed infants show different patterns of growth, as illustrated in Figure 23.13. Older studies showed that breast-fed infants gained weight particularly rapidly in the first 2 months, but that velocity then slowed relative to the old NCHS norms. Bottle-fed infants, on the other hand, showed sustained weight gain above NCHS norms throughout the first year of life.

Acknowledgement of these differences underlay the need to describe clearly the growth of breast-fed babies and create the new WHO multicentre growth standard now adopted for growth monitoring in the UK. In 2009 the UK-WHO 0–4 growth chart replaced the UK 1990 chart for clinical growth monitoring in this age group. This development should reduce significantly the number of breast-fed infants referred erroneously to secondary care, as happened because earlier charts were biased by the inclusion of artificially fed infants.

Dietary supplements in infancy

Vitamin K

All babies should receive vitamin K at birth, in order to prevent haemorrhagic disease of the newborn (HDN), a rare but potentially fatal bleeding disorder. 'Classical' HDN occurs in approximately 1/10 000 unsupplemented infants during the first week of life. It usually presents as apparently minor bleeding from, for example, the umbilicus, scalp, or gut. If unheeded, such 'warnings' may be followed by major internal (e.g. intracranial) haemorrhage with significant morbidity and mortality. More rarely, HDN can present later on in the early months of life. Unfortunately, this 'late' form often presents only after severe bleeding has already occurred. Consequently it is associated with much higher risk of death or lifelong disability. Breast-fed babies are at greater risk than bottle-fed babies, because infant formula is supplemented with vitamin K. Babies who are preterm, delivered instrumentally, or have liver disease are also more commonly affected, as are those whose mothers are taking certain drugs, notably anticonvulsants.

Vitamin K can be given orally or intramuscularly. The intramuscular route is associated with the lowest risk of both early and late HDN (about one per million births) and is therefore the most commonly adopted, particularly for those in high-risk groups. If, however, parents choose oral dosing for their baby, it must be repeated at least at the end of the first week and then monthly while exclusively breast-feeding. A number of oral-dosing regimens are in use, though their relative safeties and efficacies have not been fully determined.

A micellar preparation of the fat-soluble form of vitamin K, phytomenadione (Konakion MM), is currently used for neonatal administration. Early reports of haemolytic jaundice associated with vitamin K were associated with the water-soluble analogue acetomenaphthone, which has not been used for many years.

Vitamin drops

Supplementary vitamins A, C, and D (in the form of 'children's vitamin drops') are advised for all children under 2 years of age in the UK. In the case of breast-fed babies, they should be started from about 6 months of age, but they may be deferred until 1 year of age in babies fed infant formula, because it is fortified. Vitamin D is probably the most important component of the drops, particularly among high-risk ethnic groups in whom clinical rickets is still seen. In a UK national study, some 20–30% of toddlers from Asian backgrounds had low (<25 nmol/l) plasma concentrations of 25-hydroxy vitamin D, about half of whom had levels typically associated with rickets. UK recommendations therefore suggest that vitamin drops are started much earlier in these groups, from about 1 month of age. It is also important to note that the vitamin D status of the infant during the early months of life is strongly influenced by the mother's status during pregnancy. Population data for the UK show that the prevalence of hypovitaminosis D is quite high in younger women of childbearing age, even those of white British ethnic background. Moreover, few pregnant women consume the vitamin D supplements advised during pregnancy. In such circumstances, it seems advisable

> ### Box 23.11 Dietary supplements
>
> - Infancy is a period of rapid tissue deposition: Reference Nutrient Intakes (RNIs) for certain vitamins at this age are high and may not be met by diet.
> - Vitamin supplements are therefore recommended as a safety net to catch vulnerable individuals in the population.
> - All newborn babies should be given vitamin K to prevent HDN.
> - Breast-fed babies should receive supplements of vitamins A, C, and D from 6 months or earlier until at least 2 years of age.
> - Formula-fed babies should receive them from about 1 year.
> - Vulnerable groups (e.g. dark-skinned) may benefit from commencing vitamin D from about 1 month onwards. A vitamin D supplement should also be started early if the mother did not consume a vitamin D supplement during her pregnancy.
> - Low-birth-weight infants are at greater risk of iron deficiency and should receive iron supplements with multivitamins for at least the first 6 months.

for the infant to receive a vitamin D supplement before the age of 6 months, particularly if breast-fed.

Special circumstances

Some groups of infants have special nutritional needs, including preterm and low-birth-weight infants (i.e. those born before 37 completed weeks of gestation or weighing <2.5 kg at birth). These reflect low nutrient stores, high growth potential, and the need to catch up on, for example, bone mineralisation. Such infants should receive a multivitamin supplement soon after birth, normally until at least 2 years of age.

Low-birth-weight infants are particularly vulnerable to iron deficiency in later infancy or early in the second year of life. This so-called late anaemia of prematurity arises because expansion of the blood volume with growth exhausts iron reserves present at birth. These are limited because most (about 75%) of the body iron is in the form of haemoglobin and preterm babies have both a slightly lower haemoglobin concentration and low blood volume (about 80 ml/kg of body weight). Iron supplements are usually prescribed for low-birth-weight infants from about 1 month of age and continued until complementary feeding is well established. Iron is not started earlier because it favours colonisation of the gut with coliform organisms.

Key points relating to dietary supplements are summarised in Box 23.11.

23.5 Preschool children

Children between 1 and 5 years of age remain at significant risk of under-nutrition. They are still growing rapidly but have not fully developed independent feeding skills: in the earlier years of this era, they remain totally dependent on an adult.

Common dietary problems of young children

By about a year of age, a child should be established on a pattern of three meals per day plus snacks and breast feeds. Even at this stage, breast milk (or formula/cow's milk) will be providing about a quarter of energy and about a third of protein requirements. In situations where food is short, sustained breast-feeding into the second year acts as an important nutritional safety net; indeed, cessation of breast-feeding associated with the arrival of another baby at this stage can be a factor that precipitates malnutrition. Globally, continued insufficiency of food into the second year of life is a prime cause of chronic energy deficiency, manifesting as 'stunting' or restricted linear growth. This failure to achieve growth potential as a consequence of chronic food shortage in early life remains the commonest manifestation of nutritional deficiency today (see Section 23.2).

In industrialised countries, nutritional problems of a different sort arise and commonly present to primary care services. Growth may falter ('failure to thrive') because of problems with the establishment of an appropriate eating pattern even where there is an abundance of food in the household. Parents may, for example, offer excessive amounts of milk or fruit juice, often because solids are refused. In these circumstances it is advisable to limit milk intake to <600 ml/day and continue to offer three meals. Uneaten food should merely be removed and no more offered until the next mealtime. The temptation to coax or force young children into eating should always be resisted as it is usually counter-productive and negatively reinforces eating behaviour.

Sometimes growth failure may occur even in the presence of normal meal patterns because the energy density of the diet is inadequate. Parents may be relatively affluent and deliberately offer foods which they perceive as 'healthy', for example high in fibre and low in fat. This has been labelled 'muesli malnutrition'.

Its occurrence emphasises that energy needs at this stage are still relatively high and that fat plays a role in providing a diet of sufficient energy density. The transition from the young infant's milk diet, in which 50% of energy is provided by fat, to an adult-appropriate target of <35% must occur gradually over the first 5 years. To facilitate this, full-fat milk should be used until the age of 2, when it may be replaced by semi-skimmed. Skimmed milk and low-fat spreads are unsuitable dietary items for under-5s.

Excessive consumption of fruit juice or squash is also common in toddlers. Recent evidence suggests that the 'squash syndrome' can be associated with growth failure (short, fat children) and that these drinks replace the intake of more nutritious food. This suggests that the overall dietary intake does not allow children to reach their genetic potential in height, but leads to a deposition of excess energy. Consumption of squash may even be so high as to cause diarrhoea and provoke suspicion of malabsorption. Frequent loose stools, often containing undigested vegetable material, are generally a very common problem in this age group, but almost always innocuous and associated with normal growth. This presentation is described as 'toddler diarrhoea'. It is probably related to an immature pattern of small-bowel motility and can sometimes be ameliorated by increasing dietary fat intake to enhance ileal braking.

Preschool children remain vulnerable to micronutrient deficiencies, notably of vitamin A, iron, vitamin D, and zinc. These are particularly common in resource-poor countries and are multifactorial in origin. Low birth weight (hence low stores) and chronic low intake are compounded by both increased urinary losses during recurrent acute infection and chronic gastrointestinal losses caused by parasite infestation (such as hookworm). Children in industrialised countries are not however immune to micronutrient deficiency. Iron deficiency, hypovitaminosis D, and even frank rickets are often seen, particularly amongst children from South Asian and Afro-Caribbean backgrounds.

Behavioural eating problems in young children

Eating problems are very common among toddlers, and cause much concern to parents. Some degree of faddism and food refusal can however be construed as a normal phase of toddler development, provided it does not persist or lead to overt signs of nutrient deficiency (such as growth faltering: see Section 23.7).

Sometimes more persistent eating problems are encountered. These include such things as severely selective eating (e.g. jam sandwiches, chocolate biscuits) and eating food of inappropriate texture (e.g. the child will take only liquids or pureed food and spits out lumps). Another prevalent problem in children who have required nutritional support as a result of illness early in life is difficulty withdrawing from tube feeding and establishing an eating pattern.

Problems such as these almost never have a basis in organic disease but develop out of a complex variety of aetiological factors, including:

- Early aversive experience of eating, such as vomiting or choking on particular foods, force-feeding during weaning, or using inappropriate complementary foods.
- Abnormal developmental experiences.
- Conflict with parents.

These may be reinforced by neglect, abuse, parental disagreement, and lack of support. The primary management of such problems is behavioural. A multidisciplinary-team approach is most successful, coordinating the skills of psychologist, dietitian, health visitor, and, if necessary, a speech and language therapist to assist with the assessment of swallowing. The nutritional aim is ultimately to provide normal food in sufficient quantities, not to resort to supplements or other nutritional interventions as a means of increasing intake. Indeed, to do so might actually be counter-productive and 'medicalise' the problem. Solving it can take time and persistence.

Box 23.12 Preschool children

- Preschool children are still growing relatively quickly and have high nutrient requirements.
- Successful transition to a varied diet and the establishment of eating patterns can be demanding on parenting skills.
- Behavioural eating problems are common in this age group and require multidisciplinary management. Coaxing or force-feeding must always be avoided.
- Globally, children are at high risk of chronic energy deficiency (causing stunting) and several specific micronutrient deficiencies.

Thus it may be necessary to accept suboptimal intake in the short term in the interests of long-term gain associated with establishing normal dietary patterns.

Key nutritional points concerning preschool children are summarised in Box 23.12.

23.6 Schoolchildren and adolescents

Children of this age can eat independently of a carer, and by completion of adolescence are capable of providing for themselves – indeed, capable of reproducing and caring for their offspring. The emergence of independence is associated with nutritional problems of a different sort: children are learning to make choices of their own and this has many implications. They are a population susceptible to marketing and peer-group influences, which will impact on patterns of both diet and activity. For the health educator, nutritional education at this age has the potential, at least, to influence habits for life. Many of the overt problems which present to health services during this era of development represent behavioural extremes, for example childhood overweight, obesity, and adolescent eating disorders.

National data collected in the UK show that in addition to these conditions, the diet and activity patterns of schoolchildren and adolescents are cause for concern. Low consumption of vegetables and fruit and increasing reliance on snacks, soft drinks, and fast food eaten outside the home are associated with low intakes of many micronutrients. Reduced activity levels, particularly amongst adolescent girls, can be expected to impact unfavourably in several areas: they may partially explain the increasing prevalence of overweight and obesity, and can be expected to affect adversely the attainment of peak bone mass (see Chapter 19).

Eating disorders

Although a number of disordered-eating presentations have been described in this age group, anorexia nervosa and bulimia nervosa are the most frequently encountered, the former being commonest (see Chapter 7). These syndromes share many features, particularly over-concern with body weight and shape, but are distinguished by the pattern of intake. In bulimia, food is consumed (often in large quantities – 'bingeing') and then eliminated through vomiting or purgation, whereas food refusal and pre-occupation with exercise predominate in anorexia. Children from higher socioeconomic groups are more frequently affected: often they are high achievers with perfectionist or frankly obsessive traits but lack self-esteem. Their overwhelming ambition is to be thin. Family psychodynamics are often complex and the presentation is believed to indicate the child's attempt for autonomy and self-control in some area of life. It is also argued that the illness represents an attempt to regress from puberty, but this has been questioned on the grounds that it may present before indications of puberty appear.

The prevalence of eating disorders amongst adolescents and young adults appears to be increasing in Western countries, where they appear to be more common than in the developing world. Psychosocial and media pressures stigmatising obesity and associating thinness with success may have contributed to this trend.

The classical form of anorexia described in young adults differs in an important respect from that encountered in children. When anorexia nervosa presents during (or sometimes before) puberty, it will significantly delay progression of endocrine development and the pubertal growth spurt (see Section 23.2). In most cases, recovery is accompanied by resumption of progress through puberty, with full attainment of final height, breast development, and commencement of menstruation. However, in some severe, chronic cases, puberty is arrested, with prolonged delay in appearance of menses and ultimately a deficit in final height. It is also worth remembering that although classical (post-menarchal) anorexia affects almost exclusively girls, boys are occasionally affected both before and during puberty.

The presentation of anorexia in young girls may be quite insidious. Preoccupation with exercise, calorie counting, and static weight (or loss of small amounts) may at first be viewed as normal. Overt refusal of food becomes apparent only later, often after the child has resorted to other strategies, such as hiding food, exercising in secret, or abusing laxatives. Detection at an early stage may be compatible with management in the community, but later admission to hospital may become necessary. Criteria for inpatient management include:

- weight <80% of expected weight for height;
- dehydration, electrolyte abnormalities, and cardiovascular decompensation;
- persistent vomiting (sometimes haematemesis);
- evidence of complicating psychiatric features (usually depression);
- failure of outpatient management.

The management of children with anorexia nervosa is difficult and the disease has a significant mortality over the long term, variously estimated at between 2 and 10%. It is essential that a multidisciplinary approach is followed, coordinated by the psychiatric team with input from a paediatric dietitian and a paediatrician. The general principles of nutritional management are as follows:

- Parents are made responsible for the child's eating as the key to resuming health. Initially this can cause resentment and objection on the part of the child, but it can sometimes be traded against freedom to choose in other aspects of lifestyle.
- A target weight range needs to be agreed with the child and parents (usually in the range 90–100% of expected weight for height).
- Once electrolyte deficiencies and hydration state have been corrected, refeeding is instituted (see Section 23.7). Competing needs to replete tissue versus the child's sensitivities to eating large amounts of food will need to be balanced. Attempting immediate hyperalimentation will be counterproductive and carries the risk of inducing 'refeeding syndrome'. It is safer to increase amounts of normal food more gradually. Although children can participate if they wish by discussing the daily menu, it is important not to hand over control at this early stage. A multivitamin supplement is usually given, although clinical micronutrient deficiency is not so common as might perhaps be expected given the degree of weight loss present.
- Sometimes (in the face of severe weight loss, dehydration, or persistent refusal to eat) it may prove necessary to embark on enteral nutritional support or parenteral therapy. If so, it can be made clear that the amount of support will be reduced as more oral diet is accepted.

Clearly these steps must be instituted hand in hand with psychotherapeutic measures addressing the child's underlying problems, relationships with family and friends, and continuing education (bearing in mind that absence from school may be prolonged).

Key nutritional points concerning schoolchildren and adolescents are summarised in Box 23.13.

23.7 Under-nutrition in children

Causes of under-nutrition

Childhood under-nutrition has many origins: psychological disturbance, socioeconomic deprivation, and underlying illness. All may act in concert and the treatment of under-nutrition therefore involves more than the mere provision of nutrients. For example, interventions may be needed at the societal level to increase food supply, at the family level to improve parenting skills, and with the child to treat associated problems such as infection.

Nutritional assessment

A child's nutritional status is assessed by taking a history, performing a physical examination (including anthropometry), and, sometimes, performing special investigations (see also Chapter 2).

Key points on nutritional assessment in children are listed in Box 23.14.

History

The history should be taken from the parent, carer, or a close relative, and must be thorough because nutritional status at the time of consultation reflects what has happened since conception. For example, a

school-age child may be small because of severe foetal growth retardation, critical illness, or malnutrition in early life from which catch-up has been incomplete, leading to stunting.

Questions asked may include:

- *Pregnancy and birth.* Was the pregnancy uncomplicated or was foetal growth slow? What was the gestation at birth and the birth weight? Were there neonatal illnesses (which might have led to early postnatal growth failure)?
- *Infant feeding.* Was the child breast- or formula-fed? When was the child first given foods other than milk and what were they (specifically, when were gluten-containing foods started)? Did the child thrive in infancy? If not, when were there first concerns? Was there vomiting or diarrhoea in infancy? Were dietary supplements (such as iron or vitamins) given?
- *Developmental history.* Inquiry should be made into 'milestones' to ensure that developmental delay or motor disability have not caused feeding difficulty.
- *Current dietary history.* Recent intake of food and fluids. If breast-feeding: has there been any change in feeding pattern, and has the mother experienced any problems such as pain or mastitis? If formula feeding: what is being given, how exactly is the mother making up the feeds, and how much is consumed? For older children, enquiries should be made about change of appetite, meal patterns, behaviour disturbance, and food refusal. Is the child considered to be intolerant of particular foods, and why?
- *Family history.* How tall and heavy are the parents and siblings? Is there any family history of food intolerance or gastrointestinal problems?
- *Social history.* Who is/are the child's primary carer(s) throughout the day? What are the family's dietary habits?

- *Illness*. Ask particularly about diarrhoea and vomiting, features of malabsorption, chronic disease, and recurrent and recent acute infections.

Clinical examination

- Weight and height should be measured, recorded, and plotted on a growth chart. Head (occipitofrontal) circumference is also measured routinely in infancy, and other measurements such as mid-arm circumference, triceps, and subscapular skinfolds may be made as appropriate. Previous measurements are usually easily obtainable from sources such as the parent-held child health record (a multidisciplinary record of the child's medical care which parents in the UK are encouraged to bring to all consultations).
- Note the child's affect: malnourished children are withdrawn and miserable; 'frozen watchfulness' may signify neglect.
- Assess the child's development. Infants and toddlers who show developmental delay may fail to thrive because of difficulty communicating their needs or due to problems with handling, chewing, and swallowing food. Delay in development may also be the consequence of severe malnutrition.
- Look for signs of micronutrient deficiency, such as pallor (iron deficiency), dermatoses, cheilosis (B vitamin deficiencies), xerophthalmia (vitamin A deficiency), acrodermatitis (zinc deficiency), and goiter (iodine deficiency).
- In older children, note the pubertal stage attained: chronically undernourished children or those with growth failure attributable to chronic disease often undergo late puberty and allowance may be needed for this, particularly where cross-sectional growth references are being applied.
- Conduct a full systemic examination, looking especially for signs such as muscle wasting, abdominal distension, and heart murmurs (sometimes due to high cardiac output in anaemia).

Anthropometric measurements can provide two kinds of information: body proportions (body mass index (BMI) or weight for height) and body function (adequacy of growth – if a series of measurements is available). BMI can either be read from a chart or looked up using the weight and height centiles (Figure 23.14).

Special investigations

In circumstances where special investigations are feasible, those chosen will clearly depend on the findings of history and examination. The possibilities are numerous but they can help in assessment of status by providing information in complementary ways (see Chapter 2). Examples include:

- Assessment of nutrient balance (e.g. microscopy of stool for fat globules in infants failing to thrive).
- Assessment of body composition (e.g. haemoglobin and serum ferritin as measures of iron stores).
- Assessment of metabolic and physiological function (e.g. plasma alkaline phosphatase as an indicator of bone turnover, X-ray of wrist to assess bone age).

Screening for malnutrition

Opportunistic weighing of babies and young children is common in primary care, for example when immunisations are given during the first 6 months, but they should not be weighed too frequently if healthy as normal fluctuations in weight gain may cause unjustifiable concern. Currently in the UK it is recommended that babies are weighed in the first 2 weeks, in order to help with the assessment of feeding, but that thereafter, unless there are concerns, they be weighed no more frequently than monthly in the first 6 months, no more than 2-monthly in the second 6 months, and then no more than 3-monthly after the age of 1 year.

Foe reasons previously stated, the interpretation of weight measurements at this age can be difficult: catch-up and catch-down growth associated with 'regression to the mean' during the first year (see Section 23.2) mean that a proportion of normal babies cross weight-centile lines on the growth chart. In the case of the new UK-WHO growth chart, up to 3% of infants cross two centile spaces down. This is many fewer than was the case when the older UK 1990 growth reference was used. It follows that, where serial measurements are available, any baby who has crossed two centile spaces, particularly in less than a year, needs close assessment (see next subsection).

A good deal of thought has been given to the problem of correcting mathematically for the phenomenon of regression to the mean and thereby separating

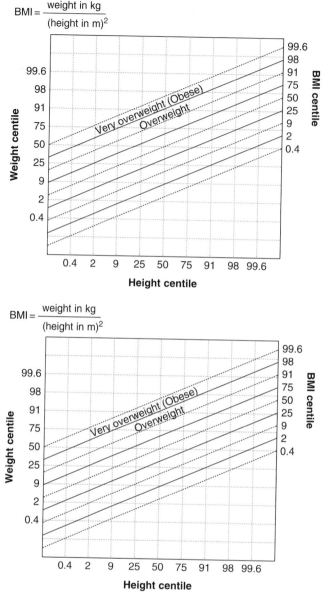

Figure 23.14 Body mass index (BMI) look-up. As an alternative to using a chart BMI can be looked up using the weight and height centile. This is accurate to within one-quarter of a centile space (see Cole 2002). Adapted by permission from Macmillan Publishers Ltd: Eur J Clin Nutr (Cole TJ. A chart to link centiles of body mass index, weight and height. Eur J Clin Nutr 56 (12); 1194–1199). Copyright (2002).

more objectively babies who are merely 'catching down' from those who are failing to thrive. Simple methods of expressing such 'conditional weight gain' include calculation of the 'thrive index' and the use of 'thrive lines' which show the 5th and 95th centiles of conditional weight-gain velocity (available from http://www.healthforallchildren.com/index.php/ shop/product/Growth+Charts/LQRmOlu5i0Iw WiOP/1 as a transparent overlay for the UK-WHO growth chart). Where only single measurements are available, any child who measures less than the 0.4th centile for weight or length on the chart requires early medical assessment: only 4 in 1000 normal children can be expected to be so small, so the chance

Box 23.15 Weight faltering in young children

- Only 2–3% of healthy infants show downward crossing of two or more centile spaces on the new UK-WHO growth chart. This is a much smaller proportion than the 5% observed using the previous UK 1990 growth reference.
- Weight faltering needs to be distinguished from other causes of centile crossing, such as catch-down growth. As a group, infants who are light at birth are much less likely to show downward centile crossing than those who are heavy at birth.
- Weight faltering may reflect underlying illness but is most commonly due to low intake of nutrients, particularly energy.
- Low intake can arise through physical illness but is most commonly a reflection of parenting difficulty.
- Sometimes weight faltering is a consequence of neglect or abuse.
- The management of weight faltering requires a coordinated multidisciplinary approach to increasing the intake of normal food. Prescription of dietary supplements alone is not the solution but may be considered as part of the management plan after assessment by a paediatric dietitian.

that an abnormality is present is quite high. A baby weighing less than the 9th centile should be weighed again after an interval of at least 2 weeks, and repeatedly until it is established that the growth trajectory is satisfactory.

Weight faltering ('failure to thrive')

Slow weight gain in the infant and young child is not in itself a diagnosis, but implies that growth (usually in weight) is faltering pathologically and does not merely reflect simple inter-individual variations.

Key points on weight faltering are listed in Box 23.15.

Weight faltering may result from many causes, simply classified as:

- inadequate intake (e.g. a breast-feeding problem, inadequate parenting, frank neglect, or abuse);
- excessive losses (e.g. vomiting and regurgitation, diarrhoea and malabsorption, high REE in acute infection, or chronic disease);
- abnormal nutrient partitioning.

Note that these factors usually operate in combination, rather than independently. For example, children with infection will become anorexic, may vomit, and often show increased urinary losses of trace minerals and vitamins. REE may be increased in the presence of fever and tachycardia, with the nutrient demands of the immune system increased. Following infec-

tion, there will be increased nutrient (particularly energy) requirements to meet the demands of catch-up growth (see Section 23.8).

It is important to recognise that growth faltering in an industrialised country is usually 'non-organic' in origin (see Figure 23.15). Low food (particularly energy) intake may result from some combination of the following:

- developmental abnormality;
- oral-motor dysfunction;
- abnormal mealtime interactions with a carer;
- feeding insufficient amounts, as the result of either parental perceptions or poor appetite in the child;
- sometimes frank neglect or physical or emotional abuse.

The management of these problems demands a multidisciplinary approach, directed at identifying and rectifying the eating problem – rather than resorting to special formulas or food. The first step is direct observation at mealtimes, preferably in the child's home environment. Video-recording can assist later review or facilitate sharing of information with other professionals. Problems can then be addressed in a coordinated fashion by appropriate disciplines. For example, a dietitian may be able to make simple recommendations about food choices to increase the nutrient density of meals. A physiotherapist or occupational therapist might advise on improving the child's positioning at mealtimes, and a speech and language therapist may be able to identify disordered oral-motor function. These aspects are particularly suitable if there is coexisting developmental delay or neuromuscular disability.

In summary, weight faltering amongst young children in industrialised countries is most commonly the result of chronic energy deficiency arising from inappropriate care practices, rather than underlying physical disease or food shortage. The treatment is predominantly behavioural and directed at rectifying the deficit in intake of normal food. Mere prescription of food supplements or nutrient-enriched formulas is neither an appropriate nor a sustainable solution in the majority of instances. Such measures should be reserved for the infant with disturbed energy balance as the result of underlying chronic illness (for example of the cardiac or respiratory system) requiring nutritional support.

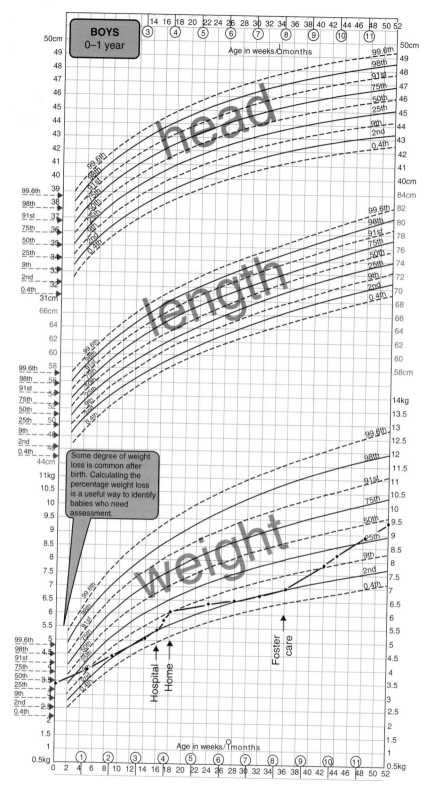

Figure 23.15 Weight faltering. The baby's weight has crossed three centile spaces downwards in the early months of life. Admission to hospital is associated with rapid weight gain followed by a further period of faltering. Rapid catch-up then occurs in foster care. This pattern of growth is typical of parental neglect. Chart developed by RCPCH/WHO/Department of Health, copyright © 2009 Department of Health.

Severe malnutrition

Severe under-nutrition in children is life-threatening. Injudicious treatment is itself dangerous and can increase mortality further. Most severe primary under-nutrition occurs in resource-poor countries, though it can occur in industrialised countries too; for example, as the result of anorexia in teenagers. It may also develop as the result of severe underlying disease. Whatever the cause, and wherever severe under-nutrition occurs, some common principles apply to its assessment and treatment. In particular, it is important that the metabolic perturbations which are associated with chronic energy deficiency are corrected at an appropriately gradual pace to prevent refeeding syndrome (see Chapter 9).

Diagnosis

Classically, two patterns of malnutrition were recognised in young children. These were known as kwashiorkor (oedematous malnutrition, most commonly in the young child) and marasmus (severe wasting, usually in infancy). Recently a more unifying treatment approach has been adopted, though weight measurements must always be interpreted carefully for two important reasons:

- Presence of oedema ('pitting' elicited by applying digital pressure over feet and ankles) will cause the child's true body weight to be overestimated.
- Absence of oedema may mean the child's low weight is due to chronic energy insufficiency (or 'stunting') rather than recent weight loss (or 'wasting'). Thus weight must be interpreted along with a measurement of length (or height if over 2 years of age).

Assessment of wasting and stunting

A 'stunted' child is below his or her appropriate height for age, whereas a 'wasted' child is under the appropriate weight for height. Severity of stunting can be calculated from the child's height as a percentage of the median (50th percentile) height for one of that age. Similarly, the degree of wasting can be expressed by calculating the child's weight as a percentage of the weight which would be appropriate for a child of that height and age. The latter can be estimated by first plotting the child's height against age on a growth chart to establish the percentile line on which it falls; the weight associated with the corresponding percentile for age is then read off the weight chart. An alternative method, less prone to errors of reading and interpolation, is simply to read the percentage weight for height from tables or a chart (Figure 23.16). This method also has the advantage that knowledge of the child's age is not required. Weight for height < 70% equates with a standard deviation score of −3 SDS and is classified as severe wasting. Likewise, a height for age < 85% represents a score of −3 SDS, viewed as severe stunting. Weight for height of 70–79% (−2 to −3 SDS) and height for age of 85–89% (−2 to −3 SDS) represent moderate malnutrition. In children over the age of 2 years, BMI is preferred to weight for height.

Treatment

A child who presents with clinical features of malnutrition has survived low food intake for a very variable period. As a result, adaptive changes in metabolism and body composition will have occurred. For example, the intracellular compartment will be more depleted than the extracellular, resulting particularly in depletion of intracellular cations such as potassium and magnesium. The extracellular compartment may even be expanded to the extent that oedema is present. This might coexist with a contracted blood volume, causing secretion of antidiuretic hormone (ADH), leading to water retention and hyponatraemia despite a normal or increased total body sodium content. It is worth noting that these changes are the converse of those observed in the child with acute diarrhoea. As a result, one of the greatest dangers in treating malnourished children is refeeding too quickly. Administering excessive amounts of fluid and/or high-energy feeds will shift fluid between the intra- and extracellular fluid compartments, which can fatally derange plasma electrolyte concentrations. Management is therefore considered to have three phases:

- resuscitation;
- stabilisation and tissue repair (the first few days);
- tissue repletion and rehabilitation (subsequent weeks to months).

Resuscitation, stabilisation, and repair

The key priorities are:

- To diagnose and treat underlying infection, for example respiratory infection, gastrointestinal infection, malaria, measles, or human immunodeficiency virus (HIV)-related illness. (Note, however,

Weight-for-length BOYS

Birth to 2 years (percentiles)

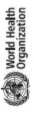
World Health
Organization

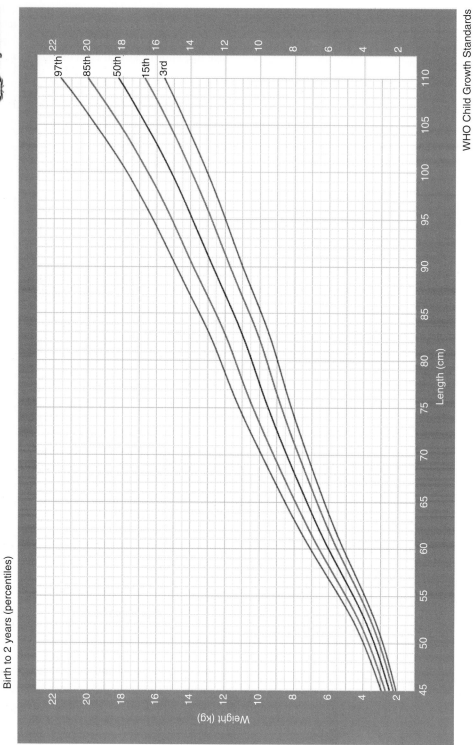

Figure 23.16 The WHO weight-for-height chart. http://www.who.int/childgrowth/standards/cht_wfl_boys_p_0_2.pdf, accessed 24 February 2012, © World Health Organization.

that physical signs such as fever may be absent in severe malnutrition. 'Blind' broad-spectrum antibiotics are therefore usually given initially to all severely malnourished children.)

- To reverse hypoglycaemia and hypothermia (often signs of infection).
- To begin the correction of fluid and electrolyte imbalance.
- To start correction of micronutrient deficiencies (which are universally present in severe protein–energy malnutrition) by administration of a multivitamin preparation with folic acid, zinc, and copper.

Small, frequent (e.g. hourly or 2-hourly) oral or nasogastric feeds are given. These are restricted to about 100 ml/kg/day if the child is oedematous; otherwise up to 130 ml/kg/day of specially formulated milk- or cereal-based feed, low in osmolality and lactose content (e.g. 'F75 starter formula'), is given. This provides about 100 kcal/kg/day of energy and 1–1.5 g/kg/day of protein, which can be supplemented by breast feeds.

Children who are both dehydrated (e.g. as the result of diarrhoea) and malnourished should be treated differently. They can be fed a solution called 'ReSoMal', which contains less sodium and more potassium and magnesium than standard oral rehydration solution (ORS). It is given orally in small amounts frequently. Intravenous therapy is reserved for shocked children; that is, those who are hypotensive with evidence of impaired peripheral circulation. These aspects are discussed further in the next section.

Repletion and rehabilitation

After about a week, the child's appetite begins to return. The aim of treatment now is to replete stores and promote catch-up growth. Energy intake is gradually increased to achieve growth rates exceeding about 10 g/kg/day. This can be achieved by using high-energy formula (about 100 kcal/100 ml) and gradually increasing the amount offered. Breast feeds should be offered after the high-energy formula to ensure that high-energy intake is maintained. Iron can now be given with the micronutrient supplement (it is usually deferred initially because of its possible effect on Gram-negative infection; see Section 23.4).

Box 23.16 Severe malnutrition

- Careful note should be taken of body proportions, to establish whether a child's low weight is attributable to wasting or stunting.
- Management comprises the resuscitation, repair, and repletion stages.

During the resuscitation and repair phase:

- Fluid and electrolyte balance need careful assessment – they influence the choice of initial feed.
- They must be closely monitored throughout treatment.
- Underlying infection and micronutrient deficiencies must be treated quickly.
- Hypoglycaemia and hypothermia must be addressed quickly.

During the repletion stage:

- Sufficient food is needed to promote catch-up growth.
- Play and stimulation are important.
- Carers will need re-education about feeding, and about other aspects of their child's healthcare.

Rehabilitating the child involves much more than feeding. Play and environmental stimulation have been shown to accelerate catch-up growth and to be associated with improved longer-term cognitive outcomes. Parents may need re-education about feeding and teaching about food preparation for their child. Sometimes abnormal behaviour such as 'frozen watchfulness', rumination, or head-banging, possibly signifying frank neglect, needs more careful assessment. This is also an opportunity to bring the child's immunisation status up to date and to diagnose and treat any chronic underlying problems, such as anaemia, parasitic infestation, or tuberculosis.

Key points on severe malnutrition (see Chapter 5) are summarised in Box 23.16.

Micronutrient deficiencies

Deficiencies of trace minerals (particularly iron and zinc) and vitamins (particularly vitamins A and D) are very common in young children. They occur in both industrialised and resource-poor countries. Many others are seen in specific circumstances. These include iodine deficiency, selenium deficiency, scurvy, and B-vitamin deficiency.

The underlying causes of micronutrient deficiency reflect the general vulnerabilities of children. These are:

- low body stores (e.g. as a result of low birth weight);
- low intake as a result of improper feeding practices;
- increased losses (e.g. during acute intercurrent infection).

Some deficiencies (especially selenium and iodine) occur endemically in particular geographical areas where the mineral is lacking in the earth's crust. The effects of these are particularly important in infants and young children because they impair thyroid function, which will impact adversely on development of the brain during its critical growth period, causing cretinism.

Iron deficiency

Dietary iron deficiency is the commonest cause of a microcytic, hypochromic anaemia in young children. Important differential diagnoses to consider at this age are haemoglobinopathies (usually beta-thalassaemia) and causes of malabsorption (particularly coeliac disease). Blood loss is unusual at this age in industrialised countries, though occult losses associated with hookworm and parasitic infestations are very important globally.

Concern about the effects of iron deficiency in young children relates not so much to the physiological effects of anaemia as to the possible consequences for cognitive function and development. Iron deficiency is associated with a delay in the acquisition of cognitive skills, which appears to be reversible on treatment. This concern, though still controversial, has been the principal justification for programmes aimed at the prevention, detection, and treatment of deficiency.

It has been claimed that between 10 and 20% of inner-city toddlers in the UK are iron-deficient, though one of the problems associated with determining the exact prevalence is the assessment of iron status. Although the WHO defines iron deficiency as a haemoglobin concentration $< 11\,g/dl$, many 'iron-deficient' toddlers may have a haemoglobin concentration only just below this diagnostic threshold. Consequently, if children are tested repeatedly, substantial numbers of individuals move between iron-sufficient and iron-deficient categories. These natural fluctuations in haemoglobin concentration present considerable barriers to the introduction of effective screening programmes.

Other parameters of iron status are susceptible to similar criticisms; for example, serum ferritin concentration rises in the presence of acute infection.

Factors associated with iron deficiency are: low birth weight, early introduction of whole cow's milk, vegetarian weaning, use of tea as a drink, South Asian ethnic background, and low socioeconomic status. Medicinal supplements are a useful preventive strategy for some high-risk groups (e.g. low-birth-weight infants), though concern has been expressed about the possible detrimental effects of supplements on weight gain among children who are iron-replete. It has been suggested that this may reflect reduced availability of zinc, which competes with iron and copper for absorption.

Some large controlled studies conducted amongst non-breast-fed infants have shown that continuing the use of iron-fortified infant formulas rather than cow's milk for the first 12–18 months of life is associated with reduced incidence of anaemia and, probably, some developmental advantage. Other simple measures include the use of a vitamin C source (such as fruit juice or vitamin drops), avoidance of tea, and introduction of red meat into the weaning diet. Unfortunately, at least in the UK, controlled studies have shown little benefit associated with the provision of parental education programmes designed to prevent the condition.

Vitamin D deficiency

Vitamin D deficiency is common in parts of North Africa, the Middle East, and Pakistan. It is also prevalent in ethnic-minority communities living at northerly latitudes, including the UK. In the UK, an RNI for vitamin D intake is set for infants, young children, and pregnant and lactating women. This cannot be achieved by diet, making the consumption of supplements important amongst these groups. Children from Afro-Caribbean and South Asian backgrounds are most commonly affected in the UK. Important aetiological factors are season (winter and spring), prolonged (>6 months) exclusive breast-feeding, and cultural factors (e.g. purdah and concealing clothing).

Clinical presentations of vitamin D deficiency in childhood include hypocalcaemic tetany in young infants and nutritional rickets. The latter is usually detected radiologically when the child presents with, for example, coexisting iron-deficiency anaemia and growth faltering. Frank clinical signs are now rarely seen in the UK but may include swelling of epiphyses, beading of the ribs (the 'rickety rosary'), bossing of the frontal bones, and softening of the cranium ('craniotabes'). Closure of the fontanelles and appearance of teeth may be delayed. Hypotonia may also hold back gross motor development (see Section 23.3).

Severe rickets in early life may also affect adult health: for example, linear growth and bone mineralisation may be suboptimal, and bony deformity of the lower skeleton may result. In the latter context, pelvic deformity in girls may cause later problems in childbirth.

An X-ray of the wrist is the quickest and most helpful diagnostic test (Figure 23.17). The radiological signs include a general reduction in bone density, loss of metaphyseal density with 'cupping', and a frayed appearance to the edges of the bone. These reflect increased bone turnover at the growth plate, resulting from secondary hyperparathyroidism. These

changes are not, however, diagnostic of vitamin D deficiency and can sometimes be caused by rarer inherited diseases (e.g. familial hypophosphataemic rickets, in which there is excessive tubular loss of phosphate, or vitamin D-resistant rickets, in which there is either inability to synthesise 1,25-dihydroxy vitamin D or insensitivity of the receptor) or chronic renal failure. Rickets may also be due (particularly in parts of Africa) to very low calcium intake rather than vitamin D deficiency. For this reason, it is important to confirm vitamin D status by measuring the serum concentration of 25-hydroxy vitamin D. In the UK, a level below 25 nmol/l is considered to be indicative of vitamin D deficiency, and a level in the range 25–50 nmol/l is considered 'insufficient'.

To treat vitamin D deficiency, a large dose of vitamin D (about 1000–5000 IU/day, depending on the child's age) is usually given for the first 4–6 weeks, with the aim of repleting stores. During treatment plasma calcium and phosphorus concentrations must be monitored to ensure toxicity is avoided. Gradually the plasma alkaline phosphatase concentration will return to the normal range. Thereafter, 400–1000 IU (10–25 µg) should be given as a daily supplement to continue healing and prevent recurrence. Similar daily amounts are advised for children whose 25-hydroxy vitamin D levels are in the 'insufficient' range.

Vitamin A deficiency

Vitamin A deficiency remains an important and cheaply preventable cause of early blindness globally. It is endemic in many parts of the world, particularly Africa, South East Asia, and South Asia, and is considered a public-health problem when the prevalence of night blindness exceeds 1% or when >0.05% of individuals show corneal scarring. Randomised trials in such areas have demonstrated that significant reduction in childhood mortality and infectious morbidity can be achieved by supplementation.

Factors causing vitamin A deficiency include:

- low intake of fat and fat-soluble vitamins;
- curtailment of breast-feeding;
- poverty;
- increased losses in, for example, acute infections – particularly measles and diarrhoea.

Deficiency can be documented by measuring serum retinol concentration (<0.35 µmol/l) or by detection

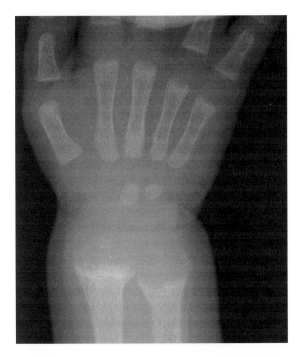

Figure 23.17 Rickets. This is the wrist X-ray of a 9-month-old baby of Asian ethnic origin. The baby was still exclusively breast-fed. Neither the mother nor the baby had consumed vitamin D supplements. Characteristic 'cupping' of the radial metaphysis can be seen, together with a 'frayed' appearance of the bone edges. These changes are the consequence of bone reabsorption caused by secondary hyperparathyroidism.

of changes in corneal-impression cytology. However, these tests are rarely practicable for clinical purposes in countries where deficiency is endemic. In such circumstances, oral vitamin A therapy should be given to all children presenting with diarrhoeal diseases, malnutrition, measles, and acute respiratory infections. If deficiency is identified in a child, it is advisable to treat any siblings and the mother as well (particularly if breast-feeding). Dietary education should also be given: foods rich in vitamin A include red palm oil, carrots, oily fish and liver, and green leaves.

Zinc deficiency

Foods high in protein, such as meat and fish, are rich sources of dietary zinc. Human milk contains zinc in a highly bioavailable form, though the zinc content of human milk falls several-fold over the first 6 months of lactation. Iron and copper compete with zinc for gastrointestinal absorption: one reason multinutrient supplements may be preferred to the use of single nutrients in populations at risk of micronutrient deficiency. Globally, diarrhoeal disease is an important precipitant of zinc deficiency. There is also a rare disorder of gastrointestinal zinc absorption known as acrodermatitis enteropathica, in which infants show faltering of growth and develop the classical skin rash of zinc deficiency.

Clinical zinc deficiency is particularly characterised by slowing in the accumulation of lean tissue. Oedema is often present, and the plasma concentration of alkaline phosphatase (a zinc metalloenzyme) falls. Eventually the characteristic rash appears as a severe desquamative eruption affecting the hands, feet, peri-oral and peri-anal areas. In view of its peripheral distribution (probably reflecting the areas of highest cell turnover), this is described as an acrodermatitis. Initiation of zinc repletion (as oral zinc sulphate) leads to rapid healing, within a week.

Zinc deficiency is extremely common in resource-poor countries and is associated with both stunting and impaired immunity. Supplementation in such circumstances has been associated with improved growth and reduced infectious morbidity, particularly from pneumonia and diarrhoea. Zinc deficiency is occasionally seen also in industrialised countries, usually among sick children. Children on parenteral nutrition may be at risk, because some commercial trace mineral solutions are relatively low in zinc concentration. Those with severe, prolonged diarrhoea are also vulnerable. Late (after about 3–4 months of age) zinc deficiency occasionally occurs in human milk-fed extremely low-birth-weight (<1000 g) preterm infants: this reflects the combined effects of low stores at birth, rapid somatic growth, and extended duration of lactation with associated fall in zinc supply.

Iodine deficiency

Iodine deficiency is important in children because globally it is a major cause of disability through impairment of thyroxine synthesis. It is endemic in some parts of the world, particularly remote mountainous areas. Deficiency encompasses a spectrum of problems, from mild cognitive impairment to cretinism, in which bone age is delayed, growth is impaired, and neurological deficit can sometimes be severe (incorporating deafness, cerebral palsy, and severe learning difficulty). Treatment after clinical presentation is associated with universally poor prognosis: even early recognition will be associated with some deficit. In view of this, much effort has been directed at population-scale prevention in affected communities. Strategies employed include food fortification (table salt is globally the commonest vehicle employed) and medicinal supplementation of pregnant women (using a single oral dose). The latter is important both because much brain development occurs before birth and because goiter (thyroid swelling) in an affected foetus may give rise to problems in labour if neck extension causes face presentation. In the UK, table salt is not fortified and milk is an important source of iodine. Recently, concerns have been expressed about the iodine status of adolescent girls and young women. This may have implications for pregnancy.

Other vitamin deficiencies

A number of B-vitamin deficiencies may occur in areas where severe malnutrition is common. These include:

- thiamine deficiency, resulting in beri beri (cardiac failure, peripheral neuropathy, and encephalopathy);
- nicotinic acid deficiency, resulting in pellagra (diarrhoea and photo-dermatosis);
- riboflavin deficiency, associated with cheilosis and anaemia.

The common coexistence of these deficiencies with severe malnutrition re-emphasises the importance of early micronutrient supplementation in treatment.

Vitamin B_{12} deficiency is much less common in children than in, for example, the elderly, but can occur rarely in breast-fed infants of vegan mothers and some vegan children. It is also sometimes seen in children who have undergone resection of the terminal ileum, usually as a consequence of necrotising enterocolitis in the neonatal period. In such circumstances, deficiency may take many years to present clinically – perhaps until puberty. This reflects the adequacy of stores in the face of low turnover rates, until stressed by the additional metabolic demands of the pubertal growth spurt.

Folic acid deficiency results in megaloblastic anaemia. It is uncommon as an isolated dietary deficiency in children and usually signifies the presence of malabsorption: commonly coeliac disease.

Vitamin C deficiency, which causes scurvy, is now rare in children in the absence of severe malnutrition. Historically it is of interest because it became endemic in the latter part of the nineteenth century, when artificial feeds were introduced. Subsequently this was found to be due to inactivation of vitamin C by heat treatment. The scorbutic child typically presents with bruising, bleeding, and bone tenderness – sometimes sufficiently marked as to cause a pseudoparesis. X-rays show severe subperiosteal haemorrhage with calcification and loss of trabecular bone mineral. The subperiosteal swellings may cause obvious swelling of the limbs and anterior ends of the ribs.

Vitamin K deficiency has been covered in Section 23.4.

Finally, vitamin E deficiency may occur in children with inherited disorders which cause severe fat malabsorption – such as abetalipoproteinaemia and cystic fibrosis. It eventually manifests as a demyelinating disorder of the spinocerebellar tracts, by which stage changes are not reversible. This observation emphasises the importance of vitamin E supplementation in such children. Rarely, it may also cause haemolytic anaemia in preterm infants.

Other trace-mineral deficiencies

Copper deficiency is rare but has been described in babies of extremely low birth weight. It causes anaemia and severe osteopaenia, sometimes giving rise to fractures.

Selenium deficiency is also rare but has been observed in a few children on long-term parenteral nutrition. As it is associated with the development of a cardiomyopathy (cf. 'Keshan disease'), it should be considered in any such child developing signs of heart failure.

23.8 Nutrition as treatment

Nutritional support for the sick child

Technical advances in the provision of techniques of nutritional support have greatly increased the prospects of survival for sick children. Some of the most striking advances have been in the field of neonatal medicine: indeed, it is of interest to note that the earliest applications of parenteral nutrition in human patients were amongst newborn infants undergoing bowel surgery.

General principles

There is one important conceptual difference between paediatric and adult medical practice in the aims of providing nutritional support. While in both there will have been tissue depletion of variable extent by presentation (depending on balance and the size of body stores), the child will additionally have undergone a period of suboptimal growth. Thus nutritional support must provide for:

- maintenance demands (as in the adult);
- tissue repletion (as in the adult);
- growth;
- catch-up growth (Figure 23.18).

Consequently, nutrient demands are much greater than they are for a healthy child of similar age and size. Moreover, they must be met within the constraints imposed by immature homeostatic systems and complicating morbidity.

Aside from this consideration, the general principles of nutritional support in adults (see Chapter 9) also apply to sick children:

- The gut should be used when it is functioning.
- Potential intake of normal food should be maximised before and during the use of commercial supplements or specialist feeds where clinically indicated.
- Careful attention to hygiene should be observed both when handling enteral feeds and when managing parenteral lines.

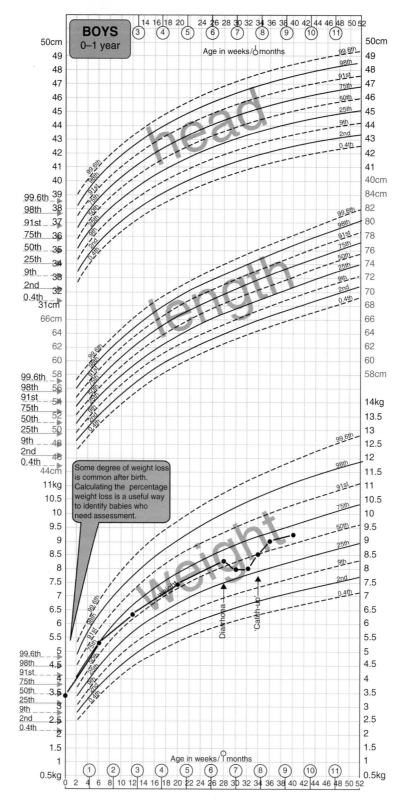

Figure 23.18 Weight loss and catch-up. An episode of protracted diarrhoea causes significant weight loss over a month. On treatment, weight gain is extremely rapid. This process of catch-up after illness is associated with very high nutritional requirements. Chart developed by RCPCH/ WHO/Department of Health, copyright © 2009 Department of Health.

- A multidisciplinary-team approach to management should be followed, both in hospital and in the community.
- Clear guidelines and care pathways must be in place to support children and parents managing nutritional support in the community.
- Nutritional support should be organised in such a way as to minimise disruption to the child's daily life (particularly schooling). In order to accomplish this in the case of children receiving long-term nutritional support, it may be necessary to make a formal statement of Special Educational Needs to the local education authority (in the UK) and consider application for benefits such as Disability Living Allowance or Attendance Allowance (UK).
- Growth, fluid balance, and plasma biochemistry must be closely monitored, because normal homeostatic controls (especially thirst and hunger) may be overridden when nutritional support is provided.

Routes of access for enteral nutritional support

The most commonly employed route at all ages is nasogastric tube feeding. Medical-grade polyvinyl chloride (PVC) or polyurethane (PU) tubes are most commonly used, particularly in young infants. If long-term tube feeding is considered, silicon tubes are softer and can be left in place for weeks. These need a guidewire to stiffen them sufficiently for introduction, but parents and adolescent children can be taught the technique. This allows them, for example, to be used for overnight feeding and removed for school. In very young infants, especially if preterm, nasogastric tubes increase upper-airway impedance and hence the work of breathing (young infants are obligate nose-breathers).

Each time a gastric tube is passed, its position should be checked by aspirating and testing for an acid reaction with indicator paper. If there is doubt, tube position should be confirmed by X-ray. This precaution is necessary to exclude accidental intubation of a bronchus, something which can happen particularly with young preterm infants, unconscious children, or those with neuromuscular disability who have a weak gag reflex.

Naso- or orojejunal tubes were once used quite commonly as an alternative to gastric tubes, particularly in preterm infants. These are weighted to facilitate passage through the pylorus, but a degree of skill is needed (sometimes it helps to stiffen the tube in a freezer first). It is also difficult to aspirate the tube and an X-ray is usually needed to confirm its position. Another, more theoretical, disadvantage is that this method of feeding seems less 'physiological' than gastric feeding. For example, the neurenteric peptide responses to feeding gastrically and jejunally are different, and feeds must be given by continuous infusion rather than by bolus as the jejunum will not tolerate such large volumes as the stomach. This may impair fat digestion. For all these reasons, jejunal feeding has declined in popularity, though it can still be particularly useful in babies who have severe gastrooesophageal reflux or who are receiving continuous positive airways pressure (CPAP) applied to the oropharynx.

Where long-term access to the gut is required, gastrostomy has become an increasingly popular procedure. Classically this was performed as a surgical procedure, an inflatable balloon being used to fix the catheter. Most gastrostomies are now, however, inserted endoscopically (percutaneous endoscopic gastrostomy (PEG)) and retained by a flat disc (or 'button'). This can be simply closed off or opened (e.g. for overnight tube feeding), which aids concealment and makes it popular with older children. A considerable disadvantage of gastrostomy is that it tends to exacerbate any gastrooesophageal reflux present, so any vomiting may worsen. Occasionally this can be so marked as to necessitate surgical fundoplication of the stomach. Gastrostomy is particularly common in the management of children with chronic feeding problems and severe neuromuscular disability, such as those with cerebral palsy.

Types of enteral feed

Breast milk (or infant formula if the mother is not breast-feeding) is used for the majority of young infants. This may be given in volumes of up to 180–200 ml/kg body weight/day, the caloric density approximating 0.7 kcal/ml. Preferably the mother's own breast milk is used. If her baby is unable to feed at the breast, the mother will need support and help to express and store her milk. She can either express manually or use a hand-, battery-, or electricity-powered pump. Whatever her preference, she will need to do this at least six times per day to maintain her supply. When a mother's own milk is not available, milk from a donor may be used. If so, it is vital to follow available guidelines about donor deferral (declining high-risk donors), serological testing (for HIV, human T-lymphotropic virus (HTLV), hepatitis, and other infections), processing (including pasteurisation), and microbiological testing in order to prevent transmission of infection. On the other hand, it is not usually necessary to microbiologically test or process a mother's own milk so long as simple hygiene instructions in relation to cleaning pumps and bottles are followed.

If there is a need to increase energy intake further, or to reduce the fluid volume administered (e.g. because of cardiac or renal disease), several options are available:

- High-fat breast milk can be obtained by showing the mother how to separate hind milk (richer in fat) when she expresses.
- Commercial supplements can be used to increase energy density to as much as 1 kcal/ml. These include glucose polymer powder, Calogen (a long-chain triglyceride emulsion), and Duocal (a combined fat/carbohydrate supplement).
- A specialist high-energy nutritionally complete formula can be chosen from the wide range commercially available.

Some infants will not tolerate a standard infant formula, for example because they have had major gut resection or have protracted diarrhoea. For these, a hydrolysate-based feed may be tried (e.g. Pregestimil), an elemental formula may be given (e.g. Neocate), or a 'modular feed' may be made, consisting of a protein source (e.g. comminuted chicken meat and/or a commercial product such as Maxipro) supplemented with carbohydrate, fat, minerals, and vitamins. It can be demanding to achieve the right nutrient balance with this approach, and it may also be difficult to keep the ingredients in suspension when an infusion pump is used. For this reason, it is generally preferable to use a commercially prepared complete feed. A variety of specially formulated enteral feeds is available for oral or tube feeding of infants and children, the composition of which is set in European Law (European Commission Directive on Foods for Special Medical Purposes 1999/21/EC).

For children over 1 year of age, a similar range of specialist feeds is available: those with a whole (milk) protein base, those with a hydrolysed protein base, and those which are elemental in composition. The chief distinction between these and specialist enteral feeds for adults is that they have higher nutrient (particularly energy) density. This is because children tolerate large volumes of feed less well than adults. The composition of these feeds is generally specified differently for children under and over 2 years of age. Children over 10 years of age will generally receive a feed of 'adult' composition.

Administration of tube feeds

Naso- and orogastric tube feeding of young infants is usually accomplished by giving small 'bolus' quantities of milk. A small reservoir (such as a 10 ml syringe) is filled and a measured amount of feed is allowed to flow into the stomach under the action of gravity. The frequency of feeding may vary from 1- to 4-hourly, the interval usually depending on the size and maturity of the baby and the volume of gastric residual when the tube is aspirated prior to each feed. 'Bolus' feeding is also suitable for older infants and young children.

The alternative is to give the same daily quantities of feed by continuous infusion at a constant rate. This is sometimes used when young infants tolerate bolus feeding poorly, and is essential when the jejunal (rather than the gastric) route is employed. The other major application is overnight feeding in older children, through either a gastrostomy or a gastric tube.

Continuous feeding in children always requires the use of a suitable pump, because both the volume prescribed and the limits of tolerance are smaller. Some pumps are battery-operated and so can offer the child mobility as feeding continues.

Parenteral feeding: general principles

The development of parenteral nutrition over the last 40 years has been life-saving for many sick children, particularly very low-birth-weight preterm infants born with minimal nutrient stores before the gut has sufficient absorptive function to supply nutrient needs. In most such children it is a therapy which can be discontinued within weeks, as the transition to enteral feeding is accomplished. However, the survival into childhood of small numbers of infants with intestinal failure originating in the neonatal period has proved that it is possible in some cases to provide adequate nutrition for growth and development. The

Age	Typical weight (kg)	Energy provision (kcal/kg/day)	Amino acid intake (g/kg/day)	Guideline fluid intake (to be adjusted according to losses)
0–3 months	5	90–100	1.5–3.0	120–150 (max. 180) ml/kg/day
4–12 months	8	90–100	1.0–2.5	120–150 (max. 180) ml/kg/day
1–2 years	12	75–90	1.0–2.5	80–120 (max. 150) ml/kg/day
3–6 years	18	75–90	1.0–2.0	80–100 ml/kg/day
7–10 years	27	60–75	1.0–2.0	60–80 ml/kg/day
11–14 years	40	30–60	1.0–2.0	50–70 ml/kg/day
15–18 years	60	30–60	1.0–2.0	50–70 ml/kg/ day

Table 23.5 Basic parenteral nutrition requirements for children of different ages (excluding preterm babies). Abstracted from Koletzko *et al.* (2005).

mortality rate of such children is high, the commonest causes of death being septicaemia related to line infection and hepatic failure consequent on cholestasis.

The aetiology of the latter is complex. Important factors are lack of gall-bladder emptying (normally provoked by enteral feeding) and hepatic steatosis. In practice, the simplest preventative measure is to provide enteral feeds whenever possible (even in subnutritional quantities) in order to promote bile flow, avoid excessive glucose load, and allow a few hours each day off parenteral nutrition in order to promote the mobilisation of hepatic fat stores. This underscores the importance of a general point made above: parenteral nutrition should be provided only if gut function remains inadequate to supply nutritional requirements once all options for enteral support described above have been exhausted. In consequence, parenteral nutrition is most commonly used in paediatrics to complement, rather than replace, enteral intake.

Access for parenteral nutrition

The options are a surgically implanted line (e.g. Hickman or Broviac) or a fine silastic catheter passed through a peripherally inserted cannula. The latter are now available in sizes sufficiently small to pass through a 25 G needle, making this approach possible even for infants 500–1000 g in weight. A peripherally inserted cannula is usually advanced to lie in the inferior or superior vena cava; if necessary, its position is radiologically confirmed by injection of contrast medium (though some lines are radio-opaque). It is essential to take care to site the cannula correctly in a high-flow central vessel, as extravasation of hyperosmolar solutions from smaller vessels has caused serious complications, including pleural effusions and ascites. The tip of a small-bore line must also be

outside the heart, as perforation with consequent tamponade has proved fatal in some neonates.

There is little place for the provision of parenteral nutrition in children through peripheral cannulas. These need frequent replacement (which is distressing for the child), and extravasation may cause severe scarring of superficial tissues. Moreover, the number of suitable infusion sites is rapidly exhausted, making a peripherally inserted central line much harder to place.

Providing parenteral nutrition

The prescription will vary with:

- age of child;
- weight;
- disease process (which may both affect requirements and place constraints on intake);
- losses (stool, fistula output, or urine).

It must therefore be tailored to the individual child.

Approximations of intake are provided in Table 23.5, which illustrates how greatly children's requirements alter with age. It does not show data for preterm infants, in whom both energy and protein requirements may be considerably higher (120 kcal/kg/day and 3.0–3.5 g protein/kg/day) as a result of rapid tissue accretion and high brain/body weight ratio. Non-protein energy is provided by glucose, a fat emulsion (such as 20% Intralipid), and nitrogen in the form of crystalline L-amino acid solutions. A number of considerations apply to the choice of preparation and the exact amount infused.

Glucose

Hepatic glucose production rates expressed per kilogram of body weight fall as a child grows, principally because brain tissue accounts for a declining proportion of body mass. The following are estimates:

- preterm infant: 4–6 mg/kg/minute;
- small-for-gestational-age infant: 6–8 mg/kg/minute;
- term infant: 3–5 mg/kg/minute;
- adult: 1–2 mg/kg/minute.

Providing glucose at these rates will suppress gluconeogenesis and maintain normoglycaemia, but not promote anabolism. To do so, it is necessary to provide increased amounts, usually starting at about 7 mg/kg/minute and increasing to about 10–12 mg/kg/minute over a week. This is achieved by increasing the concentration of glucose provided, though concentrations in excess of 10% should always be administered through a central rather than a peripheral line. Blood glucose should be monitored closely, particularly in sick preterm infants, among whom a marked counter-regulatory stress response may cause hyperglycaemia even at the minimal rates of infusion set out earlier.

Even if normoglycaemia is maintained, it is important not to exceed a total glucose intake of about 18 g/kg/day. Provision of greater amounts exceeds capacity for oxidative disposal and stimulates lipogenesis. This can have undesirable effects:

- CO_2 production is increased as the respiratory quotient rises > 1.0. This may embarrass babies with poor respiratory function.
- Plasma triglyceride concentration increases. The unwary may react to this by reducing the rate of lipid infusion, when a more appropriate response would be to cut glucose intake.

Lipid

Intravenous lipid is most commonly provided in the form of soybean oil emulsion with phospholipids and glycerol (e.g. Intralipid), though the use of marine oil formulations is increasing in popularity, as these appear to reduce the risk of cholestatic liver disease in children with intestinal failure on long-term parenteral nutrition. As well as providing energy, they are rich sources of the n-3 and n-6 essential fatty acid precursors α-linoleic and linolenic acid. Normally, fat should provide about 30–40% of the non-protein energy intake, though it is customary to commence intravenous fat emulsions in smaller amounts, starting at about 1 and building to a maximum of 4 g/kg/day in increments of 1 g/kg/day, as tolerated. Tolerance is best monitored by measuring the plasma triacylglycerol (TAG) concentration.

Somewhat counterintuitively, more-concentrated fat emulsions (20 or 30%) are more rapidly cleared from the plasma than a 10% solution. This is because lower concentrations of lipid contain greater amounts of solubilising agent relative to the quantity of fat. These agents are associated with the formation of abnormal circulating lipoproteins, which interfere with fat uptake. Other factors that may interfere with the uptake of fat through inhibition of lipoprotein lipase activity are infection, acidosis, and stress. Liver disease may also impair fat clearance. Deficiency of carnitine (necessary to transport acyl CoA across the mitochondrial membrane) can compromise fat oxidation. It is not routinely added to parenteral nutrition solutions, and supplementation sometimes augments fat clearance, though the literature on this point is conflicting.

Nitrogen

The choice of a suitable amino acid solution is particularly important for neonates and young infants, in whom there is an expanded range of essential and conditionally essential amino acids as a result of immaturity of the metabolic pathways. The latter can also affect disposal: in particular, the use of Vamin 9, a solution intended for adult parenteral nutrition, was associated in the past with levels of hyperphenylalaninaemia approaching those observed in PKU. The composition of modern solutions is based on the amino acid composition of human-milk protein or on differences in the amino acid concentrations of umbilical venous and arterial samples (which presumably reflect requirements for foetal accretion).

Nitrogen should be supplied in amounts which reflect the non-protein energy intake. This is because energy restriction will limit rates of tissue accretion, thereby reducing the nitrogen requirement. Amounts of nitrogen exceeding this will therefore add to RSL, a consideration which is particularly important in young infants. As a rough estimate, providing 1 g nitrogen per 250 kcal will be appropriate, though the exact relationship is more complex, particularly at lower protein or energy intakes.

Vitamins and trace minerals

The vitamin and trace-mineral requirements of young children are very different to those of adults, and generally much higher when calculated per unit of body weight. Accordingly, specialist paediatric solutions must be used. Trace-mineral concentrations should be regularly monitored in children on long-term parenteral nutrition. Deficiencies in zinc, copper, and selenium occur most commonly; in some centres, amounts of zinc and selenium in particular are given in addition to standard trace-mineral solutions. Selenium may be absent from commercial solutions, and zinc may be present only in small amounts in some. In contrast, hypermanganesaemia has been observed in some children (particularly preterm infants), though its clinical significance seems unclear.

In this context, it is useful to remember that copper and manganese are excreted in bile (hence liable to accumulate in cholestasis), whereas other trace minerals are eliminated in the urine. Iron provision in parenteral solutions can also be inadequate. It is considered undesirable to provide high concentrations of ferrous iron, partly because of its propensity to promote formation of the OH oxidative free radical and partly because it is thought to increase the risk of Gram-negative infection. In practice, many sick children receiving parenteral nutrition are repeatedly transfused for other reasons (e.g. to improve oxygen transport or replace blood losses) and sufficient iron is provided as blood. Where transfusion is not indicated, additional iron can be given in the form of iron dextran, either with the parenteral nutrition solutions or separately.

Key points on the nutritional support of a child are summarised in Box 23.17.

Box 23.17 Nutritional support

- When nutritional support is given to children, it is important not only to provide for maintenance and repletion (as in an adult), but to allow for continued growth and catch-up growth.
- Nutrient demands change with age, body proportions, and the nature of comorbidity.
- Enteral support is preferable to parenteral because it is safer and cheaper. A wide range of nutritionally complete enteral feeds is available for infants and children.
- Breast milk, supplemented if necessary, is the preferred feed for infants. The mother may need help to maintain lactation if her baby is sick.
- During nutritional support, growth, fluid balance, and plasma biochemistry (especially concentrations of glucose, electrolyte, and trace minerals) must be closely monitored.

The acutely ill child: diarrhoeal disease

Most acute illnesses in young children are brief and associated with rapid recovery. Although the child may be anorexic at presentation, recovery is associated with return of appetite and, often, increased intake to fuel catch-up growth. This assumes, however, that the child is optimally nourished at presentation, making it important to assess nutritionally any acutely ill child (see Section 23.7). Coexisting malnutrition may not only have contributed to pathogenesis (e.g. by increasing infection risk) but will increase the risk of complications or death.

Malnutrition, alone or in association with measles, malaria, respiratory illness, and diarrhoea, accounts for about 60% of all deaths in young children worldwide. Correct nutritional management is therefore important in the last, and may be life-saving: both under- and over-treatment are equally dangerous.

Management of diarrhoea

Globally, about 3 million children a year die of diarrhoea, most of whom are under 2 years of age. A key preventative strategy is promotion of exclusive breast-feeding for the first 6 months, with prolonged later breast-feeding as part of a diversifying diet. In older children, zinc and vitamin A supplements have been shown to reduce incidence. Dehydration caused by loss of electrolytes and water in the stool is the principal cause of death. The general principles followed in the management of diarrhoea are:

- Urgent replacement of water and electrolytes, using the right type of fluid given by the correct route. This should be achieved in the first 6–12 hours. Delay in treatment and use of the wrong fluid are major contributors to mortality.
- Early reintroduction of food, to optimise nutrient intake and prevent and treat malnutrition.
- Continued monitoring of growth, to ensure that catch-up occurs and diarrhoea does not persist.

Note particularly that antidiarrhoeal drugs should not be used to treat diarrhoeal disease in children, and antibiotics are only indicated in dysentery (passage of frequent, loose stools containing blood and mucus, usually associated with fever, abdominal pain, and other signs; most often caused by *Shigella* infection). Also bear in mind that diarrhoea and vomiting in children can be caused by non-gastrointestinal

Table 23.6 Summary of WHO guidelines for managing diarrhoea. ORS, oral rehydration solution. From the World Health Organization.

Dehydration	Rehydration	Plan
None	Not needed, but extra fluid as demanded	'Schedule A': home treatment with extra fluid as ORS, water, or food-based fluid. Continue feeding.
Some (mild or moderate)	Oral rehydration with measured amounts of ORS, depending on age and weight	'Schedule B': rehydrate with ORS over 4 hours. Continue breast-feeding. If not breast-fed, refeed within 4 hours. Continue to replace losses with extra ORS.
Severe	Intravenous rehydration with isotonic fluid	'Schedule C': rehydrate over 4–6 hours. Give ORS as soon as the child can drink. Continue to replace losses and feed as soon as possible.

infections (e.g. meningitis, pneumonia, otitis media) or 'surgical' abdominal conditions (e.g. intussusception). Thus every child needs careful examination to exclude accompanying illness.

Assessing dehydration

The degree of dehydration can be assessed clinically as follows:

- *Severe dehydration.* The child has sunken eyes and cold peripheries, is lethargic, and may be unconscious and unable to drink. Skin turgour is severely reduced: a pinched fold of skin 'tents' and may take more than 2 seconds to regain its shape. The peripheral pulses are extremely weak or impalpable, blood pressure is low, and there is no urine output. Children presenting with severe dehydration will typically have lost 10–15% of their body weight.
- *Moderate dehydration.* The child may have sunken eyes and reduced skin turgour but is thirsty, able to drink, and irritable. About 6–9% of pre-morbid weight will have been lost.
- *Mild dehydration.* The mucous membranes are dry and the child is thirsty, but skin turgour seems normal. Less than 5% weight loss will have occurred.

It is worth noting that the diagnosis of dehydration is never based on measurement of the plasma electrolyte concentrations. Clinical assessment and weight are much more valuable and treatment should never be delayed while blood results are ascertained. However, if the plasma sodium concentration exceeds 160 mmol/l, the risk of death or disability is particularly high. Rehydration in such cases must be slower and must aim to correct the electrolyte derangement over 24–48 hours.

Fluid replacement

WHO rehydration schedules for children with diarrhoea envisage three scenarios, based on the degree of dehydration at presentation (see Table 23.6).

Children presenting with signs of severe dehydration need urgent replacement of water and electrolytes or they will die (Table 23.6, Schedule C). This should be given intravenously, initially as 0.9% saline or Ringer's lactate solution. It is dangerous to give hypotonic fluids such as 5% glucose or 4% glucose with 0.18% saline as they will precipitate a rapid fall in plasma sodium concentration, with attendant risk of cerebral oedema (particularly if the child is hypernatraemic at presentation). The WHO recommends the following infusion rates for a child with severe dehydration:

- Child under 1 year: 30 ml/kg over first hour, followed by 70 ml/kg over the next 5 hours (equating to a total of 75 ml/kg body weight over the first 4 hours).
- Child over 1 year: 30 ml/kg in the first 30 minutes, and 70 ml/kg over the next 2.5 hours.

These amounts occasionally need to be repeated (for example, if the child remains unconscious with continuing high stool losses), but in most cases there is immediate improvement and the child recovers consciousness sufficiently to drink. It is important at this stage to offer additional ORS to replace the ongoing losses: roughly 1 ml of ORS will be needed for each millilitre (or gram) of loose stool. Breast-feeding may then be resumed and ORS given by mouth, aiming to provide about 5 ml/kg/hour.

If a child has features of severe malnutrition, ReSoMal should be used instead of ORS. The composition of these two fluids is compared in Table 23.7. They differ in important respects, particularly in sodium and potassium concentration. This reflects the fact that the child with malnutrition often has a surplus of extracellular fluid and hence excessive total body sodium balance (even if hyponatraemic) but is deficient in the intracellular electrolytes potassium

Table 23.7 Comparison of ReSoMal and WHO oral rehydration solutions (ORSs).

	ORS (mmol/l)	ReSoMal (mmol/l)
Sodium	75	45
Potassium	20	40
Magnesium	0	3
Glucose	75	55
Sucrose	0	69

and magnesium. The child with diarrhoea, on the other hand, has lost principally extracellular fluid and is acutely depleted in sodium.

Remember that children with malnutrition may quickly become oedematous (looking puffy in the face and eyelids) during rehydration. If this occurs, additional ORS should be stopped, but normal feeding continued. Once fluid balance is stabilised, ORS can be recommended if losses continue.

Feeding

Breast-feeding should not be interrupted and the child should be allowed to feed on demand. Infants under 6 months who are not breast-fed are given 100–200 ml of boiled water in addition to ORS during the rehydration period. Formula and other foods are reintroduced when rehydration has been completed, usually after about 4 hours. The old practice of using half-strength diluted milk and waiting for the diarrhoea to settle before 'regrading' is no longer endorsed: it led to significant reduction in nutrient intake without any improvement in the rate of recovery.

Persistent diarrhoea

Between 5 and 20% of acute diarrhoeal episodes become prolonged in resource-poor countries. If diarrhoea continues for more than 14 days, it is defined as 'persistent diarrhoea'. This is commonly associated with growth faltering, compromised immunity (especially if associated with HIV infection), and micronutrient deficiency (especially of zinc and vitamin A). It often leads to death. The cause may be persisting infection or mucosal injury that has caused intolerance to food constituents (usually lactose or cow's-milk proteins).

The important aspects of initial management are the following:

Box 23.18 Diarrhoea

- Acute and chronic diarrhoeal disease is a major cause of death, especially in children under 2.
- Most of these episodes can be prevented by exclusive breast-feeding, followed by prolonged breast-feeding as part of a more varied diet.
- The main cause of death amongst children with diarrhoea is mismanagement of fluid replacement – too little or too much too quickly.
- In uncomplicated diarrhoeal disease, the need is mainly to replace sodium and water, as principally the extracellular fluid compartment is depleted.
- The amount, rate, and route of salt and water replacement is determined by clinical assessment of the extent of dehydration.
- Breast-feeding should continue, supplemented with ORS.
- Children with diarrhoeal disease superimposed on malnutrition must be managed differently, to reduce the risk of acute extra-cellular fluid overload and to replace intracellular electrolytes.
- Persistent diarrhoea requires further investigation and further dietary management to prevent continued growth faltering.

- Correction of water and electrolyte imbalance, usually orally with ORS. Although children may not be severely dehydrated, they may be hypokalaemic and weak as a result.
- Detection and treatment of underlying systemic infections, parasitic infection (amoebiasis or giardiasis), or dysentery.
- Micronutrient supplementation and continued/frequent breast-feeding on demand.

If these are unsuccessful and the mother is not breast-feeding, a modified diet may be needed to reduce or eliminate lactose intake. A formula based on hydrolysed cow's-milk protein and sucrose (or glucose polymer) may be used when available. Sometimes it is necessary to use a modular feed based on ground chicken. An inexpensive lactose-free diet can also be made from egg (or ground chicken meat), rice, glucose, and vegetable oil.

Key points on the management of childhood diarrhoea are summarised in Box 23.18.

The chronically ill child: general remarks

A range of dietary products and delivery devices are now available for specialised enteral and parenteral nutritional support of sick children of all ages and sizes. Equally, improvements in paediatric treatment now mean that, with the exception of conditions caused by intolerance and allergy to food constituents, such as coeliac disease, dietary restriction is not used to control symptoms. For example, children with cystic fibrosis were once advised to follow strict low-fat diets to control steatorrhoea. The resulting chronic energy deficiency led to severe stunting, now rarely seen. The availability of modern pancreatic enzyme supplements, coupled with the use of high-energy diets and supplementation (if necessary by overnight tube or gastrostomy feeding), has meant that children survive longer and in most cases achieve weight and height in the normal range for age. Children with renal disease and heart disease similarly are no longer advised to follow severely restrictive diets.

It is not possible here to provide details of the nutritional management of the many chronic disorders affecting children. The general constraints which disease in various systems places upon nutrient assimilation, metabolism, and the excretion of waste products are covered in other sections of this chapter and elsewhere in the book.

Exclusion diets

Exclusion diets should not be given to children without good clinical justification. There are a number of reasons for this:

- The nutrient demands of growing children are high and the restrictive nature of exclusion diets poses a risk of specific nutritional deficiencies.
- The diet may be unpalatable and lead to energy deficiency.
- The normal development of eating patterns can be disturbed because meals are not shared with family and friends.

If an exclusion diet is prescribed, it must be supervised by a paediatric dietitian. Unfortunately, parents of young children may unjustifiably attribute causally a number of symptoms to particular foods and may introduce informal dietary restrictions. Symptoms related to food can be categorised in the following way:

- *Food aversion*. The child has a psychological objection to particular foods. Such symptoms can be distinguished from true intolerance if the food components are concealed or given in blinded circumstances.
- *Food intolerance*. There is a reproducible reaction to the food, even if the child and parents are blinded

to its presence in the diet. Food intolerances are not always 'allergic' in origin and may be due to a number of causes:

- o abnormal absorption (e.g. milk causing diarrhoea in lactase deficiency);
- o inherited abnormality of metabolism (e.g. fruits causing vomiting and hypoglycaemia in fructose intolerance);
- o presence of toxins or pharmacologically active compounds in food (e.g. histamine releasing sarcotoxins in some fish, caffeine in drinks);
- o immune reactions to food ('food allergy'); these may be of the immediate- or delayed-hypersensitivity type.

The types of diet used to manage food intolerances in children are:

- *Simple exclusion* of a food to which the child is reproducibly sensitive. Usually, but not always, the reaction is immediate, making the causal link clear. Examples include peanuts and milk. Very careful counselling is needed as even trace amounts present in commercially prepared foods can have significant consequences. One of the most widely used therapeutic exclusion diets in paediatrics is the gluten-free diet employed in coeliac disease. The principles of managing this condition are covered in Chapter 11.
- *Empirical diets*. Some diets have been shown to be effective in clinical trials for ill-understood reasons. Examples include milk and egg avoidance for eczema, additive avoidance in hyperactivity.
- *'Oligoantigenic' (few antigens) diets*. These very restrictive diets allow only a few foods and are generally used only for diagnostic purposes over short periods. New foods can be added one at a time in order to identify troublesome items.
- *'Hypoallergenic' diets*. These involve using specialised enteral feeds. They are usually bland and unpalatable, and hence may often be given by tube. They have, however, been used particularly successfully to induce remission in Crohn's disease among children. This is a great advantage because the alternative therapeutic option, corticosteroids, has a number of undesirable side effects – particularly growth suppression.
- *Densensitisation*. Recently it has been shown that children can be immunologically desensitised to dietary antigens by feeding them specified increasing amounts of the antigen concerned (most commonly

peanut protein). This specialised treatment should be offered only by paediatric allergists or clinical immunologists.

Food intolerance – suspected or proven – is an increasingly common problem in paediatric practice and a number of hypotheses have been raised to explain this trend. These issues, and further aspects of management, are covered in Chapter 8.

Inborn errors of metabolism

Genetically determined abnormalities have been recognised in virtually every metabolic pathway. Indeed, understanding these 'experiments of nature' has provided considerable insight into the phenotypical significance of particular enzyme steps. This is because a single gene deletion gives rise to a single enzyme deficiency, the great majority following an autosomal-recessive pattern of inheritance. Individually they are rare, but collectively they are quite common, affecting up to 1 in 1500–2000 children in the UK, for example. Incidence varies considerably from country to country, reflecting variation in the gene frequency; for example, PKU (the commonest of the inherited disorders of

amino acid metabolism) affects about 1 in 10 000 children in the UK but about 1 in 5000 in Ireland.

Some inborn errors are not treatable (e.g. respiratory-chain disorders) and may cause death very soon after birth. Others (e.g. PKU, type I glutaric aciduria, medium-chain acyl CoA dehydrogenase deficiency) are associated with metabolic decompensation, death, or severe neurological handicap, which is preventable if detected sufficiently early. All newborn infants in the UK have for many years received the so-called 'Guthrie test', which screens for PKU by measuring blood phenylalanine. This is usually done around the end of the first week of life, once milk-feeding has become established.

Historically it has not been cost-effective to screen for other metabolic diseases, but the development of tandem mass spectrometry has made it feasible practically to test for multiple disorders on a single small sample. The resulting worldwide escalation of multi-disease screening programmes is increasing very substantially the number of children requiring specialist nutritional management. The more common amino and organic acid metabolism disorders are summarised in Table 23.8, selected disorders of carbohydrate metabolism managed by diet are summarised in

Table 23.8 The more commonly occurring disorders of amino and organic acid metabolism managed by diet.

Metabolic disorder	Metabolic defect	Dietary treatment
Phenylketonuria	Phenylalanine hydroxylase deficiency (or, rarely, a defect in recycling of biopterin, a co-factor for the enzyme)	Restriction of dietary phenylalanine
Maple-syrup urine disease	Branched-chain 2-ketoacid dehydrogenase complex deficiency	Leucine restriction Thiamine supplementation (thiamine responsive form; 2 ketoacid dehydrogenase co-factor)
Homocysteinuria	Cystathionine beta-synthase deficiency	Methionine restriction Pyridoxine supplementation (cystathionine beta-synthase co-factor)
Tyrosinaemia (types I and II)	Deficiency of fumarylacetoacetate hydrolase (type I) or tyrosine aminotransferase (type II)	Low-phenylalanine, low-tyrosine diet
Urea-cycle disorders	Many, such as carbamoyl phosphate synthetase deficiency, ornithine carbamoyl transferase deficiency	Protein restriction Use of sodium benzoate or phenylbutyrate to facilitate alternative N-excretion pathways Arginine supplementation (to replace intermediate compounds not formed)
Propionic acidaemia; methylmalonic acidaemia (MMA)	Deficiency of propionyl carboxylase or methylmalonic acid mutase, respectively In MMA, sometimes deficiency of the enzyme cofactor adenosylcobalamin	Protein restriction Avoid fasting (to limit oxidation of fat and protein) Possible benefit from vitamin B_{12} in MMA and from use of antibiotics (metronidazole) to suppress synthesis of propionic acid by colonic flora
Isovaleric acidaemia	Deficiency of isovaleryl CoA dehydrogenase.	Protein restriction Supplementation with carnitine and glycine (to conjugate isovaleric acid and enhance urinary excretion)

Table 23.9 Selected disorders of carbohydrate metabolism managed by diet.

Metabolic disorder	Metabolic defect	Dietary treatment
Glycogen storage diseases (GSDs) (types I, III)	Glucose-6-phosphatase deficiency (type I) Amylo-1,6-glucosidase (debranching enzyme) deficiency (type III) Other steps also affected	Avoidance of hypoglycaemia by frequent (or continuous) feeding of glucose polymer/cornstarch to meet glucose-oxidation requirements
Galactosaemia	Classically deficiency of galactose-1-phosphate uridyl transferase	Total avoidance of lactose from milk and covert sources (such as medicines)
Galactokinase deficiency	Galactokinase	As galactosaemia
Hereditary fructose intolerance	Deficiency of fructose-1-phosphate aldolase	Avoidance of fructose (together with sucrose and sorbitol)
Congenital disorders of glycosylation (CDGs)	Several types: deficiencies of the glycosyltransferases and other enzymes which glycate proteins	Varies: for example, the use of mannose in CDG type Ib (phosphomannose isomerase deficiency) to circumvent the production of mannose from fructose
Fructose 1,6-biphosphatase deficiency	Ineffective gluconeogenesis leading to fasting hypoglycaemia	Diet low in fructose Otherwise, similar approach to that for GSDs, using frequent feeding and glucose polymer/uncooked cornstarch supplements Avoidance of alcohol (which also impairs gluconeogenesis)

Table 23.10 Selected disorders of lipid metabolism managed by diet.

Metabolic disorder	Metabolic defect	Dietary treatment
Disorders of beta-oxidation	Medium- and long-chain acyl CoA dehydrogenase deficiency (MCAD, LCAD) 3-hydroxyacyl-CoA dehydrogenase deficiencies Multiple acyl-CoA dehydrogenase deficiencies	High-carbohydrate diet and avoidance of fasting The patient does not have normal ketogenesis and will become hypoglycaemic Fatty acids and accumulated CoA derivatives are also toxic in LCAD, so diet aims to minimise long-chain fat intake
Abetalipoproteinaemia	Inability to make apolipoprotein B: therefore absence of chylomicra, LDLs, and VLDLs in lymph and the blood Results in severe fat malabsorption, with failure to thrive, acanthocytosis of red cells, ataxia, and retinopathy	Reduce long-chain triglyceride intake and supply energy as medium-chain triglyceride and carbohydrate
Hyperlipoproteinaemias	Many types Commonest is type IIA, resulting in high LDL concentrations and hypercholesterolaemia	Reduced fat intake to 30% of energy Increased intake of non-starch polysaccharide Drugs (statins and bile-salt chelators such as cholestyramine to reduce fat absorption)

Table 23.9, and some selected disorders of lipid metabolism managed by diet are summarised in Table 23.10.

Key points about inborn errors of metabolism are summarised in Box 23.19.

For most inborn errors, diet remains the mainstay of management despite the promise of technological advances. There are a few exceptions: for example, enzyme replacement has proven effective in some (e.g.

Gaucher's disease, Fabry's disease) and gene replacement in others (e.g. urea-cycle disorders, adenosine deaminase deficiency), at least in the short term. The general principles of dietary management are:

- To restrict the intake of precursor metabolites in order to prevent accumulation of the precursors themselves or their metabolites.

Box 23.19 Inborn errors of metabolism

- Inborn errors are individually rare, but collectively affect up to 1 in 500 children.
- The prevalence of inborn errors in cinical practice is likely to increase as more are identified by new screening technology.
- The only treatment for most is dietary modification.
- As they are single-gene disorders affecting single enzyme steps, these 'experiments of nature' have taught us much about normal metabolism.
- Dietary treatment may entail:
    - reducing the supply of precursors while ensuring sufficiency of other nutrients;
    - using supraphysiological doses of vitamin co-factors to increase the activity of vitamin-dependent enzymes ('vitamin dependency').
- High-energy feeding during illness reduces catabolism of fat and protein stores, thus minimising the unwanted release of precursors from body tissues.

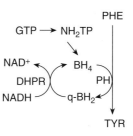

Figure 23.19 Phenylketonuria (PKU). 'Classical' PKU is caused by reduced activity in the phenlalanine hydroxyase (PH) pathway. Thus phenylalanine (PHE) cannot be converted to tyrosine (TYR). Rarely, there is instead a deficiency in the associated pathway responsible for synthesising and regenerating reduced (tetrahydro-) biopterin (BH$_4$), the enzyme co-factor. DHPR, dihydropteridin reductase; q-BH$_2$, quinoid dihydrobioptein; GTP, guanosine triphosphate; NH$_2$TP, dihydroneopterin triphosphate. This article was published in Textbook of Paediatric Nutrition, 3rd edn, McLaren DS, Burman D, Belton NR, Williams AF (eds). Copyright Churchill Livingstone, 1991.

- To augment the activity of defective metabolic pathways. Sometimes this can be accomplished by using a supraphysiological dose of the relevant vitamin co-factor. This situation is known as 'vitamin dependency' – not to be confused with deficiency. An example of such treatment is the use of vitamin B$_6$ in pyridoxine-dependent seizures.
- To provide sufficient intake of other nutrients (especially energy, trace minerals, and vitamins) in orde to meet the demands of maintenance and growth.
- To restrict the extent of catabolism during any intercurrent illness, preventing metabolic stress due to release of precursors form body stores.

Phenylketonuria

As PKU is one of the commonest inherited metabolic disorders, it is illustrative to understand some general principles of management. Classical PKU occurs when there is an absence of phenylalanine hydroxylase (Figure 23.19) or the enzyme is present in extremely low quantities. Without treatment blood phenylalanine concentrations may exceed 1 mmol/l, a level sufficient to cause cerebral damage, resulting in severe learning difficulty, seizures, and microcephaly. There is often a striking absence of skin, eye, and hair pigmentation because of the inability to convert phenylalanine to tyrosine, which is a precursor of the skin pigment melanin. Rarely, PKU is caused not by a defect in the protein structure of phenylalanine hydroxylase itself but by an abnormality in the pathway which reduces and recycles biopterin, the enzyme co-factor (Figure 23.19). Such patients need supplementation with folate and other compounds, in addition to dietary phenylalanine restriction.

The cornerstone of management in classical PKU is restriction of phenylalanine intake, titrating this against blood phenylalanine concentrations. In young infants, this can be accomplished by using a low phenylalanine formula, either alone or in combination with breast milk. As breast milk has a much lower phenylalanine concentration than cow's milk (or infant formulas), partial breast-feeding is fortunately possible in most cases. Management becomes more challenging with the introduction of complementary foods. Only very limited quantities of 'natural' dietary protein can be allowed, and staple protein sources such as meat, fish, cheese, and soya protein must be avoided completely. Those lower in protein content (such as cereals, rice, and vegetables) become the principal 'normal' components of the diet and are offered in 'exchanges' (i.e. measured portions) containing 50 mg phenylalanine. In recent years, dietary goals have become much stricter and, whereas once fruit and vegetables with low phenylalanine content were offered freely, even these are now incorporated in the 'exchange' scheme.

Such a diet might control phenylalanine intake but is grossly insufficient in total dietary protein (and hence other essential amino acids), not to mention trace minerals and vitamins. Potential dietary deficiency of protein is prevented by prescribing phenylalanine-free amino acid mixtures as substitutes for natural dietary protein. A range is available, the exact choice depending on age (which affects essential amino acid requirement). Most are complete in vitamin and essential mineral content, though these can be provided separately. Analogous products depleted in amino acids other than phenylalanine are used to treat other inherited amino and organic acidaemias. All are listed in the 'Borderline Substances' section (Appendix 7) of the *British National Formulary*, together with a range of prescribable prepared foods such as low-protein breads, pasta, confectionery bars, and so on.

Clearly, the diet of a child with PKU is very different to that of his or her peers. This can lead to substantial behavioural problems among children of all ages. Young children may ingest normal foods accidentally, whereas older ones, particularly adolescents, may rebel. The need to eat such a restrictive diet is potentially a considerable social handicap, as meals outside the home present difficulties. Food refusal can also be a major management problem.

Setting such behavioural issues aside, blood phenylalanine levels may also fluctuate for valid physiological reasons. Fasting, infection, energy, or essential amino acid deficiency and other stresses (e.g. surgery) may enhance endogenous protein breakdown, liberating phenylalanine from body protein and significantly increasing blood levels. Such effects can be minimised by maintaining a high energy intake through provision of high-carbohydrate drinks or even parenteral supplementation. On the other hand, growth spurts (e.g. at puberty or during catch-up after infections) may increase physiological demands and depress blood levels. Again, similar considerations apply to the management of other amino and organic acidaemias.

Children with PKU have always remained on their diet throughout childhood, though traditionally the diet was relaxed in adolescence and abandoned in adult life because the completion of central nervous system development was believed to eliminate the need for strict dietary control. Views on this have changed for a number of reasons:

- In the case of girls, the relative unpalatability of the diet always led to problems with regaining dietary control prior to conception and throughout pregnancy. In order to achieve a normal foetal outcome, metabolic control in such circumstances must be even tighter than in young infants. This is hard to achieve once a taste for 'normal' foods has been acquired.
- Neuropsychological studies have demonstrated superior cognitive function in well-controlled adult patients.
- Recent neuroimaging (magnetic resonance imaging, MRI) studies have demonstrated white-matter lesions in the long tracts of adults of both sexes who have relaxed their diets.
- Paraplegia, sometimes irreversible, has developed in young adults who have stopped their diet.

Most now recommend diet for life. In recent years it has been recognised that maintaining diet is associated with both improved cognitive performance in early adult life and reduced risk of the neurological abnormalities associated with white-matter changes on brain MRI scans.

Other inborn errors of metabolism

It is not possible here to give a detailed description of the management of other inborn errors of metabolism. This is a highly specialised, technically and clinically demanding subject. Tables 23.8, 23.9, and 23.10 give a glimpse of the variety of problems that may be encountered and the general principles of nutritional management.

23.9 Overweight in children: 'fatness' and 'obesity'

Defining 'obesity' in childhood

BMI changes throughout childhood, so it is impossible to follow the approach familiar in adult practice of defining overweight and obesity in terms of simple arithmetical values. BMI may be read from a chart (Figure 23.20) or calculated using a BMI look-up (Figure 23.14). The charts in common use in the UK derived from the WHO Multicentre Growth Reference Study (children 0–4 years) and the UK 1990 growth reference (children 4–18 years). There are many problems associated with the definition of overweight and obesity in children:

- First, BMI in children has undergone rapid secular change since 1990, although the year-on-year rise in proportion of children labeled as 'obese' in the UK has slowed in recent years.

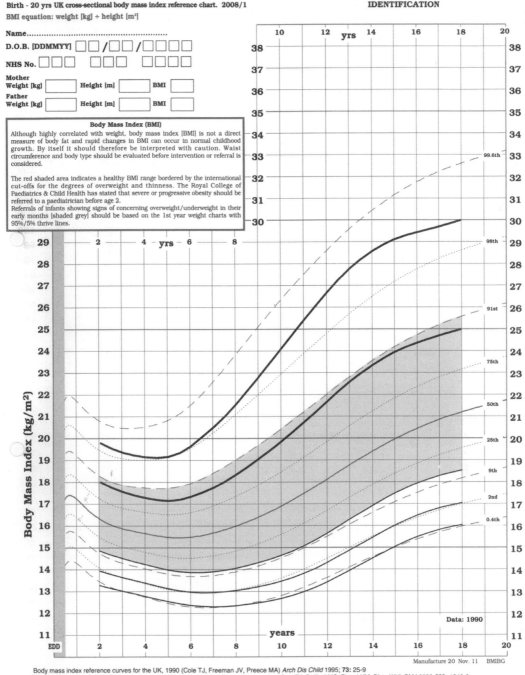

GIRLS BMI CHART

Birth - 20 yrs UK cross-sectional body mass index reference chart. 2008/1

BMI equation: weight [kg] ÷ height [m²]

IDENTIFICATION

Name...

D.O.B. [DDMMYY] ☐☐ / ☐☐ / ☐☐☐☐

NHS No. ☐☐☐ ☐☐☐ ☐☐☐☐

Mother
Weight [kg] ☐☐☐ Height [m] ☐☐☐ BMI ☐☐☐

Father
Weight [kg] ☐☐☐ Height [m] ☐☐☐ BMI ☐☐☐

Body Mass Index (BMI)

Although highly correlated with weight, body mass index [BMI] is not a direct measure of body fat and rapid changes in BMI can occur in normal childhood growth. By itself it should therefore be interpreted with caution. Waist circumference and body type should be evaluated before intervention or referral is considered.

The red shaded area indicates a healthy BMI range bordered by the international cut-offs for the degrees of overweight and thinness. The Royal College of Paediatrics & Child Health has stated that severe or progressive obesity should be referred to a paediatrician before age 2.
Referrals of infants showing signs of concerning overweight/underweight in their early months [shaded grey] should be based on the 1st year weight charts with 95%/5% thrive lines.

Body mass index reference curves for the UK, 1990 (Cole TJ, Freeman JV, Preece MA) *Arch Dis Child* 1995; **73**: 25-9
Establishing a standard definition for child overweight and obesity: international survey (Cole TJ, Bellizzi MC, Flegal KM, Dietz WH) *BMJ 2000;* **320**: 1240-3
Body mass index cut-offs to define thinness in children and adolescents: international survey (Cole TJ, Flegal KM, Nicholls D, Jackson AA) *BMJ 2007;* **335**: 194-7

Designed and Published by
© CHILD GROWTH FOUNDATION 1997/1
(Charity Reg. No 274325)
2 Mayfield Avenue,
London W4 1PW

Printed and Supplied by
HARLOW PRINTING LIMITED
Maxwell Street ◊ South Shields
Tyne & Wear ◊ NE33 4PU

Figure 23.20 Body-mass-index (BMI) charts. These charts are drawn from the UK 1990 reference. Note the earlier 'adiposity rebound' (upward inflection preceding puberty) amongst the heavier children. Note also that in the UK the UK-WHO reference is now used in preference to the UK 1990 reference for children under 4 years of age. © Child Growth Foundation, reproduced with permission. Printed supplies from www.healthforallchildren.co.uk.

BOYS BMI CHART

Birth - 20 yrs UK cross-sectional body mass index reference chart. 2008/1

BMI equation: weight [kg] ÷ height [m²]

Name...

D.O.B. [DDMMYY] ☐☐ / ☐☐ / ☐☐☐☐

NHS No. ☐☐☐ ☐☐☐ ☐☐☐☐

Mother
Weight [kg] ☐☐☐ Height [m] ☐☐☐ BMI ☐☐☐

Father
Weight [kg] ☐☐☐ Height [m] ☐☐☐ BMI ☐☐☐

Body Mass Index (BMI)

Although highly correlated with weight, body mass index [BMI] is not a direct measure of body fat and rapid changes in BMI can occur in normal childhood growth. By itself it should therefore be interpreted with caution. Waist circumference and body type should be evaluated before intervention or referral is considered.

The blue shaded area indicates a healthy BMI range bordered by the international cut-offs for the degrees of overweight and thinness. The Royal College of Paediatrics & Child Health has stated that severe or progressive obesity should be referred to a paediatrician before age 2.

Referrals of infants showing signs of concerning overweight/underweight in their early months [shaded grey] should be based on the 1st year weight charts with 95%/5% thrive lines.

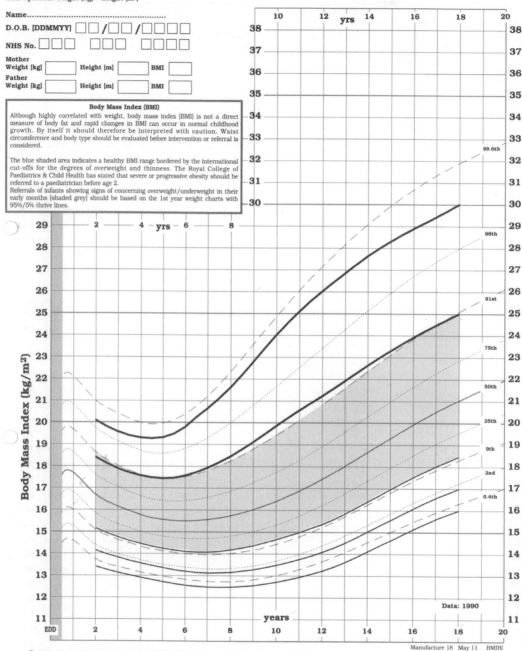

Body Mass Index (kg/m²)

years

Data: 1990

Manufacture 18 May 11   BMIBI

Body mass index reference curves for the UK, 1990 (Cole TJ, Freeman JV, Preece MA) *Arch Dis Child* 1995; **73:** 25-9
Establishing a standard definition for child overweight and obesity: international survey (Cole TJ, Bellizzi MC, Flegal KM, Dietz WH) *BMJ 2000;* **320:** 1240-3
Body mass index cut-offs to define thinness in children and adolescents: international survey (Cole TJ, Flegal KM, Nicholls D, Jackson AA) *BMJ 2007;* **335:** 194-7

Designed and Published by
© **CHILD GROWTH FOUNDATION 1997/1**
(Charity Reg. No 274325)
2 Mayfield Avenue,
London W4 1PW

Printed and Supplied by
HARLOW PRINTING LIMITED
Maxwell Street ◊ South Shields
Tyne & Wear ◊ NE33 4PU

Figure 23.20 (*Continued*)

- Second, the long-term implications of any particular BMI are much less clear for children than for adults. In other words, cut-offs cannot clearly be defined in terms of clinical risk. One solution (recommended by the International Task Force on Obesity) has been to impose on the BMI chart lines which correspond to the likely attainment of an adult BMI of 25 or 30. The lack of clear data on clinical risk and childhood BMI centile has persuaded some that the term 'fatness' is preferable to 'obesity' at this stage of life.
- Third, the charts are cross-sectional and children may change their relative position on the chart as they grow older. This raises the question of how children 'track' along particular centiles as they grow (see later). While there is a high year-on-year correlation between the centile position of any single individual, it is considerably lower over longer periods. Thus there is little relationship between fatness in adult life and infant BMI, but a much stronger relationship with BMI after puberty.

In addition to the child's position on the centile chart at any one time, other indicators that the child is at high risk of adult obesity include:

- one or two overweight or obese parents;
- early 'adiposity rebound'; that is, when the normal upwards inflection of the BMI curve preceding puberty begins relatively early.

It is important to note that in the UK the terms 'obesity' and 'overweight' are defined differently for population surveillance and clinical purposes. For population surveillance, overweight is defined by a BMI above the 85th percentile and obesity by a BMI above the 95th percentile for age. For clinical purposes, these terms are defined by BMI for age above the 91st and 98th centiles, respectively.

Complications of 'obesity' in childhood

Although much attention has been focused on the possible consequences of childhood fat mass for adult health, being overweight increases the risk of certain conditions presenting in childhood. A list is given in Box 23.20.

Currently there is particular concern about the increasing prevalence of NIDDM among children. This seems to be a greater problem in those of South Asian ethnic origin.

Box 23.20 Complications of 'obesity' in childhood

- orthopaedic (slipped femoral epiphysis, Blount's disease);
- sleep apnoea/hypoventilation;
- hyperlipidaemia;
- non-insulin-dependent diabetes mellitus (NIDDM);
- pseudotumour cerebri;
- hypertension.

Box 23.21 Less common 'medical' causes of obesity in children

- genetic;
- Prader–Willi syndrome;
- rarer syndromes;
- endocrine;
- hypothyroidism;
- Cushing's syndrome;
- growth-hormone deficiency;
- iatrogenic;
- glucocorticoid therapy;
- poorly controlled diabetes mellitus (insulin excess);
- illnesses associated with immobility (decreased energy expenditure);
- spina bifida;
- muscular dystrophy.

Less common causes of 'obesity' in childhood

Most fat children have 'simple' obesity, arising from energy imbalance. However, a few uncommon causes exist, as shown in Box 23.21. A useful general pointer to the presence of an underlying endocrine disorder is the presence of associated short stature or recent growth failure, in addition of course to physical signs specific for each condition.

The presence of learning disability, dysmorphic features, or precocious/late puberty is also of concern and should prompt referral to a paediatrician. Most 'simple' obesity in children is, however, best managed by a primary-care multidisciplinary team in the community.

Treating 'obesity' in children

Treatment is unlikely to succeed unless:

- the child and the family want to change;
- the goals set are realistic and acceptable to the child and family;
- the solution is sustainable.

The goals may include maintenance of weight or just slowing of weight gain so that height and weight centiles converge with growth. It is usually inappropriate to aim for weight loss, though if obesity is severe or complications (for example diabetes) are present it may be necessary. Even then, weight loss should be gradual – no more than 500 g per month. Rapid weight loss and strict diets are rarely appropriate for young children. Avoidance of severe energy restriction is especially important in young children and during the pubertal growth spurt, since it may lead to restriction of final height attainment.

Treatment should address the following areas:

Food and eating patterns

- Establish a regular meal pattern, avoiding 'grazing' and snacks.
- Use low-calorie drinks, spreads, and foods, to conserve as far as possible the apparent amount on the plate.
- Substitute complex carbohydrate in the form of whole grains, vegetables, and fruits for products containing fat and refined sugars, such as confectionery (these foods also have the advantage of taking more time to eat!).

Lifestyle changes

- Introduce sustainable changes in moderate activity – such as outdoor rather than sedentary pastimes.
- Increase the activity component in daily life (e.g. walking to school, using stairs).

Psychosocial adjustment

- Obese children may have low self-esteem and are frequently bullied. Dealing with these aspects may necessitate referral of the family for specialist psychological counselling.
- Bariatric surgical intervention is rarely required in childhood obesity, though it might be considered in complicated cases which have not responded to behavioural management.

Preventing obesity

The causes of the secular trend towards increasing BMI and fatness are many but particularly include:

Box 23.22 Obesity

- Defining 'obesity' in children is difficult because:
  - adiposity changes normally with age;
  - there is considerable continuing secular change in body mass;
  - there are no clear disease-risk thresholds.
- BMI charts can be used to adjust for age and sex effects.
- Obesity is associated with complications in childhood, particularly insulin resistance.
- Although most children have simple obesity, some, particularly short, fat children, have underlying disease.
- The treatment of obesity in children demands:
  - motivation of the child and family;
  - a whole-family approach to change in eating patterns;
  - a whole-family approach to change in lifestyle (activity level).
- The aim of treatment should generally be reduced rate of gain, rather than weight loss.
- Excessively strict dieting may restrict height gain and should be avoided, particularly during the adolescent growth spurt.

- A reduction in physical activity associated with increased dependence on motorised transport and indulgence in sedentary pastimes. One study in the USA, for example, showed a statistically significant correlation between BMI and the number of hours children spent watching television.
- An increase in the consumption of snack and convenience foods, high in refined carbohydrate and fat content. Media and peer pressure reinforce this behaviour.

The solutions are therefore complex and lie not just in the hands of individual parents and children but with the government and the commercial sector. Community initiatives facilitating the enhancement of exercise opportunities for children may be particularly important.

Key nutritional points on obesity in children are summarised in Box 23.22.

23.10 Concluding remarks

This chapter has described both normal and abnormal patterns of child growth and development, and touched upon the scope of nutrition as it is currently applied to the prevention and treatment of disease during childhood. Currently our understanding of the interactions between the environment, nutrients, and genes is increasing very rapidly, and this will offer new therapeutic horizons.

Within the childhood era, better understanding of the relationships between nutrition, host defence, and inflammation could enable us to make further inroads into early child mortality – a stage of life at which malnutrition and communicable diseases account for over 80% of deaths and a similar proportion of morbidity.

We will also be able to take a much longer view and turn attention to stemming the epidemic of noncommunicable diseases – such as cardiovascular disease, diabetes, and cancer – accounting for the burden of ill health in later life. In other words, we shall become more concerned with fine-tuning patterns of childhood growth and metabolic development in order to maximise lifelong metabolic fitness, thus optimising functional capacity not just throughout childhood but into the adult years. This will require:

- Specialists in clinical nutrition who can take more of a life cycle view of human growth and development, transcending boundaries of disease-based specialities such as obstetrics, paediatrics, and adult diabetology.
- Development of methods that can be used in a clinical context to measure: (i) the growth of separate body tissues and compartments; (ii) the metabolic relationships between those compartments; and (iii) the factors that control partitioning of nutrients between those compartments.
- The identification of key stages in the life cycle for nutritional interventions.
- The development of interventions that are cost-effective, recognising that the greatest burden of such disease and the accompanying disability will be borne by resource-poor countries.

References and further reading

Bhutta ZA, Ahmed T, Black RE, Cousens S, Dewey K, Giugliani E, et al. What works? Interventions for maternal and child undernutrition and survival. Lancet 2008; 371: 417–440.

Cole TJ. Do growth chart centiles need a face lift? BMJ 1994; 308: 641–642.

Cole TJ, Freeman JV, Preece MA. Body mass index reference curves for the UK, 1990. Arch Dis Child 1995; 73: 25–29.

Cole TJ. A chart to link child centiles of body mass index, weight and height. Eur J Clin Nutr 2002; 56: 1194–1199.

Cole TJ, Bellizzi MC, Flegal KM, Dietz WH. Establishing a standard definition for child overweight and obesity worldwide: international survey. BMJ 2000; 320: 1240–1243.

Dewey KG, Heinig MJ, Nommsen LA, Peerson JM, Lonnerdal B. Breastfed infants are leaner than formula-fed infants at one year of age: the DARLING study. Am J Clin Nutr 1993; 57: 140–145.

Dewey KG, Peerson JM, Brown KH, Krebs NF, Michaelsen KF, Persson LA, et al. Growth of breast-fed infants deviates from current reference data: a pooled analysis of US, Canadian, and European data sets. Pediatrics 1995; 96: 495–503.

Fomon SJ, Ziegler EE. Renal solute load and potential renal solute load in infancy. J Pediatr 1999; 134: 11–14.

Fomon SJ, Haschke F, Ziegler EE, Nelson SE. Body composition of reference children from birth to age 10 years. Am J Clin Nutr 1982; 35: 1169–1175.

Holliday MA. Metabolic rate and organ size during growth from infancy to maturity and during late gestation and early infancy. Pediatrics 1971; 47: 169–179.

Karlberg J, Jalil F, Lam B, Low L, Yeung CY. Linear growth retardation in relation to the three phases of growth. Eur J Clin Nutr 1994; 48: S25–S43.

Koletzko B, Goulet O, Hunt J, Krohn K, Shamir R. Guidelines on paediatric parenteral nutrition of the European Society of Paediatric Gastroenterology, Hepatology and Nutrition (ESPGHAN) and the European Society for Clinical Nutrition and Metabolism (ESPEN). J Pediatr Gastroenterol Nutr 2005; 41: S1–S87.

Kramer MS, Kakuma R. The Optimal Duration of Exclusive Breast-feeding: A Systematic Review. Geneva: World Health Organization, 2002.

McIntosh N, Helms PJ, Smyht RL, Logan S, editors. Forfar & Arneil's Textbook of Paediatrics, 7th edn. Edinburgh: Churchill Livingstone, 2008.

McLaren DS, Burman D, Belton NR, Williams AF, editors. Textbook of Paediatric Nutrition, 3rd edn. Edinburgh: Churchill Livingstone, 1991.

Michaelsen KF, Weaver L, Branca F, Robertson A. Feeding and Nutrition of Infants and Young Children. WHO Regional Publications, European Series, 87. Copenhagen: World Health Organization, 2000.

Ministry of Agriculture Fisheries and Food. The Infant Formula and Follow-on Regulations 1995. Statutory Instrument 77. London: The Stationery Office, 1995.

National Institute for Health and Clinical Excellence. Obesity: Guidance on the Prevention, Identification, Assessment and Management of Overweight and Obesity in Adults and Children (CG 43). London: National Institute for Health and Clinical Excellence, 2006.

National Institute for Health and Clinical Excellence. Improving the Nutrition of Pregnant and Breastfeeding Mothers and Children in Low-income Households (PH11). London: National Institute for Health and Clinical Excellence, 2008.

National Institute for Health and Clinical Excellence. Donor Milk Banks: The Operation of Donor Milk Services (CG93). London: National Institute for Health and Clinical Excellence, 2010.

Scientific Advisory Committee on Nutrition. Application of WHO growth standards in the UK. 1-51. London: The Stationery Office, 2007a.

Scientific Advisory Committee on Nutrition. Update on Vitamin D. Position statement by the Scientific Advisory Committee on Nutrition. 1-44. London: The Stationery Office, 2007b.

Scientific Advisory Committee on Nutrition. Iron and Health. London: The Stationery Office, 2010.

Scientific Advisory Committee on Nutrition. The Influence of Maternal, Fetal and Child Nutrition on the Development of Chronic Disease in Later Life. 1-192. London: The Stationery Office, 2011.

Stein C, Moritz I. A Life Course Perspective of Maintaining Independence in Older Age. Geneva: World Health Organization, 1999. pp. 1–20.

Tanner JM. Foetus into Man: Physical Growth from Conception to Maturity, 2nd edn. Ware: Castlemead, 1989.

Wells JC. A Hattori chart analysis of body mass index in infants and children. Int J Obes Relat Metab Dis 2000; 24: 325–329.

WHO, Department of Child Health and Adolescent Development. Management of the Child with a Serious Infection or Severe Malnutrition. Geneva: World Health Organization, 2000.

WHO, UNICEF. WHO child growth standards and the identification of severe acute malnutrition in infants and children. Geneva: World Health Organization, 2009.

Widdowson EM. Changes in body composition during growth. In: Scientific Foundations of Paediatrics (Davis JA, Dobbing J, eds), 2nd edn. Chapter 17. London: Heinemann, 1981.

Williams AF. Lactation and infant feeding. In: Textbook of Paediatric Nutrition (McLaren DS, Burman D, Belton NR, Williams AF, eds), 3rd edn. Edinburgh: Churchill Livingstone, 1991. pp. 26–27.

24
Cystic Fibrosis

John A Dodge

University of Swansea, UK

Key messages

- The birth incidence of cystic fibrosis (CF) is about 1 in 2500 newborns, and the carrier rate in the population is about 1 in 20 among persons of Caucasian descent, making CF the most common inherited life-shortening disease in many populations.
- The aetiology of malnutrition is complex and arises as a result of the energy imbalance caused by a combination of decreased energy intake, increased energy needs, and increased energy losses.
- Nutritional status is strongly associated with pulmonary function and survival.

- Maintenance of growth patterns as near normal as possible in children and nutritional support in adults, particularly during infection and other adverse complications, are major goals of multidisciplinary care, and along with the physician, nurse, and physiotherapist, the dietitian is one of the key members of the management team.
- Many other complications of CF may require specific nutritional intervention, including diabetes, liver disease, and osteoporosis. Fat-soluble vitamin deficiencies should be anticipated and prevented.

24.1 Introduction

Cystic fibrosis (CF) was first identified in the 1930s as an important cause of failure to thrive, malabsorption of fat, fat-soluble vitamin deficiency, and severe, recurrent, or persistent lung infection in young infants. Affected babies rarely survived beyond a year or two. Autopsy revealed fibrosis and cysts in the pancreas, hence the name. Increasing recognition, improved survival, and greater awareness of the many clinical features which may occur in CF have led to our current understanding of its genetics and pathophysiology, and to realistic hope of new treatments which will control, if not cure, CF in the foreseeable future.

In the twenty-first century, CF is a rare cause of death in infants and young children, and mean survival in western Europe and North America now approaches 40 years (see Box 24.1). In general, survival correlates well with nutritional status, although by far the most important immediate cause of death remains lung damage consequent

on chronic infection. The interaction between nutrition and lung function is complex and will be referred to throughout this chapter, but at all ages there are challenges to nutritional management. Maintenance of growth patterns as near normal as possible in children and nutritional support in adults, particularly during infection and other adverse complications, are central to the prognosis, and along with the physician, nurse, and physiotherapist, the dietitian is one of the key persons in the management team.

24.2 Definition and pathology

CF occurs as a consequence of mutations in a single gene, which codes for the cystic fibrosis transmembrane regulator protein (CFTR), a channel which conveys chloride ions through the cell membrane of epithelial cells, notably in the lungs, intestine, and pancreatic ducts. Impaired transport function of the CFTR channel explains the clinical features of the

Clinical Nutrition, Second Edition. Edited by Marinos Elia, Olle Ljungqvist, Rebecca J Stratton and Susan A Lanham-New.
© 2013 The Nutrition Society. Published 2013 by Blackwell Publishing Ltd.

Box 24.1 Factors contributing to improved survival in cystic fibrosis

- Improved nutritional status at all ages, but particularly in childhood.
- Improved antibiotic treatment.
- Survival of infants with meconium ileus, once usually fatal.
- Early diagnosis.
- Better physiotherapy techniques.
- Frequent surveillance and treatment in specialist CF clinics.
- New modalities of treatment, such as lung transplantation.

Table 24.1 Estimated frequency of CF at birth in different populations.

National group	Birth incidence
UK	1/2500
USA (white)	1/3500
USA (African American)	1/14 000
USA (Asian)	1/25 500
Sweden	1/7700
The Netherlands	1/3600
Ireland	1/1500
Finland	1/25 000
Israel	1/3300
Japan	1/323 000
Faroe Islands	1/1800

disease. Both parents of an affected child must pass on a mutated copy of the gene to their offspring: possession of only one mutation makes an individual, like the parents of a CF child, a healthy carrier (heterozygote). The incidence of CF and the predominant specific mutations of the CFTR gene vary between populations. More than 1000 different mutations have been identified, most of them very rare and some affecting only one family. In the UK the single commonest mutation, about 70% or more of the total, is known as F508del. The birth incidence of CF is about 1 in 2500 newborns, and the carrier rate in the population is about 1 in 20 among persons of Caucasian descent, making CF the most common inherited life-shortening disease. In other populations, notably in Eastern Asia, it is much less common (Table 24.1).

The CFTR channel regulates the passage of chloride through the cell membrane of secretory and absorptive epithelia. Dysfunction of CFTR results in an altered electrolyte and fluid composition of secretions, which are often dehydrated and sticky: an early name for CF, still used in some countries, was mucoviscidosis. Characteristic (but not necessarily unique) pathological features are found in the pancreas, lungs, liver, intestines, and vas deferens, among affected organs, and can superficially be attributed to blockage of small ducts by sticky secretions. Important among affected secretions is sweat, and elevated chloride content of a carefully performed standardised sweat test is the usual diagnostic criterion for CF. This is now usually confirmed by genetic analysis of DNA.

24.3 Clinical features

The clinical features of CF include intestinal obstruction with inspissated meconium in about 15% of affected newborns (meconium ileus); failure to thrive in infancy secondary to malabsorption caused by pancreatic insufficiency; repeated and eventually chronic infective and structural lung disease (bronchiectasis); atresia of the vas deferens, producing infertility in almost all CF males; and excessive salt loss in the sweat, leading to heat intolerance in warm climates or heat waves.

It is the lung disease which is the usual cause of death. Both the respiratory and the nutritional status have an effect on survival, and they are surprisingly closely associated. While progressive lung disease makes extra nutritional demands on CF patients, it may also limit their ability to increase their energy intake. Other, less constant but common clinical features of CF, which affect the patient's nutritional needs, include liver disease, cystic fibrosis-related diabetes mellitus (CFRD) and osteoporosis. The main clinical features of CF are summarised in Box 24.2.

Respiratory features

The lungs are apparently normal at birth, but in undiagnosed and untreated infants they often become infected within the first few weeks, and may go on to become seriously damaged by infection and chronic inflammation. This is the rationale for newborn screening programmes, which allow early diagnosis, with prevention and treatment of infection particularly important during this critical phase. The lungs are still growing in complexity

Box 24.2 The main features of CF

Gastrointestinal

- gastroesophageal reflux;
- pancreatitis;
- pancreatic insufficiency;
- maldigestion;
- malabsorption;
- meconium ileus (newborn infants);
- distal intestinal obstruction syndrome (DIOS);
- cholelithiasis;
- cirrhosis;
- portal hypertension;
- splenomegaly;
- fibrosing colonopathy;
- rectal prolapse.

Respiratory

- bronchiectasis (characteristic infective organisms include *Pseudomonas aeruginosa, Staph. aureus, H. influenzae, Burkholderia cepacia, Aspergillus fumigatus,* and *Stenotrophomonas maltophilia*);
- bronchitis;
- pneumonia;
- atelectasis;
- pneumothorax;
- haemoptysis;
- sinus disease.

Other

- male infertility due to atresia of the vas deferens;
- CFRD;
- osteoporosis, osteopaenia.

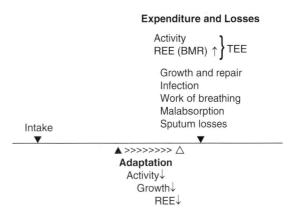

Figure 24.1 Energy balance in CF. REE, resting energy expenditure; BMR, basal metabolic rate; TEE, total energy expenditure. Adapted from Dodge & O'Rawe (1994).

during the first 2 years, and structural damage at this stage will affect lung capacity throughout life. When lung disease is established, as it is eventually in most CF patients, chronic bronchopulmonary inflammation with superimposed periods of acute infection carries an increased energy requirement, but achieving an adequate intake is hindered by breathlessness and poor appetite. Repeated coughing can cause vomiting, and large meals exacerbate shortness of breath: patients always give priority to breathing over eating. Inflamed bronchi may bleed, particularly during episodes of coughing, and frequent loss of small or large amounts of blood can lead to iron-deficiency anaemia. Most patients have chronic sinus disease, which often impairs the senses of taste and smell, which are important to appetite. Figure 24.1 illustrates how respiratory and gastrointestinal factors combine to increase energy requirements, which will produce a negative energy balance if they are not met by a correspondingly enhanced intake.

Gastrointestinal features

Pancreatic insufficiency

This is the major gastrointestinal clinical feature of CF. It results from pancreatic damage resembling chronic pancreatitis, which is usually well established even before birth. Pancreatic insufficiency occurs when more than 95% of the structure or functional capacity of the exocrine pancreas has been lost. Although some degree of pancreatic abnormality is almost universal in CF, the proportion of patients who are pancreatic insufficient (PI) varies between different populations, largely according to their particular genetic mutations. Those who retain adequate pancreatic function for normal digestion are called pancreatic sufficient (PS). In northern Europe, more than 85% of CF patients are PI, but in Mediterranean countries 60% or even more may be PS. Because slow destruction of the pancreas may continue for many years, a person who is PS in early life may become PI later, and thus require pancreatic enzyme supplements.

Pancreatic insufficiency causes maldigestion and malabsorption of macronutrients, particularly fat and protein. Fat malabsorption (steatorrhoea) makes stools bulky and greasy (in severe cases resembling melted butter), floating in water and difficult to flush. Protein malabsorption makes the stools offensive. Other symptoms include flatulence, bloating, and abdominal discomfort. Stool losses of energy – rich fat, along with less energy-dense but nutritionally essential protein – retard the growth of children and impair their ability to resist infection. Fat malabsorption is often accompanied by poor absorption of fat-soluble vitamins. In addition to pancreatic insufficiency causing maldigestion, there is a variable impairment of absorption of the products of intestinal fat digestion, such as glycerol and fatty acids, in the intestine itself, which is well documented but not completely understood. Reduced secretion of bile acids via the liver and biliary system plays a part, by limiting emulsification of lipids and reducing the surface available for attachment of pancreatic lipase.

Several direct and indirect tests are available to assess pancreatic function. Direct tests measuring enzymes and electrolytes in pancreatic secretions, following standardised stimulation, are highly specific but both invasive and occasionally dangerous, and are therefore precluded from routine use. Indirect tests include 72-hour faecal fat analysis, ideally with a known fat intake so that a coefficient of fat absorption (CFA) can be calculated. This is often referred to as a 'gold standard' test, but in practice it is not specific for pancreatic disease and not reproducible, and it is understandably unpopular with patients and laboratory staff. Recent studies have shown that although the CFA is much more consistent in healthy controls, results may vary by up to 40% when repeatedly performed in the same CF patient under identical conditions. An enzyme-linked immunosorbent assay (ELISA) for the detection of pancreatic elastase 1 in stool is useful as a sensitive and specific marker of pancreatic insufficiency, and thus for confirming whether a patient is PS or PI. It is of no value in monitoring efficacy of treatment, for which the CFA has been widely used. If the child patient is growing at a normal velocity, and the adult maintaining body weight and nutritional status, there is no need to perform repeated CFA, particularly in view of its poor reproducibility.

Serum levels of immunoreactive trypsinogen (IRT) are elevated in virtually all newborns with CF, whether they are subsequently PI or PS, indicating that at birth some degree of pancreatic function is present but that enzymes are leaking from the pancreas into the circulation. In PI babies, the IRT levels fall to subnormal or undetectable over the first weeks or months, and these low levels are an indirect confirmation of inadequate pancreatic resources. A raised IRT level in a blood spot is the basis of newborn screening programmes for CF in Europe, North America, and Australasia.

Exocrine pancreatic insufficiency is treated with oral pancreatic enzyme replacement therapy (PERT), which must be taken with all meals and snacks, apart from sugary drinks.

Pancreatitis

Acute attacks of pancreatitis may occur in PS patients, and occasionally in those regarded as PI but in whom some residual pancreatic function must remain. Pancreatitis is more common in adults than in children. Coexisting gallstones can confuse the diagnosis. Slowly progressive chronic pancreatitis is the basis of PS patients becoming PI.

Meconium ileus

This is the name given to a serious condition which affects about 15% of CF newborn infants. They present with a distended abdomen and fail to pass meconium. The colon is empty and contracted, but the small intestine proximal to the ileo-caecal valve is obstructed by thick, sticky meconium, and the small bowel has occasionally ruptured *in utero*, so that the meconium has spilled into the abdominal cavity. Uncomplicated cases can often be treated conservatively with an enema of gastrografin, a radio-opaque fluid with high osmolality, but resistant cases and those with meconium peritonitis need surgery. The convalescence is often stormy, but with modern management the great majority survive what was once a perilous presentation of CF. If extensive surgical resection is necessary, particularly if it includes the ileo-caecal valve, the child may be left with the problems of a short gut with uncertain motility, in addition to those of uncomplicated CF.

Distal intestinal obstruction syndrome

In older children and adults with CF, the distal small bowel and sometimes the proximal colon may become partially or completely obstructed by thick mucofaeculent material composed of sticky secretions and food residues. It may become so adherent to the intestinal mucosa that it cannot be removed without causing bleeding.

Contributory precipitating factors include inadequate PERT, sudden dietary changes, and dehydration. The onset may be abrupt or insidious, following a period of increasing constipation. The patient complains of abdominal cramps, pain, and distension, and a mass (which may be tender) is usually palpable in the lower-right quadrant of the abdomen. Surgeons unfamiliar with CF sometimes perform a laparotomy, suspecting an acute abdominal emergency such as appendicitis. DIOS can be treated with gastrografin, like meconium ileus, which can be given either by mouth or by enema, but the generally preferred treatment is large doses of a commercial bowel-preparation balanced electrolyte solution such as Golytely, given by mouth in the largest tolerable amounts. Following resolution, the patient must be given advice about diet, compliance with PERT, and avoidance of dehydration.

Fibrosing colonopathy

Fibrosing colonopathy (see Fitzsimmons *et al.*, 1997) is a complication of overdosing of pancreatic enzymes, almost always in children. A similar condition with thickening of the ileum is sometimes seen in adults. It may present with watery or mucousy diarrhoea, occasionally bloodstained, which reflects colitis but may be wrongly interpreted as a need for even higher doses of PERT. The condition may be clinically reversible at the colitis stage, but can progress to narrowing and shortening of the colon, with signs and symptoms of intestinal obstruction. The characteristic pathology is dense submucosal fibrosis. It must always be remembered that pancreatic enzymes are normally active in the upper small intestine, but in CF patients given PERT there is a considerable amount of potentially damaging (administered) digestive enzyme activity in the colon, and even in the stools. Fibrosing colonopathy has exceptionally been described in young (PS) CF infants who have never had PERT, following surgical intervention for meconium ileus, presumably caused by rapid transit of endogenous enzymes to the inappropriate location of the colon.

Liver disease

Some degree of fine increased biliary fibrosis is very common at autopsy in CF patients, but only about 5% have serious clinical liver disease (cirrhosis, portal hypertension, and liver failure), for reasons which are not well understood. No clear-cut genetic modifying factors have been identified which determine why it occurs in a minority of patients with common CFTR mutations. Once established, it sometimes progresses quite rapidly, out of proportion to coexisting CF lung disease. Occasionally mild obstructive jaundice occurs in young infants, apparently caused by cholestasis ('biliary sludge'), and serum liver enzymes may be raised. This is usually transient and is not a predictor of later liver disease; nor is the enlarged fatty liver sometimes observed in toddlers, usually with other evidence of poor nutrition. Although its antecedents are uncertain, patients who are going to have major liver problems usually present with appropriate symptoms by their mid-teens, and the incidence of CF liver disease does not greatly increase with improving life expectancy.

The early stages of cholestatic liver disease may be detected through elevated liver enzymes – alkaline phosphatase and γ-glutamyl transferase – and can be reversed by treatment with ursodeoxycholic acid. Gallstones are commonly found in CF and may or may not be symptomatic. Biliary cirrhosis may follow, with portal hypertension ascites and end-stage liver failure. Liver transplants have been successfully performed in CF, including heroic procedures in which liver and bilateral lung transplants were performed in the same operation.

Patients with cirrhosis and hepatosplenomegaly often find eating difficult, as a consequence of a distended abdomen with elevation of the diaphragm.

Liver disease increases the likelihood of deficiencies of fat-soluble vitamins, particularly vitamins D and K. If enteral tube feeding is needed, the presence of oesophageal varices is not a contraindication to using fine-bore soft nasogastric tubes, but gastric varices preclude percutaneous gastrostomy placement.

Gastro-oesophageal reflux

Gastro-oesophageal reflux (GOR) is common in CF. Contributory causes probably include an increased differential between abdominal and thoracic pressures as a result of 'stiff' lungs, postural drainage during physiotherapy, and abdominal distension from flatulence or enlarged liver and spleen. Reflux of acid gastric contents produces oesophagitis, with its complications of vomiting, heartburn, and aspiration into the lungs, which may complicate respiratory disease. Severe bouts of early-morning coughing in patients who had overnight nasogastric tube feeds may provoke reflux and regurgitation.

Oesophagitis is treated with drugs such as proton pump inhibitors, which inhibit acid secretion and allow the oesophageal mucosa to heal.

24.4 Malnutrition

The aetiology of malnutrition in CF is complex, but can be simplified as a combination of increased energy demands and energy losses in the presence of an often decreased dietary intake, giving rise to a negative energy balance (Figure 24.1).

The majority of patients are able to keep themselves in positive energy balance, but failure to do so results in malnutrition.

In children, malnutrition is best defined as a weight-for-height value below 90%. The corresponding definition for adults is a body mass index (BMI) below 20 kg/m^2.

Dietary intake

People with CF are advised to consume a diet high in energy, without fat restriction. Modern enteric-coated enzyme preparations ensure that most dietary fat will be digested in the intestine, although not always in the optimum location, but a variable mucosal element may still impair absorption of the free fatty acids which are the products of fat digestion. Some patients mistakenly follow dietary advice given to the general public, and some, particularly teenage girls, fear obesity and restrict their intake inappropriately.

Many factors may contribute to an inadequate intake, including respiratory infection, gastrointestinal problems, side effects of medication, nausea, reduced sense of taste and/or smell (occasionally due to zinc deficiency, often secondary to sinus disease), and social factors such as peer pressure. Management may need input from a clinical psychologist as well as the dietitian and other members of the CF clinical team.

Energy requirements

Increased oxygen consumption in CF cells in culture and a mean birth weight 0.5 SDS below the general population mean suggest that there may be an intrinsic increased metabolic demand for energy in CF. Energy requirements are also increased during periods of infection and convalescence, and continue to increase with advancing pulmonary disease. Total energy expenditure may increase in some patients, but others compensate by reducing activity. As appetite deteriorates with declining lung function, intake is reduced and a negative energy balance results, particularly during acute exacerbations of chronic pulmonary infection.

Energy losses

Malabsorption remains an important reason for increased energy losses, and even with maximised PERT it has been estimated that up to 10% of ingested energy will not be absorbed. Energy may be lost in the urine if there is poorly-controlled diabetes (CFRD). Losses of energy and protein in the sputum can be considerable, and sputum losses have been estimated to account for up to 274 kcal/day.

24.5 Other nutritional complications of CF

Cystic fibrosis-related diabetes

With steadily increasing survival in CF, the incidence of CFRD is also increasing (see Fischman & Nookala, 2008; O'Riordan et al., 2008). It is estimated that up to 50% of CF patients over 30 years of age have some degree of impaired glucose tolerance, and it is not uncommon even among CF children. Patients who have lung transplants are at particular risk of developing CFRD as a consequence of corticosteroid use for immunosuppression.

While CFRD shares common features with both type 1 and type 2 diabetes, it is a distinct clinical entity. Its primary cause is insulin deficiency caused by atrophy of insulin-producing cells that are centrally situated in the islets of Langerhans: an unusual and distinctive pathology.

The diagnostic criteria used for CFRD are similar to those of type 1 and type 2 diabetes (Box 24.3). Random glucose measurements taken in outpatient

Box 24.3 Diagnostic criteria for the diagnosis of CFRD

- 2-hour postprandial glucose level > 11.0 mmol/l during 75 g oral glucose tolerance test;
- fasting plasma glucose > 7.0 mmol/l on two or more occasions;
- fasting plasma glucose > 7.0 mmol/l and random glucose level > 11.1 mmol/l;
- random glucose level > 11.1 mmol/l on two or more occasions.

Box 24.4 Dietary advice given to patients with CFRD compared with type 1/type 2 diabetes

- High energy intake advised – calorie restriction is never advised to control blood sugars.
- High fat intake is recommended to provide extra calories, since macrovascular disease is not a concern.
- Protein restriction is not recommended because of the potential for malnutrition.
- Salt restriction is never advised.
- Flexible meal plans are necessary, to allow for periods of infection and poor intake.

Box 24.5 Risk factors for CF-related bone disease

- malnutrition;
- gonadal dysfunction;
- reduced physical activity;
- chronic respiratory acidosis;
- glucocorticoid therapy;
- vitamin D deficiency;
- vitamin K deficiency.

clinics are useful for early diagnosis, and fasting and postprandial glucose levels are needed if impaired glucose tolerance or CFRD is suspected. Glucose intolerance may be intermittent, only occurring during times of infection or steroid use.

Micro- and macrovascular complications of CFRD have been observed, and as the CF population ages, it is expected that these will become more common, although the usually rather low cholesterol levels in CF patients may be a mitigating factor.

The medical management of CFRD has usually centred around insulin therapy. Very short-acting insulins given with each meal allow for greater dietary flexibility than when longer-acting preparations are used. Recent evidence suggests that some patients with CFRD can be managed with oral agents and may not need insulin.

The nutritional management should concentrate on optimising and maintaining nutritional status. Some dietary modifications may be necessary to control blood sugar levels, and the intake of refined carbohydrate foods, particularly sugar-containing drinks and foods with a high glycaemic index, may need to be reduced in favour of complex carbohydrates and protein. The dietary advice given to CFRD patients differs significantly from that given to non-CF diabetics (Box 24.4).

Cystic fibrosis-related osteoporosis

Mean bone-mineral density of patients with CF is one or more SDs below that expected for age and sex. Although the precise cause is debatable, Box 24.5 lists some of the possible contributory factors.

Dietetic advice aimed at optimising nutritional status is crucial to the prevention of osteopaenia and osteoporosis. Good compliance with PERT is essential to maximising the absorption of fat-soluble vitamins necessary for bone health. Daily supplementation with 400–2000 IU vitamin D is recommended to keep levels at the higher end of the normal range, and should be reviewed regularly. Vitamin K is also necessary for osteocalcin production, and studies of vitamin K status in CF indicate that it is frequently low.

Steroids are sometimes used, either orally or by inhalation in the management of CF respiratory problems, as well as post-transplant. When this is the case, extra supplements of vitamin D and calcium should be considered.

For more on this subject, see Sermet-Gaudelius et al. (2007).

Eating disorders

Atypical eating patterns sometimes occur among CF patients of different ages, but particularly in young children and adolescent girls. Early identification of eating problems and management by an experienced dietitian and psychologist are essential. See Shearer & Bryon 2004).

Fertility issues

Almost all males with CF are infertile as a consequence of congenital bilateral absence or atresia of the vas deferens. Semen analysis can identify the small number with rare genotypes who may be fertile.

Fertility in females is usually normal. Women considering pregnancy are advised that it may entail a decline in lung function, with potential risk to their own health and to their ability to cope with the demands of motherhood. Pregacy counselling should include carrier screening of the partner. The best scenario for a good outcome for mother and infant is minimal lung disease and a good nutritional status before pregnancy, and if the pregnancy is planned rather than unanticipated, these should be achieved by medical and nutritional initiatives in the pre-conception period. Nutritional management during pregnancy includes folic acid supplementation, as for the general population. There should be close liaison between the CF and obstetric teams, and monitoring should be frequent, with special attention given to blood glucose levels. If weight gain is faltering during pregnancy, oral nutritional supplements should be considerd.

In women with severe CF lung disease and evidence of malnutrition, the outcome of pregnancy is usually poor for both mother and child.

Lung transplantation

Progressive lung disease remains the leading cause of mortality and morbidity in CF, but bilateral lung transplantation offers a new hope for patients with end-stage lung disease. Such patients usually have a poor nutritioonal status. Nutritional support both before and after transplantation improves the prospects of a successful outcome in terms of both survival and quality of life.

Measures which may be needed to achieve an acceptable nutritional state prior to surgery include supplementary oral or intragastric feeds, if necessary via a gastrostomy. Postoperatively, patients will be taking steroids and blood glucose levels must be closely monitored.

Successful transplantation is associated with an obvious improvement in nutritional status, but of course the previous gastrointestinal problems will remain, including the need for pancreatic enzymes and fat-soluble vitamins.

24.6 Nutritional management

The close inverse relationship between nutritional status and the severity of CF lung disease, and hence prognosis, is well established. The aim of nutritional management is therefore to achieve and maintain ideal body weight for height at all ages. Box 24.6 summarises the main goals of nutrition therapy.

Assessment of nutritional status

Body composition and anthropometry

Studies of body composition in CF have shown deficits in total body mass, lean body mass, and body fat. Generally, CF patients weigh less than age- and sex-matched controls. The reliability of electronic anthropometric measurements is poor, perhaps due to variations in body water content, so they are not used in CF except in a research context. Total body potassium (TBK) measurements as a proxy for protein status have identified unsuspected deficits. Bone-mineral density is also reduced, as a result of many contributing factors (Box 24.5).

Height and weight should be measured at every CF clinic visit, and in patients up to 20 years of age the results should be recorded on a growth centile chart. Weight in adults should be expressed as a percentage of the ideal weight for height, and the BMI should be calculated. Categories of weight-for-height measurements ranging from acceptable to severe malnutrition, proposed in an important North American Consensus document on nutrition in CF, are useful (Table 24.2). For BMI, the aim is to keep the CF patient within the normal range of 20–25.

Assessing energy requirements

Some, but not all CF patients have a raised basal metabolic rate (BMR)/resting energy expenditure (REE), which may depend in part on their specific genotype. Despite an elevated REE, total energy expenditure (TEE) may not be increased during

---

Box 24.6 Goals of nutrition therapy in CF

- Achieve and maintain optimal growth in children.
- Achieve and maintain ideal body weight in adults.
- Maximise the potential of the immune system to fight infection.
- Modify nutritional advice in light of related conditions.

Table 24.2 Categories of malnutrition. Ramsey *et al.* (1992).

Category	Percentage of ideal body weight
Acceptable	90–110
Underweight (early malnutrition)	85–89
Mild malnutrition	80–84
Moderate malnutrition	75–79
Severe malnutrition	<75

Box 24.7 Calculation of nutritional requirements

- 150 kcal/kg actual weight for infant;
- REE×1.5 (no acute illness, mild CF lung disease);
- REE×1.75 (infection, recent weight loss, moderate CF lung disease);
- REE×2.0 (acute illness, severe wasting, significant malabsorption);
- Recommended Dietary Allowance (RDA) for age×1.3 (moderate lung disease);
- RDA for age×1.5 (severe lung disease).

---

healthy periods if activity is reduced. Actual energy requirements depend upon TEE. However, in adults with moderate to severe lung disease a high energy and protein intake should be maintained during healthy intervals between infective episodes, to allow for repletion of fat and lean body mass. Infection, stress, and activity make additional demands for energy, and this is reflected in a practical template used in CF (Box 24.7). These calculations of energy requirements do not take account of energy losses though malabsorption, in sputum, or in glycosuria.

Dietary assessment

An annual detailed dietary assessment by an experienced dietitian is a routine component of CF care, and any deficiencies should be addressed. Computerised dietary analysis is a useful aid to calculation of nutritional adequacy. The weight, BMI, and height velocity in children should be documented.

At the same interview, PERT should be reviewed and adjusted in light of the patient's symptoms, including a description of the stools. The untreated PI patient has stools which are both greasy and

offensive. Greasy stools suggest that significant amounts of fat are being excreted, and offensive stools suggest that protein is being lost. If the maximum dose of PERT has been reached (10 000 lipase units/kg/day) and gastrointestinal symptoms persist, further investigations are needed before the dose is increased or adjunct treatment prescribed, because not only do higher doses of PERT carry a risk of fibrosing colonopathy, they rarely improve documented fat absorption (see later).

The Consensus document referred to above provided useful guidelines for when further nutritional intervention is needed and how it should be delivered, which are determined by the patient's clinical progress. In this analysis, the emphasis is on the category and intensity of the intervention indicated (Table 24.3). The various nutritional tools available will be discussed individually next.

Nutritional support

Diet and nutritional supplements

General dietary advice to CF patients is to consume a high-protein, high-calorie diet, without restriction of fat. The importance of maintaining a normal velocity of gain in weight and height during childhood, and maintaining body weight in adults, is emphasised. Patients are encouraged to eat frequent and regular meals and snacks, with appropriate PERT in each case, through individual and specific dietary advice. Early pre-emptive advice and information are needed when extra energy needs can be anticipated, such as puberty in children, participation in active sports – which is to be encouraged – and pregnancy in young women.

If this general dietary regime proves inadequate, supplementary high-energy feeding is needed and the patient has entered the third category in Table 24.3, requiring supportive intervention with energy-rich supplements either by mouth or by enteral tube feeding.

There are many oral preparations available to boost calorie intake. Ideally in CF, a product which also provides extra protein is advised, but most importantly it should be palatable and acceptable to the patient, to ensure compliance. In the short term, oral supplements have been shown to produce weight gain and hasten recovery from acute exacerbations of infection.

Table 24.3 Categories for nutritional management of patients with CF. Adapted from Am J Clin Nutr (1992; 55: 108–116), American Society for Nutrition.

Category	Target group	Goals
Routine management	All CF patients	Nutritional education, dietary counselling, PERT (PI patients), vitamin supplements
Anticipatory guidance	Patients at risk of energy imbalance Frequent pulmonary infections Periods of rapid growth, but maintaining a weight/height index > 90% ideal weight	Further education to prepare patients for increased energy needs, increased monitoring of dietary intake, increased caloric density of diet as needed, behavioural assessment and counselling
Supportive intervention	Patients with decreased weight velocity and/or a weight/height index < 90% of ideal weight	All of the above plus oral supplements as needed
Rehabilitative care	Patients with a weight/height index consistently < 85% of ideal weight	All of the above plus nocturnal enteral supplementation via nasogastric tube or gastrostomy
Resuscitative and palliative care	Patients with a weight/height index < 75% ideal weight or progressive nutritional failure	All of the above plus continuous enteral feeds or total parenteral nutrition (TPN)

Enteral nutrition

When diet and oral supplements fail to achieve or maintain desired nutritional goals, supplementary enteral feeding should be considered. When weight falls below 85% ideal weight for height, or the BMI falls to 19 kg/m² or below, overnight enteral feeding via a nasogastric tube or percutaneous gastrostomy should be recommended. If the nutritional setback is likely to be temporary, the nasogastric route may be preferred, but most often it is likely to be a longer-term measure and the gastrostomy approach will prove more comfortable for the patient. Experience shows that sustained weight gain and stabilising or reduction of decline in lung function can be expected, but only if the decision to embark on enteral feeding is taken in good time. As a rule of thumb, enteral feeding should be discussed with the patient as soon as the suggestion is raised by a member of the CF team, and results are better the earlier it is instituted. Gastrostomy tubes can be inserted endoscopically or surgically, and are generally well tolerated with few complications. Low-profile 'button' devices are the most acceptable to patients and the least cosmetically obtrusive of options. GOR can be a problem after overnight feeds, particularly with morning physiotherapy and coughing, but adapting gastrostomy tubes with a post-pyloric jejunal extension allows feeds to be given more distally. The type of feed given must be carefully planned. Whole-protein polymeric feeds can be successful in some patients, and clearly require PERT for digestion in PI patients – the great majority. Semi-elemental formulas are popular, and

include nutrients which are relatively easily digested and absorbed, such as medium-chain triglycerides, thus allowing smaller doses of PERT to be used. Fully elemental formulas can also be used when necessary. Enteral feeds are usually given overnight, allowing the patient full mobility during the day, during which a full normal diet should be taken as before. The PERT is usually taken by mouth in divided doses at the beginning and end of the infusion, in amounts calculated according to the type and quantity of the feed. Like steroid treatment, enteral feeding sometimes precipitates development of CF-related diabetes, and for those with impaired glucose tolerance or CFRD, blood sugar levels must be monitored carefully and extra insulin given as needed to avoid hyperglycaemia (see Morton, 2009).

Pancreatic enzyme therapy

Some degree of pancreatic dysfunction probably affects all people with CF, but not all need supplementary replacement enzymes. Patients are divided into two categories: PS and PI. In the UK and northern Europe (and populations elsewhere of northern European origin), PI patients comprise the great majority, and they need PERT with all meals and snacks. PS patients, on the other hand, are in the majority among CF populations of southern European and Mediterranean origin, and retain enough exocrine pancreatic function to be able to digest meals adequately without PERT.

The recommended dose of enzymes is individualised according to response, but should not exceed

Box 24.8 Some factors influencing the effectiveness of PERT

- age of product since manufacture;
- composition of meal;
- dissolution of enteric coating;
- rate and pattern of gastric emptying;
- gastric lipase secretion;
- duodenal pH;
- residual exocrine pancreatic secretion;
- intestinal mucus;
- intestinal motility;
- mucosal uptake of products of digestion;
- differential efficacy of lipase and protease;
- bile-acid secretion;
- concomitant medication.

Box 24.9 Recommendations for PERT (IU lipase)

- infants/milk 2500–3000 IU lipase/120 ml;
- meal 500–2500 IU lipase/kg;
- snack 250–1250 IU lipase/kg;
- dietary fat 500–4000 IU lipase/g;
- maximum dose/kg body weight/day 10 000 IU lipase;
- maximum total dose/day up to 250 000 IU lipase.

Source: Borowitz *et al.* (2002), Shearer & Bryon (2004).

2500 lipase units per kilogram body weight per main meal, or 10 000 units/kg/day. Some CF centres adjust the PERT dose to the fat content of the meal. It must be remembered that the effectiveness of enzymes is modified by many dietary and physiological variables, which make precise dosage impossible (Box 24.8).

The pattern of gastric emptying varies between individuals: passage of enzymes from the stomach into the duodenum may precede, follow, or ideally accompany passage of partially digested food. Also, some patients appear to digest and absorb fat quite efficiently, but excrete a significant amount of protein, while in others the opposite is the case. All of these observations are based on research studies, and we do not know whether the same patients would follow the same patterns of gastric emptying or relative efficacy of fat and protein absorption if the same studies were repeated. A further problem with attempting precise PERT dosage is that most currently available products are unstable. They are essentially particles of desiccated hog pancreas (microspheres) which have been enteric coated, to protect them from inactivation by gastric acid, and put into gelatine capsules. During the course of their shelf life, the enzymes gradually degrade, which means that in order to deliver the dose of lipase and protease stated on the package when their shelf life expires, they must be overfilled when they leave the factory 18 months earlier. This overfilling can be in excess of 50%, so that the patient may be taking 150% of the dose which the physician prescribed if a fresh batch has been dispensed. The pragmatic approach is to ensure that the patient is taking enough capsules of

the prescribed strength, but not too many, and to accept that PERT, unlike other prescribed pharmaceuticals, is inevitably approximate rather than precise (see Box 24.9 for recommended doses). If children are growing normally, and if adults are maintaining their body weight, they are absorbing enough macronutrients for their needs. A caution about exceeding the recommended maximum dose of enzymes has been given, and higher doses should be prescribed only if quantitative tests, such as a CFA (with all its limitations), demonstrate substantially improved absorption. Enzymes are best given at the beginning and during the course of a meal. Capsules may be opened if they cannot be swallowed whole, but enzymes should then be swallowed from a spoon, mixed with a little food if necessary. The microsphere contents should not be crushed or chewed.

Alternative sources of enzymes

Attempts have been made to develop 'artificial' PERT products using single and multiple lipases and proteases derived from bacterial, fungal, or other sources. Such enzymes are more stable, but they have the serious theoretical disadvantage that they do not include the quantitatively minor but possibly important other enzymes, such as elastase, which are present in animal pancreatic secretions. Overall, they have proved disappointing in clinical research trials and have not been accepted for routine use. A more promising initiative is improving the stability of hog-pancreas products.

24.7 Vitamin supplementation

The earliest clinical description of CF was published under the heading 'Vitamin A Deficiency in Children', and there have been many subsequent reports of fat-soluble vitamin deficiencies as a presenting or complicating feature. It is primarily a direct result of fat malabsorption caused by pancreatic insufficiency, but there may be increased demands for the antioxidant vitamin E and other vitamins as a consequence of organ involvement in CF.

With modern PERT and the routine use of multivitamin preparations in CF, clinical evidence of deficiency states is rare, but careful clinical monitoring may still reveal unsuspected night blindness as a feature of vitamin A deficiency, and biochemical tests may indicate deficiency of vitamin D in asymptomatic patients. CF patients are at particular risk of developing clinical or subclinical vitamin deficiencies if:

(1) The diagnosis is made late; even infants diagnosed within the first weeks of life often have subclinical deficiency of vitamin E and occasionally vitamin A.
(2) They have had previous bowel resection, usually for meconium ileus or intestinal atresia.
(3) There is poor compliance with PERT or vitamin supplements.
(4) There is liver disease.

The European Consensus statement on nutrition in patients with CF, published in 2002, made recommendations for vitamin supplements (Table 24.3), which are summarised in Table 24.4.

Serum levels of the fat-soluble vitamins A, D, and E should be checked at least annually, and more frequently if abnormal, and doses of supplements regulated accordingly. This applies to PS patients as well as those who are PI, because low levels might indicate that pancreatic function has deteriorated and the patient may need PERT.

Vitamin A and beta-carotene

'Vitamin A' (retinol) includes retinoids and carotenoids. One of the first symptoms of vitamin A deficiency is night blindness, which may be unreported unless specifically sought. Deficiency also causes dryness and roughening of epithelial surfaces, including the skin and conjunctiva (xerophthalmia), and increases susceptibility to respiratory infections.

In the digestive tract, vitamin A and carotenoids aggregate with digested lipids into globules (micelles), which are absorbed into enterocytes in the upper small intestine. Malabsorption of vitamin A is therefore an expected consequence in PI patients who are inadequately treated with PERT. After absorption into the enterocytes, vitamin A is transported to the liver and stored, before being bound to a specific protein (retinol-binding protein, RBP) and released into the circulation for transport to other tissues. RBP synthesis in the liver cells is often poor in CF, and may be related to zinc deficiency or general protein depletion. A paradoxical situation is then seen, in which serum levels of retinol are low, but large amounts are stored in the liver and unable to get out. If the low serum levels of vitamin A are automatically treated with extra supplements, toxic levels in the liver may follow. This is of particular importance when dealing with pregnant women with CF, because excessively high vitamin A concentrations are harmful to the developing foetus.

Beta-carotene is a precursor of retinol and is also effective as an antioxidant in its own right. Plasma levels of beta-carotene are low in almost all PI patients. The consensus view is that routine supplementation of beta-carotene may reduce lipid peroxidation of cell membranes and help to preserve their essential fatty acids. Multivitamin products designed for CF patients (such as ADEKs and Aquadeks) include beta-carotene. The recommended dose of vitamin A varies between 4000 and 10 000 IU/day, given as a single dose in the form of a water-soluble preparation if possible. Daily doses of more than 20 000 IU should be avoided if RBP is low.

Table 24.4 Current recommendations for vitamin doses. RDA, Recommended Dietary Allowance. Reprinted from J Cystic Fibrosis, vol 1, Sinaasappel M *et al.* Nutrition in patients with cystic fibrosis: a European Consensus, p51–75. Copyright 2002, with permission from Elsevier.

Vitamin	CF patients needing supplements	Recommended dose
Vitamin A	PI	4000–10 000 IU daily
Vitamin D	PI (and PS in northern countries)	400–800 IU daily
Vitamin E	PI and PS	100–400 IU daily
Vitamin K	PI, cholestasis, all(?)	0.1 mg/week to 1 mg/day (no consensus)
Water-soluble vitamins	PI and PS	200% RDA

Vitamin D

Observations of increased prevalence of low bone density and osteoporosis among CF patients have renewed interest in vitamin D deficiency. Contributory factors include malabsorption of fats and fat-soluble vitamins, inadequate calcium intake, inadequate exposure to sunlight, and, in a minority of cases, CF liver disease.

Vitamin D levels should be maintained towards the upper end of the normal range to ensure optimum bone health, but this cannot always be achieved by routine supplementation at the recommended standard dosage.

The consensus standard recommendation for vitamin D supplementation in CF is 400–800 IU/day, but serum levels must be monitored and supplements adjusted accordingly. Up to 2000 IU/day may be needed, particularly in patients with liver disease. Bone health should also be monitored by occasional DEXA scans, particularly when low levels of vitamin D are noted on routine testing.

Vitamin E

'Vitamin E' includes several fat-soluble tocopherols, of which alpha-tocopherol is the most bioactive form, and the one routinely measured in CF. Like vitamin A, it is an antioxidant and is utilised in the quenching of damaging free oxygen radicals released during inflammation. Turnover of vitamin E is increased in CF, including in PS patients, and low levels have been noted within the first weeks of life. Chronic deficiency of vitamin E results in irreversible damage to spinocerebellar tracts in the central nervous system, which has been observed in CF patients who were not taking supplements. It may also ameliorate the progression of damage to bronchial and alveolar cell membranes in the lungs, caused by free radicals released by neutrophils as part of the host inflammatory response. In young infants, particularly in those born prematurely, vitamin E deficiency is a cause of haemolytic anaemia, and this is occasionally seen in CF infants. Correction of the deficiency results in increased erythrocyte survival time and a rise in haemoglobin levels.

The recommended dose of vitamin E is within the range of 100 to 400 IU/day, ideally given as a water-miscible preparation at mealtimes, with PERT.

Standard multivitamin preparations do not contain sufficient amounts of vitamin E so additional supplements are needed, and there are no serious toxicity issues.

Vitamin K

Vitamin K is necessary for prothrombin synthesis. It is also a co-factor in carboxylation of osteocalcin, during bone formation, and its deficiency may be an important factor in osteopaenia and osteoporosis in CF. It is particularly likely to be deficient in patients with liver disease, and its absorption can be impaired by broad-spectrum antibiotics, which are widely used in CF. It is therefore not surprising that investigations have shown that more than 75% of CF patients with PI are deficient in vitamin K. Unfortunately, its measurement in blood samples, using the protein induced in vitamin K absence test (PIVKA II), is a difficult laboratory procedure that is not widely available for routine monitoring. The need for routine prescription of vitamin K in CF is now generally accepted (see Conway et al., 2005).

Water-soluble vitamins

There are occasional reports of water-soluble vitamin deficiencies in CF, but these are usually subclinical. An exception is vitamin B_{12} deficiency, which may occur in patients who have needed resection of the terminal ileum in the course of surgery for meconium ileus or later in life. With that exception, routine prescription of water-soluble vitamins should not be needed if the patient is taking a good mixed diet.

Multivitamins

Good medical practice is to supplement vitamins singly and only when they are shown to be deficient. An exception is made for CF because multiple deficiencies can be anticipated and patients take so many medications that compliance is easier if several can be usefully combined. Various products are available but none is universally suitable for the needs of every patient, and it cannot be assumed that vitamin levels will be satisfactory unless they are regularly monitored and adjustments are made as indicated (see Sagel et al., 2011).

24.8 Minerals

The minerals most likely to need supplementation in CF are iron, zinc, and selenium.

Iron

Iron deficiency, defined by low serum ferritin levels, is not uncommon in CF and may affect up to a third of patients. It may be a consequence of poor intake, chronic infection, or bleeding from oesophageal varices or another intestinal or pulmonary source. PERT can interfere with iron absorption.

Haemoglobin and ferritin levels should be regularly reviewed, but because iron is an essential substrate for the growth of *Pseudomonas aeruginosa*, a major CF pathogen, supplementation is advised only if there is evidence of iron deficiency.

Zinc

Zinc is a component of many important body enzymes, and its deficiency adversely affects growth. In normal situations, zinc absorption from the diet is in the region of 25–30%. Zinc absorption is affected by diarrhoea, intestinal mucosal abnormalities including short bowel syndrome, and malnutrition, so it may be compromised in patients with CF. Nutritional deficiency of zinc in non-CF children adversely affects linear growth, puberty in males, and wound healing. Zinc absorption is improved by PERT. Zinc status appears to deteriorate when CF lung disease worsens and it has an apparent but not fully understood relationship to essential fatty acid status. Serum and plasma levels of zinc are a notoriously unreliable indicator of total body zinc, and are affected by the acute-phase response, regardless of nutrition. Zinc is included in proprietary multivitamin products for CF and further supplementation should be considered in CF children and adolescents with growth retardation and delayed puberty.

Selenium

Small supplements of selenium are included in commercial multivitamin preparations, and are probably beneficial, but large overdoses of selenium can be fatal. Selenium is an essential component of the antioxidant glutathione peroxidase, which is secreted on to the bronchial and other epithelial surfaces, including the pancreatic duct, like chloride, through the CFTR channel. Glutathione secretion is therefore absent or much reduced in CF, and may explain the vulnerability of the bronchial mucosa to infection and oxidative damage, as well as the increased requirement for vitamin E as a replacement antioxidant. Dietary selenium deficiency is a rare but well-documented cause of cardiomyopathy, and it occurs in some regions where there is a lack of selenium in the soil (Keshan disease). There is no evidence to support additional selenium supplementation as a routine in CF, because the problem is one of secretion of selenium-containing glutathione, not its deficiency. The cell-membrane 'essential' polyunsaturated fatty acids include arachidonic acid (AA), from the *n*-6 series, and docoso-hexaenoic acid (DHA), from the *n*-3 series, and an imbalance between these constituents has been observed in CF patients and experimental animal models. This may be explained by differential oxidation caused by the absence of glutathione secretion, but some early reports, though not all, suggest clinical benefit from *n*-3 dietary supplements. At the present time there is no consensus recommendation.

24.9 Infant feeding

European and North American recommendations are that whenever possible infants with CF should be breast fed. Exclusive breast feeding of both PI and PS babies seems to delay colonisation of the lungs with *P. aeruginosa* and promote normal growth, but after 2 months' breast feeding, PI infants may need additional formula supplements to maintain weight gain. Special considerations apply to babies with meconium ileus, particularly if they have had surgery. Fat-soluble vitamin supplements should be started as soon as the diagnosis is made, irrespective of the need for PERT. See Colombo *et al.* (2007).

24.10 Concluding remarks

In the foreseeable future, it is unlikely that the nutritional approaches used in the management of CF will change significantly, although techniques and products will continue to improve. CF is a genetic condition which cannot be cured, but there are very real prospects of new drugs which will control the effects of CFTR dysfunction on the lungs (and possibly any remaining functioning exocrine pancreas), although whether such drugs might safely be given to an unborn foetus is questionable. The deleterious effect of lung disease on nutrition would then be mitigated.

Nutritional support of young children with pancreatic insufficiency established at birth will therefore continue to be a priority, helped by early diagnosis of CF through neonatal screening, which is now widely practised in relevant countries.

Acknowledgements

This chapter has been revised and updated by John A Dodge, based on the original chapter by Olive Tully and Julie Dowsett.

References and further reading

Aldámíz-Ecchevarria L, Prieto JA, Andrade F, Elorz J, Sojo A, Lage S, et al. Persistence of essential fatty acid deficiency in cystic fibrosis despite nutritional therapy. Pediatr Res 2009: 66: 585–589.

Borowitz D, Baker RD, Stallings V. Consensus report on nutrition for pediatric patients with cystic fibrosis. J Pediatr Gastroenterol Nutr 2002; 35: 246–259.

Colombo C, Costantini D, Zazzeron L, Faelli N, Russo MC, Ghisleni D, et al. Benefits of breastfeeding in cystic fibrosis: a single-centre follow-up survey. Acta Paediatr 2007; 96: 1228–1232.

Conway SP, Wolfe SP, Brownlee KG, White H, Oldroyd B, Truscott JG, et al. Vitamin K status among children with cystic fibrosis and its relationship to bone mineral density and bone turnover. Pediatrics 2005; 115: 1325–1331.

Dodge JA. Pancreatic enzyme therapy in cystic fibrosis Expert Rev Resp Med 2008; 2: 681–683.

Dodge JA, O'Rawe AM. Energy requirements in cystic fibrosis. In: Cystic Fibrosis – Current Topics, vol. 2 (Dodge JA, Brock DJH, Widdecombe JH, eds). London: John Wiley & Sons, Ltd, 1994.

Dodge JA, Turck D. Cystic fibrosis: nutritional consequences and management. Best Practice & Research Clinical Gastroenterology 2006; 20: 531–546.

Dowsett J. An overview of nutritional issues for the adult with cystic fibrosis. Nutrition 2000; 16: 566–570.

Fischman D, Nookala VK. Cystic fibrosis-related diabetes mellitus: etiology, evaluation and management. Endocrin Pract 2008; 14: 1169–1179.

Fitzsimmons SC, Burkhart GA, Borowitz D, Grand RJ, Hammerstrom T, Durie PR, et al. High-dose pancreatic-enzyme supplements and fibrosing colonopathy in children with cystic fibrosis. New Eng J Med 1997; 336: 1283–1289.

Gozdzik J, Cofta S, Piorunek T, Batura-Gabryel H, Kosicki J. Relationship between nutritional status and pulmonary function in cystic fibrosis. J Physiol Pharmacol 2008; 59(Suppl. 6): 253–260.

Kalnins D, Durie PR, Pencharz P. Nutritional management of cystic fibrosis patients. Curr Opin Clin Nutr Metab Care 2007; 10: 348–354.

Lai HJ, Shoff SM, Farrell PM. Recovery of birth weight z score within 2 years of diagnosis is positively associated with pulmonary status at 6 years of age in children with cystic fibrosis, Pediatrics 2009; 123: 714–722.

Maqbool A, Stallings VA. Update on fat-soluble vitamins in cystic fibrosis. Curr Opin Pulm Med 2008; 14: 574–581.

Morton AM. Symposium 6. Young people, artificial nutrition and transitional care. The nutritional challenges of the young adult with cystic fibrosis. Proc Nutr Soc 2009; 68: 430–440.

Munck A. Nutritional considerations in patients with cystic fibrosis. Expert Rev Respir Med 2010; 4: 47–50.

O'Riordan SM, Robinson PD, Donaghue KC, Moran A. Clinical Practice Consensus. Management of cystic-fibrosis-related diabetes. Pediatr Diabetes 2008; 9: 338–344.

Ramsey BW, Farrell PM, Pencharz P. Nutritional assessment and management of cystic fibrosis: a consensus report. Am J Clin Nutr 1992; 55: 108–116.

Sagel SD, Sontag MK, Anthony MM, Emmett P, Papas KA. Effect of an antioxidant-rich multivitamin supplement in cystic fibrosis. J Cystic Fibrosis 2011; 10: 31–36.

Sermet-Gaudelius I, Souberbielle JC, Ruiz JC, Vrielynck S, Heuillon B, Azhar I, et al. Low bone mineral density in young children with cystic fibrosis. Am J Respir Crit Care Med 2007; 175: 951–957.

Shearer JE, Bryon M. The nature and prevalence of eating disorders and eating disturbance in adolescents with cystic fibrosis J Roy Soc Med 2004; 97(Suppl. 44): 36–42.

Sinaasappel M, Stern M, Littlewood J, Wolfe S, Steinkamp G, Hiejerman HGM, et al. Nutrition in patients with cystic fibrosis: a European Consensus. J Cystic Fibrosis 2002; 1: 51–75.

Stallings VA, Stark LJ, Robinson KA, Feranchak AP, Quinton H. Evidence-based practice recommendations for nutrition-related management of children and adults with cystic fibrosis and pancreatic insufficiency: results of a systematic review. J Am Diet Assoc 2008; 108: 832–839.

25
Illustrative Cases

Simon P Allison

Formerly University of Nottingham and Queen's Medical Centre, UK

Key messages

- A simple and rapid screening process, linked to an action plan, is the first step in alerting staff to the possibility that a patient is at nutritional risk.
- A patient who screens at risk may then need a more detailed and expert nutritional assessment, taking into account anthro-
- pometry, biochemistry and haematology, clinical picture, and dietary intake.
- The results of the nutritional assessment will determine the level of nutritional support or dietary counselling required and allow a clinical management plan to be developed.

25.1 Introduction

The purpose of this chapter is to give the reader the opportunity to apply the knowledge gained from previous chapters to real clinical situations with all their challenging variety and interest. As in other branches of medicine, accurate diagnosis of nutritional problems, obtained from the full range of history, examination, and investigations, is the key to appropriate and successful treatment. Amidst the host of patients attending clinics, admitted as emergencies, or suffering the consequences of disease and its treatment, a large proportion have problems of nutritional excess, deficiency, or imbalance which affect their long-term health or the outcome of their current disease. A simple and rapid screening process, linked to action plans, is the first step in alerting staff to the possibility that the patient is at nutritional risk. You would be rightly criticised for failing to test urine or blood for glucose and missing the diagnosis of diabetes. The same principle applies to malnutrition.

A patient who screens at risk may then need a more detailed and expert assessment, leading to a clinical decision and management plan. This process will be applied to each of the patients described in

this chapter, beginning with the screening tool we use for inpatients (Box 25.1) to identify those with actual or potential protein-energy deficit or excess. This addresses the following questions:

- Where is the patient now? Body mass index (BMI) or some surrogate such as mid-arm circumference (MAC).
- Where has the patient come from? Percentage weight change over the previous 3–6 months.
- Where is the patient going? This depends on change in appetite and food intake, as well as disease severity.

In addition, micronutrient deficiencies may be suspected from the history (e.g. alcoholism or restrictive diet), and other factors need to be considered at the extremes of life (e.g. growth velocity and development in children, and poor dentition, swallowing problems, and disability in the elderly). For these reasons, illustrative growth charts are included with Case 1 and the mini nutritional screening tool for the elderly with Case 3.

Further assessment will include not only nutritional requirements but the consequences of under-nutrition (e.g. muscle weakness) and over-nutrition (e.g. complications of obesity). A similar format will

---

Clinical Nutrition, Second Edition. Edited by Marinos Elia, Olle Ljungqvist, Rebecca J Stratton and Susan A Lanham-New.
© 2013 The Nutrition Society. Published 2013 by Blackwell Publishing Ltd.

Box 25.1 Nutrition screening tool for adults

Is YOUR patient at nutritional risk?

Q1   a   **Height**

      □. □□ metres

Q2   a   **Weight**

      □ □. □ kg

Q1   b   □ Estimated or

      □ Measured

Q2   b   □ Estimated or

      □ Measured

Q3   **Body mass index** (BMI) = kg/m^2 □□

    (refer to ready-reckoner)

	Score	
Greater than 20	□	0
18–20	□	2
Less than 18	□	3

Q4   **Food intake** – has this decreased over the last month prior to admission or since the last review (or is the patient NBM)?

	Score	
No	□	0
Yes	□	1
Not known	□	2

Q5   Has the patient **unintentionally lost weight** over the last 3 months or since the last review?

    Up to ½ stone (3 kg)

    More than ½ stone (3 kg)

	Score	
No	□	0
A little	□	1
A lot	□	2

Q6   **Stress factor/severity of illness**

	Score	
None	□	0
Moderate	□	1

(Minor or uncomplicated surgery, minor infection, chronic disease, pressure sores, CVA, inflammatory bowel disease, other gastrointestinal disease, cirrhosis, renal failure, COPD, diabetes)

Severe	□	2

(Multiple injuries, multiple fractures, burns, head injury, multiple deep-pressure sores, severe sepsis, malignant disease, severe dysphagia, pancreatitis, postoperative complications)

Q7   **TOTAL SCORE**   □

Review patient in three days

Q8   **Action**

If score 0–2	Repeat screening within 7 days	□
If score 3–4	Keep food-record charts and start supplements if food intake poor	□
If score ≥ 5	Refer for expert advice	□

Reprinted with permission from Schofield (1985) © Nature Publishing Group.

therefore be applied to each case, under the following headings:

- screening;
- nutritional assessment;
- problems to be addressed;
- clinical decision;
- nutritional requirements;
- treatment;
- monitoring and outcome;
- learning points.

Cases are grouped according to problem category.

25.2 Children

Case 1

A healthy eight-year-old boy, in the 50th centile for height and weight, presented to the clinic feeling unwell with diarrhoea and abdominal pain after eating. Radiological and laboratory investigations led to a diagnosis of Crohn's disease, necessitating treatment with steroids and later with mesalazine and azathioprine. There was a series of exacerbations and remissions over the years. Between the ages of 8 and 17 years, his growth velocity fell to less than 2 cm per year, so that at the age of 17 he was below the third centile for height and weight, had no sexual development, and had a radiological bone age of only 12 years. Inflammatory markers including C-reactive protein (CRP) were raised and the serum albumin was low at 29 g/l.

Screening

Screening tools for adults are not so useful in the growing child, in whom changes in growth rate, development, and bone age are more useful. Nonetheless, at 17 years, with a BMI of 16.5 kg/m², slight weight loss of 2% over 3 months, poor appetite and diminished food intake, and moderately severe disease, he still scored 6 on the tool in Box 25.1. Considered alongside the data on growth failure, this puts him at high nutritional risk.

Nutritional assessment

The history, examination, laboratory tests, and nutritional data at the age of 17 led to a clear diagnosis of disease-related malnutrition whose main manifestation was delayed growth and development. Previously, his doctors had focused on the treatment of the underlying disease process and had ascribed growth failure largely to this and the treatment with steroids

and immunosuppressants. The doctor who saw him for the first time at the age of 17 realised that the effect of his disease on food intake and catabolic rate was the major cause of his growth failure and that this might be corrected by nutritional support.

Problems to be addressed

- Active Crohn's disease, causing low food intake and increased catabolic rate.
- Anti-anabolic effects of steroids and immunosuppressants.
- Undernutrition, causing failure of growth and development.

Nutritional requirements

These should be calculated on the basis of his biological age of 12, the repair of nutritional deficit, and the needs for growth and development catch-up. His estimated requirements were 2630 kcal (11.0 MJ) and 65 g protein per day. It was also likely that he needed vitamin and mineral supplements, including vitamin D and calcium. Elemental diets (i.e. glucose and amino acids) were shown to have benefit in Crohn's disease, but later studies have suggested that polymeric diets (oligosaccharides, fat, and whole protein) may be just as effective.

Treatment

In view of his anorexia, treatment began with the use of a nasogastric polymeric feed of 1000 kcal (4.2 MJ) and 70 g protein/l, starting slowly at 25 ml/hour and building gradually over a week to 100 ml/hour for 16 hours a day, allowing normal oral intake when desired. Once initial improvement had been obtained after 4 weeks, the nasogastric feed was discontinued and oral intake was continued using food of high energy and protein density, supported by proprietary oral supplements. The management of his underlying Crohn's disease continued in the previous manner.

Monitoring and outcome

Height, weight, growth velocity, and sexual development were used as the main criteria of response to treatment (Figure 25.1). His growth velocity returned rapidly to normal and he regained some lost ground, reaching the fifth centile for height. This illustrates the phenomenon described by Widdowson in which, with delays in growth through malnutrition, renutrition may restore growth velocity, but the patient will never reach

(a)

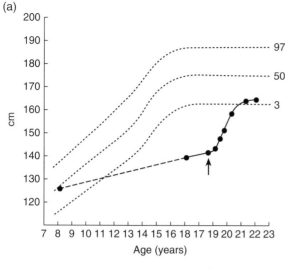

(b)

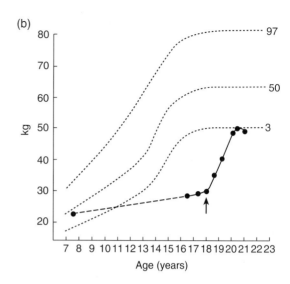

(c)

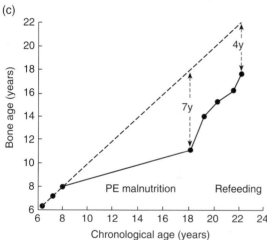

Figure 25.1 Illustrative growth charts for Case 1, showing (a) height, (b) weight, and (c) bone age compared to age.

an ultimate height commensurate with genetic potential – remember the patient started at the 50th centile.

Over the next 2 years he entered puberty, his bone age advanced, and his epiphyses closed with cessation of growth by the age of 20.

Learning points

- Failure of growth and development are the main manifestations of malnutrition in children.
- It is not always just the disease and its treatment that are responsible for the clinical manifestations of illness, but can also be the secondary malnutrition.
- Serum albumin is low because of inflammation and protein-losing enteropathy, rather than malnutrition (see later cases).

- Nutritional support, where appropriate, can be extremely effective and is an important part of management.
- Early diagnosis and treatment of malnutrition is essential if unnecessary loss of growth potential is to be prevented.

25.3 Anorexia of psychological origin and refeeding syndrome

Case 2

A young woman aged 22 had started to lose weight in her mid-teens, when anorexia nervosa was diagnosed. She was being followed up, appropriately, by a psychiatrist with a special experience in eating disorders. Her menstruation had ceased at the age of 16 as her BMI fell below 17 kg/m^2. BMI continued in the range $15–17 \text{ kg/m}^2$ until 6 months before admission, when her condition worsened. She became very weak and her family and carers feared for her life.

Screening
On admission, her height was 1.66 m and her weight 29 kg, giving a BMI of 11.0 kg/m^2. Screening score was estimated at 7 and she was referred for more detailed assessment and for nutritional support.

Nutritional assessment
Life-threatening malnutrition. Life-saving artificial nutritional support indicated.

Problems to be addressed
- severe anorexia nervosa;
- life-threatening malnutrition.

Clinical decision
She agreed to accept nasogastric feeding. Since in the UK, legally, anorexia nervosa comes under the Mental Health Act, sectioning the patient and feeding under sedation, without the patient's consent, is not only legal and ethical, but mandatory if the patient's life is deemed to be at risk, since survival below a BMI of 10 kg/m^2 in women is unusual.

Nutritional requirements
Estimated resting energy expenditure (REE) (calculated by Schofield predictive equation, see Table 25.1) was 912 kcal (3.8 MJ), although with such severe malnutrition it might be 10–15% below this. Assuming $1.5 \times \text{REE}$ for weight gain, the target intake should be approximately 1500 kcal (6.3 MJ) and 1.5 g protein/kg, or 45 g protein.

Treatment
An oral multivitamin preparation and folate were prescribed. A standard polymeric enteral feed of 4.2 kJ/ml was started at 30 ml/hour and increased to 60 ml/hour over the next 3 days. Oral intake was encouraged by day.

Monitoring and outcome
After 3 days of enteral feeding using a standard polymeric feed of 4.2 kJ/ml, starting at 50 ml/hour and increasing slowly to 80 ml/hour, she had gained 2 kg in weight and oedema was observed. At the same time, potassium and phosphate levels fell (see Table 25.2), necessitating intravenous supplementation with potassium phosphate.

After a week she became more active and lively, and after 3 weeks she was transferred to the psychiatric unit for further treatment, having gained 2 kg tissue weight without oedema. One of the long-term nutritional concerns was the development of osteoporosis associated with low oestrogen, malnutrition, and low calcium and vitamin D intake.

Learning points
The refeeding syndrome consists of (i) salt and water gain due to intolerance associated with severe malnutrition (famine oedema) and (ii) a fall in serum levels of potassium, phosphate, and sometimes magnesium due to anabolism of protein and glycogen causing cellular uptake (see also Chapter 3).

- Refeeding of severely malnourished patients should begin slowly for this reason. Diarrhoea may also be provoked with too-rapid oral or enteral refeeding.
- Careful biochemical monitoring during the initial period of refeeding is important.
- A BMI below 10 kg/m^2 in women or 11 kg/m^2 in men is usually fatal.

Table 25.1 Schofield equations for basal metabolic rate (BMR). W, weight in kg. Reprinted with permission from Schofield (1985) © Nature Publishing Group.

Age (years)	BMR (male)		BMR (female)	
	kcal/day	MJ/day	kcal/day	MJ/day
10–17	17.7 W + 657	0.074 W + 2.754	13.4 W + 692	0.056 W + 2.898
18–29	15.1 W + 692	0.063 W + 2.896	14.8 W + 487	0.062 W + 2.036
30–59	11.5 W + 873	0.048 W + 3.653	8.3 W + 846	0.034 W + 3.538
60–74	11.9 W + 700	0.0499 W + 2.930	9.2 W + 687	0.0386 W + 2.875
75+	8.4 W + 821	0.035 W + 3.434	9.8 W + 624	0.041 W + 2.610

Table 25.2 Biochemical changes with enteral nutrition (Case 2). On day 3, intravenous supplements were started with potassium phosphate. Note the low serum creatinine level, reflecting a low muscle mass.

	Day 2	Day 3	Day 5	Normal values
Na (mmol/l)	131	132	135–145	
K (mmol/l)	3.6	3.1	4.0	3.5–5.3
Urea (mmol/l)	4.0	2.2	2.0–6.5	
Creatinine (μmol/l)	37	40	50–100	
Glucose (mmol/l)	5.5	6.0	3–5	
PO$_4$ (mmol/l)	0.31	0.2	0.6	0.7–1.4
Mg (mmol/l)	0.71	0.62	0.7–1.0	
Albumin (g/l)	39	37	39	35–45

Table 25.3 Nutritional data – Case 3.

Height	1.55 m
Weight	36 kg
Now	33 kg
Allowing for 3 kg oedema	51 kg
Remembered 2 years previously	35%
% weight loss	
BMI	13.8
Now	21.3
2 years previously	
Serum albumin	41 g/l
Haemoglobin	12.8 g/dl
Lymphocyte count	0.51 (normal 1.5–4.0) $\times 10^9$/l
Creatinine	40 (normal 50–100) μmol/l
Urea	1.5 mmol/l

- Medico-legally, anorexic patients may be fed against their will in some countries, and this should be undertaken if life is at risk.
- Nutrition support only improves the patient's physical condition and does not improve the basic psychiatric disease.
- Serum albumin is often normal in anorexic patients, unless there is intercurrent inflammation or dilution with retained fluid.
- Amenorrhoea usually occurs below a BMI of 17 kg/m^2. Menstruation usually returns when the BMI rises above this level. With malnutrition, the hypothalamic release of luteinising hormone-releasing factor (LHRH) is reduced, and in both sexes gonadotropin and sex hormone levels are reduced.
- Low oestrogen levels with malnutrition and low calcium and vitamin D intake predispose to the early development of osteoporosis.

25.4 Malnutrition in the older person

Case 3

A 73-year-old woman and her twin sister both developed thyrotoxicosis and lost weight due to the increased metabolic rate associated with that condition. The thyrotoxicosis was cured and the twin sister regained her normal weight. The patient, however, then developed severe depression and anorexia, leading to persistent weight loss. On admission to hospital she was cachectic, weak, and depressed, with bruising and oedema of the leg. She was severely depressed but a Mini-Mental score revealed no evidence of dementia. Her temperature was low at 35 °C. Her nutritional data are shown in Table 25.3.

Screening

Figure 25.2 shows the Mini Nutritional Assessment (MNA) validated for nutritional screening of the elderly and the scores for this particular patient. In contrast to the nutritional screening tool in Box 25.1, a low rather than a high score indicates malnutrition here, which in this case was severe.

Nutritional assessment

The screening tool was sufficient in this case to diagnose malnutrition. More detailed assessment showed profound loss of function. Not only does depression cause anorexia and weight loss, but more than 15–20% weight loss can itself cause depression, creating a vicious circle that requires not only antidepressants but nutritional support. The latter was particularly indicated in this case because few women survive a BMI below 10 kg/m^2, or men below 11 kg/m^2. Her low temperature and low lymphocyte counts were typical of the failure of thermoregulation and of immunity associated with severe weight loss. She had so-called 'famine oedema', since, with severe weight loss, the extracellular fluid volume as a percentage of body weight increases, and salt and water may be retained in excess.

Despite severe malnutrition, the serum albumin concentration was normal, in the absence of any inflammatory condition. The low blood urea reflected low protein turnover and the low creatinine her diminished muscle mass. Her food intake had been so poor in quantity and quality that multiple micronutrient deficiencies had to be presumed, which might account for some of the bruising on her legs. Measurement of vitamin and trace-element concentrations in blood are possible in specialised laboratories, but are not routine.

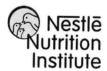

Nestlé Nutrition Institute

Mini Nutritional Assessment
MNA®

Last name:		First name:	

Sex: Female	Age: 73	Weight, kg: 36.0	Height, cm: 155	Date:

Complete the screen by filling in the boxes with the appropriate numbers. Total the numbers for the final screening score.

Screening

A Has food intake declined over the past 3 months due to loss of appetite, digestive problems, chewing or swallowing difficulties?
0 = severe decrease in food intake
1 = moderate decrease in food intake
2 = no decrease in food intake   `0`

B Weight loss during the last 3 months
0 = weight loss greater than 3 kg (6.6 lbs)
1 = does not know
2 = weight loss between 1 and 3 kg (2.2 and 6.6 lbs)
3 = no weight loss   `0`

C Mobility
0 = bed or chair bound
1 = able to get out of bed / chair but does not go out
2 = goes out   `1`

D Has suffered psychological stress or acute disease in the past 3 months?
0 = yes   2 = no   `0`

E Neuropsychological problems
0 = severe dementia or depression
1 = mild dementia
2 = no psychological problems   `0`

F 1 Body Mass Index (BMI) (weight in kg) / (height in m²) `14`
0 = BMI less than 19
1 = BMI 19 to less than 21
2 = BMI 21 to less than 23
3 = BMI 23 or greater   `0`

IF BMI IS NOT AVAILABLE, REPLACE QUESTION F1 WITH QUESTION F2.
DO NOT ANSWER QUESTION F2 IF QUESTION F1 IS ALREADY COMPLETED.

F2 Calf circumference (CC) in cm
0 = CC less than 31
3 = CC 31 or greater   ☐

Screening score
(max. 14 points)   ☐ `1`

12–14 points:	☐	Normal nutritional status
8–11 points:	☐	At risk of malnutrition
0–7 points:	☒	Malnourished

Save
Print
Reset

Ref. Vellas B, Villars H, Abellan G, *et al. Overview of the MNA® - Its History and Challenges. J Nutr Health Aging* 2006;10:456–465.
Rubenstein LZ, Harker JO, Salva A, Guigoz Y, Vellas B. *Screening for Undernutrition in Geriatric Practice: Developing the Short-Form Mini Nutritional Assessment (MNA-SF)* . J. Geront 2001;56A: M366–377.
Guigoz Y. *The Mini-Nutritional Assessment (MNA®) Review of the Literature - What does it tell us?* J Nutr Health Aging 2006; 10:466–487. Kaiser MJ, Bauer JM, Ramsch C, *et al. Validation of the Mini Nutritional Assessment Short-Form (MNA®-SF): A practical tool for identification of nutritional status.* J Nutr Health Aging 2009; 13:782–788.

For more information: www.mna-elderly.com

Figure 25.2 Mini Nutritional Assessment (MNA). Rubenstein *et al.* (2001), Guigoz (2006), Vellas *et al.* (2006), Kaiser *et al.* (2009) ® Société des Produits Nestlé, S.A., Vevey, Switzerland, Trademark Owners. © Nestlé, 1994, Revision 2009. N67200 12/99 10M. For more information, visit www.mna-elderly.com.

Problems to be addressed

- Previous thyrotoxicosis and weight loss.
- Severe depression causing anorexia.
- Profound protein-energy malnutrition, exacerbating her depression and causing major functional impairment, including failure of the thermogenic response to cold or the febrile response to infection.
- Presumed multiple micronutrient deficiencies.

Clinical decision

Ethical considerations should always inform clinical decisions, particularly at the extremes of life. Ceasing to eat and drink is a feature of dying from whatever cause, and terminal dementing illness is no exception. Artificial nutritional support in such circumstances is contraindicated since it exposes the patient to all the risks and confers none of the benefits of the treatment (for the ethical principles of beneficence and nonmaleficence, see Chapter 10). This patient, however, had two major treatable and reversible conditions: depression and malnutrition. In addition to antidepressants, therefore, she required nasogastric feeding, since her anorexia precluded sufficient feeding by mouth. The patient's permission was therefore obtained (the ethical principle of autonomy must be observed, except in anorexia nervosa) to pass a fine-bore nasogastric tube, whose position was ascertained radiologically.

Nutritional requirements

At 33 kg, her estimated resting metabolic rate was 990 kcal (4.1 MJ) (calculated by Schofield predictive equation, see Table 25.1), but with advanced starvation this was reduced by about 10%. Since the aim of treatment is first to avoid refeeding syndrome by too-rapid renutrition, second to achieve functional improvement in the short term, and third to restore body weight to normal in the longer term (i.e. over 3–6 months), continuous pump feeding was begun, using a polymeric enteral feed of 4.2 kJ/ml at an initial rate of 25 ml/hour, increasing to 40 ml/hour over 3 days (i.e. sufficient to meet 1.1×REE). Tolerance was established and over the next few days the feed was increased to achieve 1.5×REE. In the second week, the nasogastric feed was given at 100 ml/hour overnight only, allowing oral intake and activity by day. Continuous enteral feeding may disinhibit the appetite, so increasing voluntary oral intake can be used as a monitor of response to this and to the antidepressants.

Treatment

By the end of the first week, she was established on an intake of 1200 kcal (5 MJ) and 1.5 g protein/kg per day. A standard multivitamin preparation plus folate 5 mg/day was sufficient to repair deficiencies and meet her needs. Additional thiamine, potassium, and phosphate were also given. Lofepramine 70 mg daily was prescribed for her depression, since this is better tolerated by the elderly than tricyclics or selective seratonin reuptake inhibitors (SSRIs).

Monitoring and outcome

After 2 weeks of antidepressants and overnight nasogastric feeding, her voluntary oral intake had risen sufficiently to meet her requirements and there was improvement in both mental and physical function. Her oedema had resolved with a loss of 3 kg in weight, but this was partially offset by a 1 kg gain of real tissue. After the first 4 days her basal temperature had risen from 35 to 36.5 °C. She was then transferred to a convalescent unit and ultimately discharged with gradual and steady weight gain of 0.5 kg per week. Careful observations were made for any complications such as reflux, aspiration of feed, abdominal distension, diarrhoea, or tube displacement, but after some initial mild diarrhoea two to three times daily, responsive to loperamide, there were no further issues.

Learning points

- The syndrome of anorexia of psychological origin is not confined to young women. It may be difficult to treat at any age, but in the elderly it sometimes responds to antidepressants – addressing precipitating factors such as social isolation – and nutritional support.
- Refeeding should be introduced gradually by the oral and enteral route, with careful observations made for complications such as refeeding syndrome, diarrhoea, and aspiration.
- Enteral feeding overnight may help to disinhibit appetite and also allows oral intake and activity by day.

25.5 Bowel disease

Case 4

A 63-year-old patient with active Crohn's disease for 5 years was admitted with weight loss from

54 to 44 kg over a 6-month period. She developed an enterovaginal and enterovesical fistula and had oedema, suggesting a true tissue weight of <42 kg.

Screening

Nutritional screening showed a BMI of 14 kg/m², 20% weight loss, diminished food intake, and active disease, giving a high risk score of 10.

Nutritional assessment

Nutritional assessment revealed depression, apathy, and weakness, with oedema and a serum albumin of 15 g/l, reflecting inflammation and serous losses from infected fistulas.

Problems to be addressed

- gastrointestinal failure;
- gross protein-energy malnutrition;
- probable micronutrient and mineral deficiencies;
- fistula and fluid losses;
- active inflammation due to Crohn's disease and infection.

Clinical decision

Due to the intestinal fistulas, this woman clearly needed parenteral nutrition. A tunnelled subclavian line was inserted. Initial objectives of nutritional care should have been:

- Gradual introduction of feeding to avoid metabolic disturbance.
- Correction of fluid, electrolyte, mineral, and micronutrient deficiencies.
- Minimisation of bowel contents and hence fistula losses, allowing spontaneous healing of the fistula if possible.
- Improved function in the short term.
- Improvement of her general condition, to allow successful medical and surgical management of her underlying issues.
- In the long term, regaining of lost body tissue.

Nutritional requirements

Her estimated REE was approximately 1080 kcal (4.5 MJ per day, and 1.5 times this figure would be required for weight gain. Her protein needs were 1.5 g/kg or 60 g per day (9–10 g N).

Treatment

Unfortunately, she was treated with excessive enthusiasm, being infused parenterally with 2870 kcal (12 MJ) (including 400 g of glucose) and 18 g N per day. Her Crohn's was managed by a combination of medical and surgical treatment.

Monitoring and outcome

Within 24 hours she became extremely short of breath. A pulmonary embolus was suspected until the infusion rate was halved and her respirations returned to normal as her feed-induced increase in oxygen consumption and CO_2 production resolved.

She ultimately required 2 months of parenteral nutrition before her fistula closed spontaneously and bowel function returned sufficiently to allow normal oral intake. She was well at discharge, after regaining 3 kg in weight. Six months later she weighed 52 kg.

Learning points

- Parenteral nutrition is the management of gastrointestinal failure in the same sense that dialysis is the treatment of renal failure and ventilation is of respiratory failure; that is, it supports organ function until the underlying cause of the problem is resolved.
- This patient's life expectancy without nutritional support was less than 6 weeks. Survival is unlikely below a BMI of 10 kg/m² or with weight loss of more than 35%, especially in the presence of active disease. Parenteral nutrition was therefore life-saving.
- Carbohydrate and protein/amino acids cause diet-induced thermogenesis and increased demands for gas exchange. Glucose should rarely be infused at a rate greater than 0.3 g/kg/hour, since above this it merely increases CO_2 production and O_2 consumption without useful effect and may be dangerous in those with respiratory failure or those with respiratory muscle weakness due to disease or malnutrition. Her initial glucose infusion rate was 0.42 g/kg/hour, not to mention the 0.4 g N/kg per day – more than twice her requirements.

Case 5

In a 57-year-old man with a 10-year history of intestinal disease the initial diagnosis was Crohn's disease, but this was changed 4 years before admission to coeliac disease with microscopic colitis and gastritis. He was admitted in the past with extensive obstructing strictures in the duodenum and jejunum and underwent partial jejunal resection and gastrojejunostomy. His diet was gluten-free. He suffered osteoporosis from a combination of previous steroid treatment and malnutrition (with cachexia, sex-hormone levels fall). Intake and absorption of calcium and vitamin D were also impaired.

Over 4 years he took an elemental diet, but intestinal strictures, small-bowel bacterial colonisation, and protein-losing enteropathy continued to be a problem.

He was first seen in the nutrition clinic with serial measurements of weight, function, tests of mood and muscle strength, and serum biochemistry.

Screening
Height 1.7 m, weight 56 kg, BMI 19.1 kg/m². Percentage weight change in 3 months was +3 kg, although over 1 year it was −9.7 kg (score 0). Oral intake with elemental supplements appeared adequate (score 0). Disease was quiescent (score 0).

Nutritional assessment
Despite the overall picture suggesting that he might need parenteral nutrition in the long term, his recent weight gain and score of 3, combined with some anxiety as to his capacity to cope with the demands of parenteral feeding, led to a decision to rely on oral intake and to follow him in the clinic, measuring weight, muscle strength, biochemistry, and haematology. The results of his anthropometric, biochemical, and haematological measurements are shown in Table 25.4.

Table 25.4 Serial data for Case 5.

Date	Weight (kg)	BMI	Right hand grip	Albumin (g/l)	Hb (g/l)
Day 0	56.1	20	31.6		10.3
Day 7	52.6	18.7	33.5	26	9.5
Day 20	51.4	18.3	32.4		
Day 29	51.2	18.2	24	21	10.7
Day 49	48.8	17.4	23	19	
Parenteral nutrition started on Day 59					
Day 79	57.5	20.5	32.4	23	11.0
Day 130	61.2	21.8	32.6	28	12.1

Medication
- prednisolone 5 mg;
- budesonide CR 9 mg;
- lansoprazole 30 mg;
- ferrous sulphate 200 mg;
- calcichew 1 daily.

As can be seen from Table 25.4, his condition deteriorated, with declining weight, muscle strength, serum albumin, and haemoglobin. Selenium concentration was low at 0.44 mmol/l, but magnesium was normal at 0.77 mmol/l.

Problems to be addressed
- Chronic gastrointestinal failure, unlikely to improve as a result of any further medical or surgical intervention.
- Worsening malnutrition with weight loss and impaired function, with muscle weakness and fatigue, hypoalbuminaemia, anaemia, selenium depletion, and osteoporosis.
- Fluid depletion from diarrhoea.

Clinical decision
- To start parenteral nutrition to restore and maintain nutritional status, while continuing to allow oral intake at will.
- To admit for 2 weeks of training by an expert nursing team – the mechanical metabolic, thrombotic, and infectious complications of parenteral nutrition are prohibitive without an expert nutrition team to manage both short- and long-term administration.

Nutritional requirements
At 50 kg his REE (calculated by Schofield predictive equation, see Table 25.1) was 1434 kcal (6.0 MJ). Diet-induced thermogenesis will increase this by 10% and moderate activity by 40%, suggesting an approximate intake to maintain weight of 1.5 × REE; that is, 2170 kcal (9 MJ) per day. However, the aim was also to increase his weight over 2–3 months back to more than 60 kg and to restore his lean mass, meeting the energy cost of protein synthesis. It was decided to allow an extra 30% of energy over basal to meet this need, giving a total energy intake of 2870 kcal (12 MJ) per day.

To maintain nitrogen balance in a healthy man, a minimum of 0.8 g protein/kg/day is required, providing energy needs are met – a minimum of 40 g in this case. In addition, however, he had continuing protein-losing enteropathy and a requirement for lean mass restoration; that is, an intake of at least 1.5 g protein/kg/day (0.24 g N/kg/day). Micronutrient supplements and extra selenium as Na selenite were also required.

The standard ready-made all-in-one feed nearest to these requirements was one of 2.5 l containing 14 g N (87.5 g protein) and 2560 kcal (10.7 MJ – 1.5 MJ from protein, 3.8 MJ from fat, and 5.4 MJ from carbohydrate (including the glycerol component of the lipid emulsion)).

Treatment and outcome

The parenteral nutrition was given for 14 hours overnight, 7 nights per week, and supplemented by a modest oral intake. The most dramatic initial change, as always, was a large improvement in mood, energy, and muscle strength, occurring before any weight increase. Part of his initial weight gain was due to restoration of extracellular fluid deficit from diarrhoea and some gain in intracellular fluid as glycogen stores were replenished. After 2 months, the parenteral nutrition was reduced to 4 nights per week, with a reduced energy (1890 kcal/7.9 MJ) and nitrogen (11 g) composition. In combination with oral intake, this was sufficient to maintain his weight, function, and quality of life. Despite initial apprehensions, he managed his parenteral nutrition perfectly and had no complications during 2 years of follow-up.

Learning points

- Function is an even more important criterion of nutritional status than changes in body composition. It correlates well with malnutrition and responds rapidly to refeeding even before gain in tissue mass.
- Home parenteral nutrition is the management of chronic gastrointestinal failure causing malnutrition.
- The parenteral nutrition prescription should take account of likely requirements for tissue regain and maintenance, and compensate for fluid, electrolyte, mineral, and micronutrient losses or deficiencies.
- Steroids which are catabolic with respect to bone, connective tissue, and muscle should be kept to the minimum dose necessary.

- Cachexia causes impaired gonadotropin and sex-hormone secretion. Alongside poor nutrient absorption, including of Ca and vitamin D, this causes osteopaenia, which must be treated.
- A parenteral nutrition service requires an expert nutrition team.

Case 6

A 55-year-old man, height 1.73 m, weight 6 months previously 52 kg (BMI 17.4 kg/m²) presented with a current weight of 45 kg (including oedema, BMI 15.0 kg/m²). He had a history of high alcohol intake (more than one bottle of whiskey daily) and poor food intake, and developed acute confusion, dysuria, and fever 38.5 °C. On examination he was jaundiced, with spider nevi, bruising, small testes, ankle oedema, liver enlarged 5 cm below the costal margin, no enlargement of the spleen, and distended bladder.

Investigations

- haemoglobin 13.6 g/dl;
- international normalised ratio (INR) 1.6;
- mean cell volume (MCV) 121.8 fl = macrocytosis;
- total white cell count 9.25×10^9/l;
- erythrocyte sedimentation rate (ESR) 58 mm/hour;
- blood glucose low at 3.0 mmol;
- blood urea elevated at 8.1 mmol/l;
- sodium 145 mmol/l, potassium 4.4 mmol/l, magnesium 0.59 mmol/l (low), phosphate 1.58 mmol/l;
- liver enzymes elevated, serum albumin 30 g/l (low), bilirubin 45 µmol/l (high);
- urine cloudy and infected.

Screening

His nutrition screening scores are 3 for BMI of 15 kg/m², 2 for weight loss, 1 for impaired food intake, and 2 for disease severity = total score 8.

Nutritional assessment and problems to be addressed

- Alcoholic hepatitis, causing liver failure, hypoglycaemia, hypoalbuminaemia, and hypomagnesaemia.
- Urinary retention and infection secondary to prostatic hypertrophy, causing fever and postrenal failure and precipitating hepatic encephalopathy.

- Gross protein-energy malnutrition through anorexia and low intake. Interestingly, one bottle of 40% whiskey (75 cl) containing 300 g alcohol (31.5 kJ/g) provides 2270 kcal (9.5 MJ) energy.
- Impaired immunity secondary to protein-energy malnutrition and liver disease.
- Probably multiple vitamin deficiencies, particularly thiamine, absence of which causes Wernicke's encephalopathy.
- Low prothrombin level secondary to liver disease, requiring vitamin K.

Nutritional requirements

It takes a 3 l salt and water overload before oedema is manifest, so this man's real weight is a maximum of 42 kg. REE was therefore 1360 kcal (5.7 MJ)/day. Allowing a 10% increase for diet-induced thermogenesis and a 13% increase per 1 °C rise in temperature, this gives a total energy requirement of 1860 kcal (7.8 MJ)/day to maintain zero energy balance. Once his catabolic phase is over, however, he will need another 480 kcal (2 MJ)/day to meet the cost of restoring lost tissue. Cirrhotic patients without infection also have a raised REE, at 10% over estimated for weight and height. Although branched-chain amino acid preparations are available for either enteral or parenteral use and can help to reverse encephalopathy, they are unbalanced in their amino acid profile. Standard polymeric feeds are therefore preferred in most cases of malnutrition secondary to liver disease. Remarkably, increasing protein intake, up to a point, does not usually worsen encephalopathy in most cases. In this case, 0.2 g N/kg?day would be a reasonable starting point, increasing as tolerated up to 0.3 g/kg/day during recovery (52 g protein, increasing to 78 g per day).

Treatment

- Intravenous antibiotics and urinary catheterisation.
- Thiamine 100 mg×3 daily and oral multivitamin preparation.
- Vitamin K 1 mg.
- Enteral nutrition via nasogastric tube using a standard polymeric diet (as in European Society of Parenteral and Enteral Nutrition, ESPEN guidelines).
- Later, counselling concerning alcohol intake.
- Chlordiazepoxide to cover alcohol-withdrawal symptoms.

Monitoring and outcome

Despite starting a 4.2 kJ/ml (1 kcal/ml) enteral feed at only 30 ml/hour, increasing to 80 ml/hour over 5 days, his serum magnesium fell from 0.59 to 0.49 mmol/l (0.74–1.0), his serum phosphate from 1.58 to 0.31 mmol/l (0.8–1.5), and his serum potassium from 5.5 to 2.9 mmol, necessitating intravenous administration of magnesium sulphate and potassium phosphate in dextrose. This refeeding syndrome (see Case 2) is typical of the response to feeding in extremely cachectic individuals and may be fatal if untreated. For a further 3 weeks, the patient received 2150 kcal (9 MJ) and 12.4 g N per day enterally before beginning oral intake. As this increased, so his enteral feeding was limited to the night hours, and then withdrawn. Overnight enteral feeding usually disinhibits appetite. After 45 days of admission, he was discharged weighing 50 kg. He subsequently stayed off alcohol, his liver function returned to normal, and his weight gradually rose over 6 months to >60 kg.

Learning points

- Liver disease is associated with anorexia, poor food intake, protein-energy malnutrition, increased metabolic rate, and multiple vitamin deficiencies.
- In acute liver failure secondary to alcoholism, give thiamine in therapeutic doses as well as a multivitamin preparation. Vitamin K may be required if INR (international normalised ratio, an indicator of clotting ability) is prolonged.
- True weight loss may be marked by oedema and/or ascites.
- If oral intake is inadequate, enteral feeding using a standard polymeric feed is the treatment of choice.
- The feed should be introduced slowly, and gradually increased to meet targets.
- Electrolyte, phosphate, and magnesium levels should be monitored for refeeding syndrome, and any falls in concentration should be corrected.

25.6 Catabolic illness

Case 7

A man aged 45 years underwent arthroscopy of the knee. A week later he developed pain in the thigh, which worsened over 2 weeks, accompanied by fever and malaise. He then underwent drainage of osteomyelitis of the right femur and received antibiotics for a *Streptococcus milleri* infection. One month later he developed a large abscess of the thigh, with fever of 38 °C, and underwent further drainage, with antibiotics in the form of penicillin and metronidazole. His premorbid weight had been 70 kg and he now weighed 59 kg but with marked oedema. He was anorexic and nauseated, managing an energy intake of only 240 kcal (1 MJ)/day despite all attempts at oral intake, including supplements.

Screening

Height 1.7 m, weight 59 kg (real weight 54 kg after resolution of oedema). Based on 54 kg, his BMI was 19 kg/m^2 (score 2). Percentage weight loss was 20% (score 3). Grossly reduced intake (score 2). Disease severity (score 2). Total 9, indicating high nutritional risk.

Nutritional assessment

In view of his poor intake with nausea and vomiting, the nutrition team was asked to see him to provide parenteral nutrition. His symptoms, however, appeared disproportionate to his underlying disease, and suspicion fell on the side effects of his drugs. Albumin 29 g/l, haemoglobin 9.7 g, secondary to sepsis.

Problems to be addressed

- Sepsis and abscess, causing increased metabolic rate (+13% per 1 °C rise in temperature).
- This, combined with decreased intake, resulted in 20% weight loss, weakness, and immobility.
- Nauseating effect of metronidazole, preventing adequate oral intake.

Clinical decision

- Treat infection by drainage and penicillin.
- Stop metronidazole.
- Observe oral intake.

Nutritional requirements

At least 1.5×REE for weight gain and 1.5 g protein/kg/day.

Monitoring and outcome

With successful treatment of the infection his fever subsided. After stopping metronidazole all his nausea and anorexia disappeared and his spontaneous oral

intake rose to over 2400 kcal (10 MJ) daily. He regained weight rapidly, mobilised, and was discharged 3 weeks later.

Learning points

- Trauma, infection, and inflammation increase metabolic rate, accelerating weight loss and protein catabolism. Cytokines released by inflammation also depress appetite.
- First treat the underlying catabolic disease to reduce rate of weight loss, for example by draining an abscess.
- Drugs have many side effects that can affect nutritional status. Always consider the nutritional effects of medications.
- Use oral feeding where possible.

Case 8

A man of 36 years (weight 70 kg, height 1.8 m, BMI 21.6 kg/m^2) and previously fit suffered burn injury of 50% of his body surface (half being full thickness and half partial). He also suffered smoke inhalation, necessitating ventilation in the intensive-care unit (ICU) for a period of 2 weeks. After the initial 24-hour resuscitation period, the question of feeding arose.

Screening

Although zero food intake and a disease severity score of 2 gave a total score of 4, this does not reflect the severity of the metabolic problem. Like all measurements, therefore, screening must be interpreted intelligently in the light of the clinical circumstances and a knowledge of the likely natural history of the disease.

Nutritional assessment

Although nutritionally normal at the time of injury, his subsequent catabolic illness and inability to eat would necessitate artificial nutritional support, preferably by the oral and enteral route.

Problems to be addressed

- Prolonged catabolic illness with consequent wasting of lean body mass, which can be reduced but not abolished by feeding.
- Prolonged immobility, enhancing muscle wasting.
- Sepsis, ventilatory failure, and repeated surgical procedures.

- Additional micronutrient requirements due to excess loss of copper, zinc, and selenium and the need for extra vitamins, such as vitamin C.
- Need to design nutrient intake accurately to give maximum benefit without the problems of metabolic overload, such as increasing demand for gas exchange, hyperglycaemia, increasing risk of infection, and so on.
- Possible need for extra amounts of special substrates, such as glutamine, ornithine alpha-ketoglutarate.

Clinical decision

- To begin feeding after 24 hours, by the enteral route if possible, starting at 20 ml/hour of a 1.0 kcal/ml standard polymeric feed by the nasogastric route, aspirating every 4 hours to test gastric emptying.
- To nurse patient in a semi-recumbent position (if allowed by the distribution of burn injury) to minimise risk of aspiration.
- To supplement the feed by the parenteral route, if necessary, to meet nutritional targets.
- To give micronutrient supplements.
- To give additional glutamine.

Nutritional requirements

In the past, such a burn injury would have been associated with a total energy requirement in excess of $1.5 \times$ REE. With modern methods of management – (i) nursing in a thermoneutral environment (normal 28–29 °C, burned patients 30–32 °C); (ii) early debridement and grafting; and (iii) better management of infection, pain, and fluid balance – the formerly reported high energy expenditures are no longer seen and it is rarely necessary to give more than $1.3 \times$ estimated REE (calculated by Schofield predictive equation, see Table 25.1), which in this case was 2175 kcal (9.1 MJ)/day. Centers with facilities for daily measurement of REE can achieve more accurate energy balance, since estimated and measured REE may differ by 30% or more during critical illness.

Nitrogen intakes in excess of 0.25 g/kg/day ($\times 6.25 = 1.56$ g protein/kg/day) are converted to urea, increasing osmotic load and not contributing usefully to nitrogen balance. Energy requirements were met from 105 g protein = 430 kcal (1.8 MJ), 250 g glucose = 1000 kcal (4.2 MJ) (well below the 0.3 g/kg/hour at which gas exchange is adversely affected), and fat (for an additional 765 kcal (3.2 MJ)). There

was also a need for extra micronutrients and benefit was obtained from giving glutamine or ornithine alpha-ketoglutarate to enhance antioxidant and immune function and improve nitrogen balance. The role of immune-enhancing cocktails containing arginine, *n*-3 fatty acids, and nucleotides is controversial.

Treatment

Clear and realistic goals of evidence-based nutritional support were:

- To minimise loss of lean mass.
- To correct or prevent mineral, electrolyte, and micronutrient abnormalities.
- To support muscle (particularly respiratory) function.
- To maintain antioxidant status.
- To support gut and immune function and reduce the risk of invasive infection.
- To avoid metabolic, mechanical, or other complications of artificial nutritional support.
- To optimise healing of wounds and grafts.

Initially, gastric aspirations were high and enteral feeding was not tolerated. After the first week, however, enteral feeding could be introduced and increased to the full target of 2150 kcal (9 MJ) and 105 g of protein. Initially, therefore, parenteral nutrition was begun using a glutamine dipeptide-containing 'all-in-one' solution via a central catheter. Nutritional targets were maintained by this route until the 10th day, when parenteral feeding was tailed off as full enteral feeding became tolerated. His blood glucose rose to 12 mmol/l and a high-dose insulin infusion was therefore begun to maintain normoglycaemia (4–7 mmol/l), since insulin used in this way has been shown to improve nitrogen economy, enhance capacity to excrete excess salt and water, reduce infection, and improve survival and outcome in critically ill patients including burns.

Despite these measures, the patient lost 15% of his body weight during his 3-week stay in the ICU. On his return to the ward, someone decided to feed more aggressively and doubled his enteral protein intake. After a few days, his blood urea had risen to 30 mmol/l and he appeared dehydrated. A consultation for 'renal failure' resulted in the realisation that the problem was excessive protein intake, causing a high urea production rate and an osmotic diuresis.

The consequent fluid deficit was also exacerbated by diarrhoea. Reducing the enteral feed rate and increasing fluid intake corrected the problem. His subsequent course was uneventful, although nutritional supplements were continued, since insulin resistance and impaired protein synthesis persist for many weeks. As he became more mobile and started to eat, his energy and protein intake could be usefully increased to restore lost tissue.

Learning points

- Burn injury is the most potent cause of catabolic illness, but modern management has reduced the stress stimulus.
- Loss of lean mass can be minimised but not abolished by feeding in catabolic illness. The goals of feeding include preservation of as much lean mass as possible, maintenance of tissue function, reduced complications, and more-rapid recovery.
- Feeding should be begun as early as possible, preferably by the enteral route but supplemented parenterally if necessary, to achieve nutritional goals.
- To optimise benefit and minimise risk, avoid the complications of artificial nutrition by using strict protocols and an expert team.
- Nutritional requirements for most burned adult patients are met by supplying 1.3 × estimated REE and 0.25 g N/kg/day. Micronutrient and mineral supplementation is beneficial. The use of substrates, such as glutamine or ornithine alpha-ketoglutarate, is also helpful.
- During catabolic illness, the former hyperalimentation regimens have been abandoned in favour of a more conservative approach, with higher nutritional intakes during convalescence and rehabilitation, when high nutrient loads can be utilised.
- High-dose insulin and maintenance of normoglycaemia have metabolic and clinical benefits.

25.7 Dysphagia

When the swallowing mechanism is impaired by neuromuscular disease (e.g. motor neuron disease) or mechanical obstruction (e.g. upper gastrointestinal tract cancer), artificial enteral feeding is indicated. Early assessment and nutritional intervention should be undertaken before significant weight loss occurs. Since gastrointestinal function is usually intact, apart from swallowing, enteral feeding via a gastrostomy or jejunostomy is the preferred feeding method, although nasogastric feeding may be employed for short periods.

Case 9

A 60-year-old woman presented with dysarthria and dysphagia due to bulbar manifestations of motor neuron disease. At first she was able to swallow semi-solids and could maintain her weight. This became an increasing struggle and she began to choke on liquids and solids and was unable to swallow her medication. Her weight had fallen from 55 kg to below 50 kg by the time of her referral by the neurologists to the nutrition unit.

Screening

Height 1.63 m, weight 49 kg, BMI 19 kg/m² (score 2). Weight loss >3 kg (score 2). Food intake decreased (score 1). Disease severity (score 2). Total 7.

Nutritional assessment and clinical decision

In view of her worsening dysphagia, she would clearly die of starvation or aspiration pneumonia without artificial feeding. Since, at this stage, she had well-preserved limb function, she was advised to have a percutaneous endoscopic gastrostomy (PEG) placed to allow self-administration home enteral nutrition and a reasonable quality of life.

Nutritional requirements

Estimated REE (calculated by Schofield predictive equation, see Table 25.1) was 1120 kcal (4.7 MJ). Since she was mobile and needed weight gain, a target of 1.5 × REE was set at 1670 kcal (7 MJ). Protein requirement was estimated to be 1.5 g/kg initially for weight gain, falling to 1.0 g/kg for maintenance. Care was needed to ensure that the dose of proprietary enteral feed used to achieve these targets also contained sufficient micronutrients to meet her requirements.

Treatment

A PEG was inserted without complications and following strict management protocols. Over the next week she was trained to give herself overnight enteral feeding at between 100 and 125 ml/hour. Rates greater than this may induce reflux, especially in the horizontal position, and may increase diet-induced thermogenesis and demand for gas exchange. In the presence of respiratory muscle weakness (as in motor neuron disease), this can induce shortness of breath. Additional bolus feeding was also given by day, with additional water. Care was taken to avoid tube blockage by flushing with water after each period of feeding.

Monitoring and outcome

She managed her feeds extremely well for 18 months, until muscle weakness developed and a carer had to administer them. Weight was restored to 53 kg and maintained at this until the terminal phase. She died of her condition 2 years after initial presentation.

Learning points

- Home enteral feeding using a gastrostomy or jejunostomy may maintain life of reasonable quality in dysphagic patients. It has been shown to confer benefit in about 25% of patients with motor neuron disease, particularly when bulbar symptoms predominate.
- Combine overnight pump with daytime bolus feeding, avoiding rates of administration in excess of 125 ml/h to avoid reflux with aspiration or excessive diet-induced thermogenesis.
- Best results are obtained by an expert team using strict protocols and a programme of training, hot-line contact, and follow-up for the patient and carers.

25.8 Obesity

Case 10

A 23-year-old man with learning difficulties admitted to hospital with a respiratory infection.

Screening

Morbidly obese (height 1.6 m, weight 180 kg, BMI 62 kg/m²). Fever 37.8 °C. Cough and purulent sputum. Cyanosed. Dependent oedema and raised jugular venous pressure, indicating right heart failure.

Investigations

- haemoglobin 18 g/l;
- Pao_2 9 kPa;

- Pco_2 7.3 kPa;
- HCO_3 32 mmol/l;
- blood glucose 15.0 mmol/l.

These tests may be interpreted as showing a chronic anoxic state (compensatory polycythaemia) and chronic CO_2 retention (compensatory increase in HCO_3). The random blood glucose >11.0 mmol (15 mmol) showed that he was already developing type 2 diabetes from insulin resistance caused by obesity.

Nutritional assessment

Screening data with a BMI of 62 kg/m² showed morbid obesity. (Obesity is defined as BMI > 30 kg/m² and morbid obesity as BMI > 40 kg/m².) History from his mother revealed constant eating.

Problems to be addressed

- Morbid obesity, causing impaired ventilation with respiratory failure (Pickwickian syndrome), secondary pulmonary hypertension, and right heart failure.
- Exacerbation of respiratory problems by acute infective bronchitis.
- Huge food intake.

Treatment and outcome

Five-day course of antibiotics and physiotherapy for his acute bronchitis.

Long-term food restriction and exercise programme. Since he had no independent access to food and his mother was his sole carer, it was possible to ensure dietary compliance, which is not usually the case in morbidly obese patients. Additional measures could include drugs, such as sibutramine (appetite suppressant) or orlistat (intestinal lipase inhibitor, to cause fat malabsorption). Bariatric surgery is the most successful form of treatment and can be undertaken in suitable cases if all else fails (see Chapter 4).

This patient was able to lose 50 kg in 9 months as a result of dietary restriction and exercise under supervision. His blood glucose fell to normal and his respiratory and cardiac failure resolved to the point where his exercise tolerance was virtually normal.

Learning points

- Morbid obesity (BMI > 40 kg/m²) is a dangerous condition with many complications, including diabetes, hypertension, arterial disease, cardiorespiratory failure, increased cancer risk, and crippling arthritis.

- Obesity of any degree is identified by routine screening, allowing appropriate referral and treatment.
- Obesity is difficult to treat by diet alone, except in highly motivated patients. The same applies to exercise. Additional drug support is effective. Bariatric surgery used appropriately is the most effective.
- The prevalence of obesity in the UK has increased from 6 to 20% over 20 years and represents a major health problem for the future.

References and further reading

Guigoz Y. The Mini-Nutritional Assessment (MNA®) review of the literature – what does it tell us? J Nutr Health Aging 2006; 10: 466–487.

Kaiser MJ, Bauer JM, Ramsch C, Uter W, Guigoz Y, Cederholm T, et al. Validation of the Mini Nutritional Assessment short-form (MNA®-SF): a practical tool for identification of nutritional status. J Nutr Health Aging 2009; 13: 782–788.

Rubenstein LZ, Harker JO, Salva A, Guigoz Y, Vellas B. Screening for undernutrition in geriatric practice: developing the short-form Mini Nutritional Assessment (MNA-SF). J Geront 2001; 56A: M366–377.

Schofield WN. Predicting basal metabolic rate, new standards and a review of previous work. Hum Nutr Clin Nutr 1985; 39C(Suppl. 1): 5–41.

Vellas B, Villars H, Abellan G, Soto ME, Rolland Y, Guigoz Y, et al. Overview of the MNA® – its history and challenges. J Nutr Health Aging 2006; 10: 456–465.

Useful Web links for core nutrition journals

American Journal of Clinical Nutrition. http://www.ajcn.org.

British Journal of Nutrition. http://journals.cambridge.org/BJN.

Clinical Nutrition. http://www.elsevier.com/locate/clnu.

European Journal of Clinical Nutrition. http://www.nature.com/ejcn/.

Journal of Human Nutrition and Dietetics. http://eu.wiley.com/WileyCDA/WileyTitle/productCd-JHN.html.

Journal of Nutrition. http://www.nutrition.org.

Journal of Pediatric Gastroenterology and Nutrition. http://www.jpgn.org.

Journal of the American Dietetic Association. http://www.adajournal.org.

Nutrition in Clinical Practice. http://ncp.sagepub.com.

Nutrition Research. http://www.journals.elsevierhealth.com/periodicals/NTR.

Nutrition. http://www.journals.elsevierhealth.com/periodicals/nut.

Proceedings of the Nutrition Society. http://journals.cambridge.org/PNS.

PubMed. http://www.ncbi.nlm.nih.gov/pubmed/.

Index

Note: Page numbers in *italics* refer to Figures; those in **bold** to Tables.

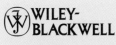
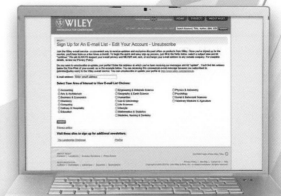